Pathophysiology: Concepts of Altered Health States

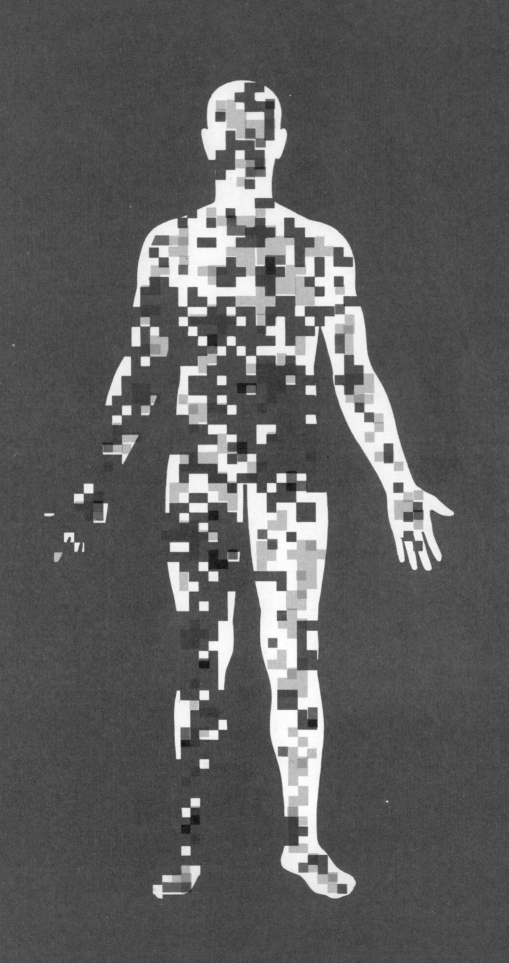

Pathophysiology

Concepts of Altered Health States

Carol Porth

R.N., M.S.N., Ph.D. (Physiology)

Associate Professor
School of Nursing
University of Wisconsin-Milwaukee

Adjunct Assistant Professor
Department of Physiology
Medical College of Wisconsin
Milwaukee, Wisconsin

With six contributors

With many original drawings by
Carole Russell Hilmer

J. B. Lippincott Company
Philadelphia   Toronto

6 5 4 3 2 1

Library of Congress
Cataloging in Publication Data

Porth, Carol.
    Pathophysiology, concepts of altered
health states.

    Bibliography.
    Includes index.
    1. Physiology, Pathological. 2. Nursing.
I. Title. [DNLM: 1. Disease—Nursing texts.
2. Pathology—Nursing texts. 3. Physiology—
Nursing texts. QZ 4 P851p]
RB113.P67   616.07   81-15653
ISBN 0-397-54252-6   AACR2

The authors and publisher have exerted
every effort to ensure that drug selection and
dosage set forth in this text are in accord with
current recommendations and practice at the
time of publication. However, in view of
ongoing research, changes in government
regulations, and the constant flow of
information relating to drug therapy and
drug reactions, the reader is urged to
check the package insert for each drug for
any change in indications and dosage
and for added warnings and precautions.
This is particularly important when the
recommended agent is a new or infrequently
employed drug.

Contents

Unit IV
Alterations in Genitourinary Function
335

Debbie Lynn Cook, R.N., B.S., M.S.N., C.N.M.
Certified Nurse Midwife
Rhinelander, Wisconsin

Robin L. Curtis, Ph.D.
Associate Professor of Anatomy and
    Physical Medicine and Rehabilitation
The Medical College of Wisconsin
Milwaukee, Wisconsin

Sheila M. Curtis, R.N., M.S.
Assistant Professor
School of Nursing
University of Wisconsin-Milwaukee
Milwaukee, Wisconsin

Janet Krejci, R.N., M.S.N.
Consultant in Nursing Care of the Emotionally Disturbed
Mount Sinai Green Tree Health Care Center
Milwaukee, Wisconsin

Stephanie MacLaughlin, R.N., M.S.N.
Assistant Professor
School of Nursing
University of Wisconsin-Milwaukee
Milwaukee, Wisconsin

Mary Wierenga, R.N., Ph.D.
Assistant Professor
School of Nursing
University of Wisconsin-Milwaukee
Milwaukee, Wisconsin

Consultant in pharmacology

Mary S. Rice, Pharm. D.
Director of Drug Information
Columbia Hospital
Milwaukee, Wisconsin

Contributors

The meaning of pathophysiology, or altered health as it is referred to in this book, reflects not so much the pathologic processes that take place as the physiologic changes that occur. It is these physiologic changes that produce the signs and symptoms, and it is these changes that determine, to a large extent, whether the disease will or will not be disabling. Furthermore, it is with the maintenance of adequate levels of functioning that most health care professionals concern themselves.

This book, intended primarily for nurses and nursing students, evolved from lectures in pathophysiology and the lecture notes that students have shared. The book is general enough to be used in other health care disciplines.

The aims in writing this book were twofold. The first was to relate an understanding of normal body functioning to the physiologic changes that occur as the result of illness, as well as the body's remarkable ability to compensate for these illness-related changes. In further accord with this objective, a conceptual model that integrates epidemiology and the preventive as well as the pathologic aspects of disease was used. The book includes concepts from human development and presents alterations in health that occur throughout the life cycle.

The second objective was to present the content in a manner that could easily be understood. The book builds on previous learning in the related sciences, yet may be used by persons who have not had extensive studies in these fields. Concepts from anatomy, cell biology, biochemistry, and physics have been integrated into appropriate sections of the book in order to minimize the frustration that occurs when a reader does not have the background necessary to understand essential content. Diagrams designed to aid in visualizing the content have been used liberally throughout the text. The same is true of tables, which have been devised to identify and summarize essential information.

The book has been divided into units. The first deals with the cellular aspects of disease, and the others with alterations in organ and system function. The book provides the rationale, but not the "how to's," of nursing care, the specifics of drug therapy, or the particulars of diagnostic methods. It is assumed that those using the book will have access to more complete reference sources in these areas than this book could provide.

In writing a comprehensive book that is nevertheless of a manageable size, I found it extremely difficult to decide what should be included and what could safely be omitted. The selection of content was influenced by my experience in the clinical setting and by the reported needs of colleagues and students. No doubt, others would have made different choices. Therefore, any comments regarding specific errors and omissions are most welcome, as are general impressions and suggestions.

It is hoped that the textbook will be helpful to both students

Preface

and teachers as they work together in studying the physiologic changes that occur with altered states of health.

At the end of each chapter is to be found a section called Study Guide. These guides have been purposefully placed to serve as both a quick review of chapter contents and a statement of chapter objectives.

Carol Porth, R.N., M.S.N., Ph.D.

It is difficult to envision writing a textbook such as this without the help of many people—family, colleagues, and students. To my children, Richard C. and Susan, I give special thanks for their patience and encouragement. I particularly appreciated the interest, suggestions, and support that my colleagues provided during the long months that it took to prepare the manuscript. The part that students played in the creation of this book also deserves recognition, for they inspired the writing of the book and through their interest in the subject provided encouragement when the task was most difficult.

A number of persons were kind enough to review parts of the text and to make helpful suggestions: Jill Barney, Kit Besag, Patricia Burke, David J. Carlson, M.D., Kathleen V. Cowles, Diane Duffy, Marcia Etu, Kathryn Gaspard, Cathy Mary Halloran, Karel Kotrly, M.D., Gordon E. Lang, M.D., Helena Kecman Lorbeck, Betty Pearson, Irene Schreck, David F. Stowe, Darlene Thornhill, Ann Taubenheim, Madeline Wake, and Linda Zwirlein. Mary Gainer provided several original drawings for Chapters 12 and 16.

The contributors to the book also deserve special mention, for they worked long hours to supply essential content. In preparation of Unit VI, Alterations in Neuromuscular Function, the assistance of The Evan and Marion Helfaer Foundation was most appreciated.

A special recognition is reserved for one person who, without question, gave service well above and beyond the call of duty: my research assistant, Joyce Myers. To Lee Ann Dzelkalna, Terry Konecke, and Sharon Krueger a word of appreciation for the long painstaking hours spent in typing the manuscript.

The acknowledgments would not be complete without a special tribute to Bernice Heller, Developmental Editor, for her support and assistance. Her organizational and editorial skills played an essential role in the development of the book. Mary Murphy, secretary to Bernice Heller, also deserves special commendations for her part in organizing and keeping track of all the various chapters and figures that were often submitted in a less-than-orderly sequence.

Acknowledgments

Pathophysiology:
Concepts
of Altered
Health States

1

Prologue: Introduction to Health and Adaptation

Health can be described as a dynamic state that includes various aspects of both wellness and illness. Although most of us perceive ourselves as being healthy, few of us can say that we have never been sick. For the most part, health includes (1) well-health, in which wellness may be periodically interrupted by acute illness, (2) modified well-health, in which aspects of chronic illness have been incorporated into a pattern of wellness functioning, and (3) consistent ill-health, which causes marked alterations in body functioning. The discussion in this chapter focuses on disease, or what this book terms altered health, and physiologic adaptation to states of altered health.

:Disease: A State of Altered Physiologic Functioning

Disease, from a practical point of view, describes a condition of impaired body function. Engel defines disease as failures or disturbances in the growth, development, function, and adjustment of the organism, either as a whole or of any of its systems.[1] Although disease usually includes alterations in body structures or in the composition of body fluids, it is the manifestations of these bodily changes that impair function and lead to an awareness of illness. Likewise, it is the return of normal function that usually marks recovery from illness.

A disease can be acute, subacute, or chronic. An *acute* disorder is one that is relatively severe, but self-limiting. *Chronic* disease refers to a continuous, long-term process. A chronic disease can run a continuous course or it can present with *exacerbations* (aggravation of symptoms and severity of the disease), and *remissions* (a period of time where there is a lessening of severity and a decrease in symptoms). *Subacute* disease is intermediate between acute and chronic; it is not as severe as acute and not as prolonged as a chronic illness.

Manifestations of Disease

Signs and symptoms are terms that are used to describe the structural and functional changes that accompany disease. A *symptom* is regarded as a subjective complaint that is noted by the person afflicted with the disorder, whereas a *sign* is a manifestation that is noted by an observer. Pain, difficult breathing, and a feeling of lightheadedness are symptoms of disordered function. On the other hand, an elevated temperature, a swollen extremity, and changes in pupil size are objective signs that can be observed by someone other than the person with the disorder. Signs and symptoms may be related to the primary disorder, or they may represent the body's attempt to compensate for the altered function caused by the pathologic condition. For our purposes, physiologic coping mechanisms refer to physiologic responses that counteract or compensate for conditions that tend to disrupt body function. "Anyone who has worked in the health professions for any length of time is aware that most pathological states are not observed directly—one cannot see a sick heart or a failing kidney. What one can see is the body's attempt to compensate for the change in structure and function."[2]

It is important to recognize that a single sign or symptom is frequently associated with a number of different disease states. For example, an elevated temperature can indicate the presence of infection, myocardial infarction, brain injury, or any of a large number of other disorders. A differential diagnosis that describes the origin of a disorder usually requires knowledge of a number of signs and symptoms. The presence of fever, a reddened sore throat, and a positive throat culture, for example, describes a "strep throat" infection, whereas, the previously mentioned presence of fever gave little information about the cause of the alteration in temperature. A syndrome is a *compilation* of signs and symptoms that are characteristic of a specific disease state. One example of a syndrome is the syndrome of inappropriate antidiuretic hormone (SIADH), described in Chapter 22.

Morphologic changes refer to changes in cell or tissue structure and *physiologic* changes refer to changes in body function. A demonstrable structural change is sometimes called a *lesion*. Quantitative measurements of structural and functional changes can be obtained through the use of physical measuring devices (thermometer or scale), laboratory tests, x-ray studies, and other scientific methods.

Causes of Disease

The causes of disease are known as the *etiological* factors while the method by which the lesions or disease develops is its *pathogenesis*. Etiology describes what sets the process in motion, and pathogenesis, how the motion evolves. Although the two terms have quite different meanings, they are often used interchangeably. For example, atherosclerosis is often cited as the cause (or etiology) of a heart attack, while in reality, the atherosclerotic changes that appear in the coronary vessels describe the pathogenesis of the disease—the etiology of atherosclerosis is still largely uncertain. The term *epidemiology* comes from the word epidemic and refers to the study of diseases in large populations. Epidemiologic studies look for patterns, such as the age, sex, race, or geographic location of persons affected with a particular disorder.

Developmental and acquired causes of disease

One way to view the factors that cause disease is to group them into categories according to whether they were present at birth or whether they were acquired following birth. The conditions that are present at birth include those that are *inherited* (due to genetic make-up) and *congenital* (due to errors in development). Not all genetic disorders are evident at birth; many take years to develop. *Acquired* defects result from conditions that occur after birth. These include trauma, exposure to injurious physical, chemical, and microbial agents; deficient food and oxygen supplies; immune responses; and neoplasia.

Multifactorial origins of disease

Most disease-causing agents are *nonspecific* and many different agents can cause disease of a single organ. For example, lung disease can result from trauma, infection, exposure to physical and chemical irritants, or neoplasia. With severe lung involvement, each of these agents has the potential to cause respiratory failure. On the other hand, a *single* agent or traumatic event can lead to disease or dysfunction of a *number* of organs and systems. An example of multisystem involvement occurs in severe circulatory shock when the blood flow to many different organs is decreased. The complications of circulatory shock can, therefore, affect a number of systems. These complications may include respiratory distress syndrome, renal failure, gastrointestinal ulcerations, and disseminated intravascular clotting.

Although a disease agent can affect more than one organ and a number of disease agents can affect the same organ, it is important to recognize that most disease states do not have a single cause. Rather, most diseases are *multifactorial* in origin. This is particularly true of diseases such as cancer, heart disease, and diabetes. The multiple factors that predispose to a particular disease are often referred to as *risk factors*.

Stress as a cause of disease

It was pointed out in the previous paragraph that most often a number of factors contribute to the cause and progression of a single disease and there is little doubt that both *physical* and *emotional stress* function as risk factors in the development of many illnesses. For example, the reader can undoubtedly identify the stresses associated with the "catching of" the common cold. Although it is generally agreed that the cold is caused by a virus, the persons most apt to develop a cold are those that have been exposed to the stresses of cold weather or wet feet, or are tired and "run down." Retrospectively, many persons can relate the actual onset of illness to the occurrence of a recent, particularly stressful event. Whether the stress contributed to the illness or the stressful event became more impressive because of its relationship to the illness is a question that remains unanswered.

Stress takes many forms and exerts its effect on many levels. There are changes in neural function, hormone release, and cardiorespiratory responses. Although the effect of stress on health is beyond the scope of this book, it is mentioned here because of its effect on physiologic functioning and its influence on the development of disease.

:Adaptation to Alterations in Function

Health is a dynamic state that requires a continual expenditure of energy. Much of this energy is used to recruit physiologic behaviors that oppose or compensate for changes that are perceived as threats to maintenance of the internal environment. In this respect, the human body is truly an amazing structure. It is able to withstand exposure to a variety of environmental stresses while maintaining its internal environment within the narrow confines of what is termed "normal." For example, we have been able to put men on the moon and send them to the depths of the ocean, yet their vital functions, as reflected by body temperature, blood pH, and heart rate, remained remarkably similar to those observed under normal environmental conditions.

The need to adapt is essential because minute changes in the internal environment can be lethal. For example, the normal range of blood pH is between 7.35 and 7.45 and even small deviations from these values can cause death. Adaptation is affected by a number of factors including impairment of capacity due to age, disease, or a *sudden* need to adapt. It is most effective when there is no impairment of adaptive capacity due to age or disease, and when the need for adaptation is a gradual process.

Generally speaking, adaptation affects the whole person. When adapting to stress the body uses those behaviors that are most efficient and effective—the body will not "use a baseball bat to kill a mosquito." Nor will the body use long-term mechanisms when short-term adaptation is sufficient. The increase in heart rate that accompanies a febrile illness is a temporary response designed to deliver additional oxygen to the tissues during the short period of time that the elevated temperature increases the metabolic needs of the tissues. On the other hand, hypertrophy of the left ventricle is a long-term adaptive response that occurs in persons with chronic hypertension.

Adaptation is further affected by the availability of adaptive responses and flexibility in selecting effective responses. The greater the number of available responses, the more effective the capacity to adapt. Adaptive capacity is decreased with extremes of age and when disease conditions limit the availability of adaptive responses. The immaturity of the infant impairs the ability to adapt as does the decline in functional reserve that occurs in the elderly. For example, the infant has difficulty concentrating urine due to the immaturity of the renal tubular structures and is, therefore, less able than an adult to cope with decreased water intake or exaggerated water losses. Similarly, persons with pre-existing diseases of the heart are less able to adapt to stresses that require recruitment of cardiovascular responses.

As indicated, adaptation is most efficient when the changes that occur in body function are gradual rather than sudden. It is possible, for instance, to lose a liter of blood through chronic gastrointestinal bleeding over a period of a week without developing signs of shock. However, a sudden hemorrhage that causes the loss of an equal amount of blood is apt to cause hypotension and shock.

In summary, disease is usually manifested by an alteration in body function. It is this alteration in function associated with the disease and the body's attempt to compensate for the altered function that causes the signs and symptoms that are associated with specific disease states.

:Study Guide

After you have studied this chapter, you should be able to meet the following objectives:

: : State an inclusive definition of *health*.

: : State and give examples of the terms used to describe changes that accompany a disease.

: : State an example of a hereditary disorder; a congenital disorder; an acquired disorder.

: : State the rationale for describing cancer as a disease of multifactorial origin.

: : State a general definition of *adaptation*, and give one example of adaptation to an alteration in function.

:References

1. Engel GL: A unified concept of health and disease. Perspect Biol Med 3:459, 1960
2. Porth CM: Physiological coping: a model for teaching pathophysiology. Nurs Outlook 25, No. 12:781, 1977

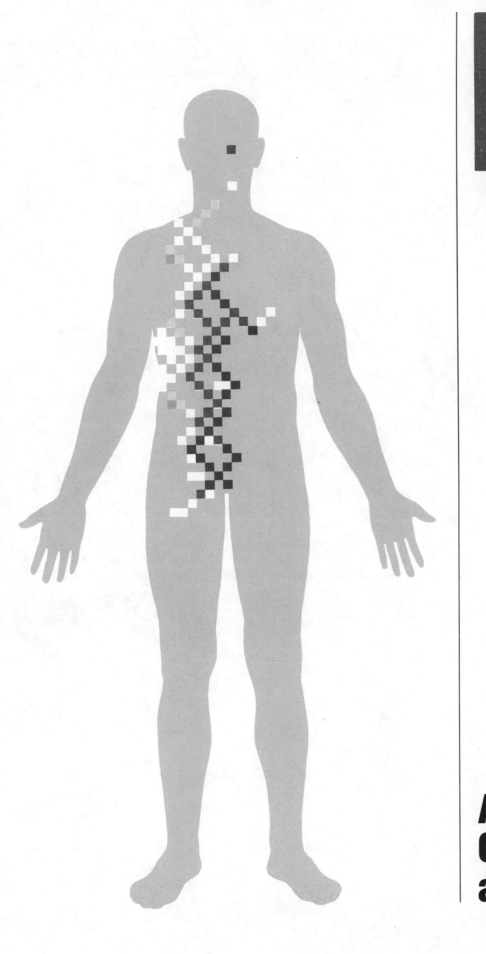

Alterations in Cell Structure and Function

From conception to death, a continuous process of human development proceeds, despite changes from within and outside the body. The ability to adapt and develop in a world of continuous stress is dependent upon both genetic endowment and the nature of the environmental stresses to which an individual is exposed. Within limits, the body is able to change cell structures so that they can survive—and even thrive—under less-than-optimal conditions. The body is able to resist attack by foreign agents and is able to repair tissue damage that accompanies the normal stresses of living. Only a fine line separates the normal, healthy adaptive responses that allow one to withstand the ravages of everyday life from the exaggerated or defective responses that cause disease.

This unit discusses (1) normal cell structure and function, (2) cellular responses to stress and injury, (3) inflammation and repair, (4) immune responses, (5) genetic and congenital influences on health, and (6) neoplasia.

2

Cell
and Tissue
Characteristics

The cell is the basic functional unit of the body. Cells, in turn, are organized into larger functional units called tissue. It is tissue that forms body structures and organs. To understand the function of the body, its various organs, and altered function that occurs with disease, it is necessary to understand the basic organization and function of the individual cells and the characteristics of the various tissue types.

:Cell Structure and Function

Although the cells of different organs vary in both structure and function, there are certain general characteristics that are common to most cells. When seen under a light microscope, three major components become evident—nucleus, cytoplasm, and cell membrane (Fig. 2-1). Within the cytoplasm are a number of physical structures generally called organelles. These are the inner organs of the cell.

The Nucleus

The nucleus controls cellular activity. Inside the *nuclear membrane* is the *nuclear sap* and *chromatin* that contains the chromosomes. The *chromosomes* contain the *genes*, which are made up of *deoxyribonucleic acid* (DNA). Genes not only control cellular replication, but they also control cellular activity by determining the type of proteins that are made by the cell.

Cell activity is largely determined by cell enzymes that are proteins.

Not all genes are active at all times, nor are the same genes active in all cell types. On the contrary, only a small, select group of genes is active in protein synthesis and this group varies from one cell type to another. This difference can be noted in the different types of proteins and enzymes that are found in different tissues of the body. Gene activity and protein synthesis can be altered by hormone actions and by stresses imposed on the cell. Many of the cellular adaptations that are discussed in the latter part of this chapter are mediated by changes in gene expression.

Although DNA determines the type of protein that is synthesized in a cell, the transmission of this information and the synthesis of proteins are carried out by the *ribonucleic acid* (RNA). The nucleus contains one or more rounded bodies known as the nucleoli (Fig. 2-1) and it is within these bodies that RNA is synthesized. There are three types of RNA. *Messenger RNA (mRNA)* is the template for protein synthesis; it carries the information coded on DNA into the cytoplasm. There is an mRNA molecule that corresponds to each gene or group of genes being expressed in the nucleus. *Transfer RNA (tRNA)* transfers the message from mRNA to the ribosomes; it selects and carries the appropriate amino acids to the ribosomes. *Ribosomal RNA (rRNA)* is the major component of the ribosomes in which protein synthesis takes place. These relationships are indicated in the chart on the facing page.

Figure 2–1. A composite cell designed to show, in one cell, all of the various components of the nucleus and cytoplasm.

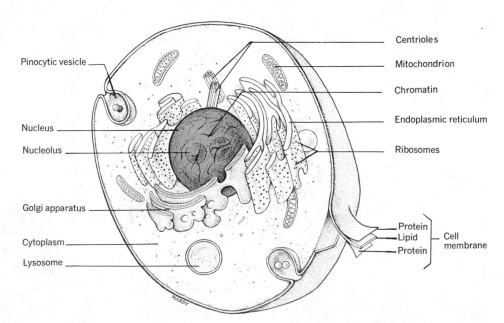

Pinocytic vesicle

Nucleus

Nucleolus

Golgi apparatus

Cytoplasm

Lysosome

Centrioles

Mitochondrion

Chromatin

Endoplasmic reticulum

Ribosomes

Protein
Lipid — Cell membrane
Protein

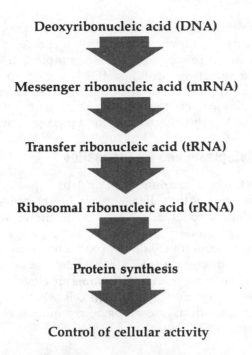

Deoxyribonucleic acid (DNA)

Messenger ribonucleic acid (mRNA)

Transfer ribonucleic acid (tRNA)

Ribosomal ribonucleic acid (rRNA)

Protein synthesis

Control of cellular activity

The nuclear contents are surrounded by a double walled *nuclear membrane*. The large number of nuclear pores in this membrane permit diffusion of fluids, metabolites, mRNA, and tRNA to move between the nuclear and cytoplasmic compartments.

The Ribosomes

The ribosomes serve as sites of protein synthesis in the cell. As previously mentioned, the ribosomes are small particles of nucleoproteins (rRNA and proteins) that are synthesized in the cell nucleus and can be found as free ribosomes or attached to the wall of the endoplasmic reticulum (see Fig. 2-2). The free ribosomes are singly scattered in the cytoplasm or are joined to form functional units called polyribosomes.

The Endoplasmic Reticulum

The endoplasmic reticulum (ER) is an extensive system of paired parallel membranes that connect various parts of the inner cell. There are two types of ER—rough and smooth. The rough ER is studded with ribosomes and functions in synthesis of proteins (Fig. 2-2).

Hormone synthesis by glandular cells and plasma protein production by liver cells takes place in the rough ER. The smooth ER is free of ribosomes, but is often attached to the rough ER. Functions of the smooth ER vary in different cells. The sarcoplasmic reticulum of skeletal and cardiac muscle cells

is a form of smooth ER. Calcium ions needed for muscle contraction are stored and released from cisterns located in the sarcoplasmic reticulum of these cells.

In the liver, the smooth ER is involved in glycogen storage and drug metabolism. There is an interesting form of adaptation that occurs in the smooth ER of the liver cells responsible for metabolizing certain drugs such as phenobarbital. It is known that repeated administration of phenobarbital leads to a state of increased tolerance to the drug, such that the same dose of drug no longer produces the same degree of sedation. This response has been traced to increased drug metabolism due to increased synthesis of drug-metabolizing enzymes by the ER membrane. This system is sometimes called the microsomal system because the ER can be fragmented in the laboratory, and when this is done, small vesicles called microsomes are formed. The microsomal system responsible for metabolizing phenobarbital has a cross-over effect that influences the metabolism of other drugs that use the same metabolic pathway.

The Golgi Complex

The Golgi complex consists of flattened, membranous saccules and cisterns that communicate with the ER, and acts as a receptacle for hormones and other substances that the ER produces. It then collects and packages these substances into secretory granules and vesicles. The secretory granules move out of the Golgi complex, into the cytoplasm, and, following an appropriate signal, are then released from the cell through the process of exocytosis or

Figure 2–2. Diagram of the endoplasmic reticulum and related ribosomes. (Chaffee EE, Lytle IM: Basic Physiology and Anatomy, 4th ed. Philadelphia, JB Lippincott, 1980)

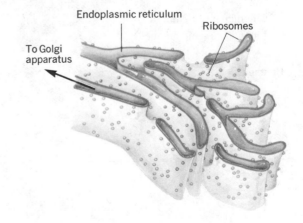

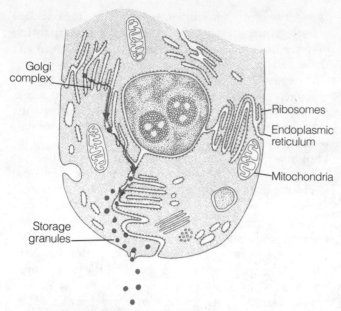

Figure 2–3. Schematic diagram for hormone secretion. The hormone is synthesized by the ribosomes. It moves from the rough endoplasmic reticulum to the Golgi complex where it forms secretory granules. These leave the Golgi complex and are stored within the cytoplasm until released from the cell in response to an appropriate signal.

Figure 2–4. Diagram of a mitochondrion. The inner membrane forms transverse folds called the cristae. It is here that the enzymes needed for the final step in ATP production (oxidative phosphorylation) are located. (Chaffee EE, Lytle IM: Basic Physiology and Anatomy, 4th ed. Philadelphia, JB Lippincott, 1980)

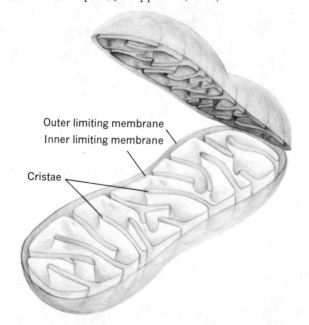

reverse phagocytosis. Figure 2-3 is a diagram of the synthesis and movement of a hormone through the endoplasmic reticulum and Golgi complex. In addition to secreting proteins, the Golgi complex is thought to produce some of the large carbohydrate molecules that are needed to combine with proteins produced in the rough ER to form glycoproteins.

The Cytoplasm and Its Organelles

The cytoplasm surrounds the nucleus and it is here that the work of the cell takes place. The cytoplasm is essentially a colloidal solution that contains water, suspended proteins, neutral fats, and glycogen molecules. Although they do not contribute to the cell's function, there are pigments that may also accumulate in the cytoplasm. The cytoplasm contains the organelles, or inner organs of the cell, which include the mitochondria, lysosomes, microtubules, microfilaments, and centrioles.

The mitochondria

The mitochondria are literally the "power plants" of the cell, for it is here that energy from foodstuffs is transformed into an energy-rich compound, adenosine triphosphate (ATP), which powers the various activities that take place within the cell. The mitochondria capture energy contained in glucose, fatty acids, and amino acids through both the tricarboxylic acid or Krebs cycle and the electron-transport system that requires the presence of oxygen for its operation (see Chap. 34 for discussion of metabolic process). The mitochondria are encased in a double membrane. An outer membrane encloses the periphery of the mitochrondria and an inner membrane is enfolded to form the cristae which aid in the production and temporary storage of ATP (Fig. 2-4). The mitochrondria are located close to the site of energy consumption in the cell, i.e., near the myofibrils in muscle cells. The number of mitochrondria in a given cell type is largely determined by the type of activity that the cell performs and the amount of energy that is needed to perform this activity.

The lysosomes

The lysosomes essentially form the digestive system of the cell. The lysosomes consist of small vesicles or sacs which contain hydrolytic enzymes capable of breaking down worn-out cell parts and foreign material that enters the cell. The enzymes contained in the lysosomes are so powerful that they are often called "suicide bags" because under abnormal conditions their contents can be released, causing lysis and the destruction of cellular contents. Under other conditions their contents can be released into the extracellular spaces, destroying the surrounding cells. One of the theories of irreversible shock suggests that this stage of shock is caused, at least in part, by widespread release of lysosomal enzymes from cells that have been damaged by lack of oxygen.

The microtubules and microfilaments

Because they control cell shape and movement, the microtubules and microfilaments are often called the cytoskeletal system.

The *microtubules* are long, rigid, threadlike structures that are dispersed throughout the cytoplasm and are usually arranged in bundles. In cilia and sperm, the microtubules occur in doublets. The centrioles, which will be discussed next, contain microtubules arranged in triplets. It appears that microtubules can be rapidly assembled and disassembled according to the needs of the cell. The assembly of microtubules is halted by the action of the plant alkaloid, colchicine. In the laboratory this compound is used to halt cell mitosis, and it is also used in the treatment of gout. It is thought that the drug interferes with microtubular function and leukocyte motility and, therefore, leads to a decrease in the inflammatory reaction that occurs with this condition.

The *microfilaments* occur in association with the microtubules. The contractile proteins—actin, myosin, and troponin—are examples of microfilaments found in muscle cells.

Abnormalities of the cytoskeletal system may constitute important causes of alterations in cellular function. Robbins suggests that in certain disease conditions, such as diabetes mellitus, alterations in

leukocyte mobility and migration may interfere with the inflammatory response and predispose to the development of bacterial infection.[1]

The centrioles

The centrioles, found in cells capable of reproducing themselves, are composed of nine bundles of microfilaments, each of which contains three microfilaments. The microfilaments aid in movement of the chromosomes during cell division.

The Cell Membrane

The cell is enclosed in a thin membrane that separates the intracellular contents from the extracellular environment. To distinguish it from the other cell membranes, such as the mitochondrial or nuclear membranes, the cell membrane is often called the plasma membrane. In many respects, the plasma membrane is one of the most important parts of the cell. The functions of the cell membrane include (1) acting as a semipermeable membrane that separates the intracellular and extracellular environments, (2) carrying receptors for hormones and other biologically active substances, (3) participating in the electrical events that occur in nerve and muscle cells, and (4) aiding in the regulation of growth and proliferation. It is also thought that the cell membrane may play an important role in the cancerous behavior of cells,[2] which function will be discussed in Chapter 7.

The cell membrane consists of an organized arrangment of lipids, carbohydrates, and proteins (Fig. 2-5). According to current theories, the lipids

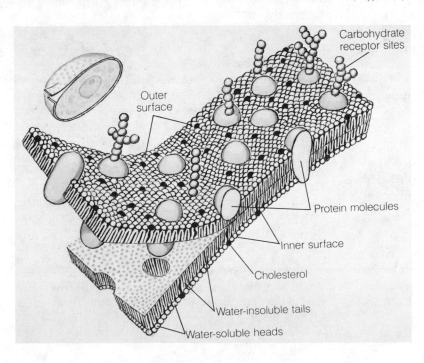

Figure 2–5.   Diagram of a cell membrane. The right end is intact, but the left end has been split along the plane of the lipid tails. (Chaffee EE, Lytle IM: Basic Physiology and Anatomy, 4th ed. Philadelphia, JB Lippincott, 1980)

form a bilayer structure that is essentially impermeable to all but the lipid-soluble substances. It is believed that globular proteins are embedded in this lipid bilayer and that these proteins participate in the transport of lipid-insoluble particles. According to this schema, some of the globular proteins move within the membrane structure acting as carriers, some are attached to either side of the membrane, and others pass directly through the membrane, communicating with both the inside and the outside of the cell. It is probable that these latter proteins form channels that permit passage of substances such as water and specific ions such as sodium, hydrogen, and chloride.

The cell surface has been observed, under the electron microscope, to be surrounded by a fuzzy-looking layer called the cell coat or *"glycocalyx."* This layer is made up of glycolipid and glycoprotein molecules (Fig. 2-5) that participate in cell membrane interactions. The cell coat contains the sites for hormone recognition, the ABO blood group, and other tissue antigens.

Microvilli are elongated protrusions of the cell membrane that are arranged as a series of tubular extensions. These extensions greatly increase the surface area of the cell membrane. This specialized cell membrane arrangement facilitates the absorption of fluids and other materials. Microvilli are found in the lumen of the small intestine.

Cilia are long protuberances of the cell membrane with the tapered ends that are characteristic of many cell types, particularly the epithelium. They are anchored in the cytoplasm by a structure similar to the centriole, and extending from this structure is a series of microtubules that are surrounded by the cell membrane. By sliding the microfilaments on each other, the cilia are capable of a sweeping type of movement. Longer cilia are called flagella. The cilia provide a mechanism for cell movement, or if the location of the cell is fixed, as in the respiratory tract, for the movement of adjacent fluids.

Membrane transport

There is a constant movement of molecules and ions across the cell membrane. This movement is facilitated by diffusion, osmosis, facilitated diffusion, active transport, and pinocytosis. Each of these mechanisms is depicted in Figure 2-6.

Diffusion refers to the process whereby molecules of gases and other substances move from an area of higher to lower concentration, and become equally distributed across the cell membrane. Lipid-soluble molecules such as carbon dioxide cross the cell membrane rapidly by diffusion.

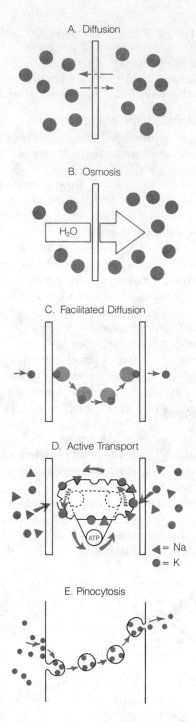

Figure 2–6. Mechanisms of membrane transport. Figure *A* represents diffusion in which the molecules are equally distributed across the membrane. In figure *B* the osmotically active particles regulate the flow of water. In figure *C*, facilitated diffusion uses a carrier system. Figure *D* represents active transport in which selected molecules are transported across the membrane using the energy driven (ATP) pump. The membrane forms a vesicle in *E* that engulfs the particle and then transports it across the membrane where it is released. This is called pinocytosis.

Osmosis is concerned with the passage of water across the semipermeable membrane. Osmosis is regulated by the concentration of osmotically active particles that are present on either side of the membrane (see Chap. 21).

Facilitated diffusion involves a carrier system. Substances that are not lipid-soluble and cannot pass readily through the cell membrane depend on their ability to combine with special carriers for transport across the membrane.

Active transport moves substances through the cell membrane against a concentration gradient (from a lower to a higher concentration). Active transport requires expenditure of ATP. The sodium and potassium membrane transport system, sometimes called the sodium and potassium pump, is an example of active transport. The sodium concentration within the cell is about 14 times less than the extracellular concentration, and the potassium concentration outside the cell is about 28 times less than that within the cell. The sodium and potassium pump extrudes sodium from the cell and then returns potassium to the cell. Were it not for the activity of the sodium and potassium pump, sodium would accumulate within the cell, and the cell would swell as water movement into the cell increased.

Pinocytosis is a mechanism by which the cell membrane engulfs particles and forms a pinocytic vesicle. The vesicle then breaks away from the inner surface of the cell membrane and moves into the cytoplasm where it is eventually freed by the action of lysosomes or other cytoplasmic enzymes. Pinocytosis is important to the transport of proteins and strong solutions of electrolytes.

Endocytosis is a mechanism for secretion of intracellular fluid into the extracellular spaces. It is the reverse of pinocytosis in that a fluid-filled vacuole fuses to the inner side of the cell membrane and an opening occurs to the outside of the cell surface, allowing the contents of the vacuole to be released into the extracellular fluid.

Phagocytosis is a mechanism similar to pinocytosis, except that larger indentations occur in the cell membrane, allowing the cell to ingest large particles such as bacteria and cell debris.

Intercellular junctions

Intercellular attachments join cell membranes of adjacent cells to form a unit. *Desmosomes* serve as a "spot weld" to hold the cell membranes of two cells together. The zonula occludens or *tight junction* is another form of intercellular junction by which the cell membranes are actually fused together. A less common form of intercellular adhesion involves the close approximation of the cell membranes with the formation of apparent pores between the cytoplasms of the two cells. These junctions or *nexus* possess low electrical-resistance properties and permit electrical communication between cells. The type of cell junction varies with the function of the tissue type. Tissues that facilitate absorption of fluids usually have cells that are connected by desmosomes. The intercalated discs that join the myocardial fibers of the heart are nexus with low resistance properties.

In summary, the cell is a remarkably autonomous structure that functions in a manner strikingly similar to that of the total organism. Cells are separated from their external environment by a semipermeable cell membrane that aids in regulating the osmotic and ionic homeostasis of the cells' interior. The cell nucleus controls cell function and is the master-mind of the cell, while the cytoplasm contains the cell's inner organs and is the cell's work site. The cell transforms foodstuffs into a high-energy chemical compound, ATP, and uses ATP as a power source for its functions. Cells contain other structures such as microtubules and microfilaments that are needed for the specific functions which they perform.

:Tissue Types

In the preceding section we discussed the individual cell. Although cells are similar, their structure and function vary according to the needs of the tissues. While an extensive discussion of tissue types is beyond the scope of this text, a brief overview is offered in preparation for understanding the subsequent chapters in this unit.

Cell Differentiation

The formation of different types of cells and the disposition of these cells into tissue types is called cell differentiation. Following conception, the fertilized ovum divides and subdivides and ultimately forms over a hundred different cell types. The process of cell differentiation normally moves forward and is irreversible, producing cells that are more specialized than their predecessors. This means that once differentiation has occurred, the tissue type does not move backward to an earlier stage of differentiation.

Although most cells proceed through differentiation into specialized cell types, many tissues contain a few cells that apparently are only partially differentiated. These cells are still capable of cell division and serve as a stem cell source for continued production of specialized cells throughout the life span of the organism. This is one of the major processes by which regeneration is possible in some but not all tissues. Skeletal muscle, for example, has relatively few undifferentiated cells to serve as a reserve supply. Cancer cells can originate from stem cells, or, in special cases, from cells that undergo undifferentiation or revert to earlier stages of differentiation (see Chap.7 for further discussion).

The Embryonic Origin of Tissue Types

The four basic tissue types are often described in terms of embryonic origin. The very young embryo is essentially a three-layered tubular structure (Fig. 2-7). The outer layer of the tube is called the ectoderm, the middle layer, the mesoderm, and the inner layer, the endoderm. All of the adult body tissues originated from these three cellular layers. Epithelium has its origin in all three embryonic layers, connective tissue and muscle develop from the mesoderm, and nervous tissue develops from the ectoderm. Mesenchymal tissue is a precursor to connective tissue and has its origin in the mesoderm. The epithelial lining of the gut, the respiratory tract, and much of the urinary system is derived from the endoderm.

Figure 2–7. Diagram of the embryonic tissue layers.

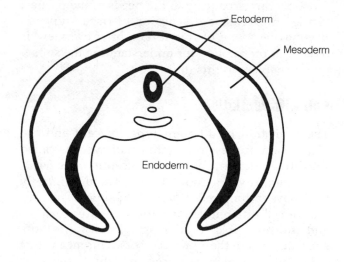

Four Types of Tissue

All of the more than 100 different types of body cells can be classified under four basic or primary tissue types: epithelium, connective, muscle, and nervous. Each of the primary tissue types has various subdivisions. The four tissue types and the major subdivisions are summarized in Table 2-1.

Table 2–1   Classification of Tissue Types

Tissue Type	Location*
Epithelium	
Covering and lining of body surfaces	
Simple epithelium	
squamous	Lining of blood vessels and body cavities
cuboidal	Covering of ovaries and thyroid gland
columnar	Lining of intestine and gall bladder
Pseudostratified epithelium	Trachea and respiratory passages
Stratified epithelium	
squamous keratinized	Skin
squamous nonkeratinized	Mucous membranes of mouth, esophagus, and vagina
transitional	Bladder
Glandular	
Endocrine	Pituitary, thyroid, adrenal, others
Exocrine	Sweat glands and glands in gastrointestinal tract
Connective Tissue	
Loose	Fibroblasts, adipose tissue, endothelial vessel lining
Hematopoietic	Blood cells, myeloid tissue (bone marrow), lymphoid tissue
Supporting tissues	Connective tissue and cartilage, bone and joint structures
Muscle	
Striated	Skeletal muscles
Cardiac	Myocardium
Smooth	Gastrointestinal tract, blood vessels, bronchi, bladder, others
Nervous Tissue	Central and peripheral nerves

*Not inclusive

Epithelium

Epithelial tissue covers the body's outer surface, lines the internal surface, and forms the glandular tissues. The epithelium protects (skin and mucous membranes), secretes (glandular tissue and goblet cells), absorbs (intestinal mucosa), and filters (renal glomeruli). The epithelial cells are avascular, that is, they have no blood vessels of their own and must receive oxygen and nutrients from the capillaries of the connective tissue upon which the epithelium rests. To survive the epithelial cells must be kept moist. Even the seemingly dry skin epithelium is kept moist by a nonvitalized waterproof layer of keratin which prevents evaporation of moisture from the deeper living cells. Epithelium is able to quickly regenerate when injury occurs.

The epithelium can be divided into three types: simple, stratified, and pseudostratified. The terms squamous (thin and flat), cuboidal (cube shaped), and columnar (resembling a column) refer to the cell shapes (Fig. 2-8).

Simple epithelium contains a single layer of cells. *Simple squamous epithelium* is adapted for filtration; it is found lining the blood vessels, lymph nodes, and alveoli of the lung. *Simple cuboidal epithelium* is found on the surface of the ovary and in the thyroid. *Simple columnar epithelium* lines the intestine. One form of simple columnar epithelium has hairlike projections called *cilia*, and another produces mucus and is called a *goblet* cell.

Stratified epithelium contains more than one layer of cells and is designed to protect the body surface. *Keratin* is a tough fibrous protein that is formed from flattened dead cells. *Stratified squamous keratinized epithelium* makes up the epidermis of the skin and *nonkeratinized cells* are found on wet surfaces such as the mouth and tongue.

Pseudostratified columnar epithelium is a mixture of columnar cell types. As some of these do not reach the surface of the tissue, it gives the appearance of stratified epithelium. Pseudostratified columnar ciliated epithelium with goblet cells forms the lining of most of the upper respiratory tract.

Glandular epithelium can be divided into two types: exocrine and endocrine. The *exocrine glands* have ducts and discharge their secretions directly onto the epithelial surface where they are located. Sweat glands and alveolar glands are examples of exocrine glands. The *endocrine glands* produce secretions that move directly into the blood stream.

Connective tissue

Connective tissue is the most abundant tissue in the body. As its name indicates, it connects and holds

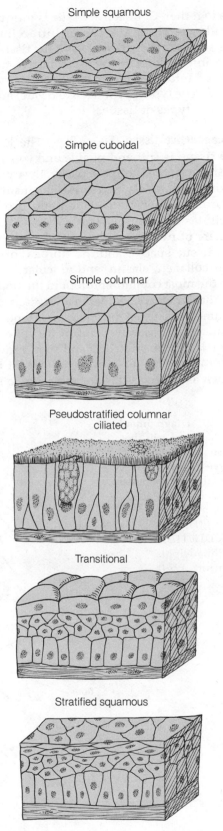

Simple squamous

Simple cuboidal

Simple columnar

Pseudostratified columnar ciliated

Transitional

Stratified squamous

Figure 2–8. Representation of the various epithelial tissue types.

tissues together. Connective tissue is unique in that it includes nonliving forms of intracellular substances such as collagen fibers and the tissue gel that fills the intercellular spaces. Connective tissue can be divided into three types: loose connective tissue, hematopoietic types of connective tissue, and strong supporting types of tissue.

Loose connective tissue (Fig. 2-9).   The loose connective tissue is soft and pliable and consists of fibroblasts, mast cells, adipose tissue, the intracellular lining of blood vessels, and intracellular substances. The fibroblasts secrete collagen and produce the intracellular substances. These intracellular substances are of two types: the *amorphous type* which fills the tissue spaces, and the fibrous form which includes collagen, elastin, and reticular fibers. *Collagen* is the most common protein in the body; it is a tough, nonliving, white fiber that serves as the structural framework for skin, ligaments, tendons, and numerous other structures. *Elastin* acts like a rubber band for it can be stretched and then return to its original form. Elastin fibers are abundant in structures such as the aorta that are subjected to frequent

stretching. *Reticular fibers* form networks that join connective tissue to other tissues. Loose connective tissue supports the epithelial tissues and provides the means by which these tissues are nourished. In an organ that contains both epithelial and connective tissue, the term *parenchymal* tissue refers to the functioning epithelium in contradistinction to its connective tissue framework.

Hematopoietic tissue.   The hematopoietic types of connective tissue include the blood cells, bone marrow, and lymphatic tissue. The role of the hematopoietic system in inflammation and immunity is discussed in Chapters 4 and 5; the reticulocyte or red blood cell is discussed in Chapter 20.

Strong supporting connective tissue.   The third form of connective tissue—the strong supporting form—consists of dense connective tissue, cartilage, and bone. The dense connective tissues form the tendons and ligaments that join muscle to bones and bones to bones. A layer of dense connective tissue also forms a capsule for many organs and body structures such as the kidney and heart. Dense connective tissue

Figure 2–9. Diagrammatic representation of cells that may be seen in loose connective tissue. The cells lie in an intercellular matrix that is bathed in tissue fluid that originates from capillaries. (Ham AW, Cormack DH: Histology, 8th ed. Philadelphia, JB Lippincott, 1979)

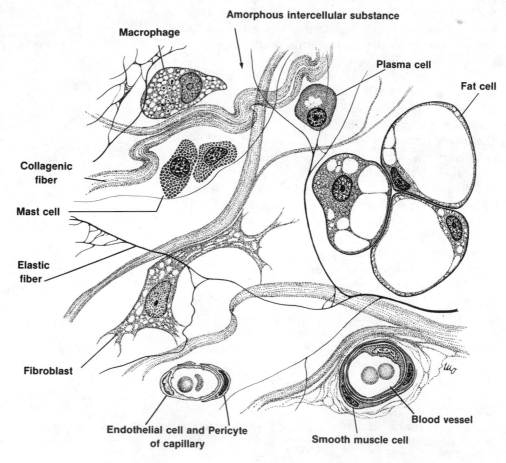

does not require many capillaries because it is composed largely of nonliving collagen fibers.

Cartilage and bone are special types of dense connective tissue in which the individual cells (chondrocytes and osteocytes) are housed in little lakes called *lacunae*. There are no blood vessels in cartilage and bone and therefore the lacunae provide a system for the diffusion of cellular nutrients and wastes. Both cartilage and bone are covered by a membrane, the perichondrium and periosteum, from which the loose connective tissue cells that form the cartilage (fibroblasts) and bone (osteoblasts) are formed. Disruption of this membranous covering interferes with regeneration of bone and cartilage.

Cartilage differs from bone in that its intercellular substance consists of a mucopolysaccharide material that has a plastic, rather than rigid, consistency. Cartilage provides the means for bone growth in both the prenatal and postnatal periods; covers the articulating surfaces of the joints; makes up the flexible structure of the rib cartilage, the nose, and larynx; and forms the spongy fibrocartilage of the intervertebral discs and the semilunar discs in the knee joint.

Bone is osseous connective tissue. It resembles cartilage in that its cells (osteocytes) are located in lacunae. The intercellular substance of bone consists of two fundamentally different components—an organic matrix and mineral salts. The organic intercellular substance of bone is secreted by the osteoblasts in a manner similar to that by which fibroblasts secrete collagen fibers. The reabsorption of bone is performed by cells called the osteoclasts (see Chap. 4 for a discussion of the function of the osteoblasts and osteoclasts in bone repair).

Muscle tissue

Muscle tissue is highly developed for contractility. Its cells contain the contractile elements actin and myosin. There are three types of muscle tissue: striated, cardiac, and smooth. In *striated muscle* the actin and myosin filaments are arranged in striations which give the muscle a striped appearance. Striated muscle is found in skeletal (voluntary) muscles. It receives its innervation from the central nervous system. *Cardiac muscle* is found in the myocardium. Myocardial muscle is designed to pump blood continuously; it has the inherent properties of automaticity, rhythmicity, and conductivity. The pumping action of the heart is controlled by impulses originating in the cardiac conduction system and is modified by blood-borne neural mediators and impulses from the autonomic nervous system (see Chap. 12).

Smooth muscle is found in many organs; it is sometimes called involuntary muscle because it is controlled by the autonomic nervous system. It contols the action of blood vessels, the gastrointestinal tract, the urinary bladder, the iris of the eye and the tubes (ureters, bile duct, others) that connect many organs. Neither skeletal nor cardiac muscle is able to undergo the mitotic activity and regeneration needed to replace injured cells. Smooth muscle, however, may proliferate and undergo mitotic activity. Some increases in smooth muscle are physiologic, such as occurs in the uterus during pregnancy. Others, such as the increase in smooth muscle that occurs in the arteries of persons with chronic hypertension, are pathologic.

Nervous tissue

Nervous tissue is a specialized form of tissue designed for communication purposes. The nervous tissue develops from the ectoderm of the embryo and includes the neurons, the supporting cells of the nervous system, and the ependymal cells that line the ventricular system. The structure and organization of nervous tissue is discussed in Chapter 40.

In summary, body cells are organized into four basic tissue types: epithelial, connective, muscle, and nervous. The epithelium covers the body surfaces and forms the functional components of the glandular structures. Connective tissue supports and connects body structures; it forms the bones and skeletal system, the joint structures, the blood cells, and the intercellular substances. Muscle tissue is a specialized tissue that is designed for contractility. There are three types of muscle tissue: skeletal, cardiac, and smooth. Nervous tissue is designed for communication purposes and includes the neurons, the supporting neural structures, and the ependymal cells that line the ventricles of the brain and the spinal canal.

:Study Guide

After you have studied this chapter, you should be able to meet the following objectives:

: : List the components of the cell nucleus and the function of each.

: : State the composition of the ribosomes.

: : Differentiate rough ER and smooth ER according to function.

: : State the function of the Golgi complex.

: : State the composition of the cytoplasm.

: :   Explain why the mitochondria are described as the power plants of the cell.

: :   State a possible role of the lysosomes in irreversible shock.

: :   Define *microtubule*, *microfilament*, and *centriole* on the basis of function.

: :   State four functions of the cell membrane.

: :   State the mechanisms of membrane transport.

: :   Explain the function of the intercellular junctions.

: :   Describe the process of cell differentiation.

: :   Explain why the basic tissue types are described in terms of their embryonic origin.

: :   Define the three types of epithelium.

: :   State the function of each of the three types of connective tissue.

: :   Describe the properties of muscle tissue.

: :   State the general function of nervous tissue.

:References

1. Robbins SL, Cotran RS: Pathologic Basis of Disease, 2nd ed, p 11. Philadelphia, WB Saunders, 1979.
2. Robbins SL, Cotran RS: Pathologic Basis of Disease, 2nd ed, p 2. Philadelphia, WB Saunders, 1979.

3

Cell Injury and Death

When confronted with stresses that tend to disrupt its normal structure and function, the cell undergoes adaptive changes that permit survival and maintenance of function. When the challenge to adapt exceeds the cell's capabilities, retrogressive changes begin to take place. These changes can be sublethal and *reversible* or they can become *irreversible*, causing cell death. In the end, the effect that cell injury exerts on overall body function is determined by the tissue type and by the location and extent of the injury. This chapter addresses cellular responses to stress, injury, and death.

:Cellular Adaptation

Cells adapt to changes in the internal environment just as the total organism adapts to changes in the external environment. Cells may adapt by undergoing changes in size, number, and type. These changes, acting singly or in combination, may lead to atrophy, hypertrophy, hyperplasia, metaplasia, and dysplasia. In contrast to abnormal cell changes, normal adaptive responses occur in response to need and an appropriate stimulus. Once the need or stimulus has been removed, the adaptive response ceases.

Figure 3–1. High-power photomicrograph of a human nerve ganglion. Two ganglion cells may be seen in the picture; their cytoplasm contains numerous granules of lipofuscin pigment. (Ham AW, Cormack DH: Histology, 8th ed. Philadelphia, JB Lippincott, 1979)

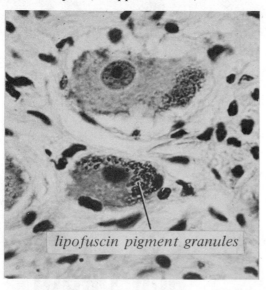

lipofuscin pigment granules

Atrophy

Atrophy refers to a decrease in the size of a body part brought about by shrinkage in the size of its cells. The size of all the structural components of the cell usually decreases as the cell atrophies. When confronted with a decrease in work demands or adverse environmental conditions, most cells are able to revert to a smaller size, and a lower and more efficient level of functioning which is compatible with survival.

The general causes of atrophy are grouped into the following categories: (1) decreased nutrition, (2) disuse, (3) denervation, (4) ischemia, and (5) lack of endocrine stimulation. When there is a prolonged period of interference with general nutrition, such as occurs during starvation or other disease conditions, the body undergoes a more or less generalized wasting of tissue mass. Localized atrophy, for example, that which appears in extremities affected by peripheral vascular disease, is often observed in association with ischemia. Disuse atrophy is seen in muscles of paralyzed limbs and in extremities that have been encased in plaster casts. Lack of endocrine stimulation causes the involutional changes that occur in the reproductive structures during menopause.

In some situations, a collection of yellow–brown pigment called lipofuscin accompanies the retrogressive changes that occur with atrophy (Fig. 3-1). This form of atrophy is referred to as *brown atrophy*. The pigment is thought to represent an accumulation of indigestible residues from within the cell. It is seen more commonly in heart, nerve, and liver cells than in other forms of tissue. The amount of lipofuscin increases with age and is sometimes referred to as the "wear and tear" pigment.

Hypertrophy

Hypertrophy is an increase in the amount of functioning tissue mass of an organ or part caused by an increase in cell size. Hypertrophy may be either physiologic or pathologic. The increase in muscle mass associated with exercise is an example of physiologic hypertrophy. Pathologic hypertrophy may be adaptive or compensatory. Examples of adaptive hypertrophy are the thickening of the urinary bladder due to long-continued obstruction of urinary outflow, and myocardial hypertrophy that results from valvular heart disease or hypertension. Compensatory hypertrophy is the enlargement of a remaining organ or tissue after a portion has been surgically removed or rendered inactive. For instance, if one kidney is removed, the remaining kidney enlarges to compensate for the loss. In hypertrophy there is an increase in the functional components of the cell that allows equilibrium between demand and the functional capacity of the cell to be reached. For example, as muscle cells hypertrophy there is synthesis of additional microfilaments, cell enzymes, and ATP.

Hyperplasia

Hyperplasia is an increase in the number of cells of a part. Hyperplasia occurs in cells which are capable of mitotic division, such as those of the epidermis, intestinal epithelial layer, and glandular tissue. Nerve cells and skeletal and cardiac muscle do not divide and therefore have no capacity for hyperplastic growth. As with other normal adaptive cellular respones, hyperplasia is a controlled process that occurs in response to an appropriate stimulus and ceases once the stimulus has been removed. There are two types of stimuli that are generally associated with hyperplasia—physiologic and nonphysiologic. Breast and uterine enlargement during pregnancy is an example of a physiologic hyperplasia that is hormonally regulated. An example of a nonphysiological form of hyperplasia occurs in response to abnormal hormonal stimulation of target cells. Hyperplasia of target cells in the endometrium occurs with excessive estrogen production; the abnormally thickened uterine layer may bleed excessively and frequently.

Metaplasia

Metaplasia is the conversion from one adult cell type to another adult cell type. It allows for substitution of cells that are better able to tolerate environmental stresses. The conversion of cell types never oversteps the boundaries of the primary groups of tissue (epithelial or connective). In metaplasia, one type of epithelial cell may be converted to another type of epithelial cell, but not to a connective tissue cell. An example of metaplasia is the adaptive substitution of stratified squamous epithelial cells for the columnar ciliated epithelial cells in the trachea and large airways in the person who is a habitual cigarette smoker. Metaplasia of epithelial tissue occurs in chronic irritation and inflammation. For unknown reasons, a vitamin A deficiency tends to cause squamous metaplasia of the respiratory tract. Metaplasia occurs in response to a stimulus and is potentially reversible.

Dysplasia

Dysplasia is deranged cell growth that results in cells with variations in size, shape, and appearance. Minor degrees of dysplasia occur in association with chronic irritation or inflammation. Although dysplasia is abnormal, it is adaptive in that it is potentially reversible once the irritating cause has been found and removed. Dysplastic tissue changes may progress to neoplastic disease, and it is at this point that dysplasia gains its importance.

In summary, cells adapt to changes in their environment and in their work demands by changing size, number, and character. Normal adaptive changes are consistent with the needs of the cell and occur in response to an appropriate stimulus. The changes are reversed once the stimuli have been withdrawn.

:Cell Injury

When cells are injured or the need to adapt becomes overwhelming, degenerative changes begin to appear. Degeneration is a retrogressive process in which there is cellular deterioration, along with changes in both the chemical structure and microscopic appearance of the cell. Degeneration can follow many paths, and eventually leads to either reversible or irreversible cell changes. Irreversible changes consist of necrosis (cell death) and tissue dissolution. Frequently, however, the final outcome is not reached because somewhere along the way the process is *reversed*, allowing cells and tissues to return to their normal state.

Causes of Cell Damage

There are many ways in which cell damage can occur. The common forms of injury tend to fall into several categories: (1) hypoxia, (2) physical injury, (3) radiation, (4) chemical injury, (5) effect of biologic agents, (6) inflammation and immune responses, (7) genetic derangements, and (8) nutritional imbalances.

Hypoxia
One of the most common causes of tissue injury is *hypoxia*. Hypoxic cell injury occurs with impairment of blood flow (development of a blood clot in an artery that supplies the brain); interference with the oxygen-carrying capacity of blood (carbon monoxide poisoning); failure to adequately oxygenate

blood (respiratory failure); failure of the heart as a pump (cardiac arrest); or poisoning of the oxidative phosphorylation system in the cell that is needed for generation of ATP (cyanide poisoning).

Hypoxia literally causes a power failure within the cell and leads to cessation of ATP-dependent activities. This includes the function of the sodium and potassium membrane pump that is needed to maintain the cell's osmotic and ionic homeostasis. The length of time that cells can survive without oxygen is determined by the tissue type and the metabolic needs of the cell. It is a well-known fact that brain cells begin to die within four to six minutes after the onset of anoxia. Damage to other cell systems, such as those of the skin, takes considerably longer to occur.

Hypoxia also serves as the ultimate cause of cell death in other forms of injury. For example, toxins from certain microorganisms interfere with cellular use of oxygen, and physical agents, such as cold, cause severe vasoconstriction and impaired blood flow.

Physical agents

Physical agents include mechanical injuries, extremes of temperature, and electrical forces. *Mechanical injuries* may actually disrupt cell contents and injure the cell membrane. The major consequences of mechanical injuries often are inflammation and disruption of blood flow. *Extremes of heat and cold* cause damage to the cell, its organelles, and its enzyme systems. Heat coagulates tissue proteins, and freezing crystallizes the cytoplasmic contents. Furthermore, extremes of temperature induce vascular changes that interfere with blood flow. *Electrical injuries* are mainly caused by heat generated from the current that passes through the tissues.

Radiation

Radiation injury includes the effects of ultraviolet radiation (sunlight) and ionizing radiation (x-rays and gamma rays). All cells are susceptible to ionizing radiation, but the degree of this susceptibility varies. Rapidly proliferating cells of both the bone marrow and the gastrointestinal epithelium are proportionately more susceptible than other cells to the effects of ionizing radiation. To the extent that ionizing radiation is selectively destructive to rapidly proliferating cells, it can be used in the treatment of malignant disease.

Chemical agents

Chemical agents are numerous and can cause injury to the cell membrane and other cell structures; can block enzymatic pathways; can cause coagulation of cell proteins; and can disrupt the osmotic and ionic balance of the cell. Even simple table salt (sodium chloride) can cause cell damage by disrupting the cell's osmotic and ionic homeostasis. Chemicals can destroy cells at the site of contact. Corrosive substances such as strong acids and alkalies destroy cells as they come into contact with the body. Other chemicals may injure cells in the process of metabolism or elimination. Carbon tetrachloride (CCl_4), for example, causes little damage until it is metabolized to a highly reactive free radical (CCl_3) by liver enzymes. Carbon tetrachloride is extremely toxic to liver cells. Still other types of chemicals are selective in their sites of action. Carbon monoxide has a special affinity for the hemoglobin molecule.

Biologic agents

Biologic agents differ from other injurious agents in that they are able to replicate and thus can continue to produce their injurious effects. These agents range from submicroscopic viruses to the larger parasites. Biologic agents cause cell injury by a number of diverse mechanisms: viruses enter the cell and disrupt the intracellular environment. Certain bacteria elaborate exotoxins that interfere with cellular production of ATP. Other bacteria such as the gram-negative bacilli release endotoxins that cause profound blood vessel changes. Still other microorganisms produce their effects through inflammatory or immune mechanisms.

Inflammation and immune responses

Although inflammation and immune responses are normally protective in nature, they can and do cause cell injury and death. Inflammation is discussed in Chapter 4 and immunity in Chapter 5.

Genetic derangements

Genetic derangements may cause a predisposition to cell injury. Many genetic defects cause an abnormal accumulation of intracellular materials. Lysosomal storage diseases are relatively rare genetic disorders in which an enzyme deficiency causes accumulation of materials that would normally be metabolized in lysosomes. Tay–Sachs disease is one such disorder. In this disorder there is an accumulation of gangliosides in many tissues, including the neurons of the central and autonomic nervous systems.

Nutritional imbalances

Both nutritional excesses and deficiencies predispose to cell injury. Obesity, and diets high in lipids and carbohydrates, are thought to predispose to atherosclerosis. Dietary deficiencies can occur in the form of starvation in which there is a deficiency of all nutrients and vitamins, or it may occur because of a selective deficiency of a single nutrient or vitamin. Iron deficiency anemia, scurvy, beriberi, and pellagra are examples of injury caused by the lack of specific vitamins or minerals. The protein and calorie deficiencies that occur with starvation cause widespread tissue damage.

Effects of Cell Injury

The extent to which any injurious agent can cause cell injury and death is dependent, to a large measure, on the intensity, the duration, and the type of cell that is involved. Cell injury can be sublethal and cause reversible tissue damage or it can be irreversible and cause cell death and tissue necrosis.

Sublethal cell injury
The manifestations of reversible cell injury fall into three main categories: cellular swelling, fatty changes, and intracellular accumulations.

Cellular swelling.   An accumulation of water within the cell is an early manifestation of almost all types of cell injury. When this happens the cytoplasm of the cell develops a cloudy appearance (*cloudy swelling*). It has been postulated that the swelling is caused by a decrease in ATP and impaired function of the sodium pump, which leads to an accumulation of intracellular sodium and subsequent water-logging of the cell. Vacuoles appear if water continues to accumulate. These vacuoles probably represent the collection of water in the endoplasmic reticulum. The term *hydropic degeneration* refers to the more severe type of cellular swelling.

Fatty changes.   Fatty cellular changes are linked to intracellular accummulation of fat. When fatty changes occur small vacuoles of fat disperse throughout the cytoplasm. The process is usually more ominous than cloudy swelling, and although it is reversible, its presence usually indicates severe injury. These fatty changes may occur because normal cells are presented with an increased fat load or because injured cells are unable to metabolize the fat properly. In obesity, fatty infiltrates often occur within and between the cells of the liver and heart due to an increased fat load. Impairment of metabolic pathways for fat metabolism may occur during cell injury and fat may accumulate within the cell as production exceeds use and export. The liver, where most fats are synthesized and metabolized, is par-

ticularly susceptible to fatty change, but fatty change may also occur in the kidney, the heart, and other organs.

Other intracellular accumulations
Many other materials can accumulate in cells. These accumulations can occur because of altered metabolic pathways or because the cells are exposed to abnormal pigments. There are a number of genetic disorders that cause abnormal intracellular accumulations. In Wilson's disease, copper deposits accumulate within the cells of the liver, brain, and cornea, causing cell destruction. There are at least ten inborn errors of glycogen metabolism, most of which lead to accumulation of intracellular glycogen stores. Similarly, other enzyme defects lead to accumulation of other materials.

Pigments, either endogenous or exogenous, may also accumulate within cells. *Icterus*, or jaundice, is a yellow discoloration of tissue caused by the retention of endogenous bile pigments. This condition may result from increased bilirubin production due to red blood cell destruction; to the obstruction of bile passage into the intestine; or from toxic diseases that affect the liver's ability to remove bilirubin from the blood. One of the best examples of exogenous pigmentation is the pigmentation due to consumption of large amounts of carotene-containing foods (such as carrots and turnips). Inhalation of foreign materials also causes exogenous pigmentation. This type of pigmentation is associated with a lung condition called *pneumoconiosis*. Pigmentation associated with coal dust is termed *anthracosis* and with silica dust, *silicosis*. The formation of the "blue lead line" along the margins of the gum is one of the diagnostic features of lead poisoning.

Irreversible cell injury and death
Necrosis means death of the cell, organ, or tissue that is still a part of the body. Widespread necrosis can occur without somatic (body) death. With cell death there are marked changes in the appearance of both the cytoplasmic contents and the nucleus. These changes are often not visible, even under the microscope, for hours following cell death. The dissolution of the necrotic cell or tissue can follow several paths: the cells can undergo liquefaction (liquefaction necrosis); it can be transformed to a gray, firm mass (coagulation necrosis); or it can be converted to a cheesy material by infiltration of fatlike substances (caseous necrosis). *Liquefaction necrosis* occurs when some of the cells die, but their catalytic enzymes are not destroyed. An example of liquefaction necrosis

is the softening of the center of an abscess with discharge of its contents. During *coagulation necrosis*, acidosis denatures the enzymatic proteins along with the structural proteins of the cell. This type of necrosis is characteristic of hypoxic injury and is seen in infarcted areas. An infarction occurs when the artery that supplies an organ or part of the body becomes occluded and no other source of blood supply exists. As a rule, the infarct is conical in shape, and corresponds to the distribution of the artery and its branches. An artery may be occluded by an embolus, a thrombus, disease of the arterial wall, or pressure on the vessel from without. *Caseous necrosis* is associated with tubercular lesions.

Gangrene

The term gangrene is applied when a considerable mass of tissue undergoes necrosis (Fig. 3-2). Gangrene may be classified as either dry or moist. Dry gangrene is usually due to interference with arterial blood supply to a part without interference of venous return. Strictly speaking, it is a form of coagulation necrosis. Moist, or wet, gangrene is primarily due to interference with the venous return from the part. Bacterial invasion plays an important role in the development of wet gangrene and is responsible for many of its prominent symptoms. Dry gangrene is confined almost exclusively to the extremities, whereas moist gangrene may affect either the internal organs or the extremities.

In dry gangrene, the part becomes dry and

Figure 3–2.   Photograph of a foot with dry gangrene of the first four toes. Note the sharp line of demarcation between the normal and necrotic tissue. (Courtesy of M. Wagner, M.D. The Anatomy Department, Medical College of Wisconsin)

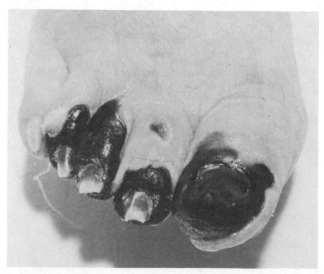

shrinks; the skin wrinkles, and its color changes to dark brown or black. The spread of dry gangrene is slow and its symptoms are not as marked as those of wet gangrene. The irritation caused by the dead tissue produces a line of inflammtory reaction (line of demarcation) between the dead tissue and the gangrenous area, and the healthy tissue. If bacteria invade the necrotic tissue, dry gangrene is converted to wet gangrene.

In moist gangrene, the area is cold, swollen, and pulseless. The skin is moist, black, and under tension. Blebs form on the surface, liquefaction occurs, and a foul odor (due to bacterial action) is present. There is no line of demarcation between the normal and diseased tissues and the spread of tissue damage is rapid. Systemic symptoms are usually severe, and death may occur unless the condition can be arrested.

Gas gangrene is a special type of gangrene that is due to infection of devitalized tissues by one of several clostridial bacteria. These anaerobic bacteria produce toxins that cause shock, hemolysis, and death of muscle cells. Characteristic of this disorder are the bubbles of gas that form in the muscle. Gas gangrene is a serious and potentially fatal disease. Treatment includes administration of gas gangrene antitoxin. Because the organism is anaerobic, oxygen is sometimes administered in a hyperbaric chamber.

In summary, cell injury can be caused by a number of agents. The injury may produce sublethal and reversible cellular damage, or may lead to irreversible cell injury and death. Necrosis refers to cell death. There are three forms of cell necrosis: (1) liquefaction necrosis, which occurs when cell death does not result in inactivation of intracellular enzymes, (2) coagulation necrosis which occurs with ischemia, and (3) caseous necrosis which is associated with tubercular lesions. Necrosis of large areas of tissue leads to gangrene. Gangrene can be classified as dry or wet gangrene. Dry gangrene is essentially a form of coagulation necrosis, and wet gangrene is due to bacterial invasion of the necrotic area.

:Study Guide

After you have studied this chapter, you should be able to meet the following objectives:

: :   State five general causes of atrophy.

: :   Distinguish between physiologic hypertrophy and pathologic hypertrophy.

: :   State the conditions under which hyperplasia may occur.

:: Differentiate between metaplasia and dysplasia.

:: State a general definition of cellular degeneration.

:: Explain the pathologic basis of hypoxia.

:: State an example of each of the following causes of cellular damage: a physical agent, radiation, a biologic agent, a chemical agent.

:: Describe the manifestations of reversible cell injury.

:: Describe an example of a disease due to the accumulation of abnormal substances in the cell.

:: Contrast liquefaction necrosis and coagulation necrosis.

:: Name and define the two chief types of gangrene.

:Suggested Readings

Anderson WAD, Kissane JM: Pathology, 7th ed, p 90. St Louis, CV Mosby, 1977

Hill RB, LaVia MF: Principles of Pathobiology, 3rd ed, p 21. New York, Oxford University Press, 1980

Jennings RB, Ganote CE, Reimer KA: Ischemic tissue injury. Am J Pathol 81:179, 1975

Robbins SL, Cotran RF: Pathologic Basis of Disease, 2nd ed, p 1. Philadelphia, WB Saunders, 1979

Widmann FK: Pathobiology: How Disease Happens, p 1. Boston, Little, Brown, 1978

4

Inflammation

:Overview of Inflammation and the Inflammatory Response

The ability of the body to sustain injury, resist attack by microbial agents, and repair damaged tissue is dependent upon the inflammatory reaction, the immune response, tissue regeneration, and fibrous tissue replacement. This chapter focuses on the local manifestations of acute and chronic inflammation, the repair process, systemic signs of inflammation, and selected disease states that affect the inflammatory cells. Chapter 5 discusses the immune response.

Inflammation is the local reaction of vascularized tissue to injury.[1] Although the effects of inflammation are often viewed as undesirable because they are unpleasant and cause discomfort, the process is essentially a beneficial one that allows a person to live with the effects of everyday stress. Without the inflammatory response, wounds would not heal and minor infections would become overwhelming. On the other hand, inflammation also produces undesirable effects. The crippling effects of rheumatoid arthritis, for example, have their origin in the inflammatory response.

Purpose of the Inflammatory Response

The inflammatory response is closely intermeshed with wound healing and reparative processes. This process acts to neutralize or destroy the offending agent, restricts the tissue damage to the smallest possible area, alerts the individual to the impending threat of tissue injury, and it prepares the injured area for healing. Wound healing and tissue repair begin during the active stages of inflammation and serve to repair the damage caused by the injurious agent.

Causes of Inflammation

The *causes* of inflammation are *many* and *varied*. Although it is quite common to equate inflammation with infection, it is important to recognize that almost all types of injury are capable of inciting the response and that only a small number of inflammatory responses are related to infections. The injurious agents that cause inflammation can arise from outside the body (*exogenous*) or they can originate from within the body (*endogenous*). Common causes of inflammation are trauma, surgery, infection, caustic chemicals, extremes of heat and cold, immune responses, and ischemic damage to body tissues.

Characteristics of the Inflammatory Response

Though the inflammatory response can be initiated by a wide variety of injurious agents, the sequence of physiologic events that follow is remarkably the same. Characteristic of the inflammatory response is that it involves *a sequence of specific physiologic behaviors that occur in response to injury by a nonspecific agent*. An acute inflammatory response will follow the same course, whether the injury is caused by a streptococcal infection or by tissue necrosis associated with myocardial infarction. The extent of the injury will vary and the site of inflammation will be different, but the tissue response and systemic manifestations will be similar. The body will, however, *use only those behaviors in the sequence that are needed to minimize tissue damage*. A small area of local swelling and redness may be sufficient to prevent injury from a mosquito bite, whereas other, more serious conditions, such as appendicitis, may incite leukocytosis, fever, and formation of an exudate.

Nomenclature Related to Inflammation

Inflammatory conditions are *named* by adding the suffix *"itis"* to the affected organ or system. For instance, neuritis refers to inflammation of a nerve, pericarditis to inflammation of the pericardium, and appendicitis to inflammation of the appendix. A further description of the inflammatory process might indicate whether the process was acute or chronic and what type of exudate was formed, e.g. acute fibrinous pericarditis.

Types of Inflammation

Inflammation can be acute or chronic. Acute inflammation is the typical short-term response that is associated with all types of tissue injury. It involves hemodynamic changes, formation of an exudate, and the presence of granular leukocytes. Chronic inflammation follows a less uniform and more persistent pattern. It involves the presence of nongranular leukocytes and usually results in more extensive formation of scar tissue and deformities.

:Acute Inflammation

Hemodynamic Changes

The classical description of acute inflammation has been handed down through the ages. In the first century A.D., the Roman physician Celsus described the local reaction to injury in terms of what has come to be known as the cardinal signs of inflammation. These signs are *rubor* (redness), *tumor* (swelling), *calor* (heat), and *dolor* (pain). In the second century A.D., Galen added a fifth cardinal sign, *functio laesa* or loss of function.

The manifestations of acute inflammation can be divided into two categories, *hemodynamic* and *white blood cell responses*. At the biochemical level, many of the responses that occur during acute inflammation are associated with the release of chemical mediators. Both the hemodynamic responses and white blood cell responses contribute to the *inflammatory exudates* that characterize the acute inflammatory response. Each of these aspects of acute inflammation is discussed separately.

The hemodynamic, or vascular, changes that occur with inflammation begin almost immediately following injury, and are initiated by a momentary constriction of small vessels in the area. This momentary period of vasoconstriction is immediately followed by vasodilation of the arterioles and venules that supply the area. As a result, the area becomes congested and warm—the *redness* and *warmth* that are characteristic of acute inflammation. Accompanying this hyperemic response is an increase in capillary permeability that allows fluid to escape into the tissue and to cause *swelling*. *Pain* and *impaired function* occur as the result of tissue swelling and release of chemical mediators. The reader can simulate the hemodynamic responses that occur with acute inflammation by running the sharp edge of a fingernail or lead pencil along the inner aspect of the arm. The response has been termed the triple response.[2] Within seconds the line becomes reddened. The second response is a red flare that develops on both sides of the line and which represents the hyperemic phase of the inflammatory response. Within several minutes, the line usually becomes slightly raised, because of swelling caused by an increase in capillary permeability. The flare response that occurs with this type of stimulus is highly variable; some persons will have only a slight response while others will have an exaggerated one.

The hemodynamic changes that occur during the early stages of inflammation are beneficial in that they aid in controlling the effects of the injurious agent. During this stage, the exudation of fluid out of the capillary into the tissue spaces helps *dilute* the toxic and irritating agents. Sometime later, white blood cells accumulate in the area and leave the capillary as part of the exudate. As fluid moves out of the capillary, there is *stagnation* of flow and *clotting* of blood in the small capillaries that supply the inflamed area. This aids in *localizing* the effects of the injury.

Patterns of Response

According to the severity of injury, the hemodynamic changes that occur with the inflammatory reaction follow one of three patterns of response. The first is an immediate transient response that occurs with minor injury. The second is an immediate sustained response that occurs with more serious injury and continues for several days. With this response there is actual damage to the vessels in the area. The third type of response is a delayed response—the increase in capillary permeability is delayed for a period of 4 to 24 hours. A delayed response often accompanies radiation types of injuries, such as a sunburn.

White blood cell response
The cellular stage of acute inflammation is marked by movement of white blood cells (leukocytes) into the area of injury. This stage includes (1) the margination or pavementing of white blood cells, (2) emigration of white blood cells, (3) chemotaxis, and (4) phagocytosis. A description of white blood cells precedes the discussion of cellular events that occur in acute inflammation.

Leukocytes
The leukocytes, or white blood cells, develop from the primordial stem cells that are located in the bone marrow and lymphoid tissue. The leukocytes are larger and less numerous than the red blood cells. There are two types of white blood cells, granular and nongranular leukocytes. The different types of leukocytes are illustrated in Figure 4-1.

Granular leukocytes. The granular leukocytes are identifiable because of their cytoplasmic granules and are commonly referred to as granulocytes. In addition to their cytoplasmic granules, these white blood cells have distinctive multilobar nuclei (Fig. 4-1). The granulocytes are divided into three types (neutrophils, eosinophils, and basophils) according to the staining properties of the granules.

The *neutrophils*, which constitute 60% to 70% of the total number of white blood cells, have granules that are neutral and hence do not stain with either an acid or a basic dye. Because these white cells have nuclei that are divided into three to five lobes, they are often called *polymorphonuclear leukocytes*

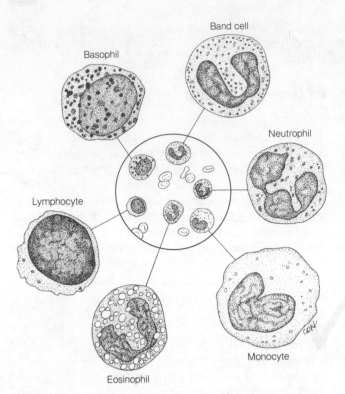

Figure 4–1.   White blood cells that are involved in the inflammatory response.

(PMNs). The neutrophils are the first cells to arrive at the site of inflammation, usually appearing within 90 minutes of injury. Neutrophils increase greatly during the inflammatory process. When this happens, immature forms of neutrophils are released from the bone marrow. These immature cells are often called *bands* or *stabs* because of the horseshoe shape of their nuclei. The neutrophils have a life span of only about 10 hours and therefore must be constantly replaced if their numbers are to be adequate.

The cytoplasmic granules of the *eosinophils* stain red with the acid dye eosin. These leukocytes constitute 1% to 3% of the total number of white blood cells, and increase during allergic reactions and parasitic infections. It is thought that they detoxify the agents or chemical mediators associated with allergic reactions and assist in terminating the response.

The granules of the *basophils* stain blue with a basic dye. These cells constitute only about 0.3% to 0.5% of the white blood cells. The granules in the basophils contain heparin and histamine and are similar to those of the mast cells. It is thought that the basophils are involved in allergic and stress responses.

Nongranular lymphocytes.   There are two groups of nongranular lymphocytes, the monocytes and the lymphocytes. The *monocytes* are the second order of cells to arrive at the inflammation site and their arrival usually requires 5 hours or more. Within 48 hours, however, the monocytes are usually the predominant cell type in the inflamed area. Monocytes are the largest of the white blood cells, constituting about 3% to 8% of the total leukocyte count. The circulating life span of the monocyte is 3 to 4 times longer than that of the granulocytes, and these cells survive for a longer period of time in the tissues. The monocytes, which are phagocytic cells, are often referred to as *macrophages*. The monocytes engulf larger and greater quantities of foreign material than the neutrophils. These leukocytes play an important role in chronic inflammation and are also involved in the immune response. When the monocyte leaves the vascular system and enters the tissue spaces it becomes known as a *histiocyte*. Histiocytes function as macrophages in the inflamed area. They can also proliferate to form a capsule enclosing foreign material that cannot be digested.

The *lymphocytes* constitute 20% to 30% of the white blood cell count. There are two types of lymphocytes, B cells and T cells. The B cells form plasma cells. The B cells are concerned with antibody formation and the T cells with cell-mediated immunity. Both types of lymphocytes play a major role in immunity and are discussed in Chapter 5.

Margination and pavementing of leukocytes

During the early stages of the inflammatory response, fluid leaves the capillaries of the microcirculation, causing blood viscosity to increase. As this occurs the leukocytes begin to *marginate* or move to the periphery of the blood vessel. As the process continues, the marginated leukocytes begin to adhere to the vessel lining in preparation for emigration from the vessel. The cobblestone appearance of the vessel lining due to margination of leukocytes has led to the designation of the term "pavementing."

Emigration of leukocytes

Emigration is a mechanism whereby the leukocytes extend *pseudopodia* (false feet), pass through the capillary walls by ameboid movement, and then migrate into the tissue spaces. The movement of red and white blood cells through the wall of the capillary is called *diapedesis*. Along with the emigration of leukocytes, there is also an escape of red cells from the capillary. The red cells may escape singly, or in small jets at points where the capillaries have become distended.

Chemotaxis

The leukocytes, after emigrating through the vessel wall, wander through the tissue space being guided by the presence of bacteria and cellular debris. The process by which leukocytes are attracted to bacteria and cellular debris is called *chemotaxis*. Chemotaxis can be positive or negative, meaning that it can act to either attract or repel the leukocytes. Many substances are capable of acting as chemotaxic agents, including infectious organisms, plasma-protein fractions (complement), and tissue debris.

Phagocytosis

In the final stage of the cellular response, the neutrophils and monocytes engulf and degrade the bacteria and cellular debris in a process called *phagocytosis* (Fig. 4-2). The neutrophils are sometimes called *microphages* because they concentrate on the phagocytosis of bacteria and small particles. The monocytes, or *macrophages*, remove tissue debris and larger particles from the area of inflammation.

Leukocytosis

Leukocytosis refers to an increase in white blood cell numbers. Acute inflammatory conditions, particularly those of bacterial origin, are accompanied by marked increases in white blood cell numbers with a disproportionate increase seen in the neutrophilic count. A differential blood count measures both the total number of white blood cells and the percentage of each type of blood cell. Table 4-1 compares the normal white blood cell count with that sometimes seen in an acute infection.

The Reticuloendothelial System

In addition to the mobile white blood cells that circulate in the blood stream, there are nonmobile phagocytic cells that are widely scattered throughout the body. This group of cells is collectively referred to as the reticuloendothelial system. The Kupffer cells in the liver sinusoids and the macrophages located in the spleen and bone marrow, and those that line the lymph channels and lymph nodes are all part of the reticuloendothelial system, as are the phagocytic histiocytes that wander through the tissue spaces.

Chemical Mediators

Although inflammation is precipitated by injury and cell death, its signs and symptoms are produced by chemical mediators such as histamine, the plasma

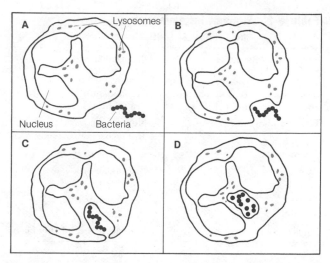

Figure 4–2.   Diagram of phagocytosis by a neutrophil. In *A*, the neutrophil has emigrated from the capillary, in *B* it is attached to the bacteria through chemotaxis, and in *C* it engulfs the bacteria. In the final stages of phagocytosis (*D*), the bacteria are degraded by the enzymes and digestive materials that are contained in the cytoplasmic granules of the neutrophil.

proteases, prostaglandins, slow-reacting substance of anaphylaxis, and other neutrophil and lymphocyte factors. Other mediators have been identified, but their role in the inflammatory process is still unclear. The chemical mediators are stored in inactive form in various body cells such as neutrophils, basophils, mast cells, and platelets. The process of mediator activation requires a number of sequential steps that control the reaction and prevent the process from occurring by chance. If this were not true, most of us would be constantly covered with swollen and reddened areas over much of our body. Table 4-2 describes the prominent manifestations of inflammation and the chemical substances that mediate their occurrence.

Table 4–1   Example of a Normal White Blood Count (WBC) Compared with White Blood Cell Count During an Acute Infection

	Normal	Acute Infection
Total WBC (cells per mm³)	5 to 10,000	16 to 18,000
Polymorphonuclear leukocytes (PMNs, %)	69	85
Stabs (% of PMNs)	—	12
Lymphocytes (%)	29	14
Monocytes (%)	2	1

Table 4–2 Signs of Inflammation and Chemical Mediators

Inflammatory Response	Chemical Mediator
Swelling, redness, and tissue warmth (vasodilatation and capillary permeability)	Histamine Prostaglandins Bradykinin
Tissue damage	Neutrophil, macrophage, and lysosomal enzymes
Chemotaxis	Complement fractions
Pain	Prostaglandins Bradykinin
Fever	Prostaglandins Endogenous pyrogens
Leukocytosis	Leukocyte-stimulating factor

Histamine

Histamine is widely distributed throughout the body. It can be found in platelets, basophils, and mast cells. Histamine causes dilatation of arterioles and enhanced permeability of capillaries and venules. It is the first mediator in the initial inflammatory response. Antihistamine drugs suppress this immediate transient response that is induced by mild injury.

The plasma proteases

The plasma proteases consist of the kinins, complement and its fractional components, and the clotting system. One of the kinins, bradykinin, causes increased capillary permeability and pain. The complement system consists of a number of component proteins and their cleavage products. These substances interact with the antigen–antibody complexes and mediate immunologic injury and inflammation (see Chap. 5). The clotting system is discussed in Chapter 11.

Prostaglandins

The prostaglandins are ubiquitous tissue proteins composed of lipid-soluble acids derived from the arachidonic acid that is present in the membranes of many cells. Prostaglandins contribute to vasodilatation, capillary permeability, and the pain and fever that accompany inflammation. Prostaglandins are present in high concentrations in the synovial fluid of inflamed joints, such as in rheumatoid arthritis. Drugs such as aspirin and indomethacin inhibit prostaglandin synthesis and are used in the treatment of arthritis. The glucocorticoid hormones secreted from the adrenal cortex (or given as a drug) are known to somehow curtail the availability of arachidonic acid for prostaglandin production.[3] The glucocorticoids have come to be known as anti-inflammatory drugs because of their ability to suppress the inflammatory response.

Slow-reacting substance of anaphylaxis (SRS-A)

Slow-reacting substance of anaphylaxis is released from mast cells during anaphylaxis. It increases vascular permeability and is thought to cause constriction of the bronchial smooth muscle.

Neutrophil and lymphocyte products

The neutrophils and lymphocytes contribute a number of mediators to the inflammatory process. The neutrophils release mediators that increase vascular permeability, act as a chemotactic factor for monocytes, and cause tissue damage. Much of the tissue damage done during the acute inflammatory process is caused by the lysosomal enzymes of the neutrophil. The lymphocytes release mediators called the lymphokines. These mediators have numerous actions including chemotaxis of macrophages, neutrophils, and basophils.

Inflammatory Exudates

Characteristically the acute inflammatory response involves production of exudates. These exudates can vary in terms of fluid, plasma protein, and cell content. Acute inflammation can produce serous, fibrinous, membranous, purulent, and hemorrhagic exudates. Inflammatory exudates are often composed of a combination of these types.

Serous exudate

The initial exudate that enters the inflammatory site is largely plasma. Serous drainage is a watery exudate that is low in protein content. A blister contains serous fluid. A catarrhal inflammation is one that affects the mucous membranes and is associated with an increase in watery secretions and desquamation of the epithelial cells. Hay fever is an example of a catarrhal inflammatory response.

Fibrinous exudate

Fibrinous exudates contain large amounts of fibrinogen and form a thick and sticky meshwork, much like the fibers of a blood clot. Fibrinous exudates are frequently encountered in the serous cavities of the body. Acute rheumatic fever often causes development of a fibrinous pericarditis. A fibrinous exudate must be removed through fibrinolytic activity of enzymes before healing can take place. Failure to remove the exudate leads to ingrowth of fibroblasts and subsequent development of scar tissue and adhesions. A fibrinous exudate may be beneficial in that it tends to glue the inflamed structures together thereby preventing the spread of infection. In appendicitis, for example, the initial formation of a fibrous exudate serves to localize the organisms in the region of the appendix and thus prevents generalized spread of the infection to the peritoneal cavity.

Membranous exudate

Membranous or pseudomembranous exudates develop on mucous membrane surfaces. The development of a membranous exudate occurs as necrotic cells become enmeshed in a fibropurulent exudate that coats the mucosal surface. *Diphtheria* was known for its ability to produce a membranous exudate on the surface of the trachea and major bronchi. *Thrush* is a monilial infection of the oral cavity that produces patches of membranous inflammation. *Membranous enterocolitis* is a severe membranous inflammatory condition of the bowel mucosa that is related to a disturbance in the normal bowel flora due to treatment with a variety of broad-spectrum antibiotics.

Purulent exudate

A purulent (suppurative) exudate contains pus, which is composed of the remains of white blood cells, proteins, and tissue debris. Purulent infections are caused by a number of pyogenic or pus-forming bacteria. An *abscess* is a localized collection of pus. Abscesses may occur at the site of injury, or they may develop as the result of metastatic spread of infectious organisms and tissue debris through the blood stream. An abscess is encapsulated in a so-called pyogenic membrane that consists of layers of fibrin, inflammatory cells, and granulation tissue. An abscess may need to be incised and the pus removed before healing can occur.

Cellulitis, or phlegmonous inflammation, is a subgroup of suppurative infections that involve massive necrosis of tissue along with production of purulent infiltrates. Instead of producing small, localized collections of pus, certain pyogenic organisms (usually the streptococci) elaborate a large amount of spreading factor, the *hyaluronidases*, which break down the fibrin meshwork and other barriers designed to localize the infection.

Hemorrhagic exudate

A hemorrhagic exudate occurs in situations in which severe tissue injury causes damage to blood vessels or when there is diapedesis of red blood cells from the capillaries. Often a hemorrhagic exudate accompanies other forms of exudate. A serosanguineous exudate describes a combination of serous and hemorrhagic exudates.

Resolution of Acute Inflammation

Acute inflammation can be resolved in one of three ways: (1) it can undergo resolution, with the injured area returning to normal or near-normal appearance and function, (2) it can progress, and suppurative processes may develop, or (3) it can proceed to the chronic phase. In the process of responding to injury, the body will use only those behaviors in the inflammatory sequence that are necessary to prevent or halt the destruction of tissue.

:Chronic Inflammation

To this point, we have discussed acute inflammation associated with a self-limiting stimulus, such as a burn or infection which is rapidly controlled by host defenses. Chronic inflammation, on the other hand, is self-perpetuating and may last for weeks, months, or even years. The persistence of chronic inflammation may occur because of the nature of the irritant or because the body defenses are inadequate. In most cases, chronic inflammation involves an immune response. Lymphocytes and plasma cells are the predominant white cells in chronic inflammation. When the irritant is nonantigenic, such as lipid or insoluble substances, macrophages (giant cells) are usually present in large numbers. Chronic inflammatory conditions usually involve proliferation of fibroblasts and vascular structures rather than the development of exudates. As a result, there is usually considerably greater risk of scarring and deformity development than there is with acute inflammation.

Granulomatous Inflammation

A granulomatous lesion is a form of chronic inflammation. A granuloma is typically a small, 1- to 2-mm lesion in which there is a massing of macrophages that are surrounded by lymphocytes. These modified macrophages resemble epithelial cells and are sometimes called *epithelioid cells*. Like other macrophages, the epithelioid cells that form a granuloma are derived from blood monocytes. Granulomatous inflammation is associated with foreign bodies such as splinters, sutures, silica, and talc particles, and with microorganisms such as those that cause tuberculosis, syphilis, sarcoidosis, deep fungal infections, and brucellosis. These types of agents have one thing in common—they are poorly digestible and are usually not easily controlled by other inflammatory mechanisms.

The epithelioid cells in granulomatous inflammation may either clump in a mass (granuloma) or they may coalesce, forming a large multinucleated giant cell which attempts to surround the foreign agent. Some giant cells may contain as many as 200 nuclei. A giant cell is usually surrounded by granuloma cells and a dense membrane of connective tissue eventually encapsulates the lesion and isolates it. A tubercle is a granulomatous inflammatory response to the tubercle bacillus. Peculiar to the tuberculosis granuloma is the presence of a caseous (cheesy) necrotic center. In the past, surgical gloves were dusted with talc so they could be slipped on easily, but particles of talc frequently ended up in the surgical field and caused granulomatous lesions to develop. Surgical gloves are now dusted with an absorbable starch that does not cause this problem.

In summary, inflammation describes a local response to the tissue injury and can present as an acute or chronic condition. Acute inflammation is the local response of tissue to a nonspecific form of injury. The classic signs of inflammation are redness, swelling, local heat, pain, and loss of function. Acute inflammation involves a hemodynamic phase in which blood flow and capillary permeability is increased, and a cellular phase during which there is an increase in white-cell movement in the area. While acute inflammation is usually self-limiting, chronic inflammation is more prolonged and is usually caused by persistent irritants, most of which are insoluble and resistant to phagocytosis and other inflammatory mechanisms. Chronic inflammation usually involves the presence of lymphocytes, plasma cells, and macrophages.

:Tissue Healing and Repair

The degree to which body structures return to their normal state following injury is largely dependent on the body's ability to replace the parenchymal cells and to arrange them as they were originally. Repair can assume one of two forms: regeneration, or fibrous scar-tissue replacement. Regeneration describes the process by which cells are replaced with cells of a similar type and function so that there is little evidence that injury has occurred. Healing by fibrous replacement, on the other hand, involves the substitution of a fibrous–connective tissue scar for the original tissue.

Regeneration

The ability to regenerate varies with tissue types. Body cells are divided into three types according to their ability to undergo regeneration: (1) labile, (2) stable, or (3) permanent cell types.

Labile cells are those that continue to regenerate throughout life. These cells include the surface epithelial cells of the skin and mucous membranes of the gastrointestinal tract. A constant daily turnover of cells occurs with these tissue types.

Stable cells are those that normally stop dividing when growth ceases. These cells are capable, however, of undergoing regeneration when confronted with an appropriate stimulus. In order for stable cells to regenerate and restore tissues to their original state, the underlying structural framework must be present. When this framework has been destroyed, the replacement of tissues will be haphazard. The reader will recall that epithelial tissue relies on the blood supply from the underlying connective tissues for nourishment. The hepatocytes of the liver are one form of stable cells and the importance of the structural framework to regeneration is evidenced by two forms of liver disease. In viral hepatitis, for example,

Figure 4–3. Diagram of events that follow skin and subcutaneous tissue injury.

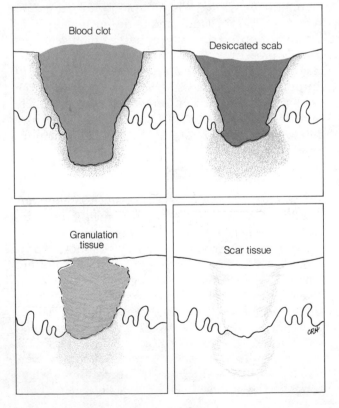

there is selective destruction of the parenchymal liver cells while the structural cells remain unharmed. Consequently, once the disease has subsided, the injured cells regenerate and liver function returns to normal. On the other hand, in cirrhosis of the liver, fibrous bands of tissue form and replace the normal structural framework of the liver, causing disordered replacement of liver cells and disturbance of liver function.

Permanent, or *fixed cells*, are those that cannot undergo mitotic division. The fixed cells include nerve cells, as well as skeletal and cardiac muscle cells. As will be discussed later, the nerve axon can regenerate under certain conditions in which the nerve-cell body is uninjured.

Soft Tissue Repair

The sequence of events that occurs with laceration of the skin and underlying tissues is familiar to most readers. This type of injury is followed almost immediately by bleeding into the area and the development of a blood clot (Fig. 4-3). Within several hours, the clot loses fluid and becomes a hard, dehydrated scab that serves to protect the area. At about the same time, phagocytic white blood cells begin to enter the injured area and begin breaking down and removing the inflammatory debris. Shortly thereafter, cells called fibroblasts arrive and begin to build scar tissue by synthesizing collagen fibers and other proteins. Meanwhile, the epithelial cells at the margin of the wound begin to regenerate and move toward the center of the wound, forming a new surface layer that is similar to that destroyed by the injury. When healing is complete, the scab falls off. With the exception of the desiccated scab, repair of injury to internal structures follows a similar pattern.

The primary objective of the healing process is to fill the gap created by tissue destruction and to restore the structural continuity of the injured part. When regeneration cannot occur, healing by fibrous-tissue substitution provides the means for maintaining this continuity. Although scar tissue fills the gap created by tissue death, it does not repair the structure with functioning parenchymal cells.

Scar tissue repair

Healing by fibrous substitution begins during the early stages of inflammation as macrophages invade the area and begin to digest the invading organisms and the cellular debris. The *fibroblasts* are connective-tissue cells that are responsible for the formation of *collagen* an other *intercellular elements* needed for wound healing.

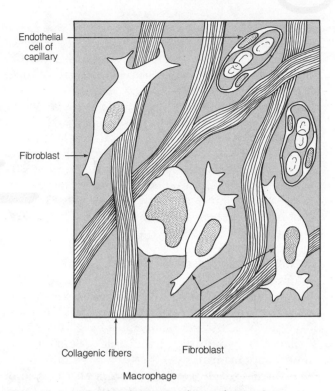

Figure 4–4.   The development of granulation tissue. Collagen fibers and vascular endothelial cells usually begin to enter the wound area around the third to sixth day following injury.

As early as 24 hours following injury, fibroblasts and vascular endothelial cells begin to enter the area, and by the third to the fifth day there is proliferation of both fibroblasts and small blood vessels (Fig. 4-4). As this happens, the area becomes filled with a specialized form of soft, pink granular tissue called *granulation tissue*. This tissue is edematous and bleeds easily because of the numerous newly developed fragile and leaky capillary buds. At times there may be formation of excessive granulation tissue, sometimes referred to as "proud flesh." This excess granulation tissue protrudes from the wound and prevents re-epithelization from taking place. Surgical removal or chemical cauterization of the defect allows healing to proceed.

As the process of scar-tissue development progresses, there is a further increase in extracellular collagen and a decrease in active fibroblastic function. The small blood vessels become thrombosed and degenerate. As this happens the collagen fibers begin to mature and shorten, and a dense devascularized scar is formed. *Wound contraction* contributes heavily to the healing of surface wounds. As a result, the scar that is formed is considerably smaller than the original wound. Cosmetically, this may be desirable because it reduces the size of the visible defect. On the other hand, contraction of the scar tissue that has developed over joints and other body structures tends to limit movement and to cause deformities.

As a result of loss of elasticity, scar tissue that is stretched fails to return to its original length. Most wounds do not regain their original tensile strength once healing has occurred. Most wounds begin to increase in strength beginning between 10 and 14 days following injury; after this there is a rapid increase in strength and by the end of three months they have reached a plateau—at about 70% to 80% of their unwounded strength.[4]

Healing by first or second intention

Wounds can be divided into two types—those in which there is minimal tissue loss and which heal by *first intention* and those which have significant tissue loss and heal by *second intention* (Fig. 4-5). Both visible skin wounds and invisible wounds of the internal organs heal by either first or second intention. A sutured surgical incision is an example of healing by first intention (healing directly, without granulations). Visible wounds that heal by second intention are burns and decubitus ulcers. When healing by second intention occurs, there is pro-

Figure 4–5. Healing by first and second intention.

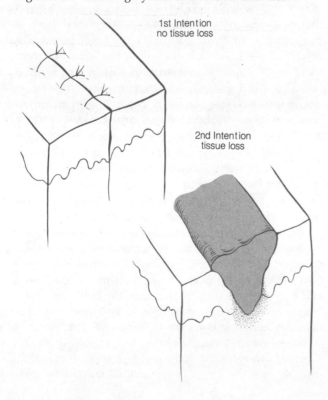

1st Intention
no tissue loss

2nd Intention
tissue loss

liferation of granulation tissue into the injured area. The granulation tissue fills the defect and allows re-epithelization to occur, beginning at the wound edges and continuing to the center, until the entire wound is covered. Healing by second intention is slower than healing by first intention and results in the formation of more scar tissue. A wound that might otherwise have healed by first intention may become infected and then heal by second intention.

Keloid formation

An abnormality in healing by scar tissue repair is *keloid* formation. Keloids involve excessive production of bulging tumor-like scar-tissue masses. The tendency to develop keloid-scars is more common in blacks and seems to have a genetic basis.

Factors that affect wound healing

There are many factors, both local and systemic, which influence wound healing. Science has not found any way to hasten the normal process of wound repair, whereas there are many factors that impair healing.

Age. The rate of skin replacement slows with aging. Healing of open wounds and epithelization of skin takes longer in the elderly.

Nutrition. Adequate nutrition that includes essential amino acids, vitamins A and C, and zinc is essential for normal wound repairs. Cystine, an amino acid, is needed for synthesis of the mucopolysaccharides by the fibroblast. Vitamin C aids in collagen formation and capillary development. Zinc is thought to be an enzyme cofactor. In animal studies, zinc has been found to aid in re-epithelization. It is of interest that while a zinc deficiency tends to impair healing, zinc therapy does not seem to improve healing.[5]

Infection. Infection tends to impair wound healing. Both wound contamination and host factors that increase susceptibility to infection predispose to wound infection. Increased susceptibility to infection is associated with conditions that lead to a deficiency in leukocytes or impaired leukocyte function. Neutrophils in the diabetic, for example, have diminished chemotaxic and phagocytic ability. This may explain why diabetics are highly vulnerable to bacterial wound invasion.

Hormonal influences. The therapeutic administration of adrenal corticosteroids is known to influence the inflammatory process and to delay healing.

These hormones decrease capillary permeability during the early stages of inflammation, impair the phagocytic property of the leukocytes, and inhibit fibroblast proliferation and function.

Blood supply. In order for healing to occur, wounds must have adequate blood flow to supply the necessary nutrients and to remove the resulting waste, local toxins, bacteria, and other debris. Impaired wound healing due to poor blood flow may occur as a result of wound conditions, such as swelling, or may be caused by pre-existing conditions. Arterial disease and venous pathology are well-documented causes of impaired wound healing.

Wound separation. Approximation of the wound edges, i.e., suturing of an incision type of wound, greatly enhances healing and prevents infection. Epithelization of a wound with closely approximated edges occurs within one to two days. Large gaping wounds tend to heal more slowly because it is often impossible to effect wound closure with these types of wounds.

Presence of foreign bodies. Foreign bodies tend to invite bacterial contamination and delay healing. Fragments of wood, steel, glass, and the like may have entered the wound at the site of injury and can be difficult to locate when the wound is treated. Sutures are also foreign bodies and although needed for the closure of surgical wounds, they are an impediment to healing. This is why sutures are removed as soon as possible after surgery.

Bone Repair

Bone is an osseous form of connective tissue. There are three forms of bone cells: osteoblasts, osteocytes, and osteoclasts. *Osteoblasts* are bone-building cells that secrete collagen and other materials needed for production of bone. *Osteocytes* are bone cells that develop from osteoblasts. The osteocytes are surrounded by an intercellular matrix of bone salts (largely calcium phosphate) that provides strength and stability for bone. *Osteoclasts* are cells that reabsorb and cause breakdown of bone. There is usually a slow, but continuous, turnover of bone. Osteoclasts are continually reabsorbing and breaking down bone, while osteoblasts are busy rebuilding bone. This turnover allows for the continual remodeling of bone that is consistent with the stress placed on the skeletal structures.

Bone repair is best understood if discussed in relation to healing of a fracture. Bone repair is carried out in three stages: (1) formation of procallus, (2) development of the fibrocartilaginous callus, and (3) conversion of the fibrocartilaginous callus to osseous bone.

The initial stage of bone healing is similar to the healing that occurs in soft tissue. During this initial stage, there is bleeding into the surrounding tissues and between the bone fragments with development of a blood clot or hematoma. As with soft-tissue repair, a form of granulation tissue, in this case *procallus*, develops at the site of hematoma formation. In the course of about five days, depending on blood supply and other host conditions, the osteoblasts begin to enter the area and to form the fibrocartilaginous structure called *callus*. This tissue may also be called *osteoid tissue*; its structural arrangment resembles that of osteoid tissue, but it lacks the calcium salts in its matrix. By the end of the first week following an uncomplicated fracture injury, the osteoid tissue becomes rather abundant and is able to act as a splint to immobilize the fragments of the fracture. Some of the callus that forms is external, ensheathing the bone ends; some is intermediate, forming a union between the fractured surfaces; and some is internal, filling the marrow cavity. The internal and external callus is eventually removed by the osteoclasts as the bone undergoes a process of remodeling to realign the bone to meet new stresses. In the final stage of bone repair, calcium salts are laid down and the fibrocartilaginous callus is replaced with osseous callus. The osseous callus is eventually remodeled so that the bone returns to its original state.

If the gap between the bone parts is not bridged by osteogenic cells within a short period of time following the fracture, fibroblasts will enter the area and fill the gap with fibrous tissue which has no affinity for calcium. When this occurs, there is nonunion of the fracture ends.

Nerve Repair

Nerve tissue is composed of highly differentiated permanent cell types and exemplifies the general principle that the more specialized the function of a tissue the less able it is to regenerate. Cell division in neurons ceases at birth, and when a nerve cell dies it cannot be replaced. It is possible, however, for a nerve-fiber extension of a peripheral nerve to regenerate as long as the cell body of the nerve remains viable. This is not true of nerve fibers that are located in the central nervous system (brain and spinal cord).

Each peripheral nerve, such as the radial nerve, contains hundreds or thousands of sensory and motor fibers that can be interrupted at the time of injury. The changes described below occur in each of the injured nerve units.

Following injury, the cell body and its attached nerve fiber undergo temporary changes—the production and flow of protoplasm down the nerve fiber ceases. At about the same time, the Schwann cells that surrounded the nerve fiber, along with other phagocytic cells in the area, begin to remove the debris from the degenerating portion of the injured fiber. Following this clean-up operation, the cell body begins heightened production of the protoplasm and proteins that are needed for nerve-fiber regeneration. These proteins move from the cell body, down the fiber, and out into the injured stump. The outgrowth of the regenerating fiber occurs at a rate of 1- to 2-mm per day. Nerve fibers are encased in a fine collagen tube called the endoneurial sheath. Successful nerve regeneration requires that the regenerating portion of the nerve fiber makes contact with, and grows down, the endoneurial sheath that connects with the tissue originally innervated by the fiber. If a crushing injury occurs and the endoneurial tube remains intact, the outgrowing fiber will grow down the tube to its former target. Trauma due to a cut may be quite a different matter, because connective tissue forms rapidly and often prevents the regenerating nerve fibers from making contact with the intact distal nerve segment. Function of the part supplied by the injured nerve is restored when motor fibers make contact with the appropriate muscle fibers and sensory fibers connect with sensory receptors.

Not all peripheral nerves are able to recover from injury. Recovery does not occur when the cell body is damaged or when the injury is close to the cell body. Recovery is also dependent upon the way nerve ends are united following injury. Careful realignment and prevention of infection and formation of scar tissue favor recovery. Nerve injury and repair is discussed in greater detail in Chapter 39.

In summary, the ability of tissues to repair damage due to injury is dependent upon the body's ability to replace the parenchymal cells and to organize them as they were originally. Regeneration describes the process by which tissue is replaced with cells of a similar type and function. Healing by regeneration is limited to tissue that has cells that are able to divide and to replace the injured cells. Body cells are divided into types according to their ability to regenerate: (1) labile cells, such as the epithelial cells of the skin and gastrointestinal tract, which continue to regenerate throughout life; (2) stable cells, such as those in the liver, which normally do not divide but which are capable of regeneration when confronted with an appropriate stimulus; and (3) permanent or fixed cells, such as nerve cells, which are unable to regenerate. Scar-tissue repair involves the substitution of fibrous connective tissue for injured tissue that cannot be repaired by regeneration.

:Systemic Signs of Inflammation

Although inflammation is classically described as a local phenomenon, there are a number of systemic manifestations that accompany its presence. Among the most commonly mentioned manifestations are leukocytosis, increased erythrocyte sedimentation rate (ESR), and fever.

Erythrocyte Sedimentation Rate

Leukocytosis was described in an earlier part of the chapter. The ESR is a laboratory test that measures the speed at which the erythrocytes settle when an anticoagulant is added to the blood. In this test, the blood to which the anticoagulant has been added is placed in a long narrow tube and the speed at which the cells settle is observed. Alterations in the plasma components that occur with inflammation are thought to increase the rate at which the red cells settle.

Variation in Body Temperature

Fever is an elevated body temperature and is an almost universal response to infection and inflammation. Body temperature is usually maintained within a range of 35.8°C to 37.4°C (96.5°F to 99.3°F). There are diurnal variations in body temperature, with the temperature reaching a high in late afternoon or evening, and a low in the early-morning hours (Fig. 4-6).

Regulation of body temperature
Body temperature is essentially the difference between body *heat production* and *loss of heat* from the body.

$$\text{Body Temperature} = $$
$$\text{Body Heat Production} + \text{Body Heat Losses}$$

Heat production. The body's main source of *heat production* is metabolism. There is a 1°F increase in body temperature for every 7% increase in metabolism. Much of the heat production takes place in the

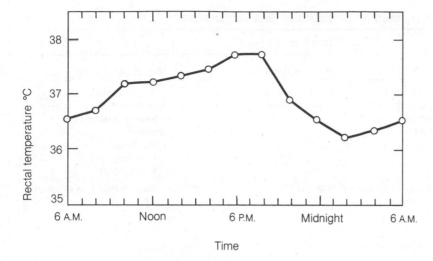

Figure 4–6.   Graph showing diurnal variations in body temperature.

inner portions of the body (inner core); this heat is carried by the blood to the skin surface where it is dissipated into the surrounding environment.

Heat loss.   Heat losses occur from the surface of the body, mainly through the skin. There are a number of arteriovenous (A–V) shunts, under the skin surface, which allow blood to move directly from the arterial to the venous system. These A–V shunts are much like the radiators in a heating system. When the shunts are open, body heat is freely dissipated to the skin and surrounding environment and when the shunts are closed heat is retained in the body. The opening and closing of these superficial vessels is regulated by the temperature control center in the hypothalamus.

There are four mechanisms that aid in dissipation of body heat from the skin surface: conduction, radiation, evaporation, and convection.

Conduction is the direct transfer of heat from one molecule to another. Blood carries or conducts heat from the inner core of the body to the skin surface. Normally only a small amount of body heat is lost through conduction to a cooler surface. Cooling blankets, or mattresses that are used for reducing fever, rely on conduction of heat from the skin to the cool surface of the mattress. Heat can also be conducted in the opposite direction—from the external environment to the body surface. For instance, body temperature may rise slightly after a hot bath.

Radiation is the transfer of heat through the air or a vacuum. Heat from the sun is carried by radiation. Normally about 60% to 70% of body heat is dissipated by radiation.

Evaporation describes heat losses that occur as the result of energy used for vaporizing water on the skin surface. Sweating increases evaporative losses and 0.58 calorie is lost from the body for each gram of water evaporated.[6]

Convection refers to heat transfer that occurs because of air currents. Normally there is a layer of heat that tends to remain near the body's surface; convection causes continual removal of this heat layer and replaces this air with that from the surrounding environment. The wind-chill factor that is often included in the weather report combines the effects of convection due to wind with the actual still-air temperature.

Body temperature is regulated by temperature-regulating centers in the hypothalamus. These centers integrate input from the various thermal receptors located throughout the body with output responses that either conserve body heat or increase its dissipation. The thermostatic centers in the hypothalamus are set so that the temperature of the body is regulated within the normal range of 35.8°C to 37.4°C. When body temperature begins to rise above the normal range, heat-dissipating behaviors are initiated, and when the temperature falls below that range heat production is increased. Heat-conservation and production responses as well as heat dissipation behaviors are described in Table 4-3. Shivering increases metabolism through movement of the skeletal muscles. Release of epinephrine and norepinephrine acts at the cellular level to shift metabolism so that energy production (ATP) is reduced and heat production is increased. This may be one of the reasons that fever tends to produce feelings of weakness and fatigue. Thyroid hormone increases cellular metabolism, but this response usually requires several weeks to reach maximum effectiveness.

Table 4–3   Heat Loss and Heat Gain Responses Used in Regulation of Body Temperature

Heat Gain		Heat Loss	
Body response	Mechanism of action	Body response	Mechanism of action
Vasoconstriction of the superficial blood vessels	Restricts blood flow to the outer shell of the body, with the skin and subcutaneous tissues acting as insulation to prevent loss of core heat	Dilatation of the superficial blood vessels	Delivers blood containing core heat to the periphery where it is dissipated through: Radiation Conduction Convection
Piloerection (contraction of the piloerector muscles that surround the hairs on the skin)	Reduces the heat loss surface of the skin	Sweating	Increases heat loss through evaporation
Assumption of the "huddle" position with the extremities held close to the body	Reduces the heat loss area of the body		
Shivering	Increases heat production by the muscles		
Increased production of epinephrine	Increases the heat production associated with metabolism		
Increased production of thyroid hormone	Is a long-term mechanism that increases metabolism and heat production		

Fever

Fever may be caused by infections, tumors, infarction, tissue necrosis, hemolytic responses, hypersensitivity reactions, brain injury, dehydration, and metabolic disturbances. The role of fever in the inflammatory process is still unclear. It is possible that elevation of body temperature may decrease resistance of selected infectious agents to host defenses. It is also possible that the increased metabolism and blood flow associated with fever may enhance healing.

Pyrogens.   Pyrogens are fever-producing substances. Leukocytes release endogenous pyrogens during inflammation. Pyrogens may also be released from other tissues. For example, in Hodgkin's disease the malignant cells reportedly produce endogenous pyrogens.[7] It is thought that pyrogens act directly on the hypothalamic temperature control center, increasing its set-point so that body temperature is regulated within a new and higher range.

The reactions that occur as body temperature is increased during fever usually consist of four stages: a prodrome, a chill during which the temperature rises, a flush, and defervescence.[8] During the prodromal period, there are nonspecific complaints such as mild headache and fatigue, general malaise,

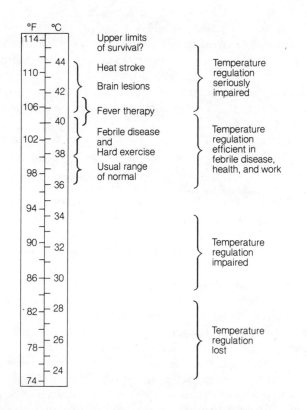

Figure 4–7.   Body temperatures under different conditions. (Dubois EF: Fever and the Regulation of Body Temperature. Springfield, Charles C Thomas, 1948)

and fleeting aches and pains. Vasoconstriction and piloerection usually precede the onset of shivering. At this point the skin is pale and covered with "goose pimples." There is a feeling of being cold and an urgency to put on more clothing or covering and to curl up in a position that conserves body heat. This is followed by a generalized shaking chill, and even as the temperature rises, there is the uncomfortable sensation of being chilled. When the shivering has caused body temperature to reach the new set-point of the temperature control center, the shivering ceases, and a sensation of warmth develops. At this point, cutaneous vasodilatation occurs and the skin becomes warm and flushed. The defervescence phase of the febrile response is marked by the initiation of sweating.

Harmful effects of fever.   Fever can be damaging to body cells; delirium and convulsions often occur when the temperature reaches 40°C. Convulsions are more common in children than adults. When the temperature goes above 41.1°C there is damage to the internal structures of many cells, including those in the brain. At this level of body temperature, regulation by the hypothalamic control center becomes impaired, and the body is no longer able to maintain the responses that increase heat loss (Fig. 4-7).

Treatment of fever.   Antipyretic drugs, such as aspirin and acetaminophen, are pharmacologic agents that act to decrease fever by returning the thermostatic temperature control center to normal. This causes dilatation of the superficial blood vessels and profuse sweating. Fever can also be treated with the use of sponge baths that increase evaporative losses, and through the use of a cooling mattress to increase conductive losses.

In summary, fever is a common systemic manifestation of inflammation. It is caused by pyrogens that are released from leukocytes. The pyrogens cause the temperature control center in the hypothalamus to be reset at a higher level. There are usually four stages that accompany fever. The first is the prodromal stage during which there are nonspecific complaints of discomfort. The second is the chill during which body temperature is raised to the new setting of the temperature control center. When the temperature reaches the new setting, the third stage—flush—occurs. During this stage there is a feeling of warmth as the superficial blood vessels become dilated. The final stage of fever is the defervescence phase during which sweating occurs.

:Disorders of White Blood Cells

There are two types of white blood cell disorders that are discussed in this chapter: leukopenia or decrease in white blood cell number, and leukemia, a malignant neoplasm of white blood cell precursors.

Leukopenia

Leukopenia is a decrease in white blood cell number. Viruses, rickettsiae, and certain protozoal infections are associated with a decrease in white blood cells. Leukopenia is also seen in persons with debilitating diseases in which the ability to produce white blood cells is depressed.

Agranulocytosis

Agranulocytosis is a decrease in the granulocytes, mainly the neutrophils. Agranulocytosis occurs when there is either an accelerated removal of neutrophils from the blood or when there is inadequate production of neutrophils by the bone marrow. Because of the short life span of the neutrophil, agranulocytosis occurs rapidly when either condition is present.

One of the causes of agranulocytosis is acute inflammation which may remove neutrophils from the blood faster than they can be replaced. When this happens the white blood cell count decreases. Drugs can cause either depression or accelerated destruction of neutrophils. Among the drugs implicated in causing agranulocytosis are many of the anticancer drugs, chloramphenicol, sulfonamides, aminopyrine, and chlorpromazine. Agranulocytosis is also encountered as an idiosyncratic reaction to other drugs and chemical agents. In nonmyelocytic leukemia and lymphomas, the overgrowth of neoplastic cells may crowd out the bone-marrow cells that produce the granulocytes.

The white-cell count in agranulocytosis is often reduced to 1000 cells per mm³ and may decline to levels as low as 200 to 300 cells per mm³. Because the neutrophil is essential to the cellular phase of inflammation, infections are common in persons with agranulocytosis, and extreme caution is needed to protect them from exposure to infectious organisms. Infections that might go unnoticed in persons with a normal neutrophil count may prove fatal to a person with agranulocytosis. Ulcerative necrotizing lesions of the mouth are common in persons with agranulocytosis. Ulcerations may also occur in the skin, vagina, and gastrointestinal tract.

Treatment with antibiotics provides a means to control infections in those situations in which the destruction of neutrophils can be controlled, or recovery of granulopoietic function of the bone marrow is possible. The prognosis for persons with agranulocytosis is variable and depends on the cause.

Leukemias

The leukemias are a group of diseases that affect the blood-forming cells, mainly the bone marrow and lymph nodes. Leukemias strike 21,500 persons in the United States each year and cause 15,000 deaths annually.[9] The disease strikes more children than any other form of cancer, and is the leading cause of death in children ages 3 to 15.

Types

There are several types of leukemias. The current methods of classifying leukemias focus on the particular type of white blood cell involved, and on the degree of differentiation that is present. Incompletely differentiated cells predominate in acute leukemia, and in chronic forms of the disease, the cells that predominate are structurally similar to normal cells. The leukemic cells usually represent an abnormal proliferation of one of the white blood cell types, although in myelogenous leukemia, all of the marrow-cell lines (erythroid, granulocytic, monocytic, and megakaryocytic) are involved. About 90% of all cases of leukemia are caused by two types of leukocytes—the lymphocytes (lymphocytic leukemia) and the granulocytes (granulocytic leukemia). Acute lymphocytic leukemia (ALL) is the most common form of leukemia in children. Acute granulocytic leukemia is most common in young adults and chronic leukemia (granulocytic or lymphocytic) is generally seen after the age of 40. More than half of all cases of leukemia occur in persons over the age of 60.

Causes

The causes of leukemia are unknown. There is an unusually high incidence of leukemia among persons exposed to high levels of radiation. The number of cases of leukemia, in the most heavily exposed survivors of the atomic blasts at Hiroshima and Nagasaki, during the 20-year-period from 1950 to 1970 was nearly thirty times the expected rate.[10] There are hints of a genetic predisposition. It is known that persons with Down's syndrome have a higher incidence of leukemia, and leukemia has been seen in a significant number of twins. A chromosomal aberration, the Philadelphia chromosome (translocation from chromosome 22 and 9), occurs in approximately 90% of persons with chronic myelogenous leukemia. There is also an increasing interest in the role of viruses as etiologic agents in leukemia. Leukemic viruses have been identified from a number of animal species.

Manifestations

Leukemic cells are immature and mobile forms of white blood cells. Being mobile, they are able to travel throughout the circulatory system, cross the blood–brain barrier, and infiltrate many body tissues. But being immature, they are unable to perform the functions of mature leukocytes, that is, they are ineffective as phagocytes. The rapidly proliferating malignant cells tend to crowd out the normal bone-marrow cells, including the erythroblasts and megakaryocytes that produce the thrombocytes. Anemia and bleeding tendencies are common in leukemia. The rapid growth of the malignant cells puts a great strain on the body's nutrient stores. Fever, anorexia, and weight loss are common.

Treatment

The treatment of leukemia varies with the type; chemotherapy and radiation are the most common treatment modalities. The goal of treatment is to effect a remission. In children with acute lymphocytic leukemia, the use of combination chemotherapy (multiple anticancer drugs) has produced about a 50%, 5-year-survival rate. It is hoped that these children may be cured.

In summary, there are a number of conditions that affect white blood cell numbers and function. Two of these are leukopenia and leukemia. Leukopenia occurs because of increased white blood cell destruction or impaired bone-marrow function in which there is a decrease in white blood cell production. Leukemia is a neoplastic disease of the blood-forming cells. There are several types of leukemia, identified by differences in the white blood cell type involved, and the degree of differentiation that is present. In acute leukemia, the poorly differentiated cells predominate, whereas, in chronic leukemia, the dominant cell type closely resembles the cells. Both leukopenia and leukemia impair the normal white cell response to inflammation and increase susceptibility to infection, leukopenia because there is an inadequate number of leukocytes and leukemia because the function of leukocytes is abnormal.

:Study Guide

After you have studied this chapter, you should be able to meet the following objectives:

: : Explain why the inflammatory response is beneficial to the body.

: : Identify one universal characteristic of the inflammatory response.

: : Explain the early hemodynamic changes that occur in acute inflammation.

: : State the three patterns of response that occur with an inflammatory reaction.

: : State the function of the granular leukocytes.

: : Contrast the monocytes and the lymphocytes on the basis of function.

: : Define *diapedesis*.

: : Relate chemotaxis to leukocytic activity.

: : Describe the process of phagocytosis.

: : List the components of the reticuloendothelial system.

: : State one characteristic that is distinctive of chemical mediators.

: : Contrast the five types of inflammatory exudates.

: : Describe three patterns of resolution of acute inflammation.

: : State the characteristics of chronic inflammation.

: : Define *lability* and *stability* as these terms apply to cellular regeneration.

: : Relate the sequence of events in soft tissue repair.

: : Describe the process of scar tissue development.

: : Define *first intention* and *second intention* in relation to wound healing.

: : Relate the influence of local and systemic factors on wound healing.

: : Identify the stages in bone repair.

: : Relate the sequence of events in nerve repair.

: : State the purpose of the ESR.

: : Relate heat production and heat loss to regulation of body temperature.

: : Relate the sequence of events in fever.

: : State the circumstances under which agranulocytosis occurs.

: : State the basic defect that is found in leukemia.

:References

1. Robbins SL, Cotran RS: Pathologic Basis of Disease, p 55. Philadelphia, WB Saunders, 1979
2. Lewis T: Blood Vessels of the Human Skin and Their Responses. London, Shaw, 1927
3. Tepperman Jay: Metabolic and Endocrine Physiology, 4th ed, p 189. Chicago, Year Book Medical Publishers, 1980
4. Robbins SL, Cotran RS: The Pathologic Basis of Disease, p 100. Philadelphia, WB Saunders, 1979
5. Neldner KH, Hambridge KM: Zinc therapy. N Engl J Med 292:879, 1975
6. Guyton A: Textbook of Medical Physiology 6th ed, p 888. Philadelphia, WB Saunders, 1981
7. Badel P: Pyrogen release in vitro by lymphoid tissue in patients with Hodgkin's disease. Yale J Biol Med 47:101, 1974
8. Sodeman WA, Sodeman TM: Pathologic Physiology: Mechanisms of Disease, 6th ed, p 546. Philadelphia, WB Saunders, 1979
9. American Cancer Society: Facts on Leukemia. 1978
10. Jablon S, Kato H: Studies of the mortality of A-bomb survivors. Radiat Res 50:658, 1972

:Suggested Readings

Inflammation and Wound Repair

Bruno P: The nature of wound healing. Nurs Clin North Am 14 No. 4:667, 1979

Bryant WM: Wound healing. Clin Symp 29 No. 3:1, 1977

Houck JC: Inflammation: A quarter century of progress. J Invest Dermatol 67 No. 1:124, 1976

Madden J: Wound healing: Biologic and clinical features. In Sabiston D (ed): Davis-Christopher Textbook of Surgery, 11th ed. Philadelphia, WB Saunders, 1977

Montandon D, D'Andrian G, Gabbiani G: The mechanism of wound contraction and epithelization. Clin Plast Surg 4 No. 3:325, 1977

Peacock E Jr, Van Winkle W: Wound Repair, 2nd ed. Philadelphia, WB Saunders, 1976

Ryan GE, Majno G: Acute inflammation. Am J Pathol 86 No. 1:185, 1977

Ryan G Majno G: Inflammation. Kalamazoo, A Scope Publication, Upjohn, 1977

Fever

Bernheim HA, Block LH, Atkins E: Fever: Pathogenesis, pathophysiology, and purpose. Ann Intern Med 91:261, 1979

Castle M, Watkins J: Fever: Understanding the sinister sign. Nursing '78 9, No. 2:26, 1978

Davis–Sharts J: Mechanisms and manifestations of fever. Am J Nurs 78, No. 11:1874, 1978

Rosendorff C: Neurochemistry of fever. S Afr J Med Sci 41, No. 1:23, 1976

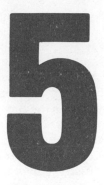

Immune
Responses

Immunology is the study of immune mechanisms and can be divided into four categories: immunity, serology, immunochemistry, and immunobiology.[1] Immunity is concerned with the prevention of infectious diseases and the growth of abnormal cells. Application of serologic procedures facilitates the diagnosis of diseases (rickettsial, viral, syphilis, and others). Immunochemistry views immune mechanisms as complex chemical reactions between antigens, haptens, antibodies, and complement. At the molecular level, immunochemistry has advanced to the point of identifying the structure of the amino-acid sequence of the immunoglobulins and other components of the immune response. Immunobiology encompasses a broader view of immunology: it proposes theories about how antibodies are formed, about how hypersensitivity develops, and about the origin of autoimmune disease. The content presented in this chapter focuses on the last-named category and presents a broad overview of immunity as it relates to the prevention and development of disease. The chapter is divided into three parts: (1) an overview of immunological concepts, (2) a discussion of the role of immunity as it relates to the production of disease, and (3) selected neoplasms of immune cells or related structures.

:Immunologic Concepts

Immunity is a normal adaptive response. It protects the body from destruction by foreign materials and invasion by microbial agents, and prevents proliferation of mutant cells, such as those involved in neoplastic growth. Basic to the normal immune response is the body's ability to recognize its own cells as self and to distinguish them from nonself.

The immune response describes the interaction between the cells of the immune system and an antigen. Alterations in immunity develop when the immune response is inadequate, inappropriate, or exaggerated. The response is inadequate when the body cannot build the immune cells or immunoglobulins needed to protect against common pathogens, and it is inappropriate when it destroys its own tissues or reacts to common substances in the environment.

Active, Passive, and Natural Immunity

Immune responses can be active or passive. *Active immunity* implies that the body has developed or acquired the ability to defend itself against a specific

agent. Active immunity is achieved through actually having had a disease or through immunization against the disease. *Passive immunity* is temporary immunity that is transmitted or borrowed from another source. An infant receives passive immunity from its mother *in utero* and from antibodies that it receives from its mother's breast milk. Passive immunity can also be transferred through injection of antiserum which contains the antibodies for a specific disease or through the use of pooled gamma globulin which contains antibodies for a number of diseases. Both antiserum and gamma globulin are obtained from blood plasma. *Natural immunity* is species specific. It is the reason that humans do not contract certain animal diseases, such as feline distemper.

Terminology

Like all other disciplines, immunology has its own terminology. An *immune response* involves an interaction between an *antigen (immunogen)* and an *antibody (immunoglobulin)* or *reactive lymphocyte*. The *immunogenicity* of an antigen refers to its ability to stimulate the immune response. *Tolerance* implies that the body does not build antibodies or reactive lymphocytes to an antigen—there is a natural tolerance to the body's own tissues. Immunologic tolerance describes the situation in which there is a failure to respond to a specific antigen. *Immunosuppression*, however, is nonspecific and refers to the body's inability to build antibodies or reactive lymphocytes to all antigens.

Antigens

An antigen or immunogen* is any substance recognized as foreign that stimulates the immune response. Not all foreign substances are antigenic. The immunogenicity of a substance is determined by its foreignness, chemical complexity, molecular size, and the method of administration. As a general rule, the more foreign a substance is to the body, the more antigenic it is. In terms of identifying a substance as foreign, the immune system recognizes certain chemical groups (antigenic determinant sites) on the antigen. Therefore, large proteins and polysaccharides make good antigens because of their com-

---

*The terms antigen and immunogen are both used in describing a foreign substance that stimulates an immune response. Although the term antigen has been used for a number of years, the newer term immunogen is becoming more widely preferred. This text uses both terms interchangeably.

plex chemical structure. On the other hand, amino acids and small molecules (those with a molecular weight of less than 10,000) all look alike to the immune system and are usually poor antigens. There are some substances that cannot act as antigens by themselves, but which have antigenic determinant sites and which can combine with a *carrier* substance and then act as an antigen. These substances, which usually have a low molecular weight, are called haptens. House dust, animal danders, and plant pollens are haptens.

The site of access to the body may influence the antigenic strength of a substance. For example, the digestive enzymes often hydrolyze and destroy the antigenic quality of otherwise fully antigenic materials. When these same substances are given parenterally (injected), greater amounts of the antigen are available for interacting with the antigen-processing cells. The oral polio vaccine is one exception; when taken into the gastrointestinal tract, it invades the lining of the intestine and reproduces itself.[2]

Histocompatibility antigens

Histocompatibility refers to the sharing of transplantation genes. It has been found that all nucleated cells in the body contain surface antigens (histocompatibility antigens) which are genetically determined. In humans, these antigens are called the human leukocyte antigens (HLA) because they were first detected on the leukocyte. The histocompatibility antigens are similar in many respects to the ABO antigens that are found on the red blood cell and which must be matched for transfusion purposes.

The histocompatibility antigens are inherited as part of the genetic makeup of an individual. There are five closely linked gene loci—HLA–A, HLA–B, HLA–C, HLA–D, HLA–DR—that have been identified at the time this text was written. These gene loci are located on the sixth chromosome. Each of the five loci is occupied by multiple alleles or genes that code the development of each cell surface antigen. There are at least 20 gene products or antigens for the A loci and 30 antigens for the B loci. Each of the antigens is numbered, HLA–A1, HLA–A2, and so on. Table 5-1 lists the major histocompatibility antigens.

Each individual receives a pair of genes, one from each parent. The pairs of genes that are inherited dictate a person's HLA type (Table 5-2). Because

Table 5–1   Major Human Histocompatibility Loci, 1977*

HLA-A	HLA-B		HLA-C	HLA-D	HLA-DR
HLA-A1	HLA-B5	HLA-Bw42	HLA-Cw1	HLA-Dw1	HLA-DRw1
HLA-A2	HLA-B7	HLA-Bw44	HLA-Cw2	HLA-Dw2	HLA-DRw2
HLA-A3	HLA-B8	HLA-Bw45	HLA-Cw3	HLA-Dw3	HLA-DRw3
HLA-A9	HLA-B12	HLA-Bw46	HLA-Cw4	HLA-Dw4	HLA-DRw4
HLA-A10	HLA-B13	HLA-Bw47	HLA-Cw5	HLA-Dw5	HLA-DRw5
HLA-A11	HLA-B14	HLA-Bw48	HLA-Cw6	HLA-Dw6	HLA-DRw6
HLA-Aw19	HLA-B15	HLA-Bw49		HLA-Dw7	HLA-DRw7
HLA-Aw23	HLA-Bw16	HLA-Bw50		HLA-Dw8	
HLA-Aw24	HLA-B17	HLA-Bw51		HLA-Dw9	
HLA-A25	HLA-B18	HLA-Bw52		HLA-Dw10	
HLA-A26	HLA-Bw21	HLA-Bw53		HLA-Dw11	
HLA-A28	HLA-Bw22	HLA-Bw54			
HLA-A29	HLA-B27				
HLA-Aw30	HLA-Bw35				
HLA-Aw31	HLA-B37				
HLA-Aw32	HLA-Bw38				
HLA-Aw33	HLA-Bw39				
HLA-Aw34	HLA-B40				
HLA-Aw36	HLA-Bw41				
HLA-Aw43					
	HLA-Bw4				
	HLA-Bw6				

*The practice of applying "w" (workshop) prefixes is used to designate antigens that are only provisionally accepted by the International Histocompatibility Workshops. (Announcement: New Nomenclature for the HLA System. *J Immunol* 116, No. 2:573, 1976)

(From Fudenberg HH et al: Basic and Clinical Immunology, 3rd ed. Copyright 1980 by Lange Medical Publications, Los Altos, California. Reproduced with permission.)

Table 5-2   Genetic Transmission of HLA Antigens and Haplotypes

	A Antigens						B Antigens					
	1	2	3	9	10	11	5	7	8	12	13	14
Father	+	–	+	–	–	–	–	+	+	–	–	–
Mother	–	+	–	+	–	–	+	–	–	+	–	–
Children												
First	+	+	–	–	–	–	+	–	+	–	–	–
Second	+	–	–	+	–	–	–	+	+	–	–	–
Third	–	+	+	–	–	–	+	+	–	–	–	–
Fourth	–	+	+	–	–	–	+	+	–	–	–	–

Interpretation

	Phenotypes	Haplotypes
Father	A1, 3/ B7, 8	A1, B8/ A3, B7
Mother	A2, 9/ B5, 12	A2, B5/ A9, B12
Children		
First	A1, 2/ B5, 8	A1, B8/ A2, B5
Second	A1, 9/ B8, 12	A1, B8/ A9, B12
Third	A2, 3/ B5, 7	A3, B7/ A2, B5
Fourth	A2, 3/ B5, 7	A3, B7/ A2, B5

(From Barrett JT: Textbook of Immunology, 3rd ed, p. 388, St. Louis, CV Mosby, 1978)

Table 5-3   HLA and Disease Associations

Disease	HLA Antigen	Frequency in Patients (%)	Frequency in Controls (%)
Ankylosing spondylitis	B27	90	7
Reiter's disease	B27	76	6
Acute anterior uveitis	B27	55	8
Psoriasis	B13	18	4
	B17	29	8
	B16	15	5
Graves' disease	B8	47	21
Celiac disease (gluten-sensitive enteropathy)	D3	95	15
Dermatitis herpetiformis	B8	62	27
Myasthenia gravis	B8	52	24
Multiple sclerosis	D2	60	15
	B7	36	25
Acute lymphatic leukemia	A2	63	37
Hodgkin's disease	B5	25	16
	B1	39	32
	B8	26	22
Chronic hepatitis	B8	68	18
Ragweed hay fever			
Ra 5 sensitivity	B7	50	19
Allergen E sensitivity	Multiple (in family studies)		

(From Krupp MA, Chatton MJ (eds): Current Medical Diagnosis and Treatment. Copyright 1981 by Lange Medical Publications, Los Altos, California. Reproduced with permission.)

of the number of genes involved, the chances of common HLA types, such as persons with type A blood antigens, are unlikely.

The typing of histocompatibility antigens is important in tissue grafting and organ transplantation. The closer the matching of HLA types, the less the chance of organ or graft rejection.

It has been noted that specific HLA antigens are seen more frequently in persons with certain disease conditions (Table 5-3). For example, it has been observed that 90% of persons with ankylosing spondylitis have HLA-B27 antigen; whereas only 7% of a control group without the disease have the antigen. The mechanism responsible for the association between the HLA antigens and these diseases is not yet known.

Immune Cells

There are three types of immune cells: the macrophage, the B lymphocyte, and the T lymphocyte. The macrophage processes the antigen and transfers the antigenic determinants to the lymphocytes. The T lymphocytes are responsible for forming the sensitized lymphocytes that provide cellular immunity and the B lymphocytes for forming the antibodies that provide humoral immunity.

Lymphocytes represent 20% to 30% of the leukocytes (Fig. 5-1). They begin their life in the bone marrow as lymphoblasts and travel in the blood to many organs, but are eventually imprinted in a series of critical events that occur in either the thymus or bursal equivalent tissue. Two types of lymphocytes, the T lymphocytes and the B lymphocytes, emerge as a result of the changes that occur in these two structures.

The *T lymphocytes* are imprinted in the thymus and are the smaller of the two types. They have a life span of years, much longer than that of the B lymphocytes. Among the characteristics shared by T lymphocytes is the presence of a surface antigen called the θ (theta) antigen. T lymphocytes may be recognized by their ability to react with antitheta sera. The antitheta sera are, however, difficult to prepare and purify. A simpler method for recognizing and enumerating the T lymphocytes is through the use of sheep erythrocytes. When normal lymphocytes are incubated with sheep erythrocytes, they form rosettes which can be visualized under the microscope.

The second type of lymphocyte is called the *B lymphocyte* because in birds, its maturation and development occur in an organ located near the hind part of the gut called the *bursa of Fabricius*. At present, the location of the human equivalent of the

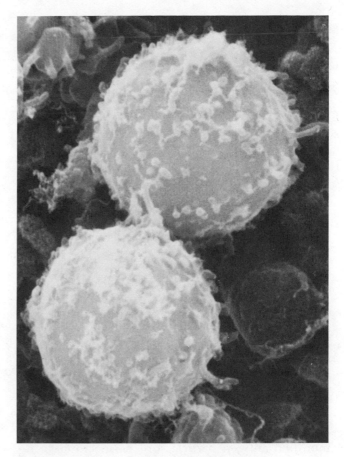

Figure 5–1. A scanning micrograph of two lymphocytes. (Courtesy of Kenneth Siegesmund, Ph.D., Anatomy Department, Medical College of Wisconsin)

bursa is not known for certain. There are indications that gut-associated lymphoid tissue serves this function. The B cells are larger than the T cells and their life span is much shorter, being only about five to seven days. Among the characteristics of the B lymphocytes is the presence of bursal (B) antigen and immunoglobulins on their surface. B lymphocytes have the capacity for transformation into plasma cells when exposed to an antigen. There are several classes of B lymphocytes, each responsible for producing one class of immunoglobulins. The B-cell population is high in certain tissues, such as the tonsil and spleen, and is low in the circulating blood.

It has been determined that the macrophages, the blood monocytes, and the tissue lymphocytes participate in the immune response by processing foreign substances and by presenting the antigen to the lymphocytes in a form that increases its immunogenicity (Fig. 5-2). In the process of phagocytosis, the macrophage ingests the foreign substance and digests it; then portions of the antigen move through

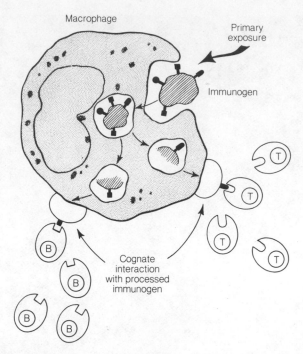

Figure 5–2. Diagram of the interaction between the immunogen (antigen), macrophage, and lymphocytes.

the cell membrane and become attached to receptors on the cell surface. The interaction between the modified antigen particles on the macrophage receptors and the lymphocyte stimulates lymphocyte differentiation and proliferation. These receptor-site interactions also appear to provide the stage for T-cell and B-cell interactions; it facilitates the helper role of the T lymphocytes in terms of B-cell function. There is also evidence to suggest participation by the T lymphocyte in humoral immunity, as well as evidence to suggest that the macrophage can act under T-cell influence to destroy bacteria and tumor cells. As will be discussed later, lymphokines that are produced by the effector T cells cause migration or activation of the macrophages.

Types of Immunity

There are two general types of immunity—humoral and cell-mediated (Fig. 5-3). Humoral immunity is dependent upon the presence of circulating antibodies that are formed by the B cells. Cell-mediated immunity is mediated by the T cells that react directly with the antigen to cause its destruction.

Humoral immunity

The B lymphocytes, which form about 20% to 30% of the lymphocyte population are capable of developing into plasma cells which produce antibodies or

immunoglobulins. Although the B cells produce large numbers of antibodies to a vast variety of antigens, each plasma cell produces only one type of antibody. It is implied that the B-cell antigen interaction results in an individual clone of plasma cells which are committed to produce the antibody for that particular antigen. Some cells in the clone are thought to produce antibodies, while others become memory cells.

The immunoglobulins are found in the globulin fraction of the plasma proteins. Only recently has the chemical structure of the immunoglobulins been identified (Fig. 5-4). Each of the immunoglobulins is composed of two heavy (H) chains and two light (L) chains. The amino-acid sequence of each of the chains has a constant (C) region and a variable (V) region. The antigen reacts with the variable region. Each of the immunoglobulins has a different amino-acid sequence in the variable region that provides it with the specificity needed to react with a single antigen. The heavy chains in each of the classes of immunoglobulins are antigenically distinctive, and it is this distinction that permits division of the immune globulins into classes through the use of immunoelectrophoresis.

Through immunoelectrophoresis, the immunoglobulins have been divided into five classes—IgG, IgA, IgM, IgD and IgE (Table 5-4). Each of these immunoglobulins is made by a different group of B lymphocytes and each varies according to the nature of the antigen. IgG (gamma globulin) is the most abundant of the immunoglobulins. It circulates in body fluids and is the only immunoglobulin that crosses the placenta. IgG activates the complement system. IgA, the second most abundant of the immunoglobulins, is found in saliva, tears, and in bronchial, gastrointestinal, prostatic, and vaginal secretions. It is a secretory immunoglobulin and is considered to be a primary defense against local infections. IgM appears to most antigens early in the immune response. Like IgG, IgM activates the complement system. IgE is involved in allergic and hypersensitivity reactions. It binds to mast cells and causes release of histamine and other mediators of allergic responses. The main function of IgD has not been determined.

There are two types of responses that occur in the development of humoral immunity (Fig. 5-5). There is a primary response that occurs when the antigen is first introduced into the body. During this primary response, there is a latent period before the antibody can be detected in the serum. This latent period involves the recognition of the antigen by the antibody and the development of a clone of plasma

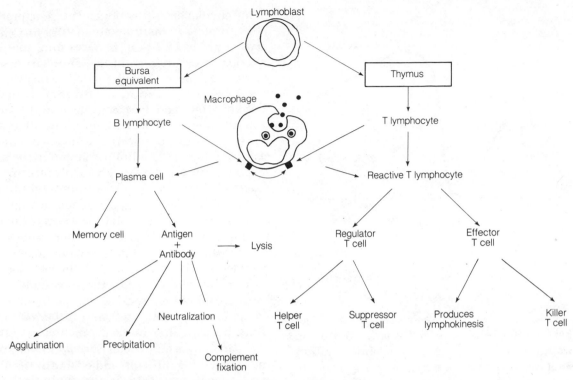

Figure 5–3. Diagram of the development of cellular and humoral immunity.

cells that will produce the antibody. This period usually takes from 48 to 72 hours, after which the detectable antibody titer continues to rise for a period of ten days to two weeks. Recovery from many infectious diseases occurs at about the time during the primary response when the antibody titer is reach-

Figure 5–4. Basic immunoglobulin structure formed from four polypeptide chains bound together. Light chains (L), heavy chains (H), constant amino acid region (C), and variable amino acid region (V). Antigens bind to the variable region of the immunoglobulin.

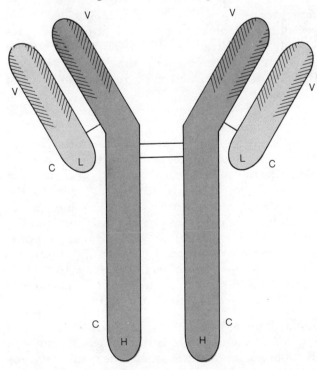

Table 5-4   Classes of Immunoglobulins

Class	Percent of Total	Characteristics
IgG	75.0	Present in majority of B cells; contains antiviral, antitoxin, and antibacterial antibodies; only immunoglobulin that crosses the placenta; responsible for protection of newborn; activates complement and binds to macrophages
IgA	15.0	Predominant immunoglobulin in body secretions, such as saliva, nasal and respiratory secretions, breast milk; protects mucous membranes
IgM	10.0	Forms the natural antibodies such as those for ABO blood antigens; prominent in early immune responses; activates complement
IgD	0.2	Action is not known; may affect B cell maturation
IgE	0.004	Binds to mast cells and basophils; involved in allergic and hypersensitivity reactions

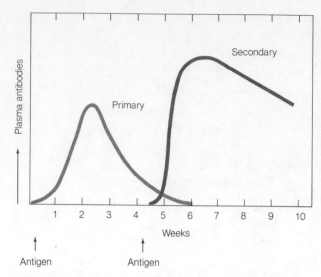

Figure 5–5. Primary and secondary responses of the humoral immune system to the same antigen.

ing its peak. The secondary response occurs on second or subsequent exposures to the antigen. During the secondary response, the rise in antibody titer occurs sooner and reaches a higher level. There are two forms of plasma cells that develop during the primary response: one produces the antibody and the other becomes a memory cell that records the information needed for antibody production. During the secondary response, the memory cell recognizes the antigen and stimulates production of plasma cells which produce the specific antibody. The "booster immunization" given for some infectious diseases, such as tetanus, makes use of the secondary response. For persons who have been previously immunized, administration of a "booster shot" causes an almost immediate rise in antibody titer to a level sufficient to prevent development of the disease.

Antigen–antibody reactions can take several forms. Combination of antigen with antibody can result in precipitation of the antigen–antibody complex; it can cause agglutination or clumping of cells, neutralization of bacterial toxins, lysis or destruction of the pathogen or cell membranes, adherence of the antigen to immunocytes or other structures, opsonization which enhances phagocytosis, and complement fixation or activation. Some of these reactions, such as opsonization occur because of complement fixation. Antigen–antibody reactions can be studied *in vitro* (in serum samples studied in the laboratory) or they can occur *in vivo* (in the body).

Complement system

The complement system is the primary mediator of the humoral immune response. The system consists of at least 20 serum proteins that are normally present

in the circulation as functionally inactive precursors. These proteins constitute about 10% to 15% of the plasma-protein fraction. In order for a complement reaction to occur, each of the complement components must be activated in the proper sequence. Only immune responses involving immunoglobulins IgG and IgM activate complement, and it is probable that complement is bound in all antigen–antibody reactions that involve these two classes of immunogolobulins. Table 5-5 lists immune responses that occur as the result of complement fixation.

There are several known abnormalities of the complement system. One of the better known defects is a condition called hereditary angioneurotic edema which is caused by a congenital deficiency of complement 1 inactivator. The uncontrolled activation of this component of the complement system leads to sporadic attacks of subcutaneous edema which are associated with minor trauma to the affected part. In extensive reactions, edema of the face, neck, and joints may occur. Edema of the throat may make breathing difficult, and edema of the abdominal organs may produce intense abdominal pain.

Other deficiencies of the complement system have been described, many of which are associated with recurrent infections.

Cell-mediated immunity

In cell-mediated immunity, the action of the T lymphocytes and the macrophages predominates. In addition to its protective effects, cell-mediated immunity is responsible for delayed hypersensitivity and transplant reactions. It is also thought to protect against tumor-cell development.

The T lymphocytes mature in the thymus and constitute about 70% to 80% of the lymphocytes.

Table 5–5   Complement-Mediated Immune Responses

Response	Effect
Cytolysis	Destruction of cell membrane of body cells or pathogens
Adherence of immune cells	Adhesion of antigen–antibody complexes to the inert surfaces of cells or tissues such as the reticuloendothelial cells that line the blood vessels and have the capacity for phagocytosis
Chemotaxis	Induces leukocyte migration from an area of lesser concentration to areas of higher concentration with the agent
Anaphylaxis	Involves degranulation of mast cells with release of histamine and other mediators
Opsonization	Modification of the antigen so that it can be easily digested by a phagocytic cell

There are two populations of T cells: regulatory T cells and effector T cells. Regulatory cells act by either enhancing or suppressing the action of the B lymphocytes. These cells are sometimes called the *T helper* cells or *T suppressor* cells. The effector cells synthesize and release immune mediators called lymphokines and cause death of target cells by contact with cell-linked antigens. The type of effector T cell that causes cell death is called the *killer T cell*.

The *lymphokines* produced by the T cell are low molecular weight proteins that are capable of influencing other inflammatory cells, including the macrophage, the neutrophil, and the lymphocyte. The lymphokines also activate or suppress the macrophage. Lymphokines can act as chemotactic factors for neutrophils, eosinophils, and basophils and can cause histamine release from mast cells. Cytotoxic factor, or lymphotoxin, causes lysis of certain target cells.

Cell-mediated immunity provides protection against viruses, cancer cells, and foreign tissue. Unlike humoral antibodies which can be injected as an antiserum, cell-mediated immunity is not readily transferred from one individual to another.

Interferons

A discussion of immune mechanisms would not be complete without mention of interferons which provide the body with antiviral protection. Interferons are a family of proteins produced by somatic cells in response to a variety of stimuli, including viral infections. The interferon is released from infected cells almost as soon as the virus is produced. Three types of interferons have been identified—fibroepithelial, leukocyte, and immune—depending on the type of cell producing each. Interferon interacts at the gene level to inhibit the translation of messenger RNAs, which regulate viral protein synthesis but not host protein synthesis. This antiviral activity can be transferred to neighboring cells without the continued presence of interferon. The actions of interferon are pathogen nonspecific, that is, they are effective against different forms of viruses. They are, however, species specific. Animal interferons will not provide protection for humans.

Techniques have been developed for producing interferon by using human leukocytes. Interferon has shown promise in the treatment of certain types of viral infections, such as the herpes viruses, and its use in the treatment of certain types of cancer is under investigation. Although interferon is now very expensive because of the production methods that must be employed, it is hoped that other methods will be found which will allow for commercial production at a more reasonable cost. There are several avenues of large-scale production of interferon that are being pursued. One is gene splicing, the combining of genes that make human interferon with bacteria which then become interferon factories; a second avenue is the quest to identify the amino-acid sequence of interferon synthetically; a third approach is to find a safe and effective chemical that could induce the human body to produce its own interferon.

In summary, the immune system provides the body with protection against foreign materials, invasion by microbial agents, and proliferation of mutant cells. The immune system relies on three types of cells—the macrophages and the T and B lymphocytes. The macrophages act to process the antigens and to interact with the lymphocytes in the immune process. The T lymphocytes are responsible for cell-mediated immunity and the B lymphocytes for humoral immunity. The mechanisms involved in both types of immunity are summarized in Figure 5-3.

:Role of the Immune Response in Production of Disease

Although the immune response is a normal protective mechanism, it can cause disease when the response is deficient (immunodeficiency disease), when the response is inappropriate (allergy and hypersensitivity), or when the response is misdirected (autoimmune disease). Each of these conditions will be discussed in the section that follows.

Immunodeficiency Disease

The immunodeficiency states include disorders in antibody (B cell) function, cellular (T cell) immunity, and complement deficiency. The immune deficiency states can range from a deficiency in one class of immunoglobulins to a lack of both humoral and cellular immunity. The deficiency states may be either primary (hereditary or developmental), or secondary (acquired as the result of some other condition that occurred following birth). The major categories of immunodeficiency disorders are summarized in Table 5-6.

Antibody (B cell) immunodeficiency

At birth a baby is partially protected by maternal IgG antibodies. During the first four to five months of life there is a gradual decline in serum IgG levels as these antibodies are destroyed; the IgG level reaches its lowest point at about five to six months. At about

Table 5-6 Immunodeficiency States

Antibody (B cell) immunodeficiency

Primary
    Transient hypogammaglobulinemia of infancy
    X-linked hypogammaglobulinemia
    Selective deficiency of IgG, IgA, IgM

Secondary
    Decreased synthesis of immunoglobulins (lymphomas)
    Increased loss of immunoglobulins (nephrotic syndrome)
    Production of defective immunoglobulins (multiple myeloma)

Cellular (T cell) immunodeficiency

Primary
    Congenital thymic aplasia (DiGeorge's syndrome)
    Abnormal synthesis (Nezelof's syndrome)

Secondary
    Malignant disease (Hodgkin's disease, and others)
    Transient suppression of T-cell production and function due to an acute
      viral infection such as measles

Combined antibody (B cell) and cellular (T cell) immunodeficiency

Primary
    Severe combined immunodeficiency (autosomal or sex-linked recessive)
    Wiskott–Aldrich syndrome (immunodeficiency, thrombocytopenia,
      and eczema)
    Immunodeficiency with ataxia and telangiectasia

Secondary
    X-radiation
    Immune suppressant and cytotoxic drugs
    Aging

Complement abnormality

Primary
    Selective deficiency in a complement component
    Angioneurotic edema (complement 1 inhibitor deficiency)

this time, the infant's immune system begins to function and the antibody level begins to rise, reaching adult levels when the infant is about 12 to 16 months of age. Some babies may, however, experience a delay in onset of gamma globulin production that may last until two to three years of age—*transient hypogammaglobulinemia*. These babies are particularly susceptible to bacterial and respiratory infections and to bronchitis. Usually, the condition is self-limiting and immunoglobulin production becomes normal sometime between the second and third year of life.

A much more serious disorder of immunoglobulin deficiency is a sex-linked, inherited condition that is restricted to males. This form of *X-linked hypogammaglobulinemia* was first described by Bruton in 1952 and is sometimes called Bruton's disease. It is thought that in these infants the bursa equivalent stem cells fail to develop and as a result there is a deficiency in both B cells and plasma cells. Symptoms of the disorder usually begin to develop at about the time that maternal antibodies have been depleted. Children with this disorder are particularly prone to develop severe recurrent episodes of pharyngitis, otitis media, and respiratory tract infections from exposure to common antigens. Treatment for the condition consists of injections of gamma globulin.

A selective deficiency of IgA is the most common form of primary immunodeficiency state known. It occurs in 1 out of every 1000 individuals and consists of a virtual lack of both serum and secretory IgA. Most individuals with the disorder are asymptomatic, although some may have repeated respiratory infections, diarrhea, and increased incidence of asthma and other allergies. The disorder is thought to consist of a defect in the terminal stage of B-cell development. Patients with IgA deficiencies may experience an anaphylactic reaction when given a blood transfusion, because IgA in the donor blood is often recognized as a foreign agent.[3]

Cellular (T cell) immunodeficiency

There are very few primary forms of T-cell deficiency. One such condition is a congenital failure of thymus gland development (*DiGeorge's syndrome*). The condition occurs as a defect associated with embryonic development of the third and fourth pharyngeal pouches. These embryonic structures are also involved in development of other parts of the head and neck, and babies born with this disorder also fail to develop the parathyroid gland and have congenital defects of the face and heart. Another condition, *Nezelof's syndrome*, is a genetically (autosomal recessive) determined disorder in which there is faulty development of the thymus gland and T-cell function, but lack of other developmental defects.

Temporary suppression of T-cell function has been reported following acute viral infections, such as measles. Secondary forms of cellular immunodeficiency occur with some diseases of the lymphoid tissue, including Hodgkin's disease, a neoplastic disease of lymphoid tissue. Persons with Hodgkin's disease have impaired T-cell function and what is called *anergy*, or the failure to respond to a variety of skin antigens, including the tuberculin test. In terms of the protective function of the T cells, persons with Hodgkin's disease have a well-defined predisposition to develop tuberculosis, fungal and yeast infections, and herpes zoster varicella.

Combined antibody (B cell) and cellular (T cell) immunodeficiency

A complete lack of both humoral and cellular immunity causes early susceptibility to infection. The deficiency state can be sex-linked or autosomal recessive. Infants with the disorder seldom survive beyond the first year of life because of poor resistance to infection. A histocompatible bone-marrow transplant is the treatment of choice.

There are several other combined forms of humoral and cellular immunodeficiency. These conditions are accompanied by other abnormalities. One of these is the Wiskott–Aldrich syndrome which is accompanied by thrombocytopenia and eczema. Another is ataxia-telangiectasia in which loss of muscle coordination and blood vessel dilatation are combined with deficits in IgA production and T lymphocytes.

In summary, immunodeficiency states describe an absolute or relative lack of immune cells or other factors, such as complement, which are involved in the immune response. Most immune deficiencies are characterized by impaired resistance to infection. The immune defect can be of a hereditary nature or can be an acquired defect and can represent an absolute or a relative lack of one or more immune cells.

Allergy and Hypersensitivity

Allergy and hypersensitivity are immune responses in which the antigen is an environmental agent, food, or drug that is not intrinsically harmful. Gell and Coombs[4] have divided allergic responses into four categories:

I. *Type I* is an IgE-mediated response that causes release of histamine and slow-reacting substance of anaphylaxis (SRS–A) from mast cells. The types of reactions seen in this category are anaphylaxis and atopic allergies such as hay fever, asthma, and urticaria (hives).
II. *Type II* is an IgG- or IgM-mediated response. It is a cytotoxic reaction which most often involves complement, but this is not a requirement. Certain drug reactions fit into this category.
III. *Type III* is an IgG- or IgM-mediated antigen–antibody complex reaction. Serum sickness is a type III response.
IV. *Type IV* is a cell-mediated response in which sensitized T lymphocytes react with an antigen to cause inflammation. Contact dermatitis is a type IV response as is the tuberculin reaction.

Type I allergic responses

The term atopy is used to describe allergic conditions that have a familial predisposition. About one out of every ten persons in the United States suffers from symptomatic allergies of this type.

Atopic immune responses result from immunoglobulin IgE activity. These immunoglobulins are sometimes called *reagins*. Reagins function only when they are attached to mast cells or basophils. Atopic reactions include anaphylaxis, seasonal pollen allergy (hay fever), allergic rhinitis, and atopic skin reactions. This discussion focuses on general concepts of atopy and seasonal pollen allergy, allergic rhinitis, and atopic skin reactions. Anaphylactic shock is discussed in Chapter 13 and bronchial asthma, in Chapter 19.

Mast cells (tissue cells) and basophils (blood cells) have granules that contain mediators involved in allergic reactions. In predisposed individuals, allergen stimulation causes IgE to bind to mast cells. On subsequent exposure, the allergen binds to the

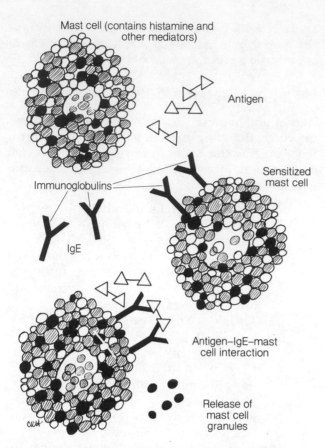

Mast cell (contains histamine and other mediators)

Antigen

Immunoglobulins

IgE

Sensitized mast cell

Antigen–IgE–mast cell interaction

Release of mast cell granules

Figure 5–6. Diagram of Type I immune response that involves an allergen (antigen), immunoglobulin (IgE) and mast cell. Exposure to the allergen causes sensitization of the mast cell with subsequent binding of the allergen which causes release of mast cell granules containing inflammatory mediators such as histamine and SRS-A.

IgE on the sensitized mast cells and this results in a series of reactions which culminate in the release of histamine and vasoactive substances from the mast cell (Fig. 5-6). There are four known mediators that are released from mast cells during an allergen IgE–mediated response: (1) *histamine*, which causes increased vascular permeability; (2) *eosinophil chemotactic factor*, which attracts eosinophils; (3) *slow-reacting substance of anaphylaxis (SRS–A)*, which causes constriction of smooth muscle, such as bronchiole smooth muscle; and (4) *platelet-activating factor*, which causes platelet aggregation and lysis.

Seasonal pollen allergy and allergic rhinitis. Seasonal pollen allergy (hay fever) is associated with sneezing, itching, and watery drainage from the eyes and nose. The conjunctiva is usually reddened and swollen and there is often an accompanying irritation and itching of the pharynx and outer ear canal. The nasal mucosa is usually pale and boggy. Nasal polyps are grapelike cystic masses that are commonly associated with allergic rhinitis. Microscopic examination of a properly stained smear of nasal secretions usually demonstrates a large number of eosinophils, whereas neutrophils predominate in infectious rhinitis.

A person with hay fever may be allergic to one or more inhalants. Common inhalants that cause hay fever are pollens from ragweed, trees, grasses, weeds, and fungal spores. There is usually a season within each geographic location in the United States during which the common trees, grasses, and weeds pollinate. It is during these seasonal periods that persons with specific allergies are expected to have symptoms. In the midwest, for example, ragweed season begins about August 15 and continues until after the first frost. Allergic rhinitis is usually a more perennial problem, caused by allergens such as house dust, animal danders, feathers, and fungal spores that are present the year around.

Diagnosis of seasonal pollen allergy and allergic rhinitis usually requires a careful history of food habits, exposure to inhalants, use of cosmetics and toiletries, presence of household pets, seasonal pattern of symptoms, and so forth. Skin tests provide a means for identifying the specific allergies. This is done by scratch or intradermal testing in which a small amount of a dilute solution of the antigen is applied to the skin; the area is then observed for edema and redness.

Treatment of hay fever and allergic rhinitis consists of avoiding the allergen when possible, treating the symptoms, and desensitization for the antigen. When an individual responds to a single allergen, such as the feathers in a bed pillow, it is often possible to eliminate the allergen. Antihistamine drugs usually provide symptomatic relief at the onset of the season, but their effectiveness often wanes as the season continues. Nasal congestants of the sympathomimetic type are effective by themselves or with antihistamines. The anti-inflammatory steroid drugs are usually reserved for severe hay fever that cannot be controlled by other methods. Desensitization involves frequent (usually weekly) injections of the offending antigen(s). The antigens, which are given in increasing doses, stimulate production of high levels of IgG, which acts as a blocking antibody by combining with the antigen before it can combine with the cell-bound IgE antibodies.

Type II cytotoxic reactions

In type II reactions IgM or IgG immunoglobulins react with cell-surface antigens and produce direct damage to the cell surface. This reaction may involve complement, but complement is not essential for the reaction. The cytotoxic reactions include transfusion reactions, hemolytic disease of the newborn, autoimmune hemolytic anemia, and certain drug reactions in which antibodies are formed to react with the drug that is complexed to the red-cell antigens.

Type III immune complex reactions

Type III reactions involve the complement-activating IgG and IgM immunoglobulins. This type of reaction is characterized by the formation of an immune complex. These complexes become attached to walls of blood vessels where they cause tissue damage by activating the complement system. Two of the more common immune complex disorders are serum sickness and the Arthus reaction.

Serum sickness develops in about 50% of persons receiving bovine or horse antitoxin against tetanus, gas gangrene, and other infections.[5] Fortunately, antitoxin therapy is infrequently used today since most individuals have been actively immunized for tetanus and because of the availability of human antisera. At present the most common cause of serum sickness is an adverse reaction to drugs such as penicillin. The symptoms of serum sickness usually appear at about 7 to 10 days following exposure to the offending antigen. The signs and symptoms that occur at this time include urticaria, patchy or generalized rash, extensive edema (usually of the face, neck, and joints), and fever. In previously sensitized individuals, severe and even fatal forms of serum sickness may occur either immediately, or within several days, after the sensitizing drug or serum is administered.

The *Arthus reaction* is a cutaneous reaction to the immune complex. It consists of vasculitis and tissue necrosis at the site of intracutaneous injection of an antigen to which there is a high level of circulating antibodies. The reaction causes erythema and swelling, which begins within several hours, and progresses to form a central area of cellular necrosis. Usually the area dries and heals within a week.

Type IV cell-mediated hypersensitivity

Cell-mediated hypersensitivity reactions involve T lymphocytes that have been sensitized to locally deposited antigens. The reaction is mediated by release of lymphokines, direct cytotoxicity, or both. Cell-mediated immunity is also called delayed hypersensitivity as compared with immediate hypersensitivity which is caused by immunoglobulins such as IgE. Two of the more common types of cell-mediated immunity are the tuberculin test and contact dermatitis.

The *tuberculin test*, in which a purified component of the tubercle bacillus is injected intrader-mally, is a good example of a delayed type of hypersensitivity reaction. In a previously sensitized individual, there is redness and swelling at the site of injection as the sensitized T-type lymphocytes interact with the tuberculin antigen. The reaction usually develops gradually over a period of 48 to 72 hours. As a point of clarification, it is important to recognize that the tuberculin test merely indicates that an individual has been sensitized to the tuberculosis bacillus through a previous exposure—it does not mean that the person has the disease.

Contact dermatitis is an acute or chronic dermatitis that results from direct contact with different chemical agents or other irritants, such as cosmetics, hair dyes, metals, and drugs applied to the skin. Two of the best known types of contact dermatitis are due to poison ivy and poison oak. When the sap from these plants comes in contact with the skin, neoantigens are formed, and sensitization develops to these new antigens. Contact dermatitis lesions usually consist of erythematous macules, papules, and vesicles (blisters). The affected area often becomes swollen and warm, with exudation, crusting, and development of a secondary infection. The location of the lesions often provides a clue as to the nature of the antigen causing the disorder.

Transplant Rejection

In transplant rejection the body recognizes the histocompatibility (HLA) antigens of the donor as foreign. In organ transplantation (*e.g.*, kidney transplant) immunosuppressive therapy is used to lessen the chance of rejection. Rejection usually involves both cell-mediated and humoral immunity and is a complex process. There are three basic patterns of transplant rejection: hyperacute, acute, and chronic.

A hyperacute response occurs almost immediately following the transplant; in kidney transplants, it can often be noted at the time of surgery. As soon as blood flow from the recipient to the donor kidney has been established, the kidney, instead of becoming pink and viable-looking, becomes cyanotic, mottled, and flaccid in appearance. Sometimes the onset of the reaction is not so sudden, but develops over a period of hours or several days. The hyperacute transplant rejection is caused by the presence of existing recipient antibodies to the graft that act at the level of the vascular epithelium to incite an Arthus type of reaction. These antibodies have usually developed in response to previous blood transfusions, pregnancies in which the mother develops antibodies that have been inherited from the father, or from infections with HLA cross-reacting bacteria or viruses.

Acute rejection is seen in the first months following transplant. In the patient with a kidney transplant, acute rejection is evidenced by signs of renal failure. Acute rejection often involves both humoral and cell-mediated immune responses.

Chronic rejection occurs over a period of months following transplant and is largely caused by cell-mediated immune responses. In renal transplant patients this rejection pattern causes a gradual rise in serum creatinine over a period of four to six months.[6]

In summary, hypersensitivity and allergic reactions are immune responses in which the antigen is an environmental agent, food, or drug usually considered harmless. There are four basic types of hypersensitivity responses: (1) a type I response that is mediated by the IgE immunoglobulins and includes anaphylactic shock, hay fever, and bronchial asthma; (2) type II cytotoxic reactions that are caused by IgG- or IgM-activated complement and include hemolytic responses due to blood transfusion reactions; (3) type III hypersensitivity reactions in which IgG or IgM reacts with an antigen to form an immune complex that causes local tissue injury; and (4) type IV cell-mediated responses in which sensitized T lymphocytes react with an antigen to cause inflammation and tissue injury.

Autoimmune Disease

Inherent in the normal immune response is the ability of the immune system to recognize body cells as self and to distinguish them from nonself. There is a normal immunologic tolerance that prevents damage to body tissues by the immune response. In autoimmune disease, there is development of self-antigens or abnormal immune cells that incite the immune response. Autoimmunity can involve abnormal or excessive activity of T cells, B cells, or the complement system.

Probable mechanisms of autoimmune disease

There are at least five probable mechanisms to explain the development of autoimmune disease. The *first* is based on the hidden antigen theory in which it is postulated that the contact of developing lymphocyte clones, with their respective antigens during fetal or early postfetal life, leads to destruction of the corresponding clones. It is also possible that circulating self-antigens, which are present throughout life, continually destroy their corresponding clones of lymphocytes before they can develop into immunocompetent cells. If this is true, autoimmune disease can develop if cells that have been hidden from the immune system during lym-

phocyte development were released. For example, trauma to the testes, with release of sperm into the tissues and circulation, has resulted in the development of sperm antibodies.[7] *Secondly*, it is possible that body cells or tissues are *altered* by chemical, physical, or biologic means so that they become self-antigens. It has been suggested that certain drugs can combine with body cells, converting them into autoantigens. Autoimmune anemia associated with such drugs as the antihypertensive medication alpha-methyldopa may result from the drug's effect on the red-cell surface.[8] A *third* potential is that similarities in exogenous antigens and self-antigens exist, and allow for *cross reactions* to occur. For example, evidence suggests that in rheumatic fever, the antibody formed to the streptococcus cross-reacts with tissues found in the heart. *Fourth*, it is possible that *mutations* or alterations in function of the immune cells develop and that these lead to inappropriate immune responses. For example, loss of T-cell suppressor function or B-cell activity and production of immunoglobulins to self-antigens has been suggested as contributing to autoimmune diseases such as systemic lupus erythematosus. A *fifth* possibility exists in that inherited immune genes which are linked to the *histocompatibility antigens* may predispose to altered immune responses and rejection of one's own tissues.

Autoimmune diseases can affect almost any cell or tissue in the body. There are known autoimmune disorders of blood cells and various body tissues, and disorders that affect multiple organs and systems. Table 5-7 describes some of the probable autoimmune diseases. Lupus erythematosus and rheumatoid arthritis are presented in this chapter as examples of autoimmune diseases. A discussion of many of the other autoimmune disorders is included in other sections of the book.

Systemic lupus erythematosus

Systemic lupus erythematosus (SLE) is a chronic autoimmune disease that affects multiple body systems. Recent studies indicate that the prevalence of the disease is about 1 in 2000.[9] The disease is seen most frequently in the 20- to 40-year-old age group, with about 85% of the affected persons being women. Blacks are affected more frequently than whites. There is a strong familial predisposition for development of the disease.

A lupus-like reaction that is indistinguishable both clinically and in the laboratory from spontaneously occurring SLE can also develop from the continual use of a number of drugs, especially the antihypertensive drug hydralazine and the anti-

Table 5-7 Probable Autoimmune Diseases

Disorder	Probable Antigens
Systemic	
Systemic lupus erythematosus	Numerous nuclear and cellular components
Rheumatoid arthritis	IgG
Dermatomyositis	Nuclear antigens, myosin (?)
Scleroderma	Nuclear antigens, IgG
Sjögren's syndrome	Salivary gland, thyroid, nuclear antigens, IgG
Mixed connective-tissue disease	Ribonucleoprotein
Blood	
Autoimmune hemolytic anemia	Erythrocyte antigens
Idiopathic thrombocytopenic purpura	Platelet surface antigens
Neutropenia and lymphopenia	Surface antigens
Other Organs	
Hashimoto's thyroiditis	Thyroglobulin
Thyrotoxicosis	Cell surface TSH receptors
Goodpasture's syndrome	Kidney and lung basement membranes
Pernicious anemia	Parietal cell antigens, intrinsic factor
Myasthenia gravis	Acetylcholine receptors, muscle
Primary biliary cirrhosis	Mitochondria, bile duct cells
Chronic active hepatitis	Liver cells, virally infected
Ulcerative colitis	Colonic mucosal cells
Autoimmune adrenalitis	Adrenal cells
Juvenile autoimmune diabetes	Islet-cell antigens
Premature gonadal failure	Cells of the ovary and testes
Sympathetic ophthalmia	Uvea
Temporal arteritis	Blood-vessel antigens
Acute idiopathic polyneuritis	Peripheral nerve myelin
Insulin-resistant diabetes	Insulin receptors

(From Robbins SL, Cotran RS: Pathologic Basis of Disease, p 293. Philadelphia, WB Saunders, 1979)

arrhythmic drug procainamide. Drug-induced reactions usually disappear once the drug has been discontinued.

One of the first cellular changes to develop in SLE of immunological origin is the presence of LE cells in the blood. The LE cells are neutrophils that contain a large LE body which has been engulfed. This LE body originates from the nucleus of certain white blood cells that have undergone nuclear changes and have been stripped of their cytoplasm by other phagocytic leukocytes. The LE factor responsible for this reaction has been identified as an anti-deoxyribonucleoprotein (anti-DNA) antibody of the IgG type.[10] The relationship between the LE factor found in the serum and the development of the body changes that occur with SLE is still obscure, particularly because the LE cells are found in about only 75% to 80% of persons with SLE, and in about 15% of persons with other collagen diseases such as rheumatoid arthritis and scleroderma.[11]

The disease affects many organs and body systems, including the skin, joints, kidney, and serosal surfaces. Its course may vary from a mild episodic disorder to a rapidly fatal illness.

The skin lesions include the classic "butterfly" rash which extends over the nose and cheeks—the sign of the red wolf for which the disease is named. There is extreme sensitivity to sunlight, and the rash appears in areas of the body that are exposed to sunlight. Dependent upon the course of the disease, the rash may resolve without problems or it may progress to form scars, hypo- or hyperpigmentation, or discoid lesions. A polyarthritis occurs in about 90% of persons with SLE; it can affect any of the joints and is often the first manifestation of the disease. The arthritis seldom causes deformities, and erosive lesions usually are not observed on x-ray films. Involvement of the serous cavities can lead to pleural and pericardial effusion and pleurisy. Renal involvement is a frequent and serious complication of SLE. The most severe type of renal lesion observed in SLE is proliferative glomerulonephritis which may be associated with nephrosis and renal failure. It is probably due to immune-complex deposition in the glomerular basement membrane. Among the other manifestations of SLE are neurological disorders such as severe depression, psychosis, and convulsions. There may also be ocular disturbances, including conjunctivitis. The disease is often called the great imitator because it affects so many body systems.

Rheumatoid arthritis

Rheumatoid arthritis is a chronic systemic inflammatory disease of connective tissue. Although it may involve the skin, voluntary muscle, heart, blood vessels, and connective tissue of other organs, the outstanding characteristic of the disease is the progressive disability that it produces. An estimated 5 million persons in the United States have rheumatoid arthritis.[12] Its incidence is higher in women than in men; and, although it affects persons in all age groups, the highest frequency of occurrence is in the fourth and fifth decades.

Although the cause of rheumatoid arthritis remains somewhat a mystery, there is sufficient evidence that immunological events play an important role. Virtually all persons with the disease have the *rheumatoid factor (RF)* in their serum. The rheumatoid factor is considered to be an antibody to an autologous (self-produced) immunoglobulin (IgG). Although most RF reacts exclusively with IgG, some RF reacts with IgA, IgE, or IgD. The question why the body would begin to produce antibodies against its own IgG cannot be answered as yet. It is possible that an infectious agent, such as a virus, could alter the immunoglobulin so that it would be recognized as foreign. Another possibility is that genetic predisposition plays a role in the genesis of the abnormal response. A large number of persons with rheumatoid arthritis have been found to have histocompatibility antigens in the HLA-DRw4 region.[13]

Rheumatoid factor has been found not only in the serum, but also in the synovial fluid and synovial membrane of affected persons. In fact, much of the RF seems to be produced by lymphocytes in the inflammatory infiltrate of the synovial tissue.[14] To partially explain the destructive changes that occur in rheumatoid arthritis, it has been suggested that the RF reacts with the antigenic IgG (or other type of antibody) to form immune complexes. This, in turn, activates the complement system which initiates the inflammatory reaction. Polymorphonuclear leukocytes, monocytes, and lymphocytes are attracted to the area by chemotaxis. These cells phagocytize the immune complexes and in the process release lysosomes, which have the capability of causing destructive changes in the joint cartilage, into the synovial fluid. The inflammatory response that follows attracts additional lymphocytes and plasma cells, setting into motion a chain of events that perpetuate the condition. Much prostaglandin E_1 has been found in the synovia of the inflamed joints, suggesting that this substance might be a mediator of the inflammatory response. This is of particular interest, inasmuch as aspirin—one of the drugs effective in the treatment of rheumatoid arthritis—is a prostaglandin inhibitor.

Pathologic changes. It is easier to understand the pathologic changes that occur in rheumatoid arthritis within the context of knowledge of normal joint structure. Most joints are freely movable or synovial joints, having synovial fluid in the cavities between two bones. Synovial fluid is secreted by the synovial membrane lining the joint cavity. The fluid is of the consistency of egg white. It serves as a lubricant for joint movement. The articular cartilage found at the ends of joints cushions the ends of the bones. The strong fibrous tissue capsule, attached to both bones, surrounds the joint and holds the bones in place. In the knee and other joints that require additional support, there are ligaments within the joint.

Early on, there are inflammatory changes of the synovial membrane. The synovial cells become hypertrophied and the subsynovial tissue undergoes a reactive hyperplasia. In the process, the synovial lining is replaced by an edematous and painful mass.[15] In larger joints, such as the knee, this mass may become as much as an inch thick.[16] In time, the inflammatory process erodes into the articular cartilage and extends to the joint capsule and surrounding ligaments, weakening the joint support and contributing to the dysfunction that is typical of the disease. With destruction of the articular cartilage, the bone is left unprotected—naked. In the late stages, there may be fibrous adhesions and ankylosis (fusion of the joint).

The *manifestations* of rheumatoid arthritis are often insidious in onset and are characterized by complaints of fatigue, malaise, and low-grade fever, before there is evidence of joint involvement. Joint involvement usually consists of symmetrical joint swelling with associated stiffness, pain, tenderness, and warmth. Characteristically, the *pain* and *stiffness* are worse in the *morning* and subside during the day with moderate joint use. Multiple joints are usually affected, particularly the small joints of the hands and feet, wrists, ankles, and knees. The overlying skin is often shiny, red, and atrophic. Muscle changes are common. Atrophy may become evident within weeks of onset, and contributes to the deformities that arise. In the late stages, joint deformities and contractures are seen.

One specific manifestation of rheumatoid arthritis is rheumatoid nodules, the granulomatous lesions that develop around small blood vessels. The nodules are not tender. They vary in diameter from 2 to 3 mm to 2 to 3 cm. Typically, they are found over pressure points such as the extensor surfaces of the ulna and, less commonly, in structures such as the sclera of the eye, the lungs, the spleen, and the septal, valvular, or pericardial structures of the heart. In many instances a nodule biopsy confirms the diagnosis.

The progression of the disease is variable. Ten to twenty percent of patients have a complete remission. After 10 to 15 years over 50% remain fully employed, and only 10% are totally incapacitated.[17] Features associated with an unfavorable outcome are (1) onset before age 30, (2) sustained symmetrical polyarthritis of over 1 year's duration, (3) subcutaneous nodules and extra-articular manifestations, and (4) sustained high RF titers.[17]

The *diagnosis* is usually based on history, physical findings, and laboratory tests which include a test for rheumatoid factor. The criteria established by a subcommittee of the American Rheumatism Association are frequently followed to establish the diagnosis (Table 5-8).[18] At least seven of the criteria must be positive to make a definite diagnosis, three for probable rheumatoid arthritis, and two for possible rheumatoid arthritis. Some of the criteria require minimum periods of observation by a physician.

Table 5-8   Abridged Diagnostic Criteria for Rheumatoid Arthritis*

A. *Classical Rheumatoid Arthritis*
This diagnosis requires seven of the following criteria. In criteria 1 through 5 the joint signs or symptoms must be continuous for at least six weeks. (Any one of the features listed under "Exclusions" will exclude a patient from this and all other categories.)
  1. Morning stiffness.
  2. Pain on motion or tenderness in at least one joint (observed by a physician).
  3. Swelling (soft tissue thickening or fluid, not bony overgrowth alone) in at least one joint (observed by a physician).
  4. Swelling (observed by a physician) of at least one other joint (any interval free of joint symptoms between the two joint involvements may not be more than 3 months).
  5. Symmetrical joint swelling (observed by a physician) with simultaneous involvement of the same joint on both sides of the body (bilateral involvement of proximal interphalangeal, metacarpophalangeal, or metatarsophalangeal joints is acceptable without absolute symmetry). Terminal phalangeal joint involvement will not satisfy this criterion.
  6. Subcutaneous nodules (observed by a physician) over bony prominences, on extensor surfaces or in juxta-articular regions.
  7. Roentgenographic changes typical of rheumatoid arthritis (which must include at least bony decalcification localized to or most marked adjacent to the involved joints and not just degenerative changes). Degenerative changes do not exclude patients from any group classified as rheumatoid arthritis.
  8. Positive agglutination test—demonstration of the "rheumatoid factor" by any method which, in two laboratories, has been positive in not over 5% of normal controls—or positive streptococcal agglutination test. [The latter is now obsolete.]

  9. Poor mucin precipitate from synovial fluid (with shreds and cloudy solution).
  10. Characteristic histologic changes in synovium with three or more of the following: marked villous hypertrophy; proliferation of superficial synovial cells often with palisading; marked infiltration of chronic inflammatory cells (lymphocytes or plasma cells predominating) with tendency to form "lymphoid nodules"; deposition of compact fibrin either on surface or interstitially; foci of necrosis.
  11. Characteristic histologic changes in nodules showing granulomatous foci with central zones of cell necrosis, surrounded by a palisade of proliferated macrophages, and peripheral fibrosis and chronic inflammatory cell infiltration, predominantly perivascular.

B. *Definite Rheumatoid Arthritis*
This diagnosis requires five of the above criteria. In criteria 1 through 5 the joint signs or symptoms must be continuous for at least six weeks.

C. *Probable Rheumatoid Arthritis*
This diagnosis requires three of the above criteria. In at least one of criteria 1 through 5 the joint signs or symptoms must be continuous for at least six weeks.

D. *Possible Rheumatoid Arthritis*
This diagnosis requires two of the following criteria and total duration of joint symptoms must be at least three weeks.
  1. Morning stiffness.
  2. Tenderness or pain on motion (observed by a physician) with history of recurrence or persistence for three weeks.
  3. History or observation of joint swelling.
  4. Subcutaneous nodules (observed by a physician).
  5. Elevated sedimentation rate or C-reactive protein.
  6. Iritis [of dubious value as a criterion except in the case of juvenile rheumatoid arthritis.]

(*From *The Primer on the Rheumatic Diseases*, 1973, prepared by the American Rheumatism Association. Used with the permission of the Arthritis Foundation.)

Some 20 factors, such as the butterfly rash of systemic lupus erythematosus, clinical rheumatic fever, and clinical gouty arthritis, rule out rheumatoid arthritis.[18]

The goals of *treatment* are designed to minimize pain and stiffness, suppress the progress of the disease, and preserve joint function as far as possible. Planned rest periods and range-of-motion and muscle-strengthening exercises are prescribed to preserve function. Usually complete inactivity is discouraged. Light-weight splints may be prescribed for immobilization, to maintain correct joint position and relieve pain, particularly at night. Aspirin is the mainstay of medication. During the active stage of the disease it is given daily, rather than as needed for pain relief, the usual dose being 600 to 900 mg four times a day. This regimen not only relieves pain but reduces inflammation as well. Aspirin and nonsteroidal anti-inflammatory drugs are believed to exert their action by inhibiting production of prostaglandins. Since the analgesic dose of aspirin is often less than the anti-inflammatory dose, persons with rheumatoid arthritis are often tempted to take less than the prescribed anti-inflammatory dose. Gastrointestinal symptoms, which may arise in some patients, are usually remedied by taking the medication with food, milk, or antacids. Enteric-coated tablets are also available. Other nonsteroidal drugs including ibuprofen, indomethacin, fenoprofen, sulindac, tolectin, and naprosyn may be substituted for aspirin by those who experience adverse effects from aspirin or those whose pain and inflammation are not controlled by aspirin. Penicillamine, gold salts, antimalarial drugs, and immunosuppressive drugs may be prescribed, also. These drugs are believed to induce a remission. The corticosteroids do relieve the inflammation and associated symptoms but are limited in use because of the frequent side-effects.

Felty's syndrome. Felty's syndrome is a variant of rheumatoid arthritis. It is characterized by splenomegaly and associated hematologic disorders. Ulcers of the leg are a frequent finding.

Juvenile rheumatoid arthritis. Juvenile rheumatoid arthritis, sometimes called Still's disease, occurs in children under 16 years of age with a peak incidence between 1 and 3 years of age. Girls are affected more frequently than boys. It is thought that the disease may represent a different group of rheumatic disorders from rheumatoid arthritis. Usually it is marked by an acute febrile onset and RF is not present. Generalized lymph node involvement and hepatomegaly are common. This form of rheumatoid arthritis is more unpredictable than the adult form. In some cases only one joint or only a few joints are affected, whereas in others—particularly those with an acute febrile onset—multiple joint deformities develop.

In summary, autoimmune disease represents a disordered immune response in which the body "recognizes" its own tissues as foreign. Autoimmune disorders can involve the T cells, B cells, or the complement system and can affect any of the body cells and tissues. Among the theories that have been used to explain the origin of autoimmunity are the (1) hidden antigen theory which suggests that autoimmunity develops due to release of substances that were sequestered from the immune system during the fetal or early postfetal period when the developing lymphocyte clones for autoantigens were being destroyed by their corresponding antigens, (2) development of an altered body antigen that comes about by chemical, physical, or biologic means, (3) occurrence of a cross reaction in which an exogenous antigen and a body tissue or cell type share antigenic properties, (4) establishment of a mutation of immune cells which leads to an inappropriate immune response, and (5) influence of the HLA antigens in rejection of a person's own tissues.

:Neoplasms of Immune Cells or Related Structures

There are a number of malignant neoplasms that affect immune cells or related structures. Two of these malignancies, multiple myeloma and Hodgkin's disease, will be discussed in this section.

Multiple myeloma

Multiple myeloma is the uncontrolled proliferation of an abnormal clone of plasma cells, usually of the IgG or IgA type. Approximately 8800 persons in the United States develop multiple myeloma each year and of these about 6100 die of the disease annually. Most cases of multiple myeloma occur in persons between the ages of 65 and 79.[19]

In multiple myeloma, plasma cells that are seldom found in healthy bone marrow proliferate and erode into the hard bone, predisposing to pathologic fractures and hypercalcemia due to bone dissolution. Bone pain, concentrated in the back, is often one of the first symptoms present in this form of cancer. Bone destruction also impairs the production of erythrocytes and leukocytes and predisposes to anemia and recurrent infections. There is often weight loss and a feeling of weakness. In some forms of the disease, synthesis of light and dark chains for the immunoglobulins is unbalanced and there is excess production of the light chains; proteinuria develops as these chains are excreted in the urine. These chains are called *Bence Jones proteins*. The most effective treatment for multiple myeloma is chemotherapy.

Hodgkin's disease

Hodgkin's disease is a malignant neoplasm of the lymphatic structures, named after an English physician, Thomas Hodgkin, who first described the disorder in 1832. More than 7000 persons develop Hodgkin's disease each year and about 2600 die from the disease annually.[20] The disease is seen with some frequency in the 15- to 34-year-old group, but is more common in persons over the age of 50. Recent reports suggest that, in contrast to many other types of cancer, the majority of cases of Hodgkin's disease can be cured with appropriate therapy if diagnosed in an early stage.[21]

Hodgkin's disease is characterized by painless and progressive enlargement of lymphoid tissue, usually a single node or a group of nodes. It is believed to originate within one area of the lymphatic system and if unchecked will spread throughout the lymphatic network. Splenic enlargement usually occurs early in the course. The proliferating cells may invade almost any area of the body and may produce a wide variety of symptoms. Low-grade fever, night sweats, unexplained weight loss, fatigue, pruritus, and anemia are indicative of disease spread. Pain in the involved lymph nodes may follow alcohol ingestion.[22] In advanced stages the liver, lungs, digestive tract, and occasionally the central nervous system may be affected.

As the disease progresses, the rapid proliferation of abnormal lymphocytes leads to an immunological defect, particularly in cell-mediated responses, rendering the person more susceptible to bacterial, viral, fungal, and protozoal infections.

Lymph-node biopsy is used to diagnose the disease. Characteristic is the presence of a distinctive giant tumor cell known as the *Reed–Sternberg (RS) cell*, which can be detected on microscopic examination.

The cause of Hodgkin's disease is unknown. There has been a long-standing suspicion that the disease might begin as an inflammatory reaction to an infectious agent.[23] This belief has been supported by epidemiologic data that include the clustering of the disease among family members and among students who have attended the same school. There also seems to be an association between the presence of the disease and a deficient immune state. As with other forms of cancer, it is likely that there is not a single agent that is responsible for the development of Hodgkin's disease.

Treatment focuses on careful staging and use of combined radiation and chemotherapy. Diagnostic surgery (laparotomy) followed by splenectomy may be done during the early stages.

In summary, there are a number of neoplasms that affect the lymphatic structures and immune system. One of these is multiple myeloma which results in the uncontrolled proliferation of plasma cells, usually a single clone of IgG or IgA immunoglobulins. Hodgkin's disease is one form of lymphoma. It usually begins in a single lymph node or group of lymph nodes and if unchecked invades the spleen and other lymphatic structures. At present the prognosis for persons with Hodgkin's disease is good with early detection and appropriate therapy.

:Study Guide

After you have studied this chapter, you should be able to meet the following objectives:

:: Differentiate among active, passive, and natural immunity.

:: State a general definition of *antigen*.

:: Define *histocompatibility antigen*.

:: Explain the origin of the T lymphocyte and the B lymphocyte.

:: Contrast humoral immunity and cell-mediated immunity.

:: Describe the role of interferons in immunity.

:: List the most important categories of immunodeficiency disorders, and state one example of each category.

:: Explain the pathogenesis of Type I allergic responses.

:: List the possible causes of serum sickness.

:: Define the Arthus reaction.

:: Explain the pathogenesis of Type IV cell-mediated hypersensitivity.

:: Describe the three patterns of transplant rejection.

:: Describe three or more postulated mechanisms underlying autoimmune disease.

:: Describe the pathologic changes that are characteristic of rheumatoid arthritis.

:: State the significance of the LE factor in systemic lupus erythematosus.

:: Describe the pathogenesis of multiple myeloma.

:: Describe the characteristics of Hodgkin's disease.

:References

1. Barrett JT: Textbook of Immunology, 3rd ed, p 3. St. Louis, CV Mosby, 1978
2. Barrett JT: Textbook of Immunology, 3rd ed, p 54. St. Louis, CV Mosby, 1978
3. Sodeman WA, Sodeman TM: Pathologic Physiology: Mechanisms of Disease, p 125. Philadelphia, WB Saunders, 1979
4. Gell RGH, Coombs RRA, Lachman PJ (eds): Clinical Aspects of Immunology, 3rd ed. Oxford, Blackwell Scientific Publications, 1975
5. Barrett JT: Textbook of Immunology, 3rd ed, p 344. St. Louis, CV Mosby, 1978
6. Robbins SL, Cotran RS: Pathologic Basis of Disease, 2nd ed, p 291. Philadelphia, WB Saunders, 1979
7. Hëckman A, Rumke P: Autoimmunity and isoimmunity against spermatozoa. In Miescher PA, Miller–Eberhard HJ (eds): Textbook of Immunopathology, Vol II, 2nd ed, p 947. New York, Grune & Stratton, 1976
8. Robbins SL, Cotran RS: Pathologic basis of disease, 2nd ed, p 295. Philadelphia, WB Saunders, 1979
9. Engleman EP, Shearn MA: Arthritis and allied rheumatic disorders. In Krupp, Marcus A, Chatton MJ (eds): Current Medical Diagnosis and Treatment, p 501. Los Altos, 1980
10. Barrett JT: Textbook of Immunology, 3rd ed, p 430. St. Louis, CV Mosby, 1978
11. Fye KA, Talal N: Rheumatic diseases. In Fundenberg HH et al: Basic and Clinical Immunology, 3rd ed, p 443. Los Altos, Lange Medical Publishers, 1980
12. Arthritis; Out of the Maze. Vol I, The Arthritis Plan. Report of the Congress of the United States. National Commission on Arthritis and Related Musculoskeletal Diseases. U.S. Department of Health, Education, and Welfare. Public Health Service. National Institute of Health. DHEW Publ No. (NIH) 70–1150
13. Stastny P: Association of B-cell alloantigen DRw4 with rheumatoid arthritis. N Engl J Med 298, No. 16:869, 1978
14. Williams RC: Immunopathology of rheumatoid arthritis. Hosp Pract 13, No. 2:58, 1978
15. Williams RC: Rheumatoid arthritis. Hosp Pract 14, No. 6:57, 1979
16. Robbins SL, Cotran RS: Pathologic Basis of Disease, 2nd ed, p 1517. Philadelphia, WB Saunders, 1979
17. Christiansen CL: Diseases of the joints. In Beeson PB, McDermott W, Wyngaarden JB (eds): Cecil Textbook of Medicine, 15th ed, p 185. Philadelphia, WB Saunders, 1979
18. Arthritis Foundation: Primer on Rheumatic Diseases, 7th ed, p 137. National Office, 3400 Peachtree Road N.E., Atlanta, GA, 1973
19. American Cancer Society: Facts on Lymphomas and on Multiple Myelomas, p 13, 1979
20. American Cancer Society: Facts on Hodgkin's Disease, p 3, 1978
21. Rosenberg SA: The management of Hodgkin's disease. N Engl J Med, 299 No. 22:1246, 1978
22. Bolin RH, Auld M: Hodgkin's Disease. Am J Nurs, 74 No. 11:1982, 1974
23. Robbins SL, Cotran RS: Pathologic Basis of Disease, 2nd ed, p 777. Philadelphia, WB Saunders, 1979

:Suggested Readings

Benacerraf Baruj: Suppressor T cells and supressor factor. Hosp Pract 13, No. 4:65, 1978
Bobrove AM, Fuks Z, Strober S et al: Quantification of T and B lymphocytes and cellular immune function in Hodgkin's disease. Cancer 36, No. 1:169, 1975
Bridgewater SC, Voignier RR, Smith CS: Allergies in children: Recognition. Am J Nurs 78, No. 4:613, 1978
Dharan M: The immune system: Immunoglobulin abnormalities. Am J Nurs 76, No. 10:1626, 1976
Donley DL: The immune system: Nursing the patient who is immunosuppressed. Am J Nurs 76, No. 10:1619, 1976
Fruth R: Anaphylaxis and drug reactions: Guidelines for detection and care. Heart Lung 9, No. 4:662, 1980
Groenwald SL: Physiology of the immune system. Heart Lung 9, No. 4:645, 1980
Ishizaka K: Structure and biologic activity of immunoglobulin e. Hosp Pract 12, No. 1:57, 1977
Lind M: The immunologic assessment: A nursing focus. Heart Lung 9, No. 4:658, 1980
McAdams CW: Interferon the penicillin of the future? Am J Nurs 80:714, 1980
McLeod BC: Immunologic factors in reactions to blood transfusions. Heart Lung 9, No. 4:675, 1980
Nysather JO, Katz EE, Lenth JL: The immune system: Its development and functions. Am J Nurs 76, No. 10:1614, 1976
Rana AN, Luskin A: Immunosuppression, autoimmunity, and hypersensitivity. Heart Lung 9, No. 4:651, 1980
Sasazuki T, McDevitt HO: The association between genes in the major histocompatibility complex and disease susceptibility. Annu Rev Med 28:425, 1977
Shahinpour N: The patient with systemic lupus erythematosus: Prototype of autoimmunity. Heart Lung 9, No. 4:682, 1980
Starr MS, Weinstock M: Studies in pollen allergy. Int Arch Allergy Appl Immunol 38:514, 1970
Stiller CR, Russel AS, Dossetoer JB: Autoimmunity: Present concepts. Ann Intern Med 82, No. 3:405, 1975
Torbett MP, Ervin JC: The patient with systemic lupus erythematosus. Am J Nurs 77:1299, 1977
Unanue ER: The macrophage as a regulator of lymphocyte function. Hosp Pract 14, No. 11:61, 1979
Voignier RR, Bridgewater SC: Allergies in children: Testing and treating. Am J Nurs 78:617, 1978

6

Genetic and Developmental Defects

Genetic and congenital disorders are important at all levels of health care because they affect all age groups and can involve any of the body organs and tissues. Recent statistics indicate that an estimated 15 million Americans have birth defects of varying degrees. Eighty percent of birth defects are estimated to arise as the result of genetic disorders and the remaining 20% represent the effects of agents such as infection, drugs, and physical injury to the fetus. Major congenital defects are present in about 2% to 4% of all live births, and at least 40% of all infant mortality results from genetic factors.[1]

This chapter is designed to provide an overview of genetic and congenital defects and is divided into five parts: (1) patterns of inheritance, (2) disorders of genetic inheritance, (3) chromosomal disorders, (4) developmental defects, and (5) diagnosis and counseling. Specific genetic and congenital defects are integrated into appropriate chapters in the book.

:Patterns of Inheritance

Each individual represents a unique compilation of inherited traits from a long list of ancestors. Some of these traits are undoubtedly more desirable than others. For example, we all know families in which a particular desirable trait such as musical or mathematical talent is transmitted from parent to child. The transmissibility of hereditary information through succeeding generations has been recognized since ancient times, but only during the last half century have the mechanisms involved in this transmission become relatively clear.

The main feature of inheritance is predictability: given certain conditions, the likelihood of the occurrence or recurrence of a specific trait is remarkably predictable. The units of inheritance are the genes, and the pattern of single gene expression can be predicted using Mendel's laws, with some modification as the result of knowledge accumulated since 1865, the date of Mendel's publication.

Genes

The word "gene" is defined somewhat differently by the various scientific disciplines. There are the breeding genetic units, a cellular chromosomal or cytogenetic gene, a functional polypeptide gene, a nucleoprotein structural unit gene, and others. In all of these, the word *gene stands for the fundamental unit of hereditary information storage*. This information is stored in the structure of an extremely stable macromolecule within the nucleus of each cell. Because of this stable structure, the genetic information survives the many processes of gamete (ovum and sperm) formation, fertilization, and the many cell divisions involved in the formation of a new organism from the single-celled zygote that forms from the union of an ovum and a sperm.

The nuclei of all cells in an organism contain the same accumulation of genes derived from the gametes of the two parents. This means that liver cells contain the same genetic information as do skin cells and muscle cells. For this to be true, the molecular code must be duplicated prior to each succeeding cell division, or mitosis. Theoretically, although not yet achieved for the adult, any of the highly differentiated cells of an organism could be used to produce a complete genetically identical organism (clone). From this it becomes evident that each particular tissue uses only some of the information that is stored in the genetic code, while information required for the function of other types of tissues is repressed, although it is still present.

Gene structure

The stable molecule storing the information of the genes within the cell nucleus is *deoxyribonucleic acid (DNA)*. This very long molecule is composed of nucleotides arranged in a *double-stranded helix* (Fig.6-1). A *nucleotide*, in turn, consists of a nitrogenous base, a sugar, and one or more phosphate groups. Alternating groups of sugar and phosphate groups form the "backbone" of the molecule, with the bases protruding to the sides of each sugar molecule. The purine or pyrimidine bases of the DNA molecule are *adenine, thymine, guanine*, and *cytosine*. The spatial sequence of these four bases along the sugar-phosphate backbone make up the alphabet of the genetic code, and a sequence of *three bases* constitutes a fundamental *triplet code*. Thus, the sequence of bases on one strand of the DNA molecule contains areas in which triplet-code words serve to control the sequence of amino acids that are used in the synthesis of polypeptides within the cell. These triplet-code words are separated by "nonsense" code sequences. Some of the polypeptides produced within the cell are enzymes and others are structural proteins. Among the enzymes are some that are involved in the synthesis of the code-reading machinery of the cell. Other polypeptides can repress the use of parts of the code or suppress the formation of certain other polypeptides.

The DNA molecule is a double-stranded helix with precise pairing of the bases; adenine is paired with thymine, and guanine with cytosine. Of these two, only one of the strands of the DNA molecule is used in transcribing the information for the cell's polypeptide-building machinery. If the triplet-code sequence of one strand is meaningful, then the complementary code of the other strand will somehow not make sense and will therefore be ignored. Both strands are involved, however, in DNA duplication. Prior to cell division, the two strands of helix separate and a complementary molecule is organized next to each original strand. Thus two strands make four strands, with each strand joined to a new complementary strand. During cell division, the newly duplicated double helix molecules are separated and placed in each daughter cell by the mechanics of mitosis. As a result, each of the daughter cells again contains the meaningful strand and the complementary strand, joined in the form of a double helix. The very long DNA molecule is surrounded by a specific class of proteins called histones, and this makes up a chromosome.

Mutations

Rarely, accidental errors in duplication or destruction of parts of the genetic code occur. Such changes are called *mutations*. Many of these mutations are caused by environmental agents, chemicals, and radiation. If the duplicating cell line that contains such a change forms gametes, or germ cells, then the mutation can be transmitted to the offspring. Much more frequently, the affected cell line differentiates into one or more of the many tissues of the body and thus is not transmissible to the next generation. These are *somatic mutations* and result in genetic differences between the cells and tissues of the same organism, producing what is called a *genetic mosaic*. Occasionally, a person is born with one brown eye and one blue eye as a result of a somatic mutation. The change or loss of gene information is just as likely to affect the fundamental processes of cell function or organ differentiation. Such somatic mutations in the early embryonic period can result in embryonic death or congenital malformations. Somatic mutations are important causes of cancer and other tumors in which cell differentiation and growth get out of hand. Fishermen, farmers, and others who are excessively exposed to the ultraviolet radiation of sunlight have an increased risk of developing skin cancer due to potential radiation damage to the genetic structure of the skin-forming cells.

Mendel's Laws

At a particular part of the DNA molecule, the genetic code may be capable of controlling the production of an observable trait. Such a segment of the DNA molecule is called a *gene locus*. Alternative forms of

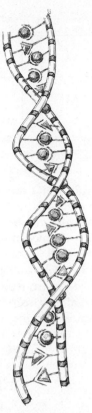

Figure 6–1. Schematic representation of a long, double-stranded DNA molecule which is a repeating arrangement of nucleotides. It is thought that from 500 to 1000 nucleotides make up a single gene and that there are over 1000 genes in a chromosome. (Chaffee EE, Lytle IM: Basic Physiology and Anatomy, 4th ed. Philadelphia, JB Lippincott, 1980)

the gene code are possible and each form may produce a different aspect of the trait. Alternative codes at one gene locus are called *alleles*. A cell contains two and only two alleles at each locus.

It was Mendel who, in 1865, discovered the basic pattern of inheritance by conducting carefully planned experiments with simple garden peas. From his experiments with wrinkled and round peas, Mendel proposed that inherited traits are transmitted from parents to offspring by means of independently inherited factors—now known as genes—and that these factors are transmitted as recessive and dominant traits. Mendel labeled dominant factors (his round peas) "A" and recessive (his wrinkled peas) "a." Geneticists continue to use capital letters to designate dominant traits and lower-case letters to identify recessive traits. The possible combinations that can occur with transmission of single-gene dominant and recessive traits can be described by constructing a figure using capital and lower-case letters (Fig. 6-2).

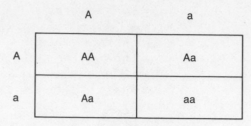

Figure 6–2. Possible combinations for dominant, A, and recessive, a, observable traits.

The observable traits are inherited from one's parents. During maturation, the germ cells (sperm and ovum) of both parents undergo meiosis, or reduction division, in which the number of chromosomes is divided in half (from 46 to 23). At this time, the two alleles from a gene locus separate so that each germ cell gets one allele from each pair. According to Mendel's laws, the alleles from the different gene loci segregate independently and then recombine in a random fashion in the zygote that is formed by the union of the two germ cells (Fig. 6-3). Individuals in

whom the two alleles of a given pair are the same (AA or aa) are called *homozygotes*. *Heterozygotes* have different (Aa) alleles at a gene locus.

A *recessive trait* is one that is expressed only in a homozygous pairing; a *dominant trait* is one that is expressed in either a homozygous or a heterozygous pairing. All persons with a dominant allele inherit that trait. A *carrier* is a person who is heterozygous for a recessive trait and does not manifest the trait. For example, if the genes for blond hair were determined to be recessive and those for brunet hair dominant, then only persons with a genotype with two alleles for blond hair would be blond, and all persons with either one or two brunet alleles would have dark hair.

Pedigree

A pedigree is a graphic method for portraying a family history of an inherited trait (Fig. 6-4). It is constructed from a carefully obtained family history, and is useful for tracing the pattern of inheritance for a particular trait.

Figure 6–3. Schematic diagram of the segregation of gene pairs during meiosis and the possible recombinations in the zygote. If *A* was a dominant mutant gene, then 50% of the offspring would present with the trait. If *a* represents a recessive mutant gene then only 25% of the offspring will be affected with the trait, 50% of the offspring will be carriers.

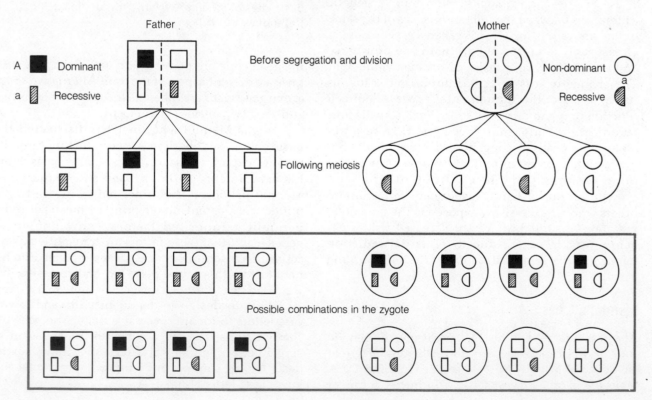

Patterns of Single-gene Inheritance

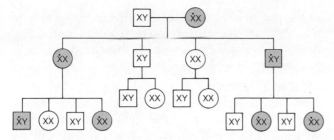

Figure 6–4.   Simple pedigree showing the inheritance of a dominant genetic trait.

Definitions

Genetics has its own set of definitions. The *genotype* of an individual is a term for the genetic information stored in the base sequence triplet code. The *phenotype* refers to the recognizable traits, physical or biochemical, that are associated with a specific genotype. There are many instances in which the genotype is not evident by available detection methods. Thus, more than one genotype may have the same phenotype. Some brown-eyed people are carriers of the code for blue eyes and other brown-eyed persons are not. Phenotypically, these two types of brown-eyed people are the same, but genotypically they are different.

When it comes to a genetic disorder, not all individuals with a mutant gene are affected to the same extent. *Penetrance* means the ability of a gene to express its function. Seventy-five percent penetrance means that only 75% of the individuals of a particular genotype will demonstrate a recognizable phenotype. *Expressivity* refers to the expression of the gene in the phenotype, which can range from mild to severe.

A locus is the location or site on a chromosome (i.e., along the DNA molecule) where an allele or group of alleles are located. When only a pair of alleles are involved in the transmission of information, the term *single-gene* is used. Single-gene traits follow the mendelian laws of inheritance. At present it appears that there are multiple alleles, or alternative codes, in about one-half of the genetic loci in humans, accounting for some of the dissimilar forms that occur with certain genetic disorders.

:Disorders of Genetic Inheritance

A mutant gene is inferred by the sudden appearance of a genotype in a demonstrably noncarrier pedigree. Genetic disorders represent changes (or mutations) in gene function or changes in chromosomal structure. A genetic disorder can involve a single gene trait or it can involve a polygenic trait. Polygenic traits are observable characteristics which result from the additive interactions of more than one, and sometimes many, gene loci. The shape of the nose, body height, native intelligence, and other characteristics, involve polygenic inheritance. Almost all of the hereditary traits that are of importance in most individuals result from the interaction between multiple, independently associated gene loci and the environment.

The expression of the effects of a genetic trait may be present at birth or may not become apparent until later in life. Huntington's chorea, for example, has its onset between 20 and 30 years of age. Some diseases tend to "run in families" and it is thought that the combined effects of a genetic predisposition and environmental factors influence the development of these diseases. This is true of some types of diabetes mellitus, hypertension, and cancer.

Every individual probably has 5 to 8 recessive genes that would cause defects if present in the homozygous state.[2] About 80 to 85% of these abnormal genes are from the pedigree and the remainder represent new mutations. Either autosomal genes (those located on the nonsex chromosomes) or those located on the sex chromosomes can be affected in single-gene disorders. At last count there were more than 2336 single-gene disorders—1218 autosomal

Table 6–1   Some Disorders of Mendelian or Single-Gene Inheritance

Autosomal Dominant

Achondroplasia (short-limb dwarfism)
Adult polycystic kidney disease
Huntington's chorea
Hypercholesteremia
Marfan's syndrome
Multiple neurofibromatosis (von Recklinghausen's disease)
Osteogenesis imperfecta
Spherocytosis
von Willebrand's disease (bleeding diathesis)

Autosomal Recessive

Color blindness
Cystic fibrosis
Glycogen storage diseases
Oculocutaneous albinism
Phenylketonuria (PKU)
Renal glycosuria
Sickle cell disease
Tay-Sachs disease
Wilson's disease

X-Linked Recessive

Bruton-type agammaglobulinemia
Classic hemophilia
Duchenne muscular dystrophy

dominant, 947 autosomal recessive and 171 X-linked disorders.[3] Table 6-1 lists some of the more common defects in each of these classifications.

Single-gene Disorders

Single-gene disorders involve dominant or recessive traits. They may involve a gene locus on an autosome (nonsex chromosome) or a sex chromosome. Disorders of the Y or male chromosome are extremely rare.

Autosomal dominant

In autosomal dominant disorders, an affected parent has a single mutant gene, which is transmitted to the offspring regardless of sex. The unaffected relatives

Figure 6–5.   Pattern of inheritance for an X-linked recessive trait. (From Department of Health, Education, and Welfare: What Are the Facts About Genetic Disease?, 1977)

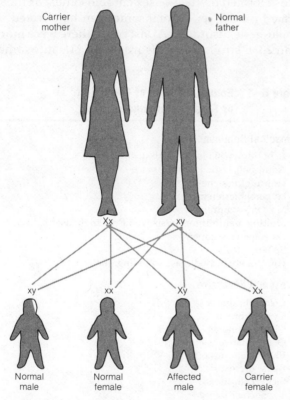

How X = Linked Inheritance Works

In the most common form, the female sex chromosome of an unaffected mother carries one faulty gene (X) and one normal one (x). The father has normal male x and y chromosome complement.

Carrier mother   Normal father

Xx   xy

xy   xx   Xy   Xx

Normal male   Normal female   Affected male   Carrier female

The odds for each *male* child are 50/50:
1. 50% risk of inheriting the faulty X and the disorder
2. 50% chance of inheriting normal x and y chromosomes

For each *female* child, the odds are:
1. 50% risk of inheriting one faulty X, to be a carrier like mother
2. 50% chance of inheriting no faulty gene

of the parent or siblings of the affected offspring do not transmit the disorder. The affected individual has a 50% chance of transmitting the disorder to each offspring (Fig. 6-4).

Autosomal recessive

Autosomal recessive disorders are manifested only when both members of the gene pair are mutant alleles. Both parents are usually unaffected, but are carriers for the defective gene. The disorder affects persons of both sexes. The recurrence risk in each pregnancy is 1 in 4 for an affected child, 2 in 4 for a carrier child, and 1 in 4 for a normal, homozygous child (Fig. 6-3).

X-linked recessive

Sex-linked inheritance is almost always associated with the X or female chromosome and is predominantly recessive. The common pattern of inheritance is seen in an unaffected mother who carries one normal and one mutant allele on the X chromosome. This means that she will have a 50% chance of transmitting the defect to her sons and that her female children will have a 50% chance of being carriers of the mutant gene (Fig. 6-5). When the affected male procreates, he will transmit the defect to all of his daughters who will then become carriers of the mutant gene. Since the genes of the Y chromosome are unaffected, the affected male will not transmit the defect to any of his sons and they will not be carriers or transmit the disorder to their children.

Manifestations of single-gene disorders

Many single-gene disorders result in inborn errors of metabolism. These biochemical defects involve the formation of abnormal structural proteins, abnormal biochemical mediators or enzymes, or abnormal diffusible or membrane-bound transport or receptor proteins.

Structural protein defects are usually manifested as autosomal dominant disorders. *Marfan's syndrome*, for example, is a disorder of the connective tissues which is manifested by changes in the skeleton, the eyes, and the cardiovascular system. Characteristics of the skeletal defects are a long, thin body, hyperextensive joints, arachnodactyly (spider fingers), and scoliosis. Defects of the eye include the upward displacement of the lens and the potential for retinal detachment. Involvement of connective tissue in the cardiovascular system may lead to mitral valve disease and a tendency for development of a dissecting aortic aneurysm. Abraham Lincoln's extremely long legs and the unequal lengths of his thumbs suggest that he may have been mildly affected by Marfan's syndrome. Both Abraham Lincoln and a distant male cousin who was diagnosed as having Marfan's syndrome are descendants of Mordecai Lincoln II. Although Mordecai almost certainly had the gene for Marfan's syndrome, he showed no signs of the disorder, probably because in him the gene had low expressivity.[4]

Primary enzyme defects are usually autosomal recessive. These enzyme defects may result in any of the following: (1) deficiency of a metabolic end-product; (2) production of harmful intermediates or toxic by-products of metabolism; or (3) accumulation of destructive substances within the cell. In *albinism*, the basic biochemical defect is the absence or nonfunctioning of the enzyme tyrosinase. This enzyme is necessary for the production of melanin, the pigment that gives skin its color. *Phenylketonuria (PKU)* is another genetically inherited primary enzyme defect. In this disorder, there is a deficiency of phenylalanine hydroxylase, the enzyme needed for conversion of phenylalanine to tyrosine, and as a result of this deficiency, toxic levels of phenylalanine accumulate in the blood. Like other inborn errors of metabolism, PKU is inherited as a recessive trait and is manifested only in the homozygote. It is possible to identify carriers of the trait by subjecting them to a phenylalanine test in which a large dose of phenylalanine is administered orally and the rate at which it disappears from the bloodstream is measured. PKU occurs once in approximately 10,000 births, and damage to the developing brain almost always results when the concentrations of phenylalanine and other metabolites persist in the blood. Presently, a screening test (the bacterial inhibition assay method of Guthrie) is widely used for detection of abnormal levels of serum phenylalanine in newborn infants. Infants with the disorder are treated with a special diet that restricts phenylalanine intake. Dietary treatment must be started early in neonatal life, because the untreated affected child may have evidence of arrested brain development by 4 months of age.[5] *Tay-Sachs disease* is caused by an accumulation of ganglioside GM_2 in body tissues due to an enzyme deficiency (hexosaminidase A), resulting in gangliosidosis. The disease is particularly prevalent among the Eastern European (Ashkenazi) Jews. Infants with Tay-Sachs appear normal at birth, but begin to manifest neurological signs at about 6 months of age. These neurologic manifestations eventually lead to muscle flaccidity, dementia, and finally death at about 2 to 3 years of age. Although there is no cure for the disease, analysis of the blood serum for a deficiency of hexosaminidase A allows for accurate identification of the genetic carriers for the disease.

Membrane associated transport defects can be either dominant or recessive. Hereditary *spherocytosis*, an autosomal dominant trait, is a form of hemolytic anemia which is caused by a defect in sodium transport in the red cell. *Renal glycosuria*, on the other hand, is an autosomal recessive trait that involves glucose transport in the renal tubules.

Polygenic Disorders

Polygenic disorders are conditions in which two or more genes or gene loci are influential in the expression of a gene trait. In some diseases, such as diabetes mellitus and essential hypertension, the genetic component is influenced by multiple environmental influences.

Polygenic traits

The exact number of genes contributing to polygenic traits is not known, and these traits do not follow the clear-cut pattern of inheritance as do single-gene disorders. Polygenic inheritance has been described as a threshold phenomenon, in which the parent's expression of a particular gene trait might be compared to the amount of water contained in a glass of a given capacity (Fig. 6-6).[6] Using this analogy, one might say that the expression of a genetic disorder occurs when the amount of the trait that is in the glass overflows.

Although polygenic traits cannot be predicted with the same amount of accuracy as the mendelian, single-gene mutations, there are characteristic patterns that exist. First, polygenic congenital malformations involve a single organ or tissue that is derived from the same embryologic developmental field. Second, the risk of recurrence in future pregnancies is for the same or a similar defect. This means that parents of a child with polygenic cleft palate defect have an increased risk of having another child with a cleft palate, but not with spina bifida. Thirdly, the increased risk (compared with the general population) among first-degree relatives of the affected person is 2 to 5%, and among second-degree relatives it is about one-half that amount.[7] Furthermore, the risk increases with increasing incidence of the defect among relatives. This means that the risk is greatly increased when a second child with the defect is born to a couple. The risk also increases with severity of the disorder and when the defect occurs in the sex not generally affected by the disorder. Some conditions which are thought to arise through polygenic inheritance include the following: allergies, anencephaly, cleft lip (palate), clubfoot, congenital dislocation of the hip, congeni-

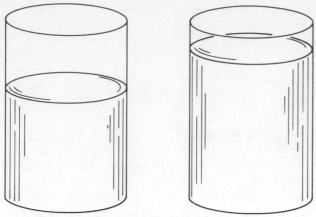

Both parents carry genes for polygenic trait

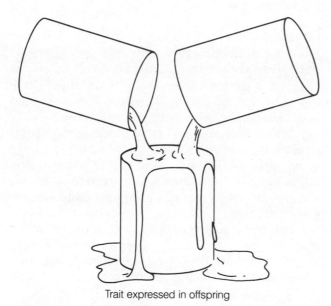

Trait expressed in offspring

Figure 6–6. Water glass analogy to explain polygenic inheritance. (Riccardi VM: The Genetic Approach to Human Disease. New York, Oxford University Press, 1977)

tal heart disease, diabetes mellitus, hydrocephalus, myelomeningocele, pyloric stenosis, and urinary tract malformation.

Chromosomal Disorders

There are 46 human chromosomes—22 pairs of autosomes and 1 pair of sex chromosomes. Each of the autosomes appears to be identical to its partner, but each pair is different in genetic content and appearance from the other pairs. The two sex chromosomes are labeled X and Y (Fig. 6-7). The X is the female chromosome and the Y is the male chromosome. All normal males have one Y and one X chro-

mosome, the Y coming from the father and the X from the mother. All normal females have two X chromosomes, one being received from each parent. It is believed that with two X chromosomes in the female only one is active in controlling the expression of genetic traits. Both X chromosomes are involved, however, in transmission to the offspring. In the female the active X chromosome is invisible, while the inactive X chromosome can be demonstrated by nuclear staining techniques as the *chromatin mass* or *Barr body*. Thus the "genetic sex" of a child can be determined by microscopic study of cell or tissue samples. The total number of X chromosomes is equal to the number of Barr bodies (inactive X chromosome) plus one (active X chromosome). For example, the cells of a normal female will have one Barr body and two X chromosomes. A male will have no Barr bodies. In the female, the decision whether the X chromosome derived from the mother or the X chromosome derived from the father is active is determined within a few days after conception and occurs randomly for each postmitotic cell line. This is called the Lyon principle (after Mary Lyon, the British geneticist who developed it).

Chromosome studies

Cytogenetics is the study of the structure and numerical characteristics of the cell's chromosomes. Chromosome studies can be done on any tissue or cell that will divide in culture. The lymphocytes from venous blood are frequently used for this purpose. Once the cultured cells have been fixed and spread on a slide, they are stained to demonstrate banding patterns so that they can be identified. The chromosomes are then photographed, and each chromosome is cut from the photograph and arranged according to the standard set by the 1971 Paris Chromosome Conference to form the *karyotype* (or chromosome picture) of the individual.[8] This arrangement is called an *idiogram*.

Mosaicism is the presence, in one individual, of two or more cell lines as the result of a chromosomal duplication accident. Sometimes mosaicism consists of an abnormal karyotype and a normal one, in which case the physical deformities caused by the abnormal cell line are usually less severe.

Chromosome defects

During the process of germ cell (sperm and ovum) formation, a special form of cell division called meiosis takes place. During this division, the *double set* of 22 autosomes and the 2 sex chromosomes (normal *diploid number*) become reduced to a *single set* (*haploid number*) in each gamete. In another form of cell division (mitosis) there is replication of the chromosomes so that each cell receives a full diploid number. At the time of conception, the haploid number in the ovum and sperm join and restore the diploid number of chromosomes.

There are essentially two types of accidental chromosomal abnormalities that can occur during meiosis—a change in number and a change in structure.

Alterations in chromosome number

A change in chromosome number is called *aneuploidy*. Among the causes of aneuploidy are failure of separation of the chromosomes during oogenesis or spermatogenesis. This can occur in either the autosomes or the sex chromosomes and is called *nondisjunction*. Nondisjunction gives rise to germ cells that have an even number of chromosomes (22 or 24). The products of conception that are formed from this even number of chromosomes will have an uneven number of chromosomes, either 45 or 47. *Monosomy* refers to the presence of only one member of a chromosome pair. The defects associated with monosomy of the autosomes are severe and usually cause abortion. Monosomy of the X chromosome (45, X/O), or Turner's syndrome, causes less severe defects. *Polysomy*, or the presence of more than two chromosomes to a set, occurs when a germ cell containing more than 23 chromosomes is involved in conception. This defect has been described for both the autosomes and the sex chromosomes. Trisomy of chromosomes 8, 13, 18, and 21 is the more common form of polysomy of the autosomes. There are several forms of polysomy of the sex chromosomes in which one or more extra X or Y chromosomes are present.

Alterations in chromosome structure

Aberrations in chromosome structure occur when there is a break in one or more of the chromosomes followed by rearrangement or deletion of the chromosome parts. Among the factors believed to cause chromosome breakage are the following: (1) exposure to radiation sources, such as x-rays; (2) influence of certain chemicals; (3) extreme changes in the cellular environment; and (4) viral infections.

There are a number of patterns of chromosome breakage and rearrangement that can occur (Fig. 6-8). There can be a *deletion* of the broken portion of the chromosome. When one chromosome is involved, the broken parts may be *inverted*. *Isochromosome formation* occurs when the centromere, or central portion, of the chromosome separates horizontally instead of vertically. *Ring formation* results

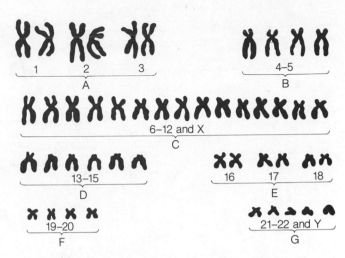

Figure 6–7.   Normal male karyotype. The first 22 pairs of chromosomes are the autosomes and the last two chromosomes are the sex chromosomes, in this case an X and Y chromosome. (Singer S: Human Genetics. San Francisco, WH Freeman, 1978)

when there is deletion followed by uniting of the chromatids to form a ring. *Translocation* occurs when there are simultaneous breaks in two chromosomes from different pairs with exchange of chromosome parts. With a translocation no genetic information is lost, and therefore persons with translocations are generally normal. These persons are, however, translocation carriers and may have both normal and abnormal children. A rare form of Down's syndrome is caused by translocation of some segment of chromosome 21 or 22 to another chromosome, often 14 or 15.

The manifestations of aberrations in chromosome structure will depend to a great extent upon the amount of genetic material that is lost. Many cells suffering unrestituted breaks will be eliminated within the next few mitoses because of deficiencies that may in themselves be fatal. This is beneficial because it prevents the damaged cells from becoming a permanent part of the organism or, if it occurs in the gametes, from giving rise to grossly defective zygotes. Some altered chromosomes, such as those that occur with translocations, will be passed on to the next generation.

Trisomy 21 (Down's syndrome)

Trisomy 21, or Down's syndrome, is the most common form of chromosomal disorder. It has an incidence of 1 in 1000 live births. The condition is usually accompanied by moderately severe mental retardation. The risk of having a baby with Down's syndrome is greater in women who are 35 years of

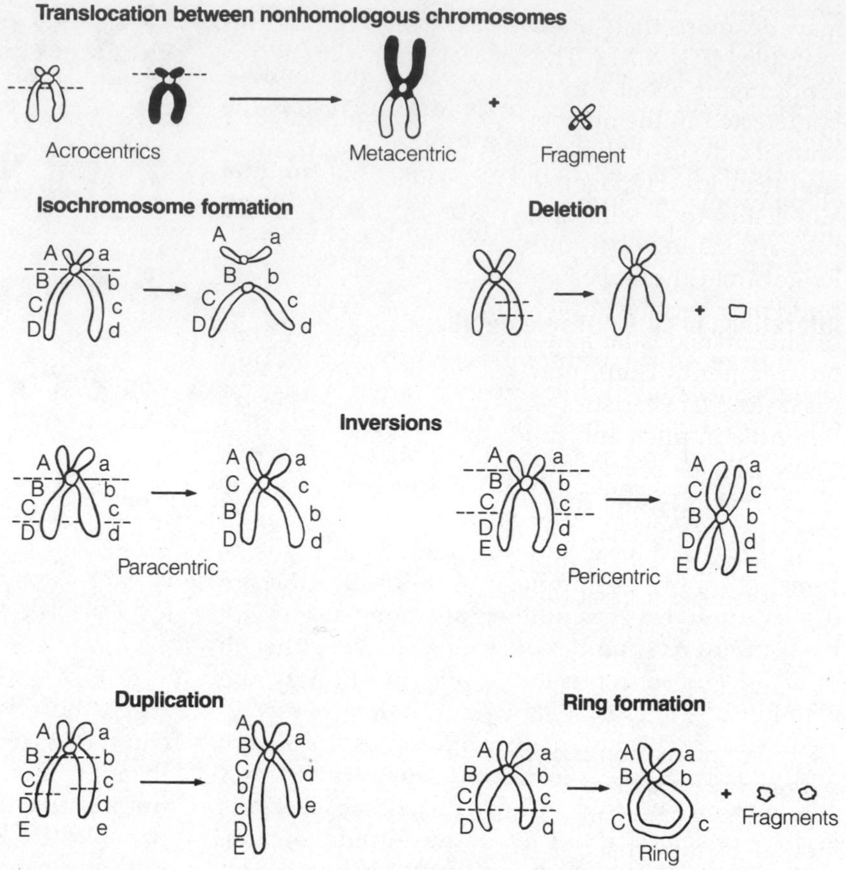

Translocation between nonhomologous chromosomes

Acrocentrics → Metacentric + Fragment

Isochromosome formation

Deletion

Inversions

Paracentric

Pericentric

Figure 6–8. Diagram showing rearrangement following breaks in chromosome structures. (Robbins SL, Angell M: Basic Pathology, 2nd ed. Philadelphia, WB Saunders, 1976)

Duplication

Ring formation

Ring + Fragments

age or older at the time of delivery (Table 6-2). The physical features of a child with Down's syndrome are distinctive and therefore the condition is usually apparent at birth. These features include a small and rather square head. There is an upward slanting of the eyes, small and malformed ears, an open mouth, and a large and protruding tongue. The child's hands are usually short and stubby with fingers that curl inward, and there is only a single palmar (simian) crease. There are often accompanying congenital heart defects. These children are usually happy and affectionate.

Table 6-2   The Relationship Between Maternal Age and the Risk of Down's Syndrome in a Newborn Child

Maternal Age	Approximate Risk of Occurrence
20-24	1 in 1,350
25-29	1 in 1,175
30-35	1 in 750
36-40	1 in 250
41-45	1 in 65
46-50	1 in 25(?)

(From Wisniewski LP, Hirschhorn K: A Guide to Human Chromosome Defects, 2nd ed. White Plains, March of Dimes Birth Defects Foundation, BD:OAS XVI(6), 1980)

Monosomy X (Turner's syndrome)

Turner's syndrome describes a monosomy of the X chromosome (45,X/O) with gonadal agenesis, or absence of the ovaries. This disorder is present in about 1 out of every 2500 live births. There are variations in the syndrome, with abnormalities ranging from essentially none to webbing of the neck with redundant skin folds, nonpitting edema of the hands and feet, and congenital heart defects (particularly coarctation of the aorta). Characteristically, the female with Turner's syndrome is short in stature, but her body proportions are normal. She does not menstruate and shows no signs of secondary sex characteristics. Administration of the female sex hormones (estrogens) may cause the secondary sexual characteristics to develop and may produce additional skeletal growth. Infertility of the affected individual cannot be restored. When a mosaic cell line (45,X/O and 46,XX or 45,X/O and 46,X/Y) is present, the manifestations associated with the chromosomal defect tend to be less severe.

Polysomy X (Klinefelter's syndrome)

Klinefelter's syndrome is characterized by an X-chromatin positive (47,X,X,Y) male and is associated with testicular dysgenesis. In rare situations, there may be more than one extra X chromosome, for example, 47,X,X,X,Y. The incidence of Klinefelter's syndrome is about 1 in 600. The condition may not be detected in the newborn. The infant usually has normal male genitalia, with a small penis and small-firm testicles. Hypogonadism during puberty usually leads to a tall stature with abnormal body proportions in which the lower part of the body is longer than the upper part. Later in life, the body build may become heavy with a female distribution of subcutaneous fat and variable degrees of breast enlargement. There may be deficient secondary male sex characteristics such as a voice that remains feminine in pitch and sparse beard and pubic hair. There may be sexual dysfunction, along with complete infertility and impotence. There may be personality problems, but the intellect is usually normal. Replacement hormone therapy with testosterone is used to treat the disorder.

:Developmental Defects

There are many nongenetic influences to which the developing embryo is subject. Following conception, development is influenced by the environmental factors that the embryo shares with the mother. The physiologic status of the mother—her hormone balance, her general state of health, her nutritional status, and the drugs she takes—undoubtedly influence the development of the unborn child. For example, diabetes mellitus is associated with increased risk of congenital anomalies. Smoking is associated with lower than normal neonatal weight. Alcohol, in the context of chronic alcoholism, is known to cause fetal abnormalities. Some agents cause early abortion. Others, such as radiation, have the potential for causing chromosomal and genetic defects as well as developmental disorders. Measles and other teratogenic agents cause developmental defects.

Period of Vulnerability

The embryo's development is most easily disturbed during the period when differentiation and development of the organs is taking place. This time interval is often referred to as the period of *organogenesis*; it extends from days 15 to 60 following conception. Environmental influences during the first two weeks following fertilization may interfere with implantation, resulting in abortion or very early resorption of the products of conception. Each organ has a critical period of time during which it is highly susceptible to environmental derangements (Fig. 6-9). Often,

the effect is expressed at the biochemical level, just prior to the time that the organ begins to develop. The same agent may affect different organ systems that are developing at the same time.

Teratogenic Agents

A *teratogenic* agent is one that produces abnormalities during embryonic or fetal development. For discussion purposes, teratogenic agents have been divided into three groups: (1) irradiation, (2) drugs and chemical substances, and (3) infectious agents. Table 6-3 lists commonly identified agents in each of these groups.

Radiation

Heavy doses of ionizing radiation have been shown to cause microcephaly, skeletal malformations, and mental retardation. At present, there is no evidence that diagnostic levels of radiation cause congenital abnormalities. Since the question of safety remains, however, many agencies require that the day of a woman's last menstrual period be noted on all radiologic requisitions. Other institutions may require a pregnancy test before any extensive diagnostic x-ray studies are performed. Radiation is not only teratogenic but also mutagenic, and there is the possibility of effecting inheritable changes in genetic materials. Administration of therapeutic doses of radioactive iodine (I^{131}) during the 13th week of gestation, the time when the fetal thyroid is beginning to concentrate iodine, has been shown to interfere with thyroid development.

Chemicals and drugs

Some of the best-documented chemical teratogens are the organic mercurials, which cause neurologic deficits and blindness. Exposure sources of mercury include contaminated food (fish) and water.

A number of drugs are suspected of being teratogens, but only a few have been documented with certainty. Perhaps the best known of these drugs is thalidomide, which has been shown to give rise to a full range of malformations, including phocomelia (short flipper-like appendages) of all four extremities. Other drugs known to cause fetal abnormalities are the antimetabolites used in the treatment of cancer, the anticoagulant drug warfarin, several of the anticonvulsant drugs, and ethyl alcohol. Some drugs affect a single developing structure; for example, propylthiouracil can impair thyroid development and tetracycline can interfere with the mineralization phase of tooth development. The progestins, which are included in many birth control pills, can cause virilization of a female fetus depending on their dosage and timing.

Highly Sensitive Periods of Development In Terms of Teratogenic Effects

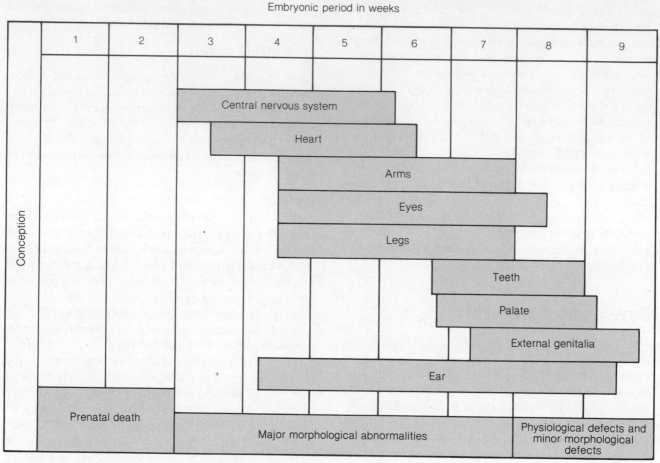

Figure 6–9. Susceptible periods during embryological development during which teratogenic agents are most likely to impair development of the various body structures. (Developed from information included in Moore KL: The Developing Human, 2nd ed. Philadelphia, WB Saunders, 1977)

Only recently have the teratogenic effects of alcohol been described in the literature. Alcohol has widely variable effects on fetal development, ranging from minor abnormalities to a unique constellation of anomalies that have been termed the "fetal alcohol syndrome." The syndrome is associated with several severe problems: (1) central nervous system dysfunction ranging from hypotonia and poor muscle coordination to moderate mental retardation; (2) craniofacial anomalies that can include microcephaly and a cluster of facial and eye defects; (3) deficient growth; and (4) others such as cardiovascular defects. Each of these can vary in severity, which probably reflects the quantity of alcohol consumed as well as hereditary and environmental influences. Evidence suggests that the consumption of 89 ml of alcohol or more per day—

equivalent to 6 hard drinks—constitutes a major risk to the fetus.[9]

Because many drugs are suspected of causing fetal abnormalities, and even those that were once thought to be safe are now being viewed critically, it seems unwise for women in their childbearing years to use drugs unnecessarily. This pertains to nonpregnant women as well as pregnant ones, because many developmental defects occur very early in pregnancy. As happened with thalidomide, the damage to the embryo often occurs before pregnancy is suspected or confirmed.

Infectious agents

Many microorganisms cross the placenta and enter the fetal circulation, often producing multiple malformations. The agents most frequently implicated

Table 6-3 Teratogenic Agents

Irradiation

Chemical Agents and Drugs

 Alcohol
 Anticoagulants
  Warfarin
 Anticonvulsants
  Paramethadione
  Phenytoin
  Trimethadione
 Cancer drugs
  Aminopterin
  Methotrexate
  6-mercaptopurine
 Progestins and oral contraceptive drugs
 Propylthiouracil
 Tetracycline
 Thalidomide

Infectious Agents

 Viruses
  Cyclomegalovirus
  Herpes simplex, type II
  Measles (rubella)
  Mumps
  Chicken pox
 Nonviral factors
  Syphilis
  Toxoplasmosis

in fetal anomalies are TOxoplasmosis, Rubella, Cytomegalovirus and Herpes simplex 2 virus—TORCH, an acronym for the screening test in which infant serum is tested for the presence of antibodies so as to identify the agent responsible for a developmental defect. These infections tend to cause similar clinical manifestations, including microcephaly, hydrocephaly, defects of the eye, and hearing problems. Cytomegalovirus may cause mental retardation and rubella virus, congenital heart defects.

Toxoplasmosis is a protozoal infection that can be contracted by eating raw or poorly cooked meat. The domestic cat also seems to carry the organism, excreting the protozoa in its stools. It has been suggested that pregnant women should avoid contact with the excrement from the family cat. *Rubella* (German measles) is a commonly recognized viral teratogen. About 15% to 20% of babies born to women who have had rubella during the first trimester have abnormalities.[10] The epidemiology of the *cytomegalovirus* is largely unknown. Some babies are severely affected at birth and others, while having evidence of the infection, have no symptoms. In some symptom-free babies, brain damage becomes evident over a span of several years. There is also evidence that some babies contract the infection during the first year of life and in some of them the

infection leads to retardation a year or two later. *Herpes simplex 2* is considered to be a genital infection and is usually transmitted through sexual contact. The infant acquires this infection either *in utero* or in passage through the birth canal.

:Diagnosis and Counseling

The birth of a defective child is a traumatic event in any parent's life. There are usually two issues that must be resolved. The first deals with the immediate and future care of the affected child and the second with the possibility of future children in the family having a similar defect. Genetic assessment and counseling can help to determine whether the defect was inherited as well as the risk of recurrence. Prenatal diagnosis provides a means of determining whether the unborn child has certain types of abnormalities.

Genetic Assessment and Counseling

Effective genetic counseling involves accurate diagnosis and communication of the findings along with the risks of recurrence to the parents and other family members who need such information. Counseling may be provided following the birth of an affected child; or it may be offered to persons at risk for having defective children (siblings of persons with birth defects). A team of trained counselors helps the family to understand the problem and stands ready to support their decisions about having more children.

Assessment of genetic risk and prognosis is usually directed by a clinical geneticist, often with the aid of laboratory and clinical specialists. A detailed family history (pedigree), a pregnancy history, and detailed accounts of both the birth process and of postnatal health and development are included. There is usually a need for a careful physical examination of the affected child and often of the parents and siblings. Laboratory work including chromosomal analysis and biochemical studies often precedes a definitive diagnosis.

The creases and dermal ridges on the palms and soles are examined in a genetic study called *dermatoglyphic analysis*. This is of value because the dermal ridges are formed by 16 weeks of gestation and any abnormalities will document the time during which the developmental defect occurred. Dermatoglyphic analysis includes examination of the patterns of the arches on the fingertips, the flexion creases of the fifth finger, and the arch pattern of the base of the great toe. One of the most readily identi-

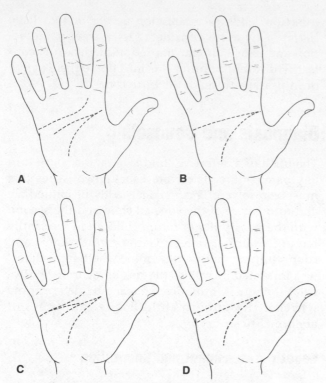

A   B

C   D

Figure 6–10. The transverse palmar crease. Hands (A) and (C) are normal. Hand (B) shows the typical transverse or simian crease. It is found in about 4% of the normal population and in about 50% of persons with Down's syndrome and certain other chromosomal defects. The sydney line (D) can be regarded as a variant of (B) and has the same significance. (Valentine GH: The Chromosome Disorders, 3rd ed. Philadelphia, JB Lippincott, 1975)

fied creases is the palmar (simian) crease (Fig. 6-10). For additional information on dermatoglyphic analysis, the reader is referred to other sources including those listed in the reference section at the end of this chapter.

Prenatal diagnosis

One form of prenatal diagnosis involves amniocentesis. The test is useful in women over 35 in whom there is an increased risk of giving birth to a baby with Down's syndrome, in parents who have another child with chromosomal abnormalities, and in situations where either parent is known to be a carrier of an inherited disorder. The procedure involves the withdrawal of a sample of amniotic fluid from the pregnant uterus by means of a needle inserted through the abdominal wall (Fig. 6-11). Ultrasound is used to gain additional information and as a guide for placement of the amniocentesis needle. The amniotic fluid cells shed by the fetus are then cultured and studied. Amniotic fluid is also useful in biochemical studies. Amniocentesis is currently useful for detecting some 60 genetic disorders, although not all hereditary or developmental defects can be detected in this way. Usually a determination can be made by the 16th to 17th week of pregnancy, and if the fetus is defective, the parents can then decide if they want to terminate the pregnancy. In most cases, the fetus is normal and the fears and anxieties of the prospective parents are relieved.

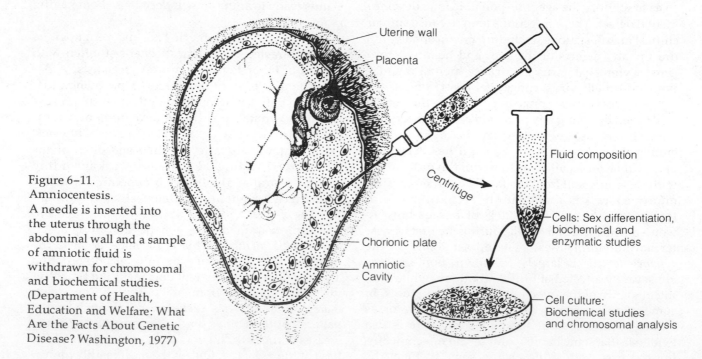

Figure 6–11. Amniocentesis. A needle is inserted into the uterus through the abdominal wall and a sample of amniotic fluid is withdrawn for chromosomal and biochemical studies. (Department of Health, Education and Welfare: What Are the Facts About Genetic Disease? Washington, 1977)

Uterine wall
Placenta
Fluid composition
Centrifuge
Cells: Sex differentiation, biochemical and enzymatic studies
Chorionic plate
Amniotic Cavity
Cell culture: Biochemical studies and chromosomal analysis

In summary, genetic and developmental defects affect all age groups and all body structures. Genetic disorders can affect a single gene (mendelian inheritance) or several genes (polygenic traits), or they can be acquired in utero as a result of exposure to environmental influences. Identification of the cause of such disorders involves an assessment of genetic risk and is usually done by a genetic counselor and a team of health care professionals, who are prepared to diagnose the disorder and assist the family in understanding the risk and in making decisions based on this knowledge.

:Study Guide

After you have studied this chapter, you should be able to meet the following objectives:

: : State a universal definition of *gene*.

: : Describe DNA.

: : Describe the pathogenesis of mutations.

: : Construct a hypothetical pedigree according to Mendel's laws.

: : Contrast genotype and phenotype.

: : Describe three types of single-gene disorders.

: : Contrast polygenic disorders with single-gene disorders.

: : Relate the significance of the Barr body to chromosomal disorders.

: : Describe two chromosomal abnormalities that demonstrate aneuploidy.

: : Describe three patterns of chromosomal breakage and rearrangement.

: : Relate maternal age to the expression of Down's syndrome.

: : Relate radiation, chemical agents, and infectious agents to teratogenicity.

: : Explain the purpose of dermatoglyphic analysis.

:References

1. National Institute of Health: What Are the Facts About Genetic Disease? Washington, D.C., U.S. Department of Health, Education, and Welfare, Public Health Service, 1977
2. Erbe RW: Principles of medical genetics. N Engl J Med 294:381, 480, 1976
3. McKusick VA: Mendelian Inheritance in Man: Catalogs of Autosomal Dominant, Autosomal Recessive, and X-linked Phenotypes. Baltimore, Johns Hopkins University Press, 1975
4. Singer S: Human Genetics, p 13. San Francisco, WH Freeman and Company, 1978
5. Vaughn VC, McKay RJ, Nelson WE: Nelson Textbook of Pediatrics, 10th ed, p 132. Philadelphia, WB Saunders, 1975
6. Riccardi VM: The Genetic Approach to Human Disease, p 500. New York, Oxford University Press, 1977
7. Riccardi VM: The Genetic Approach to Human Disease, p 92. New York, Oxford University Press, 1977
8. Paris Conference (1971): Standardization in Human Cytogenetics. Birth Defects XI, No. 9:1, 1975
9. National Institute of Alcohol Abuse and Alcoholism: Critical Review of the Fetal Alcohol Syndrome. Rockville MD, Alcohol, Drug Abuse, and Mental Health Administration, 1977
10. Dudgeon JA: Infectious causes of human malformations. Br Med J 32:77, 1976

:Suggested Readings

Chapelle CS: Development defects: Some thoughts on their causes. The National Foundation–March of Dimes Birth Defects 8:6, 1972
Clarren SK, Smith DW: The fetal alcohol syndrome. N Engl J Med 298, No. 19:1063, 1978
Davies DP, Gray OP, Elwood PC et al: Cigarette smoking in pregnancy: associations with maternal weight gain and fetal growth. Lancet 1:385, 1976
Erbe RW: Current concepts in genetics: Principles of medical genetics. N Engl J Med 294, No. 7:381, 1976
Erbe RW: Current concepts in genetics: Principles of medical genetics (part two). N Engl J Med 294, No. 9:480, 1976
Fraser FC: Current concepts in genetics: Genetics as a health care service. N Engl J Med 295, No. 9:486, 1976
Hanson JW, Jones KL, Smith DW: Fetal alcohol syndrome: Experience with 41 patients. J Am Med Assoc 235, No. 14:1458, 1976
Hanson JW, Smith DW: The fetal hydantoin syndrome. J Pediatr 87, No. 2:285, 1975
Janerich DT, Piper JM, Glebatis DM: Oral contraceptives and congenital limb-reduction defects. N Engl J Med 291, No. 14:697, 1974
Kushnick T: When to refer to the geneticist. J Am Med Assoc 235, No. 6:623, 1976
Level RR: Ethical issues arising in the genetic counseling relationship. The National Foundation–March of Dimes. Birth Defects 14:9, 1978
Marx JL: Cytomegalovirus: A major cause of birth defects. Science 190:1184, 1975

Milunsky A: Current concepts in genetics: Prenatal diagnosis of genetic disorders. N Engl J Med 295, No. 7:377, 1976

Mulvihill JJ, Smith DW: The genetics of dermatoglyphics. J Pediatr 75:579, 1969

Omenn GS: Prenatal diagnosis of genetic disorders. Science 200, No. 26:952, 1978

Shiono H, Kadowaki J: Dermatoglyphics of congenital abnormalities without chromosomal aberrations: A review of clinical applications. Clin Pediatr 14:1003, 1975

Siegel M: Congenital malformations following chicken pox, measles, mumps, and hepatitis. J Am Med Assoc 226, No. 13:1521, 1973

Tomasi TB: Structure and function of alpha-fetoprotein. Annu Rev Med 28:453, 1977

Wilson JG: Teratogenic effects of environmental chemicals. Fed Proc 36, No. 5:1698, 1977

7

Neoplasia

Cancer is the second leading cause of death in the United States. The American Cancer Society has estimated that over 54 million Americans, or one out of every four who is alive today, will develop cancer during their lifetimes. In 1981, about 805,000 persons were diagnosed as having cancer.[1] It has been estimated that, with present methods of treatment, one out of every three persons who develop cancer each year will be alive five years later. Cancer affects all age groups. It is the leading cause of death in children 3 to 14 years of age.

Cancer is not a single disease; rather, the term describes almost all forms of malignant neoplasia. As shown in Figure 7-1, cancer can originate in almost any organ, with the lung being the most common site in men and the breast, in women. This chapter provides a general overview of cancer (malignant neoplasia) along with a brief discussion of benign neoplasia. Specific forms of cancer are discussed elsewhere in this book.

The term *neoplasm* comes from the Greek word meaning *new formation*. In contrast to tissue growth that occurs with hypertrophy and hyperplasia, a neoplasm serves no useful purpose, but tends to increase in size and persist at the expense of the rest of the body. Furthermore, neoplasms do not obey the laws of normal tissue growth. For example, they do not occur in response to an appropriate stimulus, and they continue to grow once the stimulus has ceased or the needs of the organism have been met. Although the terms are not synonymous, a neoplasm is often referred to as a *tumor*. Strictly speaking, a tumor is a swelling that can be caused by a number of conditions, including inflammation and trauma. The Latin word *malus* means bad; hence a *malignant tumor* is a "bad" tumor that will cause death if it is not controlled. A *benign tumor* is a "good" tumor—it usually will not cause death unless by its location it interferes with vital functions.

Oncology is the study of tumors and their treatment.

:Concepts of Cell Growth and Replication

A basic knowledge of cell growth and replication is helpful in understanding the characteristics of neoplasms. Cell division and replication are inherent adaptive mechanisms for many body cells, and in a single day many cells are being replaced by new cells. Normally, these cells are identical in structure

Figure 7–1. Cancer deaths (1981 estimates) by site and sex. (American Cancer Society: Cancer Facts. New York, 1981)

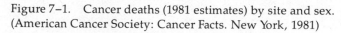
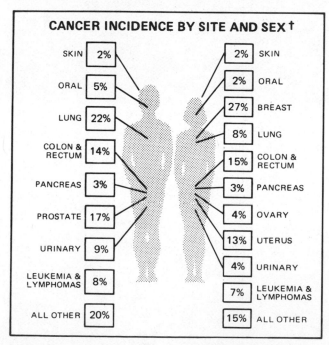
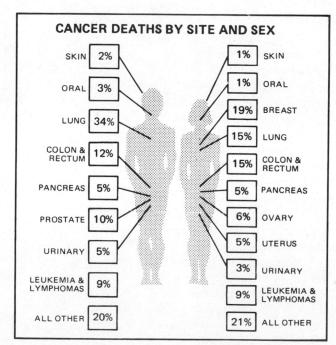

† Excluding non-melanoma skin cancer and carcinoma in situ.

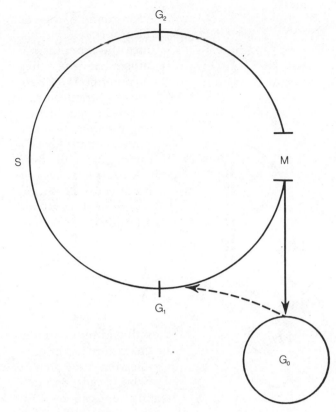

Figure 7–2. Phases of the cell cycle. The cycle represents the interval between the midpoint of mitosis to the subsequent end-point in mitosis in one daughter cell or both. Note the number of doubling times before the tumor reaches an appreciable size.

and function to the cells they replace. When abnormal or mutant cells do develop, they are usually either defective and incapable of survival or are destroyed by the body's immune system.

The life of a cell is called the *cell cycle*. It consists of the interval between the midpoint of mitosis and the subsequent midpoint of mitosis in one or both daughter cells. The cell cycle is divided into five distinct phases for which *gap* or G terminology is used (Fig. 7-2). G_1 is the first gap, the postmitotic phase during which DNA synthesis ceases while RNA and protein synthesis and cell growth take place. Toward the end of G_1, some critical event occurs that commits the cell to continue through the phases of the gap cycle, and enter mitosis. G_0 is the resting or dormant phase in which the cell performs all activities except those related to proliferation. Cells can leave G_1 and enter G_0. The time spent in G_0 varies according to the cell type, and not all cells spend time in G_0. It is believed that some special

growth signal is needed to move cells that have been dormant in G_0 back into the cell cycle. The S phase is the synthesis phase. During the S phase, DNA replication occurs, giving rise to two separate sets of chromosomes. G_2 is the premitotic phase. During this phase, as in G_1, DNA synthesis ceases while synthesis of RNA and protein continues. The M phase represents *mitosis*.

Mitosis is the period of time when cell division is actually taking place. Mitosis is subdivided into four stages: prophase, metaphase, anaphase, and telophase. During *prophase*, the centrioles in the cytoplasm separate and move toward opposite sides of the cell, the chromosomes become shorter and thicker, and the nuclear membrane breaks up so that there is no longer a barrier between the chromosomes and the cytoplasm. *Metaphase* involves the organization of the chromosome pairs in the midline of the cell and the formation of a mitotic spindle composed of the microtubules. *Anaphase* is the period during which there is splitting of the chromosome pairs with the microtubules pulling each set of 46 chromosomes toward the cell poles in preparation for cell separation. Cell division is completed during *telophase*, when the mitotic spindles vanish and a new nuclear membrane develops and encloses each of the sets of chromosomes (Fig. 7-3).

In normal tissue, cell proliferation is regulated so that the number of cells actively dividing is equivalent to the number of cells dying or being shed. Most tissues have three types of cell populations: (1) cells that continue to divide and move through the cell cycle, (2) cells that have become differentiated and are no longer able to divide, and (3) cells that leave the cell cycle and become dormant as they move into G_0. Bone marrow is a good example of tissue that has all three types of cell populations. One population of rapidly proliferating cells continues to move through the cell cycle. A second population leaves the cell cycle after a few divisions and becomes differentiated; at the end of their life span these cells die. The granulocytes are good examples of this cell type. The third group remains dormant until some event causes them to reenter the cell cycle. Stem cells belong to this cell population.

The rate of tissue growth in both normal and cancerous tissue depends on three factors: (1) the number of cells that are actively dividing or moving through the cell cycle, (2) the cell-cycle time, and (3) the number of cells that are being lost. One of the reasons that cancerous tumors often seem to grow so rapidly is related to the size of the cell pool actively engaged in cycling. It has been shown that the cell-

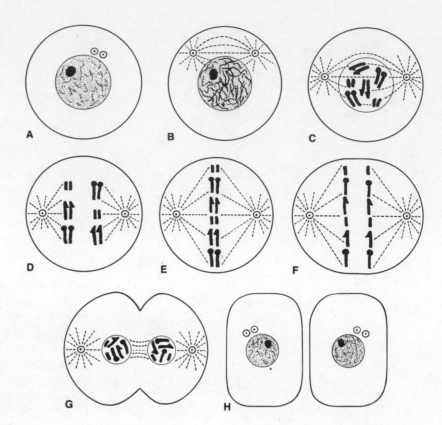

Figure 7–3. Cell mitosis. A and H represent the nondividing cell; B, C, D prophase; E metaphase; F anaphase; and G telophase. (Chaffee EE, Greisheimer EM: Basic Physiology and Anatomy, 3rd ed. Philadelphia, JB Lippincott, 1974)

Figure 7–4. Growth curve of a hypothetical tumor on arithmetic coordinates. (Collins VP et al: Observations of growth rates of human tumors. Am J Roent, Rad Ther Nuclear Med 76:988, 1956. Charles C Thomas, Publisher)

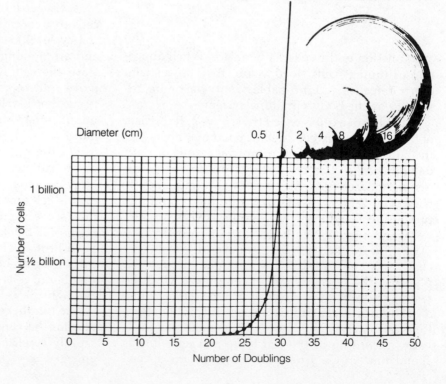

cycle time for cancerous tissue is not necessarily shorter than that for normal tissue; neither is the number of cells that are lost any smaller. Rather, it appears that the growth factors that allow cells to enter G$_0$ when they are not needed for cell replacement is lacking, and therefore there is a greater percentage of tumor cells actively engaged in cycling than usually occurs in normal tissue.[2]

The *doubling time* is the length of time that it takes for the total number of cells in a tumor to double. Figure 7-4 demonstrates the increase in the size of a tumor according to doubling time. The reader will note that it takes a long period of time before the tumor reaches a size where it is detectable, and then it seems to grow rapidly. Actually, the doubling time for each of the tumors is the same, but as the tumor increases in size the number of cells that are actively dividing has increased. This is why it is important that women do a self breast examination on a monthly basis; a tumor that was too small to be detected one month may have a doubling time such that it becomes palpable the next month.

Experimentally it is possible to measure the cell-cycle time and the percentage of cells that are cycling during a given period of time, and to estimate the doubling time. From this information, it is possible to estimate the rate of cell increase per hour for the different types of tumors. Knowledge of the cell-cycle time and the rate of cell increase is used in planning cancer therapy.

:Characteristics of Cancer Cells

Two basic characteristics of neoplasms are *autonomy* and *anaplasia*. Autonomy is the disregard of cancerous tissue for normal limitations of growth, and anaplasia is the loss of cell differentiation and function.

Abnormalities in Cell Replication

Changes in the karyotype, or organization of cell chromosomes, can be observed in many cancer cells. In normal cells, mitosis yields two identical cells, each with a normal arrangement of chromosomes. Diploid cells are double folded and when they divide, they form two identical cells. *Polyploidy* is cell division that results in more than two cells. *Aneuploidy* refers to abnormal cell division in which the daughter cell receives an uneven number of chromosomes; for example, one cell may receive 47 chromosomes and another 45. Cancerous tumors often

undergo abnormal mitosis and display polyploidy and/or aneuploidy. These cells often have multiple spindles that result in uneven division of nuclear and cellular contents. The term *pleomorphism* refers to variations in the size and shape of both cells and cell nuclei.

Abnormalities in Cell Differentiation

All tumors are made up of two types of tissue: the proliferating tumor cells that form the parenchymal component of the tumor and the supporting structures such as the connective tissue matrix and the blood vessels that supply the tumor with nourishment. It is usually the parenchymal cells that are involved in neoplastic growth.

Cell differentiation is the degree to which the parenchymal cells formed in the process of cell proliferation resemble the original tissue type in structure and function. Well-differentiated cells are identical to the cells they replace. As previously mentioned, anaplasia is lack of cell differentiation, and cancerous tissue usually displays some degree of anaplasia. The poorly differentiated tumor cells arise from the reserve or stem cells found in all specialized tissue, not from the mature parenchymal cells. In the process of becoming cancer cells, some event causes these reserve cells to develop in an undifferentiated manner. The degree of anaplasia that a tumor displays varies. Some cancers display only slight anaplasia and others are markedly undifferentiated. As a general rule, the more undifferentiated the tumor, the more numerous the mitoses and the more rapid the rate of growth.

Cell Membrane Changes

In addition to changes in cell growth and differentiation, cancer cells display alteration in surface characteristics which are related to the cell membrane. These changes include alterations in contact inhibition, cohesiveness, and adhesiveness; failure to form intracellular junctions; and impaired cell-to-cell communication. Contact inhibition is the cessation of movement once a cell comes in contact with another cell. Contact inhibition usually "switches off" cell growth by blocking net RNA and protein synthesis and by blocking new DNA synthesis. In wound healing, contact inhibition causes fibrous tissue growth to cease at the point where the edges of the wound come together. Cancer cells, on the other hand, tend to grow rampant without regard for other cells. Although in the laboratory many of the membrane changes that have been reported for cancer cells have been observed with individual cancer cells, there is reason to believe that these same properties exist in cancer cells present in the body, and these changes account for the invasive and destructive nature of cancer cell growth. There are also changes in the membrane transport of sugars and amino acids by the tumor cells. Cancer cells have been called "nitrogen traps" because they tend to rob normal cells of amino acids.

:Properties of Benign and Malignant Neoplasms

Benign and malignant neoplasms are generally differentiated by their (1) cell characteristics, (2) manner of growth, (3) rate of growth, (4) potential for metastasizing and spreading to other parts of the body, (5) tendency to recur once they have been removed, (6) ability to produce generalized effects, (7) tendency to cause tissue destruction, and (8) capacity to cause death. The characteristics of benign and malignant neoplasms are summarized in Table 7-1.

Benign Tumors

Benign tumors are made up of well-differentiated mature tissue types. For example, the cells of a uterine leiomyoma resemble uterine smooth muscle. The slow expansive growth of a benign tumor produces pressure on the surrounding tissues, leading to formation of a fibrous capsule. Figure 7-5 shows a benign encapsulated tumor. The formation of the capsule is thought to represent the reaction of the surrounding tissues to the tumor. The presence of the capsule is responsible for a sharp line of demarcation between the benign tumor mass and the adjacent tissues, so that benign tumors are usually enucleated more easily than malignant tumors. A benign tumor once removed is not likely to recur.

Benign tumors do not usually undergo degenerative changes as readily as malignant tumors and they do not usually cause death unless by their location they interfere with vital functions. For instance, a benign tumor growing in the cranial cavity can eventually lead to death by compressing the brain. Benign tumors can also cause disturbances in the function of adjacent or distant structures by producing pressure on tissues, blood vessels, or nerves.

Table 7–1 Characteristics of Benign and Malignant Neoplasms

Characteristics	Benign	Malignant
Cell characteristics	Cells resemble normal cells of the tissue from which the tumor originated	Cells often bear little resemblance to the normal cells of the tissue from which they arose; there is both anaplasia and pleomorphism
Mode of growth	Tumor grows by expansion and does not infiltrate the surrounding tissues; encapsulated	Grows at the periphery and sends out processes that infiltrate and destroy the surrounding tissues
Rate of growth	Rate of growth is usually slow	Rate of growth is usually relatively rapid and is dependent upon level of differentiation; the more anaplastic the tumor the more rapid the rate of growth
Metastasis	Does not spread by metastasis	Gains access to the blood and lymph channels and metastasizes to other areas of the body
Recurrence	Does not recur when removed	Tends to recur when removed
General effects	Is usually a localized phenomenon that does not cause generalized effects unless by location it interferes with vital functions	Often causes generalized effects such as anemia, weakness, and weight loss
Destruction of tissue	Does not usually cause tissue damage unless location interferes with blood flow	Often causes extensive tissue damage as the tumor outgrows its blood supply or encroaches on blood flow to the area; may also produce substances that cause cell damage
Ability to cause death	Does not usually cause death unless its location interferes with vital functions	Will usually cause death unless growth can be controlled

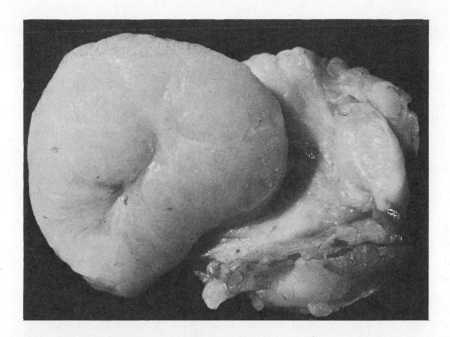

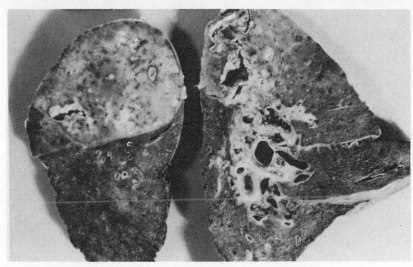

Figure 7–5. Photograph of a benign encapsuled fibroadenoma of the breast at the top and a bronchogenic carcinoma of the lung at the bottom. Note that the fibroadenoma is a discrete mass, whereas the bronchogenic carcinoma is diffuse and infiltrates the surrounding tissues.

Some benign tumors are also known for their ability to cause alterations in body function due to abnormal elaboration of hormones. Examples of hormone-secreting benign tumors are the pheochromocytomas which produce adrenalin, and parathyroid tumors which elaborate excessive parathyroid hormone.

Malignant Tumors

In contrast to benign tumors, malignant neoplasms tend to grow more rapidly, spread widely, and kill regardless of their location. The destructive nature of malignant tumors is related to changes in their rate of growth, their lack of cell differentiation, and their ability to spread and metastasize. Their malignant potential usually depends on their degree of anaplasia. Because they grow rapidly, they capture large quantities of essential amino acids and other nutrients which they rob from normal cells. This rapid growth also may cause compression of blood vessels as well as thrombosis; the tumors outgrow their blood supply liberating toxins that destroy both tumorous and normal tissue. The end result may be ischemia, degeneration, ulceration, and tissue necrosis. The generalized effects of these changes on body function are discussed later in this chapter.

Cancer in situ

Cancer in situ is a localized preinvasive lesion. Depending on its location, this type of lesion can usually be removed surgically or treated so that the chances of recurrence are small. For example, cancer in situ of the cervix is essentially 100% curable.

Spread of the tumor

The spread of cancer can take many forms: direct extension, seeding of cancer cells to adjacent structures, or metastatic spread through the blood or lymph pathways. Growth usually occurs at the tumor periphery with direct extension to or *invasion* of the surrounding tissue. The word *cancer* is derived from the Latin word meaning "crab-like," hence cancerous growth spreads by sending crab-like projections into the surrounding tissues. Unlike benign tumors, which are encapsulated, malignant tumors have no sharp line of demarcation separating them from the surrounding tissue, and this often makes complete surgical removal of the tumor difficult (Fig. 7-5). *Seeding* of cancer cells into body cavities occurs when a tumor erodes into these spaces and tumor cells drop onto the serosal surface. For example, a tumor may penetrate the wall of the stomach and its cells implant on the surfaces of the peritoneal cavity.

Metastatic spread occurs when a malignant tumor invades the vascular or lymphatic channels, and parts of the tumor break loose and travel to distant parts of the body where implantation occurs. When metastasis occurs by way of the lymphatic channels, the tumor cells lodge first in the regional lymph nodes that receive their drainage from the tumor site. The regional lymph nodes may contain the tumor cells for a time, but eventually the cells break loose and gain access to more distant nodes and to the blood steam by way of the thoracic duct. The *lungs* and the *liver* are common sites for secondary growth when a cancer gains access to the venous system. The venous blood from the gastrointestinal tract, the pancreas, and the spleen is routed to the liver through the portal vein before entering the general circulation. Therefore, the liver is a common site of metastatic growth for cancers that originate in these organs. Likewise, venous blood from all parts of the body must travel through the lungs before moving to the arterial side of the circulation. On the other hand, the *bone* and the *brain* are frequent sites of metastasis when cancer cells enter the arterial circulation. This is particularly true of lung cancer, as cells from these tumors move directly into the left heart, thence out into the systemic circulation.

To a great extent, metastatic tumors retain many of the characteristics of the primary tumor from which they had their origin. Because of this, it is possible, in some cases, to discover an unsuspected

Table 7–2   Names of Selected Benign and Malignant Tumors According to Tissue Types

Tissue Type	Benign	Malignant
Epithelial tumors		
Surface	Papilloma	Squamous cell carcinoma
Glandular	Adenoma	Adenocarcinoma
Connective tissue tumors		
Fibrous	Fibroma	Fibrosarcoma
Adipose	Lipoma	Liposarcoma
Cartilage	Chondroma	Chondrosarcoma
Bone	Osteoma	Osteosarcoma
Blood vessels	Hemangioma	Hemangiosarcoma
Lymph vessels	Lymphangioma	Lymphangiosarcoma
Muscle tumors		
Smooth	Leiomyoma	Leiomyosarcoma
Striated	Rhabdomyoma	Rhabdomyosarcoma
Nerve cell tumors		
Nerve cell	Neuroma	
Glial tissue		Glioma
Nerve sheaths	Neurilemoma	Neurilemic sarcoma
Hematologic tumors		
Granulocytic		Myelocytic leukemia
Erythrocytic		Erythroleukemia
Plasma cells		Multiple myeloma
Lymphoid		Lymphocytic leukemia

malignancy before the original primary tumor begins to produce symptoms. Some tumors tend to metastasize early in their course, while others do not metastasize until late. Occasionally, the metastatic tumor will be far advanced before the primary tumor becomes clinically detectable. Malignant tumors of the kidney, for example, may go completely undetected and be asymptomatic even when a metastasis is found in the lung.

:Classification and Nomenclature

There are two major categories of cancer—solid tumors and hematologic cancers. *Solid tumors* initially are confined to a specific tissue or organ. The cells shed from the original tumor mass travel through the blood and lymph stream. *Hematologic cancers* involve the blood and lymph systems and are disseminated diseases from the beginning.

The significance of the system of naming and classifying tumors is that it facilitates communication among researchers and health professionals. Tumors usually are identified by the addition of the suffix *-oma* to the name of the tissue type from which the growth originated. Thus, a benign tumor of glandular epithelial tissue is called an adenoma, and a

Table 7-3   TNM Classification System

T† subclasses

    Tx—tumor cannot be adequately assessed
    T0—no evidence of primary tumor
    TIS—carcinoma in situ
    T1, T2, T3, T4—progressive increase in tumor size and involvement

N‡ subclasses

    Nx—regional lymph nodes cannot be assessed clinically
    N0—regional lymph nodes demonstrably abnormal
    N1, N2, N3, N4—increasing degrees of demonstrable abnormality of regional lymph nodes

M§ subclasses

    Mx—not assessed
    M0—no (known) distant metastasis
    M1—distant metastasis present, specify site(s)

Histopathology

    G1—well-differentiated grade
    G2—moderately well-differentiated grade
    G3, G4—poorly to very poorly differentiated grade

†T = Primary tumor.
‡N = Regional lymph nodes.
§M = Distant metastasis.
American Joint Committee on Cancer: Manual for Staging of Cancer. Chicago, American Joint Committee, 1977

benign tumor of bone tissue, an osteoma. If the tumor is malignant, the word *carcinoma* is used to designate the *epithelial tissue* origin of the tumor, for example, in the case of an adenoma that became cancerous, the term adenocarcinoma is used. Malignant tumors of *mesenchymal origin* are called *sarcomas*, e.g., osteosarcoma. Table 7-2 lists the names of selected benign and malignant tumors according to their tissue type.

At present, there are two basic methods for classifying cancers: (1) grading according to the histologic or cellular characteristics of the tumor; and (2) staging according to the spread of the disease. Both are used to prognosticate the course of the disease and to aid in selecting an appropriate treatment or management plan. The clinical staging is intended to provide a means by which information related to the progress of the disease, the methods and success of treatment modalities, and the prognosis can be communicated to others. The TNM system, which has evolved from the work of the International Union Against Cancer (UICC) and the American Joint Committee on Cancer Staging and End Stage Reporting (AJCCS), is used by many cancer facilities. This system, which is briefly described in Table 7-3, quantifies the disease into stages, using three tumor components: (1) T stands for the extent of the primary tumor, (2) N refers to the involvement of the regional lymph nodes, and (3) M describes the extent of the metastatic involvement. The TNM system further defines each specific type of cancer, such as breast cancer. The rationale for use of the system encompasses the need to classify the disease at various time periods—initial diagnosis, presurgical treatment, postsurgical treatment, and so on.

:Causative Factors

Since cancer is thought not to be a single disease, it is reasonable to assume that it does not have a single cause. More likely, cancer occurs because of interaction between multiple risk factors or repeated exposure to a single carcinogenic agent. Among the factors that have been linked with the development of cancer are heredity, chemical and environmental carcinogens, cancer-causing viruses, immunologic defects, and precancerous lesions.

Heredity

Certain types of cancers seem to "run in families." Breast cancer, for example, occurs more frequently in women whose grandmothers, mothers, aunts and sisters also have had a cancerous disease. Cancer is

Table 7-4 Some Cancers and Cancer Predisposing Diseases with Mendelian Inheritance Patterns*

Dominant (Autosomal)	Recessive (Autosomal)
Adenocarcinoma (primarily colon and endometrium)	Albinism
Familial polyposis of colon	Ataxia telangiectasia
Gardner's syndrome (predisposes to colonic cancer)	Bloom's syndrome
Melanocarcinoma	Franconi's aplastic anemia
Multiple endocrine adenomatosis (MEA)	Xeroderma pigmentosum
Neurofibromatosis (von Recklinghausen's disease)	
Retinoblastoma	

*Modified from Robbins SL, Cotran RS: Pathologic Basis of Disease, 2nd ed. Philadelphia, WB Saunders, 1979
Fagin-Dubin, L: Causes of cancer. Cancer Nurs 2(6):436, 1979

found in approximately 10% of persons having one affected first-degree relative, in approximately 15% of persons having two affected family members, and in 30% of persons having three affected family members.[3]

The genetic predisposition for development of cancer has been documented for a number of cancerous and precancerous lesions that are transmitted by mendelian inheritance (Table 7-4). Fortunately, most of these neoplasms are extremely rare—probably accounting for less than 1% of the cancers that occur in the general population.[4]

Among the inherited forms of cancer are retinoblastoma and multiple polyposis of the colon. In about 40% of cases, retinoblastoma (a form of eye cancer which occurs most frequently in small children) is inherited as an autosomal dominant trait (Fig. 7-6). The penetrance of the genetic trait is high as evidenced by the fact that the risk of developing the disease is increased 100,000 times when the gene is present as compared with an occurrence rate of 1 in 30,000 in the general population.[5] Familial polyposis of the colon is another example of an autosomal dominant inheritance pattern. It is the underlying cause of precancerous pedunculated adenomatous polyps of the colon (Fig. 7-7). About 50% of persons with the polyps develop cancer by age thirty and almost all others develop the disease by age 60.[6]

Carcinogens

A carcinogen is an agent capable of causing cancer. The role of environmental agents in causation of cancer was first noted in 1775 by Sir Percival Pott,

who related the high incidence of scrotal cancer in chimney sweeps to their exposure to coal soot. In 1915, Yamagiwa and Ichikawa conducted the first experiments in which a chemical agent was used to produce cancer. These investigators found that a cancerous growth developed when they painted a rabbit's ear with coal tar. Coal tar has since been found to contain potent polycyclic aromatic hydrocarbons. Since then, literally hundreds of carcinogenic agents have been identified. In fact, it has been estimated that 80 to 85% of human cancers are associated with exposure to environmental or chemical agents (Table 7-5).

Chemical carcinogens

There are literally hundreds of chemical carcinogenic agents, some of which have been found to cause cancers in animals and others of which are known to cause cancers in humans. These agents include both natural (e.g., aflatoxin B_1) and manmade products (e.g., vinyl chloride). Usually, carcinogenic agents can be divided into three categories: (1) direct-acting agents, (2) procarcinogens which are metabolized and converted into carcinogenic agents in the body, and (3) cocarcinogens, which are not in themselves carcinogens but which augment or promote the action of other cancer-producing factors.[7] It is of interest that the site of cancer development which is based on exposure to direct-acting carcinogens coincides with the area of the body that is exposed to the chemical, e.g., the scrotum in the chimney sweep or the lungs in the heavy cigarette smoker. With the procarcinogens, cancer usually develops in the organ where the agent

Table 7-5 Some Chemical and Environmental Agents Known to be Carcinogenic in Humans

Polycyclic Hydrocarbons
Soots, tars, and oils
Cigarette smoke

Industrial Agents
Asbestos
Vinyl chloride
Arsenic compounds
Aniline and azo dyes
Nickel and chromium compounds

Food and Drugs
Sweeteners (saccharin and cyclamates)
Smoked foods
Nitrosamines (used in preservation of meats)
Aflatoxin B_1 (mold that grows in nuts and grains)
Phenacetin
Diethylstilbestrol
Oral contraceptives

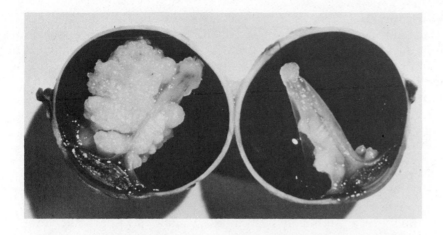

Figure 7–6. Photograph of a retinoblastoma that was removed surgically from the eye of a 2-year-old.

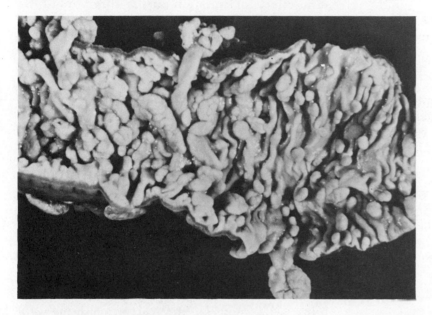

Figure 7–7. Photograph of pre-cancerous pedunculated adenomatous polyps (familial polyposis of the colon) in a segment of colon.

is metabolized or stored for elimination, e.g., in the bladder in persons exposed to analine dyes. The cocarcinogens tend to exert their effect on vulnerable body structures, such as the breast in genetically predisposed women who are exposed to the hormones contained in birth control pills.

Chemical carcinogens form highly reactive ions (electrophils) that bind with the nucleophilic residues on DNA, RNA, or cellular proteins. The action of these ions tends to cause cell mutation and/or alterations in synthesis of cell enzymes and structural proteins in a manner that alters cell replication and interferes with cell regulatory controls.

The effects of carcinogenic agents are usually dose dependent—the larger the dose or the longer the duration of exposure, the greater the risk that cancer will develop. There is usually a time delay ranging from 5 to 30 years from the time of exposure to the development of cancer. This is unfortunate, because many persons may have been exposed to

the agent and its carcinogenic effects before the association is recognized. For example, this occurred with the use of diethylstilbestrol which was widely used in the United States from the mid1940s to 1970 to prevent miscarriages. But it was not until the late 1960s that many cases of vaginal adenosis and adenocarcinoma in young women were found to be a result of their exposure to diethylstilbestrol *in utero*.[8]

Two occupational carcinogens of particular interest are asbestos and vinyl chloride.[9] Although the history of asbestos disease dates back to the early 1900s, it was not until the late 1960s that the full spectrum of the problem became evident. Exposure to asbestos is associated with cancer of the lung, cancer of the stomach, and a rare form of malignancy (mesothelioma) which affects the pleura and peritoneum. The population groups at increased risk of developing cancer due to asbestos exposure include not only those persons who work directly with the mineral but also those who live in the vicinity of industrial installations where asbestos is used in one way or another, and persons who live in the same household as the asbestos worker. The risk of cancer in these groups is increased even further if they also smoke cigarettes, which points to an additive effect. Until 1973 (when its use was banned), asbestos was frequently used as a fireproofing spray in many high-rise buildings. There is now concern that the air circulating through some buildings in which a dry type of asbestos fireproofing was applied may be contaminated with asbestos fibers. There is also concern about how exposure to asbestos is to be controlled at the time when these buildings may need to be demolished.

Vinyl chloride, which is used in the rubber industry, is associated with hemangiosarcoma of the liver. As with many other carcinogenic agents, the relationship between vinyl chloride exposure and the development of cancer was not discovered until a large number of workers had been exposed to the chemical. As of 1974, the U.S. Department of Labor has established regulations for vinyl chloride exposure in industry.

Radiation

Among the well-documented causes of cancer is radiation, including ultraviolet rays from sunlight, x-rays, radioactive chemicals, and other forms of radiation. As with other carcinogens, the effects of radiation are usually additive, and there is usually a long delay between exposure and the time that cancer can be detected. This is true of skin cancer, which is caused by overexposure to the sun and which is many years in the making. Skin cancer is an occupational hazard of farmers and sailors, particularly those who work in the southwest United States. Equally hazardous is the practice of sunbathing for the purpose of achieving a suntan.

Another example of the ultimate consequences of radiation exposure is therapeutic radiation of the head and neck—particularly in infants and small children—in which there may be a time lag as long as 35 years before a thyroid cancer is detected.[10] Probably even more dramatic have been the long-term effects of radiation on the survivors of the atomic blasts in Hiroshima and Nagasaki: between 1950 and 1970, the death rate from leukemia alone in the most heavily exposed population groups in Hiroshima was 147 per 100,000, or 30 times the expected rate.[11]

Viruses

A virus is a small particle containing genetic information (DNA and RNA) encased in a protein coat. Viruses enter a cell, called the host, and become incorporated into its chromosomal DNA, or take control of the cell's machinery for the purpose of producing viral proteins. Thus, a virus has the potential for effecting a change in the cell's function, or it can insert information into the host cell's chromosomes and thereby alter future generations of

A

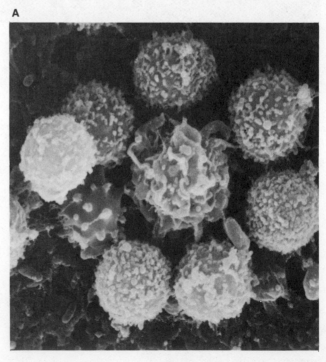

Figure 7–8.   A scanning electron micrograph showing the combination of a cancer cell and lymphocytes removed from the same patient and studied in the laboratory. Photo (*A*) shows the lymphocytes surrounding the cancer cell (60 minutes), Photo (*B*) shows the lymphocytes attacking the cancer cell (150 minutes). In Photo (*C*), the integrity of the cancer cell has been destroyed (240 minutes). (Courtesy of Kenneth Siegesmund, Ph.D. and Burton A. Waisbren Sr, M.D. The Antomy Department, The Medical College of Wisconsin)

cells. *Oncogenic viruses* are those capable of causing cancer. At present, oncogenic viruses have been demonstrated in animals, but not in humans. For example, in 1908 Ellerman, Bong and Rous were able to transmit leukemia to chickens through the use of cell-free filtrates of leukemic cells, thereby establishing the role of viral causation in fowl leukemia.

Immunologic Defects

One characteristic of mutant and cancer cells is that they develop neoantigens (neo, new) which attach to the surface of the cell. Immune surveillance is the term often used to describe the mechanism whereby an organism develops an immune response against the antigens expressed by a tumor.[12] The role of the immune system in the destruction of a cancer cell is depicted in Figure 7-8.

It has been suggested that the development of cancer might be associated with impairment or decline in the surveillance capacity of the immune system. For example, it has been observed that there is an increased incidence of cancer in persons who have immunodeficiency diseases and in renal transplant patients who are receiving immunosuppressant drugs. The incidence of cancer is also increased in the elderly, in whom there is a known decrease in immune activity. Although seemingly simple, the role of immunity in the development of cancer is still largely uncertain. At present, for example, it cannot be said with any certainty that the immune system is able to effect protection against all forms of cancer. Many growing tumors appear to suppress the immune response. Furthermore, it is well recognized that some conventional types of cancer treatment— chemotherapy and radiation—tend to suppress the immune response. *Immunotherapy*, which will be discussed later in this chapter, is a cancer treatment modality designed to heighten the patient's general immune responses so as to increase tumor destruction.

Precancerous Lesions

There are several lesions that tend to undergo cancerous transformation. One of these, multiple polyposis of the colon, was described earlier; leukoplakia, a white patchy lesion of the mucous membrane of the oral mucosa and the genitalia, is a second type of premalignant lesion. Others that may undergo cancerous transformation are fibrocystic disease of the breast, epithelial polyps of the colon, and burn scars.

:Diagnosis

Recent advances in technology provide a means whereby many forms of cancer may be successfully treated if discovered early. At present, one out of three persons diagnosed as having cancer is alive five years later. It seems likely that the five-year sur-

B

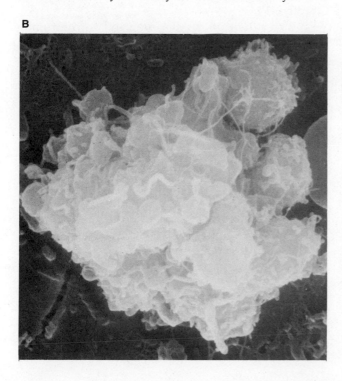

C

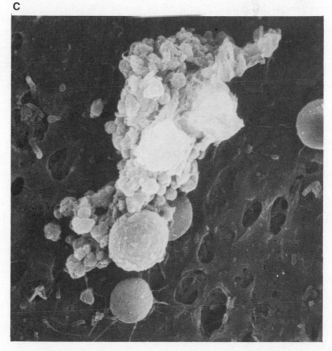

vival rate can be improved as people become aware of the early signs of cancer and seek medical attention at that time. One of the best examples of the success of treatment associated with early detection is cervical cancer, which is almost 100% curable if discovered in the in situ stage through the use of the Papanicolaou ("Pap") test. The overall death rate from cancer of the uterus has decreased more than 70% during the last 40 years, due mainly to the Pap smear and regular check-ups.[13]

Responsibility for early detection of cancer rests primarily with the individual. The American Cancer Society, in an effort to help people recognize the early signs of cancer, has developed the *seven warning signals of cancer* (Table 7-6). Since delay in diagnosis and treatment can significantly alter the course of the disease and the success of treatment, it is suggested that persons who manifest any of these signals see their physician as soon as possible. The Society also recommends that *breast self-examination* and *testicular self-examination* be done regularly on a monthly basis.

The methods used in diagnosis and staging of cancer are determined largely by the location and type of cancer suspected. Two diagnostic methods will be discussed in this chapter, the Papanicolaou (Pap) smear and tissue biopsy. The reader is referred to other sources for information regarding other diagnostic procedures.

The Pap test is an example of the type of test called *exfoliative cytology*. It consists of microscopic examination of a properly prepared slide of cells by a cytotechnologist or pathologist for the purpose of detecting the presence of abnormal cells. The usefulness of exfoliative cytology relies on the fact that the membranes of cancer cells lack the cohesive properties and intercellular junctions that are characteristic of normal tissue; therefore, they tend to exfoliate and become mixed with secretions that surround the tumor growth. The routine performance of a Pap smear (once every three years after two initial negative tests done one year apart) in women over age twenty is recommended as a means of detecting in

Table 7-6 Cancer's Seven Warning Signals

*C*hange in bowel or bladder habits
A sore that does not heal
*U*nusual bleeding or discharge
*T*hickening or lump in the breast or elsewhere
*I*ndigestion or difficulty swallowing
*O*bvious change in wart or mole
*N*agging cough or hoarseness

situ cervical cancer.[14] Exfoliative cytology can also be performed on other body secretions, including sputum, nipple drainage, pleural or peritoneal fluid, gastric washings, and others.

A *biopsy* is the removal of a tissue specimen for microscopic study. It may be obtained by needle aspiration (needle biopsy) or by endoscopic methods such as bronchoscopy or cystoscopy, which involve the passage of a scope through an orifice and into the involved structure. In some instances, a surgical incision is made, permitting the entire tumor to be removed if it is small; if the tumor is too large to be removed in its entirety, a specimen may be excised for examination purposes. Tissue diagnosis is of critical importance in designing the treatment plan should cancer cells be found.

:Effects of Cancer

There is probably not a single body function that is not affected by the presence of cancer. Table 7-7 summarizes the general associated effects of cancer. Since tumor cells replace normal parenchymal tissue, the primary area involved will manifest the cancer's effects. For example, cancer of the lung impairs respiratory function; then, as the tumor grows and metastasizes, other structures are affected. Metastasis to bone causes bone pain and predisposes the bones to fractures. (Pain, which is common to practically all types of cancer, is discussed in Chapter 41.)

Cancer disrupts tissue integrity. As the tumor grows, it compresses and erodes blood vessels, causing ulceration and necrosis along with frank bleeding and hemorrhage. For example, one early warning sign of cancer of the bowel is blood in the stool (Table 7-6). The cancer cells may also produce toxins that are destructive to cells in surrounding tissues and further disrupt tissue integrity. Tissue that has been damaged by cancerous growth does not heal normally; rather, the damaged area usually continues to increase in size. Hence the second warning signal—a sore that won't heal.

Cancer has no regard for normal anatomic boundaries—as it grows, it invades and compresses adjacent structures. Abdominal cancer, for example, compresses the viscera and causes bowel obstruction. When cancer affects the brain, it may interfere with the flow of cerebral spinal fluid as well as other cerebral functions. Cancer can penetrate serous cavities, obstructing lymph flow and causing effusion, e.g., pleural effusion and ascites.

Because of its undifferentiated nature, cancerous tissue behaves very differently from the normal tissue type. For example, bronchiogenic carcinoma may elaborate antidiuretic hormone (ADH), parathyroid hormone (PTH), adrenocorticotropin (ACTH), or other substances that have hormone-like actions. The tumor may also produce coagulation factors—which is one reason why cancer patients frequently develop venous thrombosis. Robbins uses the phrase paraneoplastic syndrome to describe symptoms—such as hyponatremia due to excess levels of ADH—that cannot be explained by either local or distant spread of the disease or by elaboration of hormones normally produced by tissue from which the tumor arose.[15] Paraneoplastic syndromes are thought to occur in about 15% of persons with advanced malignant disease.

As the cancer grows, the host wastes and becomes cachectic. *Cachexia* is a grave development, evidenced by wasting of tissues, anorexia, weight loss, weakness and malnutrition. The cancer robs normal tissues of essential nutrients, and although the patient may appear to be eating normally, he shows signs of weight loss. An unexplained weight loss may be the initial problem that causes the person with undiagnosed cancer to seek medical attention. Cachexia is undoubtedly associated with other cancer disease factors such as the depression experienced by many patients, the pain due to the cancer, and the treatment procedures.

:Cancer Treatment

The goals of current treatment methods fall into three categories: curative, palliative, and adjunctive. The most common modalities are surgery, radiation and chemotherapy, and endocrinotherapy. In recent years, immunotherapy has been added to the list of treatment modalities. Often a combination of treatment methods is used.

Surgery

For the most part, surgical intervention methods are designed for the diagnosis and staging of cancer, removal of the tumor, and, when cure cannot be effected, for palliation and relief of symptoms. The type of surgery is determined by the extent of the disease and the structures involved. It may be impossible to remove a cancer if vital tissues must be sacrificed in the process.

Table 7–7   General Effects on Body Function That Are Associated with Cancer Growth

Overall Effect	Related Tumor Action
Altered function of the involved tissue	Destruction and replacement of parenchymal tissue by neoplastic growth
Bleeding and hemorrhage	Compression of blood vessels, with ischemia and necrosis of tissue; or tumor may outgrow its blood supply
Obstruction of hollow viscera or communication pathways	Expansive growth of tumor with compression and invasion of tissues
Effusion in serous cavities	Impaired lymph flow from the serous cavity or erosion of tumor into the cavity
Inappropriate hormone production, e.g., ADH or ACTH secretion by bronchiogenic carcinoma	Production by the tumor of hormones or hormone-like substances which are not regulated by normal feedback mechanisms
Ulceration, necrosis, and infection of tumor area	Ischemia associated with rapid growth with subsequent bacterial invasion
Increased risk of vascular thrombosis	Abnormal production of coagulation factors by the tumor, obstruction of venous channels, and immobility
Anemia	Bleeding and depression of red blood cell production
Bone destruction	Metastatic invasion of bony structures
Hypercalcemia	Destruction of bone due to metastasis and/or production by the tumor of parathyroid hormone or parathyroid-like hormone
Pain	Liberation of pain mediators by the tumor, compression, and/or ischemia of structures
Cachexia, weakness, wasting of tissues	Catabolic effect of the tumor on body metabolism along with selective trapping of nutrients by rapidly growing tumor cells

Radiation

About 50% of patients with cancer receive radiation therapy, either alone or in combination with other forms of treatment. Survival rates approaching 90% have been reported with early detection and treatment of seminoma of the testes, Hodgkin's disease, and cancers of the larynx and cervix.[16] Radiation can be administered by means of either internal or external sources. If external, either an x-ray machine or radioisotopes (such as cobalt 60 or cesium 137) is used. If internal, the radioisotope is packed into needles, beads, seeds, ribbons, or catheters, which are then implanted directly into the tumor.

Ionizing radiation was discovered by Marie and Pierre Curie and Wilhelm Conrad Roentgen just before the turn of the century. Development of the first sealed vacuum x-ray tube followed during the 1920s, along with quantitative methods for measuring radiation dosage. During this same period, Claude Regaud (Foundation Curie in Paris) was able to show that fractionated—small, sublethial—doses of radiation could permanently halt spermatogenesis; whereas, no single lethal dose could do so without causing severe damage to the surrounding tissues. It was this observation that linked radiation to the treatment of cancer. Another advance in radiation therapy followed the atomic bomb with the development of radioactive cobalt. Since then, advances in technology have resulted in the development of sophisticated equipment that produces high-voltage x-ray and electronic beams capable of delivering a thereapeutic dose of radiation to the tumor without causing lethal damage to surrounding tissues.

Radiation acts at the cellular level, causing cell death as particles of radioactive energy disrupt DNA and interfere with cell activity and mitosis. Radiation exerts its greatest effect during certain phases of the cell cycle, particularly during early DNA synthesis of the S phase and in the mitotic or M phase of the cycle. To some extent, radiation is injurious to all cells, but most of all to the poorly differentiated and rapidly proliferating cells of cancer tissue. Radiation also injures such rapidly proliferating cells as those of the bone marrow and the mucosal lining of the gastrointestinal tract. Recovery from sublethal doses of radiation occurs in the interval between the first dose of radiation and subsequent doses. Normal tissue appears to be able to recover from radiation damage more readily than cancerous tissue.

The term *radiosensitivity* describes the sensitivity of cells to radiation, and it varies widely. For example, lymphomas are highly radiosensitive, whereas rhabdomyosarcomas are much less so. The radiation dose that is chosen for treatment of a particular cancer is determined by factors such as the radiosensitivity of the tumor type and the size of the tumor. The *lethal tumor dose* is defined as the dose that achieves 95% tumor control.[17] This dose is divided into a series of *smaller fractionated* doses. With the use of fractionated doses, there is a greater likelihood that the cancer cells will be dividing and in the vulnerable period of the cell cycle. This dose also allows time for normal tissues to repair the radiation damage. Selecting alternate entrance sites for radiation also helps to spare normal tissue. For example, radiation can be directed at an internal tumor from various points marked off on the front, back, and sides of the patient's body so that the maximum radiation is directed at the tumor, while the rest of the body receives only minimal radiation.

There are several factors that seem to alter the tumor's response to irradiation. One of these is tumor oxygenation, with hypoxic tumors being relatively more resistant to radiation than are well-oxygenated tumor cells. Ways to increase oxygen delivery to the tumor during radiation therapy are being studied. Another factor is radiosensitivity. Studies are being conducted in hopes of finding ways to increase the radiosensitivity of tumors, by either altering their DNA in a manner that makes it more sensitive to radiation or by finding ways to make DNA less able to repair radiation damage. Another mechanism for altering a tumor's response to radiation therapy would be to find a way to synchronize the cell cycle so that the radiation can be delivered during the most vulnerable period.

Adverse effects

Since radiation affects all rapidly proliferating cells, it usually causes some adverse effects. Tissues that are most frequently affected are the skin, the mucosal lining of the gastrointestinal tract, and the bone marrow, the radiation effects being dose dependent. With moderate doses of radiation to the skin, the hair falls out either spontaneously or when being combed, by about the 10th to the 14th day. With larger doses, erythema develops (much like a sunburn) which may turn brown; and at very high doses, the skin is denuded. Fortunately, epithelialization takes place after the treatments have been stopped. The effects of irradiation on the oral and pharyngeal mucous membranes are similar to those that occur on the skin. Radiation-induced bone marrow depression leads to a decrease in white blood cell and platelet production and thus to an increased risk of infection and bleeding tendencies. Other systemic signs associated with irradiation include anorexia, nausea, vomiting, fatigue, profuse perspiration, and even chills. These effects are temporary and reversible.

Protection from radiation is a concern of persons who are in contact with patients receiving radiation therapy. The three basic mechanisms of protection are time, distance, and shielding. *Shielding* is practiced by persons who are in contact with radiation for long periods of time, such as radiologists and radiologic technicians; they are shielded by special

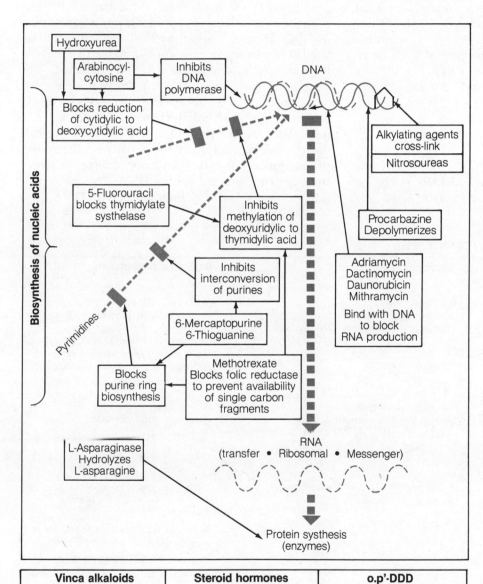

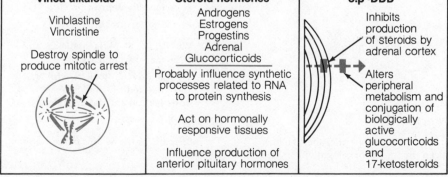

Figure 7–9. Mechanisms of action of cancer chemotherapeutic drugs. (Krakoff IH: Cancer Chemotherapeutic Agents. American Cancer Society, 1977)

walls or body coverings such as lead aprons, gloves, and throat collars. *Time* spent in contact with a radiation source increases exposure. Finally, *distance* must be considered. According to the "inverse square law" that applies to radiation exposure, one can reduce exposure from x-ray or gamma radiation to one-fourth simply by doubling the distance from the radiation source. At a distance of two feet from the radiation source, a person receives one-fourth the exposure that he would receive at a distance of one foot from the source; at a distance of four feet, the exposure is one-fourth that received at a distance of two feet.

Chemotherapy

In the past three decades, cancer chemotherapy has evolved as a major treatment modality. Drugs may be the chief form of treatment or may be used ad-junctively to other treatments. Chemotherapy is now the primary treatment for most hematologic and some solid cancers, including choriocarcinoma, acute and chronic leukemia, Burkitt's lymphoma, and multiple myeloma. Because cancer cells derive from normal cells, they retain many of the latter's properties; thus, chemotherapeutic drugs will affect both the neoplastic and the rapidly proliferating normal cells. Hence, in selecting the drug or drugs to be used, the physician will choose those that have a high affinity for and lethal effect on cancer cells but do not cause widespread destruction of normal cells.

Cancer chemotherapeutic drugs exert their effects through several mechanisms. At the cellular level, they exert their action by interrupting cell growth and replication. They do this by disrupting production of essential enzymes, damaging structural proteins, and inhibiting DNA, RNA, and protein synthesis or direct interaction with DNA (Fig.

Table 7–8   Agents Used in Cancer Chemotherapy

Agent	Mechanism of Action	Major Toxic Manifestations
Alkylating Agents		
Chlorambucil Melphalan Cyclophosphamide Busulfan	Interfere with DNA replication by attacking DNA synthesis throughout the cell cycle	Bone marrow depression with leukopenia, thrombocytopenia, and bleeding; cyclophosphamide may cause alopecia and hemorrhagic cystitis
Antimetabolites		
Methotrexate 6-mercaptopurine 5-fluorouracil Arabinocylcytosine	Structural analogs of essential metabolites and therefore interfere with synthesis of these metabolites	Bone marrow depression, oral and gastrointestinal ulceration
Antibiotics		
Adriamycin Bleomycin Dactinomycin Daunorubicin Mithramycin Mitomycin	Interfere with DNA or RNA synthesis, varying with the drug	Stomatitis, gastrointestinal disturbances, and bone marrow depression
		Adriamycin causes cardiac toxicity at cumulative doses over 500 mg/m^2
		Bleomycin can cause alopecia and pulmonary fibrosis, but only minimal bone marrow depression
Plant Alkaloids		
Vinblastine	Interfere with mitosis	Vinblastine alopecia, areflexia, and bone marrow depression
Vincristine		Vincristine neurotoxicity with ataxia and impaired fine motor skills. Constipation and paralytic ileus
Steroid Hormones		
Androgens Estrogens Progestins Adrenocorticosteroids	Cell cycle nonspecific; alter the host environment for cell growth	Specific for the actions of the hormone

7-9). By their mechanism of action, the anticancer drugs may be classified as either cell cycle specific or cell cycle nonspecific. Drugs are *cell cycle specific* if they exert their action during a specific phase of the cell cycle. For example, methotrexate, an antimetabolite, acts by interfering with DNA synthesis and thereby interrupts the S phase of the cell cycle. Drugs that are *cell cycle nonspecific* affect cancer cells through all phases of the cell cycle. The steroid hormones are considered to be cell cycle nonspecific. The administration of unphysiologic doses of some of the steroid hormones has been shown to alter the hormone environment of the host and modify the growth of some tumors that are particularly sensitive to hormonal influences. Chemotherapeutic drugs that have similar structures and effects on the cell cycle are generally grouped together, and these drugs usually have similar toxic and side-effects (Table 7-8). Because they differ in their mechanisms of action, combinations of cell cycle specific and cell cycle nonspecific agents are often used to treat cancer.

Side-effects

To understand the problems related to cancer drugs, the reader needs to appreciate what these drugs do to normal cells. The most pronounced effects are seen in the rapidly proliferating normal tissues.

Gastrointestinal tract.   Anorexia, nausea, vomiting, and diarrhea are common problems. They occur within minutes or hours of drug taking and are thought to be due to stimulation of the chemoreceptor trigger zone (vomiting center) in the medulla or the autonomic nervous system. The symptoms usually subside within 24 to 48 hours and often can be relieved by antiemetics. Some drugs cause stomatitis and damage to the rapidly proliferating cells of the gastrointestinal mucosal lining.

Bone marrow depression.   Most of these drugs suppress bone marrow function and formation of blood cells, leading to anemia, leukopenia, and thrombocytopenia. With severe granulocytopenia there is particular risk for developing serious infections.

Alopecia.   Many of these drugs impair hair follicle function with resulting loss of hair. However, the hair tends to regrow when treatment is stopped.

Germinal tissues.   The rapidly proliferating structures of the reproductive system are particularly sensitive to these drugs. Women may experience changes in menstrual flow or amenorrhea. Men may

develop oligospermia and azoospermia. Many of these agents may have teratogenic or mutagenic effects leading to fetal abnormalities.

Immunotherapy

Immunotherapy remains largely investigational and is usually used in conjunction with other forms of treatment. Immunotherapeutic methods fall into three categories. The first is *active nonspecific immune therapy*, whose purpose is to stimulate the immune response. One such agent is BCG (bacillus Calmette-Guérin), an attenuated strain of the bacterium that causes bovine tuberculosis. The second method is *specific immune therapy*, a method that is somewhat similar to immunization in that it involves the use of antigens from either the patient's tumor or from another patient with an antigenically similar tumor, as a challenge to the patient's immune system to produce immune cells against the tumor antigen. The third is *transfer of passive tumor immunity*, which is accomplished through the administration of antisera or effector substances. Transfer factor is an extract of stimulated lymphocytes that are capable of transferring specific delayed hypersensitivity to other lymphocytes.

In summary, a neoplasm is a new growth, the abnormal proliferation of a tissue type. It may be either benign or malignant. The growth of a benign tumor is restricted to the site of origin, and will not cause death unless by its location it interferes with vital functions. Cancers or malignant neoplasms, on the other hand, grow wildly and without organization, spread to distant parts of the body, and cause death unless checked. The emphasis in cancer treatment focuses on early detection, because most cancers can be successfully treated if detected early.

:Study Guide

After you have studied this chapter, you should be able to meet the following objectives:

: : Describe the five phases of the cell cycle.

: : Contrast benign and malignant neoplasms.

: : Explain the pathogenesis of metastasis.

: : State the purpose of clinical staging in cancer.

: : Relate environmental factors to the development of cancer.

: : Describe the surveillance capacity of the immune system.

: : State the significance of exfoliative cytology.

: : Describe the general effects of cancer on body systems.

: : Explain the rationale for the use of radiation to treat cancer.

: : Explain the mechanisms of chemotherapeutic agents in treatment of cancer.

:References

1. Cancer Facts. New York, American Cancer Society, 1981
2. Baserga R: The cell cycle. N Engl J Med 304:453, 1981
3. Lynch HT: Familial risk and cancer control. J Am Med Assoc 236, No. 6:585, 1976
4. Robbins SL, Cotran RS: Pathologic Basis of Disease, p 206. Philadelphia, WB Saunders, 1979
5. Knudson AG: Heredity and human cancer. Am J Pathol 77, No. 1:77, 1974
6. Robbins SL, Cotran RS: Pathologic Basis of Disease, p 202. Philadelphia, WB Saunders, 1979
7. Robbins SL, Cotran RS: Pathologic Basis of Disease, p 173. Philadelphia, WB Saunders, 1979
8. Poskanzer DC, Herbst AL: Epidemiology of vaginal adenosis and adenocarcinoma associated with exposure to stilbestrol in utero. Cancer 39, No. 4:1890, 1977
9. Nicholson WJ: Cancer following occupational exposure to asbestos and vinyl chloride. Cancer 39, No. 4:1792, 1977
10. Favus MJ et al: Thyroid cancer occurring as a late consequence of head and neck irradiation: Evaluation of 1056 patients. N Engl J Med 294:1019, 1976
11. Jablon S, Kato H: Studies of the mortality of A-bomb survivors: V. Radiation dose and mortality, 1950-1970. Radiat Res 50:649, 1972
12. Burnett FM: Immunological aspects of malignant disease. Lancet 1:1171, 1967
13. Cancer Facts and Figures, p 16. New York, American Cancer Society, 1981
14. Cancer Facts and Figures, p 16. New York, American Cancer Society, 1981
15. Robbins SL, Cotran RS: Pathologic Basis of Disease, p 190. Philadelphia, WB Saunders, 1979
16. Bloomer WD, Hellman S: Normal tissue responses to radiation therapy. N Engl J Med 293:80, 1975
17. Rubin P, Poulter C: Principles of radiation and cancer radiotherapy. In Rubin P (ed): Clinical Oncology, 5th ed, p 33. Rochester, NY, The University of Rochester School of Medicine and Dentistry, 1978

Burnett FM: Immunological aspects of malignant disease. Lancet 1:1171, 1967
Fagan-Dubin L: Causes of cancer. Cancer Nurs 2, No. 6:435, 1979
Frye RJM, Aninsworth EJ: Radiation injury: Some aspects of the oncogenic effects. Fed Proc 36, No. 5:1703, 1977
Heidelberger C: Chemical carcinogenesis. Annu Rev Biochem 44:79, 1975
Jackson B, Armenaki DW: A tumor classification system. Am J Nurs 76, No. 8:1320, 1976
Lynch HT, Brokley FD, Lynch P et al: Familial risk and cancer control. JAMA 236, No. 6:582, 1976
Lynch HT, Guirgis H, Lynch PM et al: Familial cancer syndromes: A survey. Cancer 39:1967, 1977
McGuire DB: Familial cancer and the role of the nurse. Cancer Nurs 2, No. 6:443, 1979
Nirenberg A: High-dose methotrexate. Am J Nurs 76, No. 11:1776, 1976
Regato JA, Spjut H: Ackerman and deRegato's Cancer: Diagnosis, Treatment and Prognosis. St Louis, CV Mosby, 1975
Schwind JV: Cancer: Regressive evolution. Oncology 29:172, 1974
Winters WD: Viruses and cancer. Am J Nurs 78, No. 2:249, 1978

:Additional References

Bingham CA: The cell cycle and cancer chemotherapy. Am J Nurs 78, No. 7:1201, 1978
Bloomer WD, Hellman S: Normal tissue responses to radiation therapy. N Engl J Med 293, No. 2:80, 1975

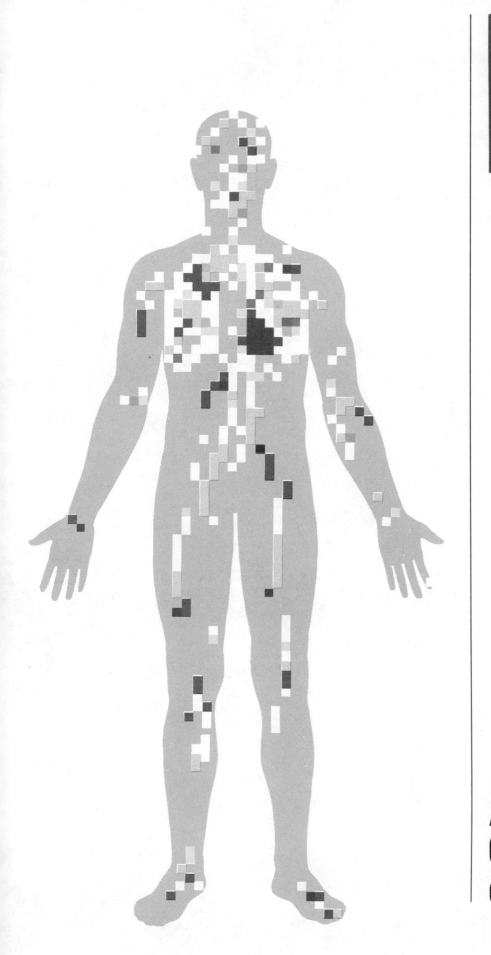

Alterations in Oxygenation of Tissues

Latest estimates indicate that over 40 million persons in the United States have cardiovascular disease. Heart attack is the nation's number one killer, having claimed 641,100 deaths in 1978. Eight out of every 1000 children are born with congenital heart defects, and rheumatic fever affects 100,000 children and 1,750,000 adults. Each year heart disease strikes many persons during the peak of their productive years. Heart and blood vessel diseases cost the nation an average of 46.2 billion dollars in 1981.[1]

In an attempt to focus on heart problems that affect otherwise healthy persons in all segments of the life cycle, this unit centers on (1) control of cardiac function, (2) coronary heart disease, (3) rheumatic heart disease, (4) congenital heart defects, and (5) congestive heart failure. It includes discussions on disorders of the blood vessels, the heart, the respiratory system, and the red blood cells.

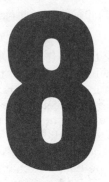

Control of Blood Flow

The blood vessels of the cardiovascular system serve as tubes through which fluids, nutrients, wastes, and other materials in the blood are transported as they travel to and from the cells. The arterial system carries blood to the cells, and the venous system transports blood back to the heart (Fig. 8-1). The capillaries connect the arterial and venous systems and it is here that the tissue exchange of nutrients and wastes occurs. This chapter focuses on vessel structure, the mechanics of blood flow, and factors that obstruct flow.

:Vessel Structure

All of the blood vessels, except the capillaries, have walls composed of three layers (Fig. 8-2). The tunica externa, or tunica adventitia, is the outermost covering of the vessel. This layer is composed of fibrous and connective tissue that serves to support the vessel. The middle layer, the tunica media, is largely smooth muscle that constricts and relaxes in order to control the diameter of the vessel. The inner layer, the tunica intima, creates a smooth and slippery inner surface of the vessel. The intima has an elastic

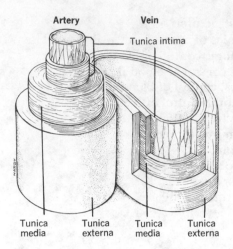

Figure 8–2.   Medium-sized artery and vein showing the relative thickness of the three layers. (Chaffee EE, Lytle IM: Basic Physiology and Anatomy, 4th ed. Philadelphia, JB Lippincott, 1980)

layer that joins the media and a thin layer of smooth epithelial cells that lie adjacent to the blood.

The layers of the vessel wall vary with the function of the vessel. Arteries are thick-walled vessels with large amounts of elastic fibers. The elasticity of these vessels allows them to stretch during cardiac systole and to recoil during diastole. The arterioles, which are predominantly smooth muscle, are the resistance vessels of the body. Sympathetic vasomotor tone enables these vessels to constrict or to relax as needed in order to maintain blood pressure.

The venules and veins are thin-walled, distensible, and collapsible vessels. The structure of the veins is such that it allows these vessels to act as a reservoir, or blood storage system. The venous system is a low-pressure system that relies on muscle pumps to help return blood to the heart. The valves within the veins prevent retrograde or backward flow of blood and help return blood to the heart.

The capillaries are microscopic, single-thickness vessels that connect the arterial and venous segments of the vascular system. Exchange of gases, nutrients, and waste materials takes place at the capillary level.

Figure 8–1.   Diagram of the arteries, arterioles; the veins, venules; and the capillaries of the circulatory system.

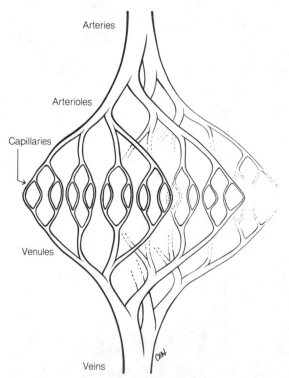

:Mechanics of Blood Flow

Blood flow is governed by many of the same factors that control fluid movement in other systems, such as in the plumbing in a house. Fluid movement is determined by four basic conditions: (1) the difference in pressure between the two ends of the tube, (2) the diameter of the tube, (3) the length of the tube, and (4) the viscosity, or thickness, of the fluid moving through the tube (Fig. 8-3). Blood flow is increased when the pressure difference between the two ends of a vessel is increased, or when the diameter of the vessel is enlarged. Conversely, flow is decreased when the length of the vessel, through which the blood must pass, is increased or when the viscosity of the blood is increased.

The velocity, or speed, at which blood flows through a vessel is determined by the cross-sectional area of the vessel (Fig. 8-4). Assuming that flow is held constant, a decrease in the cross-sectional area of the vessel will cause the velocity of flow to increase. Conversely, increasing the cross-sectional area will cause the velocity to decrease. The reader might want to relate this concept to the act of whistling—when the lips are pursed, and the cross-sectional area is reduced, the velocity of airflow is increased to the point that a whistling sound is produced.

There are two types of energy that create flow and pressure in the vascular system—kinetic (active) energy and potential (stored) energy (Fig. 8-5). Kinetic energy is involved in velocity or the forward movement of blood. Potential energy produces a lateral pressure or stretching of the vessel. Potential energy is converted to active energy when the vessel wall rebounds after being stretched. The total energy in the system is the sum of the two energies (total energy = kinetic energy + potential energy). This means that energy used for forward movement of blood (kinetic energy) cannot be stored as potential energy. Referring back to Figure 8-4, it can be seen that the velocity of kinetic energy in sections 1 and 3 is decreased, whereas the lateral pressure will be high in these segments. In section 2, however, the kinetic energy (velocity) is great, while the lateral pressure is low. In vascular disease, the diameter of blood vessels is often altered, causing disruption in blood flow.

Laminar or streamlined blood flow is smooth flow in which the blood components are layered so that the plasma is adjacent to the smooth, slippery surface of the vessel wall, and the cellular components, including the platelets, are in the center of the blood stream (Fig. 8-6). This arrangement reduces friction by allowing the blood layers to slide smoothly over each other. Structural changes in the vessel wall often disrupt flow and produce turbulence. During turbulent flow, platelets and other

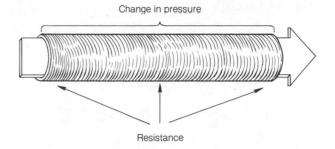

$$\text{Flow } Q = \frac{\text{Change in pressure} \times \pi \text{ radius}^4}{8 \times \text{length} \times \text{viscosity}}$$

Figure 8–3. Diagram of the factors that affect blood flow. Increasing the pressure difference between the two ends of the vessel or enlarging the diameter of the vessel causes flow to increase. Increasing the length or the viscosity of the fluid causes flow to decrease. Flow diminishes as resistance increases. Resistance is directly proportional to blood viscosity and the length of the tube, and inversely proportional to the fourth power of the radius.

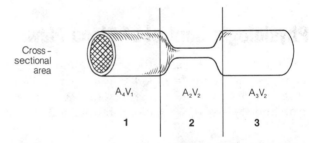

Figure 8–4. Effect of cross-sectional area on velocity of flow. In section 1, velocity is low due to an increase in cross-sectional area. In section 2, velocity is increased due to a decrease in cross-sectional area. In section 3, velocity is low again.

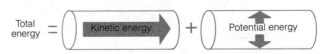

Figure 8–5. Total energy in the vascular system is spent either moving blood forward or in stretching the vessel wall.

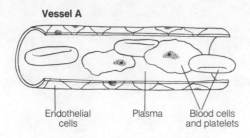

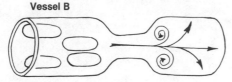

Figure 8–6. Diagram of laminar flow in blood vessels. Vessel *A* illustrates laminar flow in which the plasma layer is adjacent to the vessel endothelial layer and blood cells are in the center of the blood stream. Vessel *B* depicts the presence of turbulent flow. The axial location of the platelets and other blood cells is disturbed.

coagulation factors come in contact with the endothelial layer of the vessel and predispose to clot formation.

:Physiologic Control of Blood Flow

In the circulatory system, the pressure and resistance changes that regulate blood flow are controlled by three factors: (1) local tissue factors, (2) neural control, and (3) humoral, or blood-borne, substances.

Local Control of Blood Flow

Local control is governed largely by the nutritional needs of the tissue. For example, blood flow to organs such as the heart, brain, and kidney remains relatively constant, even though blood pressure may vary over a range of about 60 to 180 mm Hg. The ability of tissues to control their own blood flow is called autoregulation. Autoregulation of blood flow is controlled by local factors, such as oxygen lack or accumulation of tissue metabolites. It involves the selective opening and closing of capillary channels. Local control is particularly important in tissues such as skeletal muscle, which has varying blood flow requirements according to the level of activity.

An increase in blood flow to a part is called *hyperemia*. When the blood supply to an area has been occluded and then restored, local blood flow through the tissues increases within seconds to restore the metabolic equilibrium of the tissues. This increased flow is called reactive hyperemia. The ability of tissues to increase blood flow in situations of increased activity, e.g., exercise, is called functional hyperemia. Local control mechanisms rely on a continuous flow from the main arteries and, therefore, blood flow through these channels cannot increase when these vessels are narrowed. For example, if a major coronary artery becomes occluded, the opening of capillary channels supplied by that vessel cannot restore flow.

Collateral circulation is a mechanism for long-term regulation of local blood flow. In the heart and other vital structures, there are anastomotic channels between some of the smaller arteries. When a main vessel becomes occluded these anastomotic channels increase in size, and within a short period of time, blood flow through these collateral vessels greatly increases. For example, persons with extensive obstruction in a major coronary artery may rely on collateral circulation to meet the oxygen needs of the myocardial tissue normally supplied by that vessel. As with other long-term compensatory mechanisms, the recruitment of collateral circulation is most efficient when obstruction to flow is gradual rather than sudden.

Neural Control of Blood Flow

Neural control of blood flow is largely mediated through the sympathetic nervous system. The sympathetic nervous system innervates both the arterial and venous systems. Increasing sympathetic activity causes constriction of some vessels, such as those of the skin, the gastrointestinal tract, and the kidney. Skeletal muscle is innervated by both vasoconstrictor and vasodilator fibers.

Humoral Control of Blood Flow

Humoral regulation causes vessels to either constrict or dilate. For example, angiotensin and vasopressin are potent vasoconstrictors; whereas histamine and bradykinin are vasodilators.

:Obstruction to Flow

Interruption of flow in either the arterial or the venous system interferes with flow of oxygen and nutrients to the tissues. Alterations in arterial flow produce ischemia or the temporary "holding back" of blood from the tissues. Venous obstruction, on the other hand, causes congestion and edema.

Occlusion of flow within a vessel can result from (1) thrombus formation, (2) emboli, (3) vessel injury, (4) compression, (5) vasospasm, or (6) structural changes in the vessel (Fig. 8-7). Each of these mechanisms is discussed briefly in preparation for the discussion on specific alterations in arterial and venous flow.

Thrombus Formation

A thrombus is a blood clot. Blood clotting is a homeostatic mechanism intended to seal off blood vessels, to prevent bleeding, and to maintain the continuity of the vascular system. A thrombus can develop in either the arterial or the venous system and it obstructs flow. Alterations in hemostasis will be discussed in Chapter 11.

Embolus

An embolus is a foreign mass that is transported in the blood stream. Although an embolus moves freely in the larger blood vessels, it becomes lodged and obstructs flow once it reaches a smaller vessel. An embolus can be a *dislodged thrombus*, and can consist of *air*, *fat*, *tumor cells*, or *other materials*. Approximately 95% of venous emboli have their origin in the veins of the legs. These emboli move through the venous system, into the right heart, and then into the pulmonary circulation where they become

Figure 8–7.   Diagram of conditions that cause disruption of blood flow.

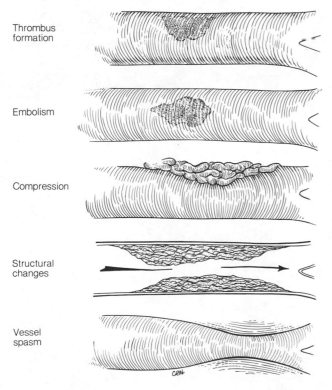

Thrombus formation

Embolism

Compression

Structural changes

Vessel spasm

lodged and obstruct blood flow. Arterial emboli commonly have their origin in the heart itself and can travel to the brain, spleen, kidney, or vessels in the lower extremity before they become lodged and obstruct flow.

Compression

Compression of the vessel lumen occurs when pressures outside the vessel exceed those within the vessel lumen. Because of the low intraluminal pressure in the venous system, these vessels are more easily compressed than are the arterial vessels. It should be emphasized, however, that application of any restrictive, circular device (elastic bandage, plaster cast, or tourniquet) to an extremity affords the potential for mechanically compressing and obstructing arterial flow. *The need for caution in situations in which such appliances are used cannot be overemphasized.* Nerve damage, loss of function, and even the need to amputate an extremity, have resulted from improper application of a cast, tourniquet, or circular bandage.

The small arteries, capillaries, and venules in the tissues covering the bony prominences are easily compressed when body weight is supported at these points. This can occur in tissues over the sacrum, scapula, and heels when a person is lying flat on the back and in tissues of the ears, shoulders, hips, and ankles when the body is on its side. The arterial and capillary pressures are such that a force of about seven pounds per square inch is often sufficient to shut off blood flow. Because the entire weight of the body is often supported by the bony prominences, it is not difficult to understand why blood flow to the tissues that cover these skeletal structures is occluded. Redness of these tissues, due to reactive hyperemia following a change in position, suggests that at least partial occlusion of blood flow to the area has occurred. Most of us move around in sleep and during other activities so that we do not experience loss of blood flow due to vessel compression over the bony prominences. For the person who is bedridden and cannot move, however, disruption of blood flow to the tissues in these areas often predisposes to tissue injury and the development of decubitus ulcers—the so-called bedsores or pressure sores.

Vasospasm

Vasospasm may result from locally or neurally mediated reflexes. Exposure to cold causes severe vasoconstriction in many of the superficial blood vessels. Fortunately, local control mechanisms produce brief periods of vasodilatation designed to maintain tissue oxygen needs. Those who have spent time on the ski slopes, or elsewhere in the cold, may have noticed the intermittent redness of their companions' noses during these periods of vasodilatation. In certain disease states, vasospasm from exposure to cold or other stimuli is excessive and may lead to ischemia and tissue injury.

Structural Changes

Structural changes in blood vessels can take many forms. Defects in venous valves may impair blood flow in the venous system causing varicose veins. Arteriosclerosis causes rigidity and narrowing of the arterioles. Aneurysms are dilatations in arteries that appear at points where the vessel wall has been weakened. Structural alterations in the arterial and venous systems are discussed in Chapters 9 and 10.

In summary, blood vessels serve as a transport system for body fluids, with the arterial system carrying fluids from the heart to the cells of the body, and the venous system carrying these fluids back to the heart. The exchange of tissue nutrients and wastes occurs at the capillary level. The flow of blood in the circulatory system can be impaired due to: (1) presence of a thrombus, (2) emboli, (3) vessel injury, (4) vessel compression, (5) vasospasm, or (6) structural changes within the vessel.

:Study Guide

After you have studied this chapter, you should be able to meet the following objectives:

: : State the factors that regulate blood flow.

: : Describe the physiologic regulation of blood flow on the basis of its local, neural, and humoral components.

: : State the contribution of thrombi and emboli to occlusion of blood flow.

: : Explain the use of restrictive devices on a body part.

:Reference

1. American Heart Association: Heart Facts. Dallas, 1981

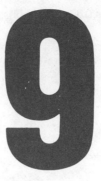

Alterations in Arterial Flow

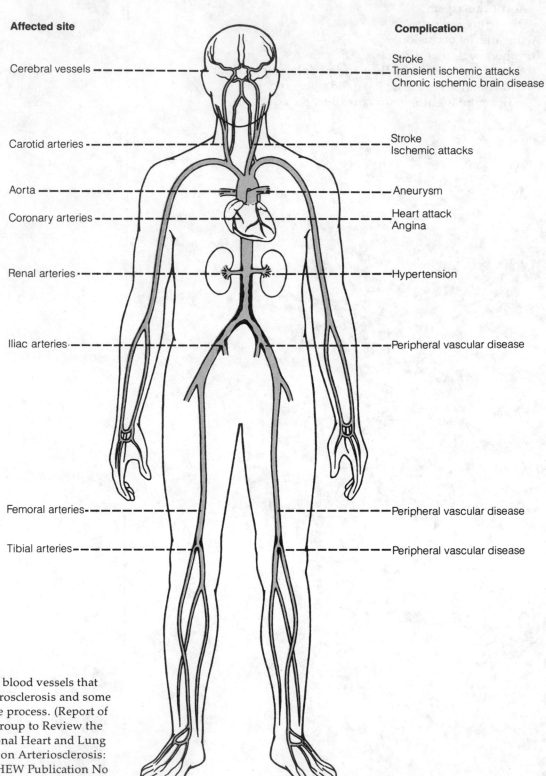

Affected site

Cerebral vessels

Carotid arteries

Aorta

Coronary arteries

Renal arteries

Iliac arteries

Femoral arteries

Tibial arteries

Complication

Stroke
Transient ischemic attacks
Chronic ischemic brain disease

Stroke
Ischemic attacks

Aneurysm

Heart attack
Angina

Hypertension

Peripheral vascular disease

Peripheral vascular disease

Peripheral vascular disease

Figure 9–1.   Major blood vessels that are affected by atherosclerosis and some complications of the process. (Report of the 1977 Working Group to Review the Report by the National Heart and Lung Institute Task Force on Arteriosclerosis: Arteriosclerosis, DHEW Publication No NIH 78–1526)

Pathology of the arterial system affects body function through impaired blood flow. Generally speaking, impairment of arterial flow results from (1) an obstruction within the lumen of the vessel, such as a thrombus or an embolus, (2) pathologic changes that produce narrowing of the vessel lumen, or (3) vasospasm or constriction of the vessel. Aneurysms are dilatations that form in a weakened vessel wall. This chapter centers on arteriosclerosis, aneurysms, acute arterial occlusion, and the peripheral vascular diseases—Raynaud's disease and Buerger's disease. Although coronary heart disease is a major manifestation of atherosclerosis, the process affects other vessels in the body, and for this reason it is discussed here.

Vascular disease is a relatively silent disorder. To be more explicit, the diseased vessel itself seldom gives rise to symptoms that warn of its presence. Rather, signs and symptoms arise because of ischemia in the body part that is served by the vessel. The angina associated with coronary heart disease, and the intermittent claudication (pain and weakness in the leg occurring with exercise), provide evidence of impaired blood flow to the lower extremities. Unfortunately, arterial disease is usually far advanced at the time that these symptoms occur.

:Arteriosclerosis

Arteriosclerosis is a general term that literally means *hardening of the arteries*. The term describes several conditions. One form of arteriosclerosis, Mönckeberg's medial sclerosis, affects the media of medium-sized arteries and is characterized by a hyaline thickening of the arterioles and small blood vessels. Because this form of arteriosclerosis does not encroach on the lumen of the vessel, there is no interference with normal flow. This chapter addresses the most common form of arteriosclerosis—atherosclerosis.

Atherosclerosis

Atherosclerosis is the leading cause of death in the United States. In 1975, 52% of all deaths were due to cardiovascular disease, and 86% of these deaths were due to complications of atherosclerosis.[1]

The lesions of atherosclerosis are found primarily in the intima of medium and large arteries—the *aorta* and its branches, the *coronaries*, and the *large vessels* that supply the *brain* (Fig. 9-1). These lesions eventually progress to affect the adjacent medial layer of the vessel. Atherosclerosis is a slow process that causes no symptoms until a critical vessel is occluded (Fig. 9-2). These vessel changes apparently begin at an early age. Among the 300 American soldiers (average age 22) killed during the Korean war, 77% were found to have gross evidence of atherosclerosis.[2]

Morphologically, atherosclerotic lesions include (1) plaques (atheroma), which consist of elevated

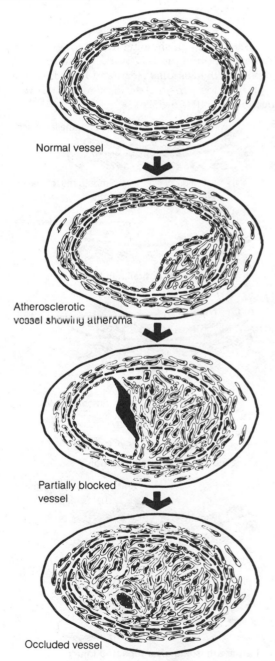

Figure 9–2.   Evolution of occlusion in an atherosclerotic vessel. (Report of the 1977 Working Group to Review the Report by the National Heart and Lung Institute Task Force on Arteriosclerosis: Arteriosclerosis, DHEW Publication No NIH 78–1526)

Normal vessel

Atherosclerotic vessel showing atheroma

Partially blocked vessel

Occluded vessel

fibrofatty infiltrates in the intima wall; and (2) complicated lesions that contain hemorrhage, ulceration, calcium deposits, and scar tissue. There is considerable controversy about whether the fatty streaks found in apparently normal vessels are precursors of atherosclerotic lesions. These fatty streaks are present in the aortas of all children at 10 years of age and in the coronary vessels during the second decade of life.[3] It has been suggested that the fatty streaks may form a vulnerable link among the various risk factors and the development of overt atherosclerotic lesions.

The mechanisms involved in the development of atherosclerosis are largely unknown. Normally, the intact endothelial layer of the vessel forms a barrier that protects the subendothelial layer. One theory suggests that injury to the endothelial layer, along with abnormal proliferation of smooth muscle cells, plays a role in atheroma formation (Fig. 9-3). Injury to the endothelial layer permits interaction of the subendothelial cells with platelets, other coagulation factors, and plasma components. This is followed by abnormal proliferation of smooth muscle cells, with accumulation of collagen, lipids, and other cell products. A number of factors are regarded as possible injurious agents, including products associated with smoking, immune mechanisms, and mechanical stress such as that associated with hypertension and chronic hyperlipidemia. If the injury is a single event, the lesion may be reversible. However, if the injury is chronic and continues for a long period of time there is less time for healing to occur and the lesions become progressive.

Figure 9–3. Diagram showing theory for evolution of atheroma. (Report of the 1977 Working Group to Review the Report by the National Heart and Lung Institute Task Force on Arteriosclerosis: Arteriosclerosis, DHEW Publication No NIH 78–1526)

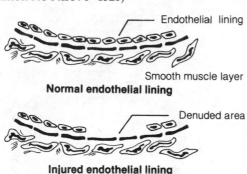

Endothelial lining

Smooth muscle layer

Normal endothelial lining

Denuded area

Injured endothelial lining

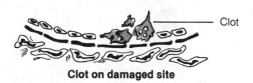

Clot

Clot on damaged site

Smooth muscle cells

Smooth muscle cells multiply

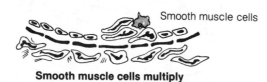

Smooth muscle, collagen, lipids, cell products

Atheroma

Site of repeated injury

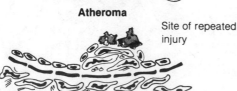

Larger atheroma after repeated injury

Risk factors

Regardless of the nature of the cellular events that occur during the development of atherosclerosis, epidemiologic studies have identified risk factors associated with its occurrence. These risk factors are listed in Table 9-1.

Established risk factors. Some risk factors are more definitively associated with atherosclerosis than others. The established risk factors include high cholesterol levels, hypertension, and smoking.

Lipoproteins. The association between high levels of cholesterol and the development of atherosclerosis

Table 9-1 Examples of Risk Factors

Established Risk Factors

> High concentration of blood cholesterol, particularly low-density lipoproteins (LDL)
> High blood pressure
> Cigarette smoking

Probable Risk Factors

> Diabetes mellitus and impaired glucose tolerance
> Stress and coronary-prone behavior
> Postmenopausal state
> Family history and genetic factors
> Contraceptive pills

Suspected Risk Factors

> Overweight
> Physical inactivity

(From: A Report by the National Heart and Lung Institute Task Force on Arteriosclerosis: Arteriosclerosis, p 19, 1977) has been appreciated for a number of years. Because lipids are insoluble in plasma, they bind to certain fat-carrying proteins—the lipoproteins—for transport in the blood. It has been suggested that it is the level of these lipoproteins, rather than the cholesterol level, that is correlated with atherosclerosis. There are three types of lipoproteins: (1) very low-density lipoproteins (VLDL); (2) low-density lipoproteins (LDL); and (3) high-density lipoproteins (HDL). The explanation for the naming of these proteins comes from the ultracentrifugation method by which the proteins are separated according to their density. The greater the ratio of lipids to protein, the lower the density; in other words, the VLDL carry large amounts of lipids compared with the HDL. The LDL are closely correlated with an increased incidence of atherosclerosis and coronary heart disease. On the other hand, a decreased incidence of coronary heart disease is seen in persons with high levels of HDL.

The liver synthesizes and secretes primarily VLDL and HDL, and the intestine may also produce VLDL. The VLDL are removed from the plasma in the capillary beds and are degraded to form triglycerides and an intermediate lipoprotein that is eventually converted to LDL. The LDL are major carriers of cholesterol. In the peripheral tissues, including the arterial walls, the cholesterol-carrying LDL enters the cell in which the protein portion of the lipoprotein is degraded, leaving the cholesterol without a carrier. Cholesterol is not metabolized in the peripheral tissues and would accumulate if there were no mechanism available for its removal. It is now believed that the HDL serve as carriers that remove the cholesterol from the peripheral tissues and transport it back to the liver for catabolism and excretion.[4] The HDL are also believed to inhibit cellular uptake of LDL. These two mechanisms help to explain the protective effect that the HDL have been observed to afford in relation to the risk of coronary heart disease. It has been observed that HDL levels are increased in trained individuals who exercise regularly, and in persons who consume a moderate amount of alcohol. On the other hand, smoking and diabetes are associated with low levels of HDL.

There are several genetic defects in lipoprotein metabolism that are associated with the increased incidence of atherosclerosis. One is a familial dysbetalipoproteinemia (type III hyperlipidemia) in which there is an accumulation of the intermediate lipoproteins formed from degradation of the VLDL. Not all of the LDL are necessarily derived from the VLDL. In another type of genetic disorder—familial hypercholesteremia—LDL is secreted directly by the liver.

The most common method for measuring lipoproteins is electrophoresis. The different classes of lipoproteins differ in their electrical charge, particle size, and adsorption to paper. In the most common procedure for electrophoresis, a drop of plasma is placed on a filter paper and put into an electrophoretic cell containing a buffer solution with albumin. The electric field created in the solution causes the lipoproteins to migrate on the paper strip and separate into distinct bands.

Blood pressure. Blood pressure levels are closely correlated with coronary heart disease. The risk of coronary artery disease in men 30 to 59 years of age with a diastolic pressure above 105 mm Hg is reported to be almost four times greater than it is when the diastolic pressure is less than 85 mm Hg.[5] Hypertension increases the risk of atherosclerosis more markedly when associated with other risk factors, such as diabetes mellitus and cigarette smoking.

Cigarette smoking. Cigarette smoking is closely linked with coronary heart disease and sudden death. The risk of death from coronary heart disease is about 60 to 70 times greater for smokers than nonsmokers.[6] The greatest effects of smoking are noted in younger men and women, particularly those below the age of 55. The effects are directly related to the number of cigarettes smoked.

Probable and suspected risk factors. The association between coronary heart disease and the probable and suspected risk factors is not as convincing as it is for the established risk factors. These factors often are linked with the established or other risk factors. For example, obesity and physical inactivity are often observed in the same individual. Furthermore, both of these situations are reported to bring about alterations in lipid levels. Likewise, smoking patterns, blood pressure levels, and other risk factors are closely associated with stress and personality patterns.

Prevention. At the present time there is no known cure for atherosclerosis; efforts are directed at its prevention and at ways to halt its progression. As was mentioned earlier, the presence of atherosclerotic changes in young soldiers killed in the Korean War suggests that the process starts at an early age. It therefore seems apparent that prevention cannot be delayed until the middle years when symptoms of atherosclerosis begin to manifest themselves. As the late Dr. Paul Dudley White so aptly stressed, prevention of atherosclerosis needs to begin at the time of conception based on wise and prudent health prac-

Berry aneurysm

Aneurysm of abdominal aorta

Dissecting aneurysm
(longitudinal section)

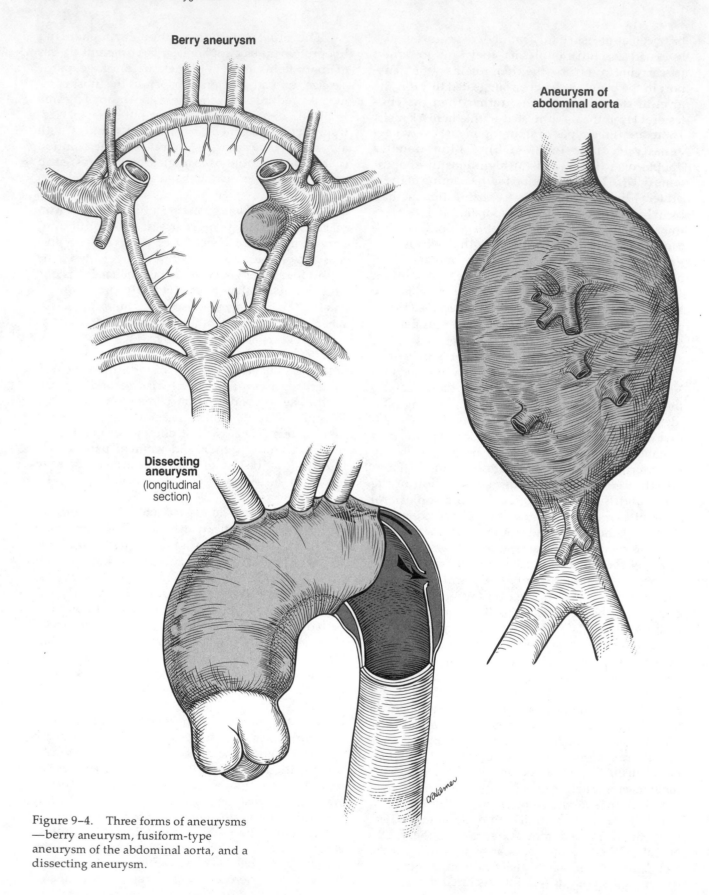

Figure 9–4. Three forms of aneurysms
—berry aneurysm, fusiform-type
aneurysm of the abdominal aorta, and a
dissecting aneurysm.

tices of the expectant mother, and it then needs to be continued after birth by the wise and careful parenting efforts of both father and mother.*

:Aneurysms

As has been stated, an aneurysm is an abnormal dilatation caused by a weakness in the arterial wall. Aneurysms can assume several forms and are classified according to their anatomic features (Fig. 9-4). A saccular aneurysm extends over part of the circumference of the vessel and is sac-like in appearance. A fusiform aneurysm involves the medial layer of the entire vessel circumference. The weakness in the vessel wall that leads to aneurysm formation may be due to any of several factors, including congenital defects, trauma, infections, and arteriosclerosis. Because it is impossible within the scope of this book to discuss all of the various types of aneurysms, the discussion is confined to berry aneurysms and aortic aneurysms.

Berry Aneurysms

Berry aneurysms are those that occur in the intracranial arteries, usually within the circle of Willis (Fig. 9-4). The lesions are typically small and balloon shaped; it is not uncommon for multiple lesions to be present. It is thought that berry aneurysms are congenital, arising from a weakening of the vessel wall which has existed for years. Approximately 10% to 15% of deaths from cerebral vascular accidents are due to rupture of a berry aneurysm. Such hemorrhages occur most often in middle-aged individuals with a history of hypertension.

Aortic Aneurysms

Aortic aneurysms were, until recently, caused largely by tertiary syphilis. Now, with better control of syphilis, atherosclerosis has advanced to become the leading cause of aneurysmal development. Although any section of the aorta can be involved, the majority of lesions affect the abdominal aorta. Multiple aneurysms may be present. Because an aortic aneurysm is of arterial origin, the affected person often complains of an awareness of a pulsating mass in the abdomen. Complications associated with aortic aneurysm depend on its location and size. The aneurysm may extend to impinge on the renal, iliac,

---

*From a speech given by Dr. Paul Dudley White which the author was privileged to attend.

or mesenteric arteries. Stasis of blood favors thrombus formation along the wall of the vessel. If the aneurysm is large, the complication most feared is rupture.

Dissecting Aneurysms

A type of aortic aneurysm that is not necessarily associated with atherosclerosis is a dissecting aneurysm. This is one in which there is destruction and necrosis of the smooth muscle and elastic tissue of the aorta. Necrosis of the media is not necessarily associated with outpouching of the vessel wall, described earlier, although such defects may be present. The cause of dissecting aneurysms is unclear, although recent evidence suggests a metabolic defect in vessel wall synthesis.

Bleeding into the necrotic area between the layers of the vessel wall is characteristic of the dissecting aneurysm. With continued bleeding, there is a longitudinal tearing apart—a dissection—of the vessel layers (Fig. 9-4). Approximately 75% of dissections have their origin in the ascending aorta. Dissection is usually bidirectional, moving proximally toward the heart, and distally into the descending aorta. When the ascending aorta is involved, expansion of the vessel wall may impair closure of the aortic valve. Although the length of the dissection varies, it is possible for the abdominal aorta to be involved, with, finally, progression into the renal, iliac, and/or femoral arteries.

A major symptom of a dissecting aneurysm is the abrupt appearance of excruciating pain, described as "tearing" or "ripping" in nature. The location of the pain may point to the site of dissection. Pain associated with dissection of the ascending aorta is frequently located in the anterior chest; whereas pain associated with dissection of the descending aorta is often located in the back. In the early stages, blood pressure is often moderately or markedly elevated. Later, both the blood pressure and the pulse become unobtainable in one or both arms as the dissection disrupts arterial flow to the arms.

Mortality due to dissecting aneurysm is high. Within the first 48 hours 50% of all untreated patients die.

:Acute Arterial Occlusion

Acute arterial occlusion usually results from a thrombus or an embolus. Trauma or arterial spasm due to arterial cannulation is another cause of acute arterial occlusion.

The signs and symptoms of acute arterial occlusion depend on the artery involved and the adequacy of the collateral circulation. Emboli tend to lodge in bifurcations of the major arteries, including the aorta and the iliac, femoral, and popliteal arteries. Occlusion in an extremity causes sudden onset of acute pain with numbness, tingling, weakness, pallor, and coldness. These changes are rapidly followed by cyanosis, mottling, and loss of sensory, reflex, and motor function. Pulses are absent below the level of the occlusion.

Treatment of acute arterial occlusion is aimed at restoring flow. Anticoagulant therapy (heparin) is usually given to prevent extension of the embolus. An embolectomy—surgical removal of the embolus—may be indicated. It is important that application of heat and cold be avoided and that the extremity be protected from hard surfaces and overlying bedclothes.

:Peripheral Vascular Disease

The peripheral vascular circulation is usually described as circulation outside the heart. For our purposes, we will consider the peripheral circulation as that outside the pulmonary and cerebral circulation. Arteriosclerosis, discussed earlier, is a major cause of peripheral vascular disorders. Two other conditions, Raynaud's disease and thromboangiitis obliterans (Buerger's disease) will serve as prototypes of peripheral vascular disease.

Assessment of Arterial Flow and Peripheral Perfusion

The volume of the peripheral pulses and capillary refill time are useful indirect methods for assessing peripheral perfusion.

Peripheral arterial pulses are palpated over vessels in the head, neck, and extremities. In situations associated with potential vessel spasm or thrombus formation, it may be necessary only to check for the presence of pulses. In many situations, however, the pulse volume provides useful information about vascular volume and the condition of the arterial circulation. Pulse volume can be graded on a scale of 0 to +4.

    0—Pulse is not palpable.
    +1—Pulse is thready, weak, and difficult to palpate; it may fade in and out, and is easily obliterated with pressure.
    +2—Pulse is difficult to palpate and may be obliterated with pressure, so light palpa-

tion is required. Once located, however, it is stronger than +1.
    +3—Pulse is easily palpable, does not fade in and out, and is not easily obliterated by pressure. This pulse is considered to have normal volume.
    +4—Pulse is strong, bounding, and hyperactive, easily palpated, and not obliterated with pressure. In some cases, such as aortic regurgitation, it may be considered pathologic.[7]

Capillary refill time is an indicator of the efficiency of the microcirculation. It is measured by depressing the nailbed of a finger or toe until the underlying skin blanches. The refill time is normal if the capillary vessels refill within 3 seconds following release of the pressure.[8]

Raynaud's disease or Raynaud's phenomenon

Raynaud's disease or Raynaud's phenomenon is a functional disorder caused by intense vasospasm of the arteries and arterioles in the fingers, and, less often, in the toes. The lack of demonstrable etiology differentiates Raynaud's disease from Raynaud's syndrome. Raynaud's disease is seen most frequently in otherwise healthy young women, and it is often precipitated by exposure to cold and by strong emotions. Raynaud's phenomenon is associated with the following: occupational trauma such as that caused by use of heavy vibrating tools, collagen diseases such as systemic lupus erythematosus, neurologic disorders, and chronic arterial occlusive disorders.

In Raynaud's disease or phenomenon, ischemia due to vasospasm causes changes in skin color that progress from pallor to cyanosis, a sensation of cold, and changes in sensory perception such as numbness or tingling. The color changes are usually first noted in the tips of the fingers, later moving into one or more of the distal phalanges. Following the ischemic episode there is a period of hyperemia with intense rubor, throbbing, and paresthesias. The period of hyperemia is followed by a return to normal color. During the attack there may be slight swelling. The nails may become brittle, and the skin over the tips of the affected fingers thickened. Nutritional impairment of these structures may give rise to nutritional arthritis. Ulceration and superficial gangrene of the fingers, although infrequent, may occur.

Treatment measures are directed toward eliminating factors that cause vasospasm and protecting the digits from trauma during an ischemic episode. Abstinence from smoking and protection from cold are first priorities. Avoidance of emotional stress is another important factor in controlling the disorder because anxiety and stress may precipitate a vascular spasm in predisposed individuals. Treatment with vasodilator drugs may be indicated, particularly if episodes are frequent, because frequency tends to encourage the potential for thrombosis and gangrene.

Thromboangiitis obliterans (Buerger's disease)

Thromboangiitis obliterans, is, as the name implies, an inflammatory arterial disorder that causes thrombus formation. The disorder affects the medium-sized arteries, usually the plantar and digital vessels in the foot, and those in the lower leg. Arteries in the arm and hand may also be affected. Although primarily an arterial disorder, the inflammatory process often extends to involve adjacent veins and nerves. The cause of Buerger's disease is unknown. It is a disease of men between the ages of 25 and 40 who are heavy cigarette smokers.

Pain is the predominant symptom. During the early stages of the disease, there is intermittent claudication of the calf muscles and the arch of the foot. In severe cases, pain is present even when the person is at rest. The impaired circulation increases sensitivity to cold. The peripheral pulses are diminished or absent, and there are changes in the color of the extremity. In moderately advanced cases, the extremity becomes cyanotic when the person assumes a dependent position. The digits may turn reddish-blue in color even when he is in a nondependent position. With lack of blood flow the skin assumes a thin, shiny look, and hair growth and skin nutrition suffer. Chronic ischemia brings thick, malformed nails. If the disease continues to progress, tissues will eventually ulcerate, and gangrenous changes will arise that may necessitate amputation.

In the treatment program for thromboangiitis obliterans, it is mandatory that the person stop cigarette smoking. Other treatment measures are of secondary importance and focus on methods for producing vasodilatation and for preventing tissue injury. Buerger's exercises take advantage of the gravitational effects of position change to improve blood flow to the affected part. The exercises consist of a cycle of approximately 2-minute positional changes: horizontal, legs elevated 45°, legs in a dependent position, and then horizontal again. The exercises are usually repeated five times and are done three times a day. Patients are usually instructed to wiggle their toes while exercising.

In summary, interruption of arterial blood flow may be temporary or permanent. In vasospasm or vessel com-

pression, the obstruction to flow is often of a temporary nature, while atherosclerosis tends to produce more permanent effects. Because the metabolic needs of the tissues determine adequacy of flow, arterial pathology can produce varying degrees of ischemia relative to the needs of the affected part. For example, a person with coronary heart disease may have adequate blood flow during normal activity, but may develop angina with exercise. Likewise, application of heat to an extremity supplied by atherosclerotic vessels may increase the metabolic needs of the tissue to the point where a previously adequate blood flow becomes insufficient.

:Study Guide

After you have studied this chapter, you should be able to meet the following objectives:

: : Describe the pathogenesis of atherosclerosis.

: : Relate the blood cholesterol level to atherosclerosis.

: : Distinguish among berry aneurysms, aortic aneurysms, and dissecting aneurysms.

: : State the signs and symptoms of acute arterial occlusion.

: : Describe gradations in pulse volume.

: : Explain the pathology involved in Raynaud's disease.

: : Explain why pain is the predominant symptom of thromboangiitis obliterans.

:References

1. Report of the 1977 Working Group to Review the Report by the National Heart and Lung Institute Task Force on Arteriosclerosis: Arterioslerosis, p 12, 1977
2. Enos WF, Beyer JC, Holmes RF: Pathogenesis of coronary heart disease in American soldiers killed in Korea. JAMA 158:912, 1955
3. Robbins SL, Cotran RS: Pathologic Basis of Disease, 2nd ed, p 604. Philadelphia, WB Saunders, 1979
4. Steinber D: Research underlying mechanisms in atherosclerosis. Circulation 60, No. 7:1559, 1979
5. McIntosh HD, Stamler J, Jackson D: Introduction to risk factors in coronary artery disease. Heart Lung 7, No. 1:126, 1978
6. Report of the 1977 Working Group to Review the Report by the National Heart and Lung Institute Task Force on Arteriosclerosis: Arteriosclerosis, p 20, 1977
7. Miller K: Assessing peripheral perfusion. Am J Nurs 78, No. 10:1674, 1978
8. Miller K: Assessing peripheral perfusion. Am J Nurs 78, No. 10:1674, 1978

:Suggested Readings

Abramson DI: Vascular Disorders of Extremities, 2nd ed. Hagerstown, Harper & Row, 1974

Barboriak JJ, Menahan LA: Alcohol, lipoproteins and coronary heart disease. Heart Lung 8, No. 4:736, 1979

Barnes RW: Axioms on acute arterial occlusion in an extremity. Hosp Med 14, No. 6:34, 1978

Barnes RW: Diagnosing vascular disease with noninvasive tests. Consultant 17:56, 1978

Bjorkerud S: Mechanisms of atherosclerosis. Pathobiol Ann 9:277, 1979

Cohen I: Role of endothelial injury and platelets in atherogenesis. Artery 5, No. 3:237, 1979

deWolfe VG: Intermittent claudication and after. Emerg Med 11:204, 1979

Dillon P, Seasholtz J: Oral contraceptives and myocardial infarction. Cardiovasc Nurs 15, No. 2:5, 1979

Fagan–Dubin L: Atherosclerosis: A major cause of peripheral vascular disease. Nurs Clin North Am 12, No. 1:101, 1977

Farrell PA, Barboriak J: The time course of alterations of plasma lipid and lipoprotein concentrations during eight weeks of endurance training. Atherosclerosis 37:231, 1980

Friedman SA: Guide to diagnosis of peripheral arterial disease. Hosp Med 15, No. 1:87, 1979

Garrison RJ et al: Cigarette smoking and HDL cholesterol—The Framingham offspring study. Atherosclerosis 30:17, 1978

Gruis M, Innes B: Assessment essential to prevent pressure sores. Am J Nurs 76, No. 11:1762, 1976

Harker L, Ross R: Pathogenesis of arterial vascular disease. Semin Thromb Hemostas 5, No. 4:274, 1979

Havel RJ: Lipoproteins and lipid transport. Adv Exp Med Biol 63:37, 1975

Hertzer NR: Abdominal aortic aneurysm: Guide to diagnosis and management. Hosp Med 15, No. 3:65, 1979

Hoffman GS: Raynaud's disease and phenomenon. Am Fam Physician 21, No. 1:91, 1980

Lee K: Aneurysm precautions: A physiologic basis for minimizing rebleeding. Heart Lung 9, No. 2:336, 1980

Margolis IB, Hayes D: Managing peripheral vascular disease secondary to arteriosclerosis. Geriatrics 32:75, 1977

Morriss NS: Dissecting aortic aneurysms. J Emerg Nurs 5:10, 1979

Mullen DC: Abdominal aortic aneurysm. Hosp Med 12, No. 1:60, 1976

Roenigk HH Jr: Leg ulcers in the elderly. Geriatrics 34:21, 1979

Sexton DL: The patient with peripheral arterial occlusive disease. Nurs Clin North Am 12:89, 1977

Shigehike S et al: Diagnosis, pathology, and treatment of Buerger's disease. Surgery 75, No. 5:695, 1974

Taggart E: The physical assessment of the patient with arterial disease. Nurs Clin North Am 12, No. 1:109, 1977

Watts RW, Brunswick RA: Management of acute dissections of the aorta. Heart Lung 9, No. 2:284, 1980

Williams R, Robinson D, Bailey A: High density lipoproteins and coronary risk factors in normal man. Lancet i: 72, 1979

10

Alterations in Venous Flow

Veins are low-pressure, thin-walled vessels that rely on the ancillary action of skeletal muscle pumps and changes in abdominal and intrathoracic pressure to return blood to the heart. Unlike the arterial system, the venous system is equipped with valves that prevent retrograde flow of blood. Although its structure enables the venous system to serve as a storage area for blood, it also renders the system susceptible to problems related to stasis and venous insufficiency. This chapter focuses on three common problems of the venous system: varicose veins, venous thrombosis, and pulmonary embolism.

:Varicose Veins

Varicose, or dilated, tortuous veins of the lower extremities, are common and often lead to secondary problems of venous insufficiency. Estimates suggest that 10% of the adult population is affected by varicose veins and another 40% or 50% have slight asymptomatic varicosities.[1] Customarily, varicose veins are described as being primary or secondary. Primary varicosities originate in the superficial saphenous veins, and secondary varicose veins result from impaired flow in the deep venous channels.

A brief review of the anatomy of the venous system of the legs explains why varicosities may develop. The venous system in the legs might well be described as being composed of two venous channels: the superficial (saphenous and its tributaries) veins, and the deep venous channels (Fig. 10-1). Perforating or communicating veins connect these two systems. Blood from the skin and subcutaneous tissues in the leg collects in the superficial veins and is then transported across the communicating veins into the deeper venous channels for return to the

Figure 10–1.   The superficial and deep venous channels of the leg. View (A) represents normal venous structures and flow patterns. View (B) illustrates varicosities in the superficial venous system that are the result of incompetent valves in the communicating veins. The arrows in both views indicate the direction of blood flow. (Modified from Abramson DI: Vascular Disorders of the Extremities, 2nd ed. New York, Harper & Row, 1974)

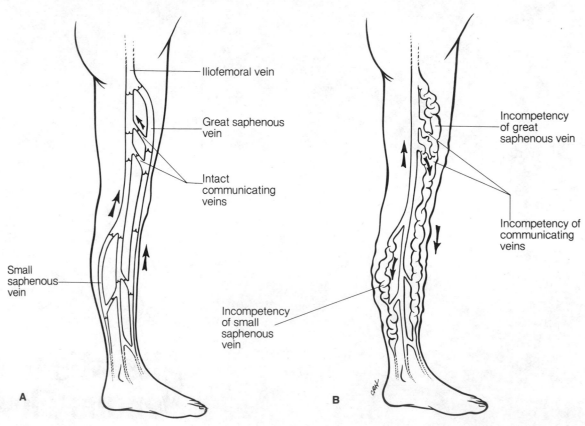

heart. When a person walks, the action of the muscle pumps produces an increase in flow in the deep channels and facilitates movement of blood from the superficial to the deep veins.

Valves present in the veins prevent the retrograde flow of blood and play an important role in the function of the venous system. Although these valves are irregularly located along the length of the veins, they are almost always found at junctions where the communicating veins merge with the larger deep veins and where two veins meet (Fig. 10-2). The number of venous valves differs somewhat from one individual to another, as does their structural competence, factors that may help to explain the familial predisposition to development of varicose veins.

Causes

Varicose veins result from prolonged dilatation and stretching of the vascular wall due to increased venous pressure. One of the most important factors in elevation of venous pressure is the hydrostatic effect associated with the standing position. When a person is in the erect position, the full weight of the venous columns of blood is transmitted to the leg veins. The effects of gravity are compounded in persons who stand for long periods of time without using their leg muscles to assist in pumping blood back to the heart. Because there are no valves in the inferior vena cava or common iliac veins, blood in the abdominal veins must be supported by the valves located in the external iliac or femoral veins. When there is an increase in intra-abdominal pressure, as there is during pregnancy, or when the valves in these two veins are absent or defective, the stress on the saphenofemoral junction is increased. The high incidence of varicose veins in women who have been pregnant also suggests a hormonal effect on venous smooth muscle, leading to venous dilatation and valvular incompetence.

Prolonged exposure to increases in pressure causes the venous valves to become incompetent so that they no longer close properly. When this happens, blood regurgitates into the superficial veins. Furthermore, once varicose veins have developed, the venous structures become deformed, promoting further dilatation.

Another consideration is that the superficial veins have only subcutaneous fat and superficial fascia for support, whereas the deep venous channels are supported by muscle, bone, and connective tissue. Therefore, obesity tends to increase the risk for varicose veins.

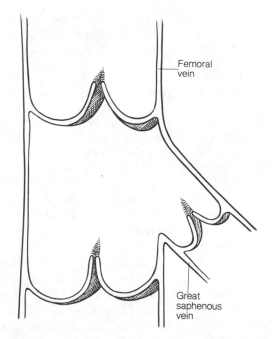

Figure 10–2.   Drawing of the venous valves that are located at the junction of the great saphenous and the common femoral veins.

Normally, about 80% to 90% of venous blood from the lower extremities is transported through the deep channels. The development of secondary varicose veins becomes inevitable when flow in these channels is impaired or blocked. Among the causes of secondary varicose veins are thrombophlebitis, congenital or acquired arteriovenous fistulas, congenital venous malformations, and pressure on the abdominal veins due to pregnancy or a tumor.

Venous insufficiency

Signs and symptoms associated with varicose veins vary. Most women complain of their unsightly appearance. In addition to their cosmetic effects, varicose veins tend to impair venous emptying, giving rise to a condition known as venous insufficiency. This often causes a sensation of progressive heaviness, and, with prolonged standing, aching legs. In contrast to the ischemia due to arterial insufficiency, venous insufficiency tends to lead to tissue congestion, edema, and eventual impairment of tissue nutrition. The edema is exacerbated by long periods of standing. In its advanced form, impairment of tissue nutrition causes stasis dermatitis and development of stasis or varicose ulcers. Stasis dermatitis is characterized by the presence of thin, shiny, bluish-brown, irregularly pigmented desquamative skin that lacks the support of the underlying subcutaneous tissues. Minor injury leads to relatively painless ulcerations that are difficult to heal. The lower part of the leg is particularly prone to develop stasis dermatitis and varicose ulcers.

Assessment Measures

Several procedures are used to assess the extent of venous involvement associated with varicose veins. One of these, the Trendelenburg test, involves the use of a tourniquet in the following manner. A tourniquet is applied to the affected leg while it is elevated and the veins are empty. The person then assumes the standing position, and the tourniquet is removed. If the superficial veins are involved, the veins distend quickly. To assess the deep channels, the tourniquet is applied while the person is standing and the veins are filled. The person then lies down and the affected leg is elevated. Emptying of the superficial veins indicates that the deep channels are patent. The Doppler ultrasonic flow probe may also be used to assess flow in the large vessels. Angiographic studies employing a radiopaque contrast medium are also used to assess venous function.

Prevention and Treatment

Ideally, preventive measures should be tried first, for once the venous channels have been repeatedly stretched and the valves rendered incompetent,

Figure 10–3. Location of internal and external hemorrhoids.

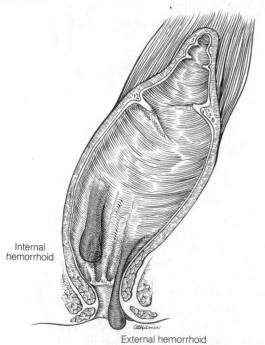

Internal
hemorrhoid

External hemorrhoid

there is little that can be done to restore normal venous tone and function. These measures center on avoiding any activities that involve prolonged elevation of venous pressure.

Treatment measures for varicose veins focus on improving venous flow and preventing tissue injury, such as avoiding prolonged standing, and providing for frequent leg elevation. When properly fitted, elastic support stockings compress the superficial veins and thus prevent distention. These stockings should be applied before the standing position is assumed, at a time when the leg veins are empty. Surgical treatment consists of removing the varicosities and the incompetent perforating veins, but it is limited to persons with patent, deep venous channels. Sclerotherapy, which is usually done on small residual varicosities, is another treatment measure; it involves injection of a sclerosing agent into the collapsed superficial veins in order to produce fibrosis of the vessel lumen.

Hemorrhoids

Hemorrhoids are varicosities of the hemorrhoidal (rectal) veins. Hemorrhoids are commonly classified as internal or external (Fig. 10-3). Both types are common and occur in about 35% of the adult population.

Internal hemorrhoids
Internal hemorrhoids are varices of the superior and middle hemorrhoidal veins and are located above the anal sphincter. They are commonly classified as first degree, second degree, and third degree. First-degree hemorrhoids do not prolapse through the sphincter; second-degree hemorrhoids may prolapse through the sphincter but recede spontaneously or can be reduced manually; and third-degree hemorrhoids are permanently prolapsed. They are usually painless, because there are no pain fibers in this area of the anal canal.

External hemorrhoids
External hemorrhoids involve the inferior hemorrhoidal vein and are located outside the anal sphincter. There are numerous nerve endings in the external anal area, so these hemorrhoids often are itching and painful. They may become swollen and thrombosed.

As is true of varicose veins in the lower extremities, it is believed that hemorrhoids result from increased pressure in the hemorrhoidal veins. Hemorrhoids, common during pregnancy, are associated with constipation. Irritation, ulceration, and bleeding are other problems. Should the hemorrhoids become strangulated and thrombosed, there will be intense discomfort and pain. In such cases, surgical excision or injection with a sclerosing agent will usually be done. That over-the-counter preparations for the relief of hemorrhoidal discomfort are very widely sold attests to the prevalence of the problem and the suffering it causes.

Esophageal Varices

Esophageal varices are dilatations of the esophageal venous plexus. They arise with persistent obstruction of blood flow through the portal vein, with development of portal hypertension; this results in diversion of blood flow to other venous channels, including the gastric and esophageal veins (Fig. 10-4). Because the esophageal veins are relatively small and inelastic, they tolerate the increased pressure poorly and are thus subject to rupture. Esophageal varices derive their clinical importance from this vulnerability, because the final outcome may be massive, often fatal, hemorrhage.

The most common cause of esophageal varices is alcohol liver disease (Laennec's cirrhosis), and persons with liver disease often have associated blood-clotting problems that interfere with hemostasis. For additional information on portal hypertension and liver disease, the reader is referred to Chapter 38.

Bleeding esophageal varices must be treated with emergency measures. The posterior pituitary hormone, vasopressin, may be administered, as it decreases splanchnic blood flow.[2] A second emergency procedure is the use of the Sengstaken–Blakemore tube. The tube is inserted in such manner that the uninflated balloon is above the bleeding vessels; the balloon is then inflated to mechanically compress the bleeding varices. Because hemorrhage is often severe and unpredictable in occurrence, surgical treatment may be indicated. Surgery involves the creation of a portal–systemic shunt—an opening between the portal vein and a systemic vein such as the vena cava—which brings about a reduction in portal hypertension with a subsequent decrease in venous distention. A more recent surgical technique has been devised in which the esophagus is resected at the site of the varices with an instrument known as the Russian circular stapling gun. With it, a ring of esophageal tissue is excised at the same time that the tissue edges are joined with tantalum staples.[3,4] Esophageal varices carry a guarded prognosis, inasmuch as they are difficult to treat, and the liver disease is usually far advanced when the varices are discovered.

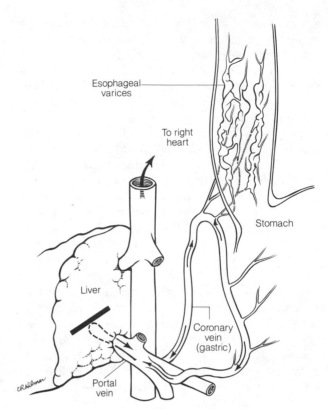

Figure 10–4. Diagram showing obstruction of blood flow in the portal circulation, with portal hypertension and diversion of blood flow to other venous channels, including the gastric and esophageal veins.

:Venous Thrombosis

In thrombophlebitis there is inflammation of a vein with subsequent thrombus formation, while in phlebothrombosis there is thrombus formation followed by inflammation. In phlebothrombosis, the clot is less firmly attached to the vessel wall than is the case in thrombophlebitis, so that embolization is a greater risk. From a clinical standpoint, it is often difficult to determine which came first—the inflammation or the clot. Therefore, this discussion treats thrombophlebitis and phlebothrombosis as one and the same.

In 1846, Virchow described the triad that has come to be associated with thrombosis: (1) stasis of blood, (2) increased blood coagulability, and (3) vessel-wall injury.[5] It is thought that two of the three factors must be present for thrombi to form. Thrombi can develop in either the superficial or the deep veins (DVT). Thrombus formation in deep veins is a precursor to venous insufficiency and embolus formation.

A number of factors may be present that promote venous thrombosis (Table 10-1). Immobilization, trauma, and surgery are definite risk factors, as are aging, heart failure, hypercoagulability states, and a previous history of venous disorders. The patient immobilized due to a hip fracture or joint replacement is particularly vulnerable to DVT. Persons in the older age groups (above 40) are more susceptible than are younger people. Although there is no single explanation for it, factors known to promote venous stasis, such as heart failure, venous pathology, and cancer occur more frequently in older individuals. Hypercoagulability is in itself a homeostatic mechanism that is invoked in conditions of stress or injury. It may be that thrombi form as a result of changes in clotting factors or in the fibrinolytic system (see Chap. 11). When because of injury or disease there is loss of body fluid, the resulting hemoconcentration will cause the clotting factors to become more concentrated. Certain malignancies are associated with increased clotting tendencies, and although the reason for this is largely unknown, it may be that substances that promote blood coagulation are released from the tissues due to the cancerous growth. In congestive heart failure and shock, there is impaired circulation with stasis of coagulation factors.

What part oral contraceptive agents play in promoting blood coagulation and as a consequence a predisposition to venous thrombosis and pulmonary embolism is controversial. Certainly, if other risk factors are present, both the risk and benefits of oral contraceptives need to be carefully weighed.

Table 10-1 Risk Factors Associated with Venous Thrombosis

Aging

Anesthesia and surgery

Circulatory failure
   Congestive heart failure
   Shock

Dehydration

Hematologic disorders
   Polycythemia
   Disorders of blood clotting
   Disorders of fibrinolytic activity

Malignancy

Massive trauma or infection

Obesity

Reproductive processes
   Pregnancy
   Parturition
   Oral contraceptive therapy

Venous disorders
   Venous insufficiency
   Vascular trauma
   Venous obstruction

Signs and Symptoms

The most common signs of thrombophlebitis are those related to the inflammatory process: pain, swelling, deep muscle tenderness, and fever. Generally, the pain is described as localized, deep, aching, and throbbing, and the pain is exacerbated with walking. A positive Homans' sign—pain in the popliteal area when the foot is forcefully dorsiflexed—suggests thrombophlebitis. Swelling of the leg usually occurs soon after the onset of pain. How much swelling there is depends on the extent to which venous flow is impaired. Fever, general malaise, and an elevated white blood cell count and sedimentation rate are accompanying signs of inflammation.

Phlebothrombosis differs from thrombophlebitis in that the early signs of inflammation are often absent. Frequently, a positive Homans' sign or manifestations of pulmonary embolism are the only evidence that thrombosis has occurred.

Early detection

The risk of pulmonary embolism emphasizes the need for early detection and treatment of thrombophlebitis. Several tests are useful for this purpose: radioactive fibrinogen (I^{125}), Doppler ultrasonic flowmeter, and electrical impedance plethysmography. At present, the most reliable test appears to be the intravenous injection of radioactive fibrinogen, which becomes incorporated into any developing thrombus. The thrombus is then detected by a scintillation counter which records the radioactivity at selected points in the extremity.

The Doppler flowmeter is a device that measures venous flow.

In electrical impedance plethysmography, blood flow is estimated by measurement of the resistance changes in the extremity.

These three methods provide means for frequent assessment of venous flow or fibrinogen accumulation, and are useful in monitoring persons at risk for developing venous thrombosis.

Venography, in which a contrast medium is injected into a vein and x-ray studies are then done, is another diagnostic procedure, but it is not done routinely.

Prevention and Treatment

Whenever possible, venous thrombosis should be prevented, in preference to being treated. Early ambulation following childbirth and surgery is one measure that decreases the risk of thrombus formation. Leg exercises and the wearing of support stockings also improve venous flow. A further precautionary measure is to avoid assuming body positions that favor venous pooling. For example, in the hospitalized patient, if both the head and knees of the hospital bed are raised, blood will tend to pool in the pelvic veins. Long, unbroken auto and plane trips also promote venous pooling and thrombus formation.

In both thrombophlebitis and phlebothrombosis, bedrest with elevation of the affected extremity is prescribed. In one study, contrast medium remained in the soleus veins, on the average, for 10 minutes in supine patients whose legs were in horizontal position.[6] This may explain why postoperative thrombus often has its inception in the soleus vein. A 20° elevation of the legs will prevent stasis.[7] It is important that the entire lower extremity or extremities be carefully extended to avoid acute flexion of the knee or hip. Heat is often applied to the leg to relieve vasospasm and to aid in the resolution of the inflammatory process. Measures are also taken to prevent the bedcoverings from resting on the leg because this increases discomfort.

Anticoagulant therapy

Two anticoagulants, warfarin and heparin, are used both to treat and to prevent thrombophlebitis. *Treatment* is usually initiated with either continuous or periodic intravenous heparin infusions. This is followed by *prophylactic* therapy with either subcutaneous minidose heparin injections or oral warfarin sodium to prevent further thrombus formation. Minidose heparin is usually injected into the subcu-

taneous tissue of the lower abdomen or laterally above the iliac crest.[8,9] Prophylactic therapy is usually continued for six to ten weeks following uncomplicated DVT and for up to 6 months following pulmonary embolism. The mechanisms of action of the anticoagulant drugs are discussed in Chapter 11.

:Pulmonary Embolism

Pulmonary embolism develops when a blood-borne substance lodges in a branch of the pulmonary artery and obstructs flow. The embolism may consist of a thrombus, air which has accidentally been injected during intravenous infusion, fat which has been mobilized from the bone marrow following a fracture or from a traumatized fat depot, or amniotic fluid which has entered the maternal circulation following rupture of the membranes at the time of delivery. This discussion is limited to the most frequent form of pulmonary embolism, thromboembolism.

Thromboembolism

In the United States there are approximately 630,000 cases of thromboembolism annually.[10] About 67,000 of these persons die within the first hour, before a diagnosis can be made and treatment instituted (Fig. 10-5). Another 120,000 deaths occur in persons in whom the condition went unrecognized. If these figures are correct, symptomatic pulmonary embolism is half as frequent as myocardial infarction.[10]

Almost all pulmonary emboli are due to DVT.

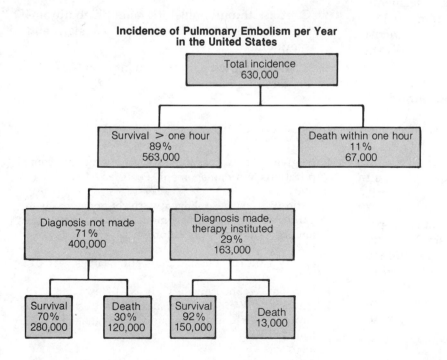

Incidence of Pulmonary Embolism per Year in the United States

Figure 10–5. Yearly incidence of pulmonary embolism in the United States. (Dalen JE, Alpert JS: Natural history of pulmonary embolism. Prog Cardiovasc Dis 17, No. 4:261, 1975. By permission.)

Therefore, persons at risk for developing venous thrombosis are the same persons who are at risk for developing thromboemboli.

The outcome of embolism on cardiopulmonary function depends on the size and location of obstruction. Small emboli that become lodged in the peripheral branches of the pulmonary artery may exert little effect, whereas, sudden death occurs when a large embolus causes total occlusion of the pulmonary artery. Dependent on size, pulmonary embolism causes (1) obstruction of pulmonary blood flow, with pulmonary arterial hypertension and right heart failure, (2) breathlessness, (3) hypoxemia, and (4) lung infarction.

Dyspnea, abrupt in onset, is the most common symptom of pulmonary embolism, and the breathing pattern is often rapid and shallow. With obstruction of pulmonary blood flow, there is severe apprehension and crushing substernal chest pain similar to that of myocardial infarction; the neck veins are distended, and cyanosis, diaphoresis, syncope, mental confusion, and other signs of shock follow. Pulmonary infarction often causes pleuritic pain that changes with respiration, being more severe on inspiration and less severe on expiration. With lung infarction there may be hemoptysis.

Diagnosis of pulmonary embolism is based on lung scan, laboratory studies, chest x-ray films and, in selected cases, angiography. The lung scan is a widely used diagnostic test. In this test, radioactive iodinated serum albumin is injected intravenously, and collects in the pulmonary circulation. A scintillation counter is passed over the chest to provide a picture of blood flow in the various lung segments. The laboratory studies and chest x-ray films are useful in ruling out other conditions that might give rise to similar symptoms. Angiography involves the passage of a venous catheter through the heart and into the pulmonary artery under fluoroscopy. An embolectomy is sometimes performed during this procedure.

There are three surgical procedures for pulmonary embolism: embolectomy, venous ligation to prevent the embolus from traveling to the lung, and vena caval plication. The plication, done with a suture, or by insertion of a clip, filter, or sieve, permits blood to flow while trapping the embolus.

Prevention focuses on (1) identification of persons at risk, (2) avoidance of venous stasis and hypercoagulability states, and (3) early detection of venous thrombosis. In patients at risk, low-dose subcutaneous heparin may be administered to decrease the likelihood of DVT, thromboembolism, and fatal pulmonary embolism following major surgical procedures.

In summary, the storage function of the venous system renders it susceptible to venous insufficiency, stasis, and thrombus formation. Varicose veins occur when there is prolonged distention and stretching of the superficial veins due to venous insufficiency. Varicosities can arise because of defects in the superficial veins (primary varicose veins), or because of impaired blood flow in the deep venous channels (secondary varicose veins). Venous thrombosis, thrombophlebitis, and pulmonary embolism are associated with three factors: vessel injury, stasis of venous flow, and hypercoagulability states. Pulmonary embolism is a serious and sometimes fatal condition that occurs when a portion of a venous thrombus "breaks loose" and travels to the pulmonary circulation where it becomes lodged and shuts off blood flow.

:Study Guide

After you have studied this chapter, you should be able to meet the following objectives:

: : Describe the anatomy of the venous system.

: : Describe the effects of gravity on the venous system.

: : State the signs and symptoms of venous insufficiency.

: : Describe the form of varicosity known as hemorrhoids.

: : Explain why bleeding esophageal varices must be treated by emergency measures.

: : Describe the pathology involved in venous thrombosis.

: : Contrast thrombophlebitis and phlebothrombosis on the basis of their respective signs and symptoms.

: : State the immediate consequent effects of pulmonary embolism.

:References

1. Lofgren KA: Varicose veins: Their symptoms, complications and management. Postgrad Med 65, No. 6:131, 1979
2. Cello JP: Gastroesophageal variceal hemorrhage—pathogenesis and management. Medical staff conference at University of California, San Francisco. West J Med 130:531, 1979
3. Cherry FM: The Russian gun. Nurs Times 74:1601, 1978
4. Johnson GW: Shooting the varix. NAT News 16:8, 1979
5. Virchow R: Weinere untersuchungen uber dic verstropfung der lungenarterie und ihre folgen. Beitr Exp Pathol Physiol 2:21, 1846

6. Nicolaides AN, Kakkar VV, Renney JTG: Soleal sinuses and stasis. Br J Surg 58:307, 1971
7. Nicolaides AN, Gordon–Smith I: The prevention of deep venous thrombosis. In Hobbs JT (ed): The Treatment of Venous Disorders, A Comprehensive Review of Current Practice in the Management of Varicose Veins and Postthrombotic Syndrome. Philadelphia, JB Lippincott, 1977
8. Caprini JA, Zoellner JL, Weisman M: Heparin therapy—Part II. Cardiovasc Nurs 13, No. 4:17, 1977
9. Chamberlain SL: Low-dose heparin therapy. Am J Nurs 80, No. 6:1115, 1980
10. Dalen JE, Alpert JS: Natural history of pulmonary embolism. Prog Cardiovasc Dis 17:259, 1975

:Suggested Readings

Varicose Veins

Baron H: Valvular incompetence and varicose veins. Hosp Med 12, No. 4:24, 1976

Thromboemboli

Coon WW: Anticoagulant therapy for venous thromboembolism. Postgrad Med 63, No. 4:157, 1978
Fitzmaurice JB: Venous thromboembolic disease: Current thoughts. Cardiovasc Nurs 14, No. 1:1, 1978
Hull R et al: Warfarin sodium versus low-dose heparin in the long-term treatment of venous thrombosis. N Engl J Med 301, No. 16:855, 1979
Kakkar VV: Deep vein thrombosis: Detection and prevention. Circulation 51:8, 1975
Nyman SJ: Thrombophlebitis in pregnancy. Am J Nurs 80, No. 1:90, 1980
Scholz P, Jones R, Sabiston D: Prophylaxis of thromboembolism. Adv Surg 13:115, 1979
Tikoff G, Prescott S: Axioms on thrombophlebitis and phlebothrombosis. Hosp Med 15, No. 4:36, 1979

Pulmonary Embolism

Douglas A: Venous thrombosis and pulmonary embolism: A disease of hospitals. Nurs Mirror 147:44, 1978
Falotico JB: Pulmonary embolism: Don't overlook these subtle warnings. RN 42:47, 1979
Gray FD: Pulmonary embolism: Avoiding the diagnostic pitfalls. Consultant 19:71, 1979
Lenig RC: Pulmonary fat embolism. J Am Assoc Nurse Anesth 47:40, 1979
Levy SE: Pulmonary embolism: Current prophylaxis and diagnosis. Hosp Med 15:65, 1979
McFarland MB: Fat embolism syndrome. Am J Nurs 76, No. 12:1942, 1976
Oldham GL, Weese WC: Fat embolism. Ariz Med 36, No. 12:885, 1979

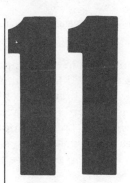

Alterations in Hemostasis

The term hemostasis refers to the stoppage of blood flow. Hemostasis is designed to maintain the integrity of the vascular system and to prevent blood from leaving its channels. Disorders of hemostasis fall into two main categories: (1) the inappropriate formation of clots within the vascular system, and (2) the failure of blood to clot in response to an appropriate stimulus.

:Mechanisms Associated with Hemostasis

Hemostasis is generally divided into five stages: (1) vessel spasm, (2) formation of the platelet plug, (3) blood coagulation or development of an insoluble fibrin clot, (4) clot retraction, and (5) clot dissolution. The steps of the hemostasis process are summarized in Table 11-1.

Vessel Spasm

Vessel spasm is the first of the stages involved in formation of a blood clot; it is caused by local and neural reflex mechanisms. Vessel spasm constricts the vessel and reduces blood flow. It is a transient event that usually lasts less than a minute.

Formation of the Platelet Plug

Platelets, or thrombocytes, are large fragments from the cytoplasm of bone stem cells called the megakaryocytes. They are enclosed in a membrane, but have no nucleus. They have a life span of only five to nine days. Platelet production is controlled by a substance called thrombopoietin. The source of thrombopoietin is unknown, but it appears that its production and release is regulated by the number of platelets in the circulation. The newly formed plate-

lets that are released from the bone marrow spend 24 to 36 hours in the spleen before being released into the blood.

The platelet plug is the second line of defense which is initiated as platelets come in contact with the vessel wall. As the platelets adhere to the subendothelial layer of the vessel wall, they become "sticky." This allows them to interact with other platelets and to form an aggregate—a process called platelet aggregation. The formation of a platelet plug usually occurs within seconds of vessel injury. There are at least two plasma factors that are needed for platelet adhesiveness and aggregation to occur: one is fibrinogen and the other is von Willebrand's factor, a protein with a structure similar to factor VIII. Persons with von Willebrand's disease are deficient in the von Willebrand factor and have bleeding problems.

During the third stage of hemostasis, the unstable platelet plug becomes cemented together with fibrin strands. When vessel injury is slight, the platelet plug may be all that is needed to close the defect, and when this happens, the formation of the fibrin clot is not needed. In addition to sealing vascular breaks, platelets play an almost continuous role in maintaining normal vascular integrity. Persons with thrombocytopenia have decreased capillary resistance and develop small skin hemorrhages which result from the slightest trauma or change in blood pressure.

Blood Coagulation

Blood coagulation is the third stage of hemostasis. It is the process by which fibrin strands form and create a meshwork that cements blood components together (Fig. 11-1). Blood coagulation occurs as a result of activation of either the intrinsic or extrinsic coagulation pathways (Fig. 11-2). The intrinsic pathway, which is a relatively slow process, occurs in the vascular system, and the extrinsic pathway, which is a much faster process, occurs in the tissues. The terminal steps in both pathways are the same and consist of the interaction between thrombin and the plasma protein fibrinogen. A final interaction for both pathways converts fibrinogen to fibrin, the material that forms the structural matrix of the clot. Both pathways are needed for normal hemostasis. Bleeding, however, when occurring because of defects in the extrinsic system is usually not as severe as that which results from defects in the intrinsic pathway. Both systems are activated when blood passes out of the vascular system. The intrinsic system is activated as blood comes in contact with the

Table 11–1 Steps in Hemostasis

Vessel spasm

Formation of the platelet plug
    Platelet adherence to the vessel wall
    Platelet aggregation to form the platelet plug

Blood coagulation
    Activation of the intrinsic or extrinsic coagulation
       pathway
    Conversion of prothrombin to thrombin
    Conversion of fibrinogen to fibrin

Clot retraction

Clot dissolution (fibrinolysis)

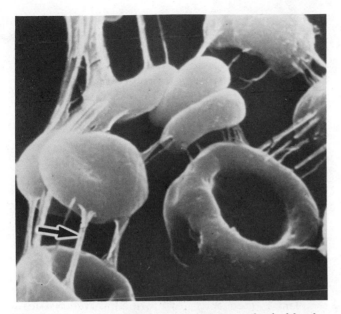

Figure 11–1. Scanning electron micrograph of a blood clot at a magnification of 5,000 times. The fibrous bridges (indicated by the arrow) that form a meshwork between red blood cells are fibrin fibers. (From Chaffee EE, Lytle IM: Basic Physiology and Anatomy, 4th ed. Philadelphia, JB Lippincott, 1980)

injured vessel wall and the extrinsic system when blood is exposed to tissue extracts.

The purpose of the coagulation process is to form an insoluble fibrin clot. This process may involve as many as thirty different substances that either promote clotting (procoagulation factors), or inhibit coagulation (anticoagulation factors). Each of the procoagulation factors is identified by a Roman numeral (Table 11-2). The decision to use Roman numerals came after it was discovered that two factors were identified by the same name. When one observes the various names that appear in Table 11-2, one can easily see how this could happen. There is no factor VI, because that number was originally assigned to what is now known to be the activated form of factor V.

Each of the procoagulation factors performs a specific step in the coagulation process. The action of one coagulation factor is usually designed to activate the next factor in the sequence (cascade effect). Some sources identify the activated form of the factor by inserting the subscript a after the factor number (factor Va). Because most of the inactive procoagulation factors are present in the blood at all

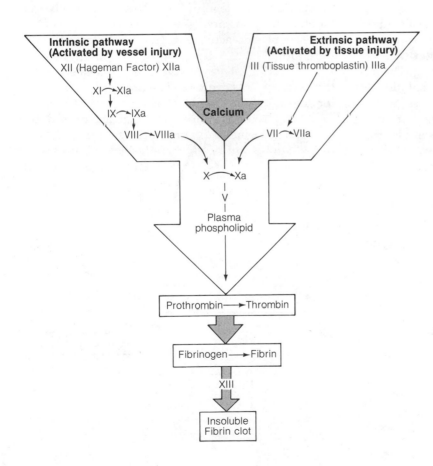

Figure 11–2. Schematic diagram of the intrinsic and extrinsic coagulation pathways. The terminal steps in both pathways are the same. Phospholipid, calcium, factors X and V combine to form prothrombin activator, which then converts prothrombin to thrombin. This interaction, in turn, causes conversion of fibrinogen into the fibrin strands that create the insoluble blood clot.

Table 11–2 Coagulation Factors

Factor I	Fibrinogen
Factor II	Prothrombin
Factor III	Tissue thromboplastin
Factor IV	Calcium
Factor V	Proaccelerin, labile factor, A-C globulin
Factor VII	Proconvertin, serum prothrombin conversion accelerator (SPCA)
Factor VIII	Antihemophilic factor (AHF)
Factor IX	Plasma thromboplastin component (PTC), antihemophilic factor B (AHF-B), Christmas factor
Factor X	Stuart factor, Stuart–Prower factor
Factor XI	Plasma thromboplastin antecedent (PTA)
Factor XII	Hageman factor
Factor XIII	Fibrin stabilizing factor

times, the multistep coagulation process ensures that a massive episode of intravascular clotting does not occur by chance. It also means that abnormalities of the clotting process will occur when one or more of the factors are deficient, or when conditions lead to inappropriate activation of any of the steps.

Calcium (factor IV) is required in all but the first two steps of the clotting process. Fortunately, the living body almost always has sufficient calcium to interact in the clotting process. The inactivation of the calcium ion is used to prevent blood that has been removed from the body from clotting. The addition of a citrate–phosphate–dextrose solution to blood stored for transfusion purposes prevents clotting by combining with the calcium ions. Both oxalate and citrate are often added to blood samples that are used for analysis in the clinical laboratory.

Clot Retraction

Clot retraction occurs immediately once the clot has formed. Clot retraction, which requires large numbers of platelets, contributes to hemostasis by pulling the edges of the broken vessel together.

Clot Dissolution (Fibrinolysis)

The dissolution of a blood clot begins shortly after its formation; this allows blood flow to be re-established and allows tissue repair to take place. The process by which a blood clot dissolves is called fibrinolysis. As with clot formation, clot dissolution requires a sequence of steps (Fig. 11-3).

Plasminogen, the proenzyme for the fibrolytic process, is normally present in the blood in its inactive form. It is converted to its active form, *plasmin*, by plasminogen activators formed in the tissues, plasma, urine, or blood clot. The plasmin formed from plasminogen digests the fibrin strands of the clot as well as other proteins. It also digests certain clotting factors such as fibrinogen, factor V, and factor VIII. Circulating plasmins are inactivated by *antiplasmins* which are normally present in the circulation in concentrations ten times those of plasmins. This high level of antiplasmins protects the blood clotting factors.

The plasma-activating factor is released from the endothelial cells by a number of stimuli, including the action of vasoactive drugs, elevated body temperature, and exercise. The tissue activation factor does not normally enter the blood unless there is extensive tissue damage, such as that caused by burns. The urine-activating factor, urinokinase, is thought to be produced by the kidney and probably

Figure 11–3.   Diagram of steps in the fibrinolytic sequence. Fibrinolysis can be initiated by tissue, plasma, urine, or clot activating factors.

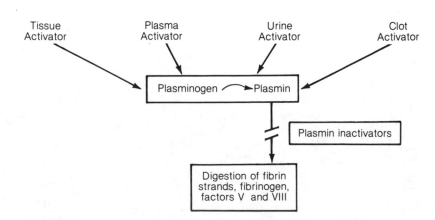

assists in maintaining the patency of the renal tract. Plasma activator is unstable and is rapidly inactivated by substances in the blood and by the liver. For this reason, chronic liver disease may cause altered fibrinolytic activity.

A number of fibrinolytic enzymes have been purified to treat thrombosis. Two of the plasminogen activators that are used are streptokinase and urinokinase. Streptokinase is antigenic and has the potential to produce an allergic reaction. Urinokinase is relatively unavailable and thus quite expensive.

:Abnormal Clotting

Blood clotting is normal when it seals a blood vessel thereby preventing blood loss and hemorrhage. It is abnormal when it causes inappropriate blood clotting or when clotting is insufficient to stop the flow of blood from the vascular compartment. The discussion of clotting disorders that follows has been divided into two groups: (1) the hypercoagulability states, and (2) bleeding diatheses (disorders).

Hypercoagulability States

All of the components or factors necessary to trigger the intrinsic coagulation pathway are present in the blood at all times. There are two general forms of hypercoagulability states: (1) conditions that create hyperactivity of the platelet system, and (2) conditions that cause accelerated activity of the coagulation system. Current evidence suggests that hyperreactivity of the platelet system results in arterial thrombosis and that increased activity of the clotting system causes venous thrombosis and its sequelae.[1] Table 11-3 summarizes conditions commonly associated with hypercoagulability states.

Hyper-reactivity of platelet function

The causes of increased platelet function tend to be twofold: (1) disturbances in flow and changes in the vessel wall, and (2) increased sensitivity of platelets to factors which cause adhesiveness and aggregation. Atherosclerotic plaques disturb flow and render the inner lining of the arterial wall more susceptible to platelet adherence. There is now considerable evidence that disturbed flow and platelet function contribute to the development of atherosclerosis as well as arterial thrombosis. It appears that platelets adhering to the vessel wall may release factors that are damaging to the underlying vessel

Table 11-3 Conditions Associated with Hypercoagulability States

Hyper-reactivity of platelets
    Atherosclerosis
    Diabetes mellitus
    Smoking
    Elevated blood lipids and cholesterol
    Increased platelet levels

Accelerated activity of the clotting system
    Pregnancy and the puerperium
    Use of oral contraceptives
    Postsurgical state
    Immobility
    Congestive heart failure
    Malignant diseases

and thereby contribute to the development and progression of atherosclerosis. Diabetes mellitus not only increases the incidence of atherosclerosis, but also appears to increase platelet adherence and aggregation. Smoking and elevated levels of blood lipids and cholesterol also appear to cause increased platelet sensitivity to factors that cause platelet adherence and aggregation.

Increased clotting activity

Factors that increase activation of the coagulation system are (1) stasis of flow, and (2) alterations in the coagulation components of the blood (either an increase in procoagulation factors or a decrease in anticoagulation factors). Venous thrombosis usually begins in regions of slow and disturbed flow. Venous thrombosis is a common event in the immobilized and postsurgical patient. Heart failure also contributes to venous congestion and thrombosis. Blood coagulation factors have been found to be increased in women using oral contraceptive agents. The incidence of stroke, thromboemboli, and myocardial infarction is more frequent among women who use oral contraceptives than among those who do not. Clotting factors are also increased during normal pregnancy, and these changes, along with limited activity during the puerperium, predispose to venous thrombosis. A third condition that predisposes to hypercoagulability is malignant disease. Many tumor cells are thought to release procoagulation factors, which, along with the increased immobility and sepsis seen in patients with malignant disease, contribute to the increased incidence of thrombosis in these patients.

:Bleeding Disorders

As with the hypercoagulability states, bleeding disorders or impairment of blood coagulation can result from defects in any of the factors that contribute to hemostasis. This includes defects in platelets and coagulation factors.

Impairment of Platelet Function

Platelet function can be impaired because of a decrease in the number of circulating platelets or because of impaired platelet function.

Platelets are produced by cells in the bone marrow and are then stored in the spleen before being released into the circulation. Consequently, a decrease in the number of circulating platelets can result from either a decrease in platelet production by

Table 11-4 Drugs That May Predispose to Bleeding

Interference with platelet production or function

Acetazolamide
Alcohol
Antihistamines
Antimetabolite and anticancer drugs
Aspirin and salicylates
Chloramphenicol
Clofibrate
Colchicine
Dextran
Dipyridamole
Diuretics (furosemide, ethacrynic acid, and the thiazide
    diuretics)
Lidocaine
Nonsteroidal anti-inflammatory drugs
Penicillins
Phenylbutazone
Propranolol
Quinine derivatives (quinidine and hydroxychloroquine)
Sulfonamides
Theophylline
Tricyclic antidepressants
Vitamin E

Interference with coagulation factors

Anabolic steroids
Coumadin
Heparin
Thyroid preparations

Decrease vitamin K levels

Antibiotics
Clofibrate

From Hansten P (ed): Drug Interactions, 4th ed. Philadelphia, Lea & Febiger, 1979

Koda–Kimble MA (ed): Applied Therapeutics for Clinical Pharmacists, 2nd ed, p 260. San Francisco, Applied Therapeutics, 1978

Packman MA, Mustard JF: Clinical pharmacology of platelets. *Blood* 50, No. 4:1977

the bone marrow, or from an increased pooling of platelets in the spleen. Replacement of bone marrow by malignant cells, such as occurs in leukemia, impairs the bone marrow's ability to produce platelets. Radiation and drugs such as those used in the treatment of cancer often depress bone marrow function and cause reduced platelet production (thrombocytopenia). On the other hand, the production of platelets may be normal, but there may be excessive pooling of platelets in the spleen. Normally the spleen sequesters about 30% to 40% of the platelets. When the spleen is enlarged (splenomegaly), however, as many as 80% of the platelets can be sequestered in the spleen.

Another cause of thrombocytopenia is the abnormal destruction of platelets that is thought to result from an autoimmune response in which the body produces antibodies against its own platelets. Often the cause of platelet destruction cannot be determined, in which case it is referred to as idiopathic thrombocytopenia. In acute disseminated intravascular clotting, discussed later, excessive platelet consumption leads to a deficiency.

Failure of platelet adherence and aggregation is seen in a number of conditions. Aspirin impairs platelet function by inhibiting platelet aggregation and is one of the most common causes of this impairment. The effect of aspirin on platelet aggregation lasts for the life of the platelet—usually about seven to eight days. The recent interest in aspirin's effect on hemostasis has been not so much on its ability to cause bleeding, but rather on its ability to prevent blood clotting. Table 11-4 describes other drugs that impair platelet function. There has been recent interest in the use of the drug sulfinpyrazone (Anturane) for reducing sudden death and recurrent infarction in persons who have had a recent heart attack.[2]

The depletion of platelets must be relatively severe (10,000 to 20,000 as compared to the normal values of 150,000 to 200,000 per mm^3) before hemorrhagic tendencies become evident. Bleeding that results from platelet deficiencies is usually spontaneous and affects the small vessels of the skin and mucous membranes. Bleeding of the intracranial vessels is also a danger with severe platelet depletion.

Coagulation Defects

Impairment of blood coagulation can result from deficiencies in one or more of the known clotting factors. Deficiencies can arise because of deficient synthesis, production of inactive factors, or increased consumption of the clotting factors.

Impaired synthesis

Coagulation factors V, VII, IX, X, XIII, prothrombin, fibrinogen, and probably XI and XII, are synthesized in the liver. Factor VIII is synthesized in the endothelial cells.

Of the coagulation factors synthesized in the liver, factors VII, IX, X, and prothrombin require the presence of vitamin K for normal activity. In liver disease there is reduced synthesis of the entire clotting factor. In vitamin K deficiency, the liver produces the clotting factor, but in an inactive form. Vitamin K is a fat-soluble vitamin that is being continuously synthesized by intestinal bacteria. This means that a deficiency in vitamin K is not likely to occur unless intestinal synthesis is interrupted or absorption of the vitamin is impaired. Vitamin K deficiency can occur in the newborn infant prior to establishment of the intestinal flora and can also occur as a result of treatment with broad spectrum antibiotics that cause destruction of intestinal flora. Vitamin K is a fat-soluble vitamin and its absorption requires bile salts. Therefore, a vitamin K deficiency may result from impaired fat absorption due to liver or gall bladder disease.

Hereditary defects in coagulation factors

Hereditary defects usually affect one factor and have been reported for each of the clotting factors. The three most common defects occur in (1) factor VIII (classic hemophilia), (2) factor IX (Christmas disease or hemophilia B), and (3) factor XI (hemophilia C). Factor VIII defects account for about 80% of the total cases of hemophilia, and Christmas disease for about 15%. The other 5% is due to defects in factor XI. Hemophilia is a sex-linked recessive disorder that primarily affects males. Although it is a hereditary disorder, there is no family history of the disorder in about one-third of newly diagnosed cases, suggesting that it has arisen as a new mutation.[3] Factor VIII is produced by the endothelial cells, and until recently it was thought that persons with hemophilia failed to produce factor VIII (or XI). It has been shown that the factor is present but in an inactive form. An individual with normal coagulation function possesses about 50% to 150% procoagulation activity for most of the coagulation factors. In hemophilia, this amount is only 1% to 20%, with 5% to 20% in mild hemophilia, 1% to 5% in moderate hemophilia, and 1% or less in severe forms of hemophilia. In mild or moderate forms of the disease, bleeding usually does not occur unless there is a local lesion or trauma. The disorder may not be detected in childhood. On the other hand, in severe hemo-

philia, bleeding is usually present in childhood (it may be noted at the time of circumcision) and tends to be both spontaneous and severe. Spontaneous hemorrhage into the joint is damaging and is a frequent cause of disability. Fortunately the coagulation factors are now available to control hemorrhage and to prevent complications.

Consumption of coagulation factors

Acute disseminated intravascular clotting (DIC) is a paradox in the hemostatic sequence in which blood coagulation, clot dissolution, and bleeding all take place at the same time. The condition begins with activation of the coagulation system with formation of microemboli and is accompanied by consumption of specific clotting factors, aggregation, and loss of platelets and activation of the fibrinolytic mechanisms responsible for clot dissolution.

Disseminated intravascular clotting is not a primary disorder; it occurs as a complication in a variety of disease conditions. The coagulation process can be initiated by activation of either the extrinsic coagulation pathway, through liberation of tissue factors, or by activation of the intrinsic pathway, through extensive endothelial damage or stasis of blood. Included among the clinical conditions known to incite DIC are massive trauma, burns, sepsis, shock, meningococcemia, and malignant disease. About 50% of individuals with DIC are patients with obstetrical complications. Table 11-5 summarizes conditions that have been associated with DIC.

Secondary activation of the fibrinolytic system is localized to the sites of intravascular clotting. Breakdown of the fibrin leads, however, to release of products that prevent conversion of fibrinogen to fibrin and thus leads to further bleeding problems.

Although the coagulation and formation of microemboli initiate the events that occur in DIC, its acute manifestations are usually more directly related to the bleeding problems that occur. The bleeding may be present as petechiae, purpura, or severe hemorrhage. Uncontrolled postpartum bleeding may indicate DIC. Microemboli may cause tissue hypoxia and damage to organ structures. The kidney is usually the most severely damaged organ, but there may also be damage to the heart, lungs, and brain. A form of hemolytic anemia may develop as red cells become damaged when they pass through vessels partially blocked by thrombus.

The treatment for DIC is directed toward the primary disease, correcting the bleeding, and preventing further activation of clotting mechanisms.

Table 11-5   Conditions That Have Been Associated with Disseminated Intravascular Clotting (DIC)

Obstetric conditions

Abruptio placentae
Dead fetus syndrome
Preeclampsia and eclampsia
Amniotic fluid embolism

Malignancies

Metastatic cancer
Leukemia

Infections

Acute bacterial infection, *e.g.*, meningococcal meningitis
Acute viral infections
Rickettsial infections, *e.g.*, Rocky Mountain spotted fever
Parasitic infections, *e.g.*, malaria

Shock

Septic shock
Severe hypovolemic shock

Trauma or surgery

Burns
Massive trauma
Surgery involving extracorporeal circulation
Snake bite
Heat stroke

Hematologic conditions

Blood transfusion reactions

Heparin may be given to decrease blood coagulation and in the process may reduce the consumption of coagulation factors.

Vascular Disorders

Vascular disorders cause easy bruising and spontaneous bleeding from small blood vessels. These disorders occur because of structurally weak vessels or vessels that have been damaged by inflammation or immune responses. Among the vascular disorders that cause bleeding are hemorrhagic telangiectasia (an uncommon autosomal dominant trait in which there are dilatations of capillaries and arterioles), vitamin C deficiency (scurvy), and Cushing's disease. Vascular defects also occur in the course of DIC as a result of the presence of the microthrombi.

Vascular disorders are characterized by easy bruising and spontaneous appearance of petechiae and purpura of the skin and mucous membranes. In persons with bleeding disorders due to vascular defects, the platelet count and other tests for coagulation defects are normal.

The Effect of Drugs on Hemostasis

A number of drugs serve to either enhance or impair hemostasis. Oral contraceptives and the corticosteroid drugs are associated with an increase in coagulation factors. Drugs that impair platelet production or function and those that interfere with coagulation are summarized in Table 11-4. There are two drugs that are commonly used as anticoagulant agents—heparin and coumadin.

Coumadin

The anticoagulant drug coumadin acts by decreasing prothrombin and other procoagulation factors that require vitamin K for biologic activity. Coumadin acts at the level of the liver and competes with vitamin K during the synthesis of the vitamin K-dependent coagulation factors. Because the relationship between vitamin K and coumadin is competitive, vitamin K is used as the antidote for coumadin overdose.

Heparin

Heparin is an anticoagulant that is found in many body cells. It is formed in large quantities in mast cells located in the pericapillary connective tissues and in the basophilic cells of the blood. Pharmacologic preparations of heparin are extracted from animal tissues. Heparin acts at several steps in the coagulation process to inhibit blood clotting. It interferes with the prothrombin activator in the intrinsic pathway and inhibits the action of thrombin on fibrinogen. Heparin also acts directly to inactivate thrombin and to increase its removal through increased absorption of fibrin.

In summary, hemostasis is designed to maintain the integrity of the vascular compartment. The process is divided into five phases: (1) vessel spasm, which constricts the size of the vessel and reduces blood flow, (2) platelet adherence and formation of the platelet plug, (3) formation of the fibrin clot, which cements the platelet plug together, (4) clot retraction which pulls the edges of the injured vessel together, and (5) clot dissolution which involves the action of fibrinolysins that dissolve the clot and allow blood flow to be re-established and healing of tissues to take place. The process of blood coagulation requires the stepwise activation of coagulation factors, which ensures that the process is not activated by chance. Bleeding disorders occur when platelet production is impaired, platelet function is altered, or when a coagulation factor is missing or inactive.

:Study Guide

After you have studied this chapter, you should be able to meet the following objectives:

: : State the five stages of hemostasis.

: : Describe the formation of the platelet plug.

: : State the purpose of coagulation.

: : State the function of clot retraction.

: : Trace the process of fibrinolysis.

: : Compare normal and abnormal clotting.

: : State the causes of platelet hyper-reactivity.

: : State two conditions that contribute to increased clotting activity.

: : State two causes of impaired platelet function.

: : Describe the role of vitamin K in coagulation.

: : State three common defects of coagulation factors and the distribution of each.

: : Describe the physiologic basis of acute disseminated intravascular clotting.

: : Describe the effect of vascular disorders on hemostasis.

: : State the mechanism by which coumadin and heparin inhibit coagulation.

:References

1. Arkin CF, Hartman AS: The hypercoagulability states. CRC Crit Rev Clin Lab Sci 10:397, 1979
2. Anturane Reinfarction Trial Research Group: Sulfinpyrazone in the prevention of sudden death after myocardial infarction. N Engl J Med 302, No. 5:250, 1980
3. Lazerson J: Prophylactic infusion therapy in hemophilia. Hosp Prac 14, No. 5:49, 1979

:Suggested Readings

Arkin CF, Hartman AS: The hypercoagulability states. Crit Rev Clin Lab Sci 10, No. 4:397, 1979
Bosl GJ, Edson JR: Intravascular coagulation. Minn Med 62, No. 7:544, 1979
Caparini JA, Zoellner J: Heparin therapy. Part II. Cardio-Vasc Nurs 13, No. 3:13, 1977
Chamberlain SL: Low-dose heparin therapy. Am J Nurs 80, No. 6:1115, 1980
Chart IS, Sanderson JH: General aspects of the blood coagulation system. Pharmacol Ther 5, No. 1–3:220, 1979
Dressler D: Understanding and treating hemophilia. Nursing '80 10, No. 8:72, 1980

Erslev AJ, Gabuzda TG: In Sodeman WA, Sodeman TM: Pathologic Physiology, 6th ed, p 741. Philadelphia, WB Saunders, 1979
Fawns HT: Vitamin K and blood clotting. Nurs Times, 74:1764, 1978
Fischbach F: Tests of coagulation and hemostasis. In A Manual of Laboratory Diagnostic Tests, p 75. Philadelphia, JB Lippincott, 1980
Franco LM: Acute disseminated intravascular coagulation. Cardio-Vasc Nurs 15, No. 5:22, 1979
Green D: Role of the von Willenbrand factor in atherogenesis. Artery 5, No. 3:262, 1979
Guyton A: Textbook of Medical Physiology, ed. 6, p 92. Philadelphia, WB Saunders, 1981
Hand J: Keeping anticoagulants under control. RN 42, No. 4:25, 1979
Kouts J, Howard M, Firkin BG: Factor VIII physiology and pathology in man. Prog Hematol 11:115, 1979
O'Brian BS: The paradox of DIC. Am J Nurs 78, No. 11:1878, 1978
Zalamas J, Simon C: Anticoagulants: Accepted treatment and current trends. Nurse's Drug Alert 3:105, 1979
Vargaftic BB, Conrad H, Samama M: Blood coagulation and platelet function. Pharmacol Ther 5, No. 1–3:225, 1979
How aspirin helps prevent thrombosis. Patient Care 13, No. 6:28, 1979

12

Control of Blood Pressure

Blood pressure is the force used to push blood through the arterial circuit of the vascular compartment. Maintenance of blood pressure is essential for adequate distribution of blood flow to the various tissues of the body, and therefore for survival. Many factors, both physiologic and psychological, exert an effect on blood pressure. The normal individual experiences many moment-by-moment fluctuations in blood pressure. Blood pressure increases during periods of fear, anger, and excitement and decreases during sleep and relaxation.

:Blood Pressure Measurement

Clinically, arterial blood pressure is usually monitored by an *indirect method*, which uses an *inflatable rubber bladder* connected to a *mercury manom-*

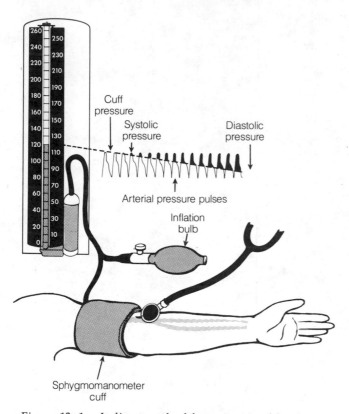

Figure 12–1. Indirect method for measuring blood pressure. When the sphygmomanometer cuff pressure is above arterial pressure no auscultatory sounds can be heard. As the cuff is deflated and the arterial pressure becomes greater than the cuff pressure, the blood spurts into the artery below the cuff, producing vibrations that can be heard through the stethoscope. The pressure at which the auscultatory sounds are first heard is called the systolic pressure. As the cuff is deflated, the sounds increase in intensity, then suddenly become muffled and finally disappear. This represents phase IV and V of Korotkoff's sounds.

eter or an *aneroid gauge* by means of rubber tubing (Fig. 12-1). Blood pressure is measured in *millimeters of mercury* (mm Hg).

In measurement of blood pressure, the uninflated cuff is wrapped around an extremity, usually the upper arm, with the rubber bladder placed superficial to the brachial artery. The cuff is then inflated to a point where its pressure exceeds that of the artery, thus occluding blood flow. The cuff is then slowly deflated until the pressure in the vessel exceeds, once again, the pressure in the cuff. At this point a small amount of blood is forced through the partially obstructed artery. By placing a stethoscope over the artery distal to the cuff, it is possible to audibly monitor the tapping sounds that are produced as blood is forced through the partially obstructed vessel.

Blood pressure is recorded in terms of both systolic and diastolic pressure, for example, 120/70 mm Hg. The *systolic pressure* reflects the initial tapping sound heard as the blood is first forced through the artery. *Diastolic pressure* reflects the point at which the sounds are no longer heard; it measures the point at which arterial pressure is sufficient to prevent vessel compression by the cuff, that is, when the vessel pressure just exceeds the cuff pressure (Fig. 12-1). The auscultatory sounds or tapping sounds heard during blood pressure measurement are often referred to as the Korotkoff sounds, after the Russian physician who first described them. Both phases IV and V have been used to describe diastolic pressures. It has been suggested that phase IV is the best indicator of diastolic pressure.[1] When there is a marked difference between phases IV and V, it is suggested that both pressures be recorded (e.g., 142/85/70). (See chart below.)

Korotkoff Sounds

Phase I: That period marked by the first tapping sounds which gradually increase in intensity.

Phase II: The period during which a murmur or swishing quality is heard.

Phase III: The period during which sounds are crisper and increase in intensity.

Phase IV: The period marked by distinct abrupt muffling or by sounds so that a soft blowing quality is heard.

Phase V: The point at which sounds disappear.

Accuracy of blood pressure measurement requires that the equipment be properly calibrated, correct cuff size be used, the arm be properly positioned, and the cuff be inflated and deflated correctly. The room should be free of distracting noises and the blood pressure gauge should be at eye level. The appropriate cuff size is essential for accurate blood pressure measurement—too large a cuff is apt to give low readings while an inappropriately small cuff may give too high a reading. In adults, the bladder of the cuff should completely encircle the upper arm (or leg) and should be long enough to cover two-thirds of the upper arm. The arm being used should be positioned so that the artery is at the level of the heart. Deflation should be slow enough so that accurate measurements can be obtained (2 mm Hg/beat).

Blood pressure can also be measured intra-arterially. Intra-arterial measurement requires the insertion of a catheter into a peripheral artery. Figure 12-4 shows a tracing of blood pressure recorded from the brachial artery.

Blood Pressure Measurement in Children

There are special methods for obtaining blood pressure measurements in infants and small children. Either the Doppler (ultrasonic) or the flush method is recommended for infants and children under one year of age. In the *Doppler method*, blood movement through the artery is interpreted audibly by a special transducer contained in the cuff. Although this method provides accurate measurement of systolic pressure, its reliability for diastolic pressures has not been established. The *flush technique* is done in the following manner: (1) a cuff of appropriate size is placed around the infant's upper arm, (2) the entire arm is elevated, (3) an elastic bandage is wrapped around the arm (from the level of the hand to the cuff), forcing blood into the upper arm, (4) at the point where the hand becomes pale, the cuff is rapidly inflated and the elastic bandage removed, (5) the cuff is slowly deflated as with the auscultatory method. The mean arterial pressure coincides with the first evidence of a flush; as with the auscultatory method, this is the point at which blood is able to move through the partially occluded vessel.

When the auscultatory method is used for children or adolescents, it is recommended that phase IV Korotkoff sounds be used as an indicator of diastolic pressure; this is because heart sounds are often audible throughout deflation of the cuff.

:Determinants of Blood Pressure

The systolic and diastolic components of the arterial blood pressure are determined by two basic mechanisms. One mechanism is the cardiac output and the other is the total resistance that is encountered in the peripheral circulation. Cardiac output is the product of the stroke volume (blood ejected from the heart with each beat) multiplied by the heart rate. The total peripheral resistance reflects the viscosity or thickness of the blood as well as the resistance to flow that is afforded by the many resistance vessels in the body, namely the arterioles. The small diameter of the arterioles contributes to their effectiveness as resistance vessels, since it takes more force to push a liquid through a small tube than through a large one.

Arterial Pressure Waves

The intermittent ejection of blood into the arterial system gives rise to what are called *pressure waves* or *pulses*. The systolic pressure occurs at the highest point of the pressure wave, and the diastolic pressure at its lowest.

The pressure or pulse wave developing when blood is ejected into the arterial system results from an impulse generated by the sudden ejection of blood into the aorta at the onset of systole. This impulse is then transmitted from molecule to molecule throughout the entire length of the vessel. It is this pressure wave that is responsible for the Korotkoff sounds heard during blood pressure measurement, and it is this impulse that is felt when the pulse is taken. The pressure wave is transmitted through the aortic blood column at a velocity of 4 to 6 meters-per-second, which is about 20 times faster than the actual flow of blood.[2] The pressure wave has little direct relationship to blood flow and it would theoretically be possible to have a pulse wave without blood flow. These pressure waves are similar to those created when water is splashed in a pan or tub.

Systolic Blood Pressure

Systolic blood pressure is determined largely by the *stroke volume*, the *distensibility* of the aorta, and the *velocity* with which blood is ejected into the aorta (Fig. 12-2). During systole the ejection of blood into the aorta raises the aortic and arterial pressure. The extent to which the systolic pressure is raised is determined by the amount of blood ejected (stroke volume) and the distensibility or elasticity of the aorta. For example, systolic pressure will increase when there is rapid ejection of a large stroke volume

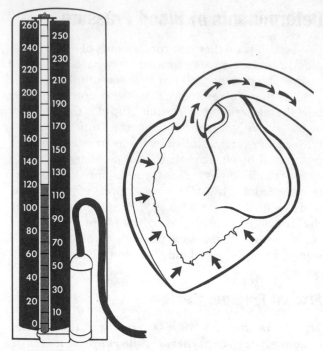

Figure 12–2.   Systolic blood pressure results from ejection of blood into the aorta during systole; it reflects the stroke volume, the distensibility of the aorta, and the velocity with which the blood is ejected.

Figure 12–3.   Diastolic blood pressure represents the pressure in the arterial system during diastole; it is largely determined by the ability of the arterial system to accept the run-off of blood that is ejected into the aorta during systole.

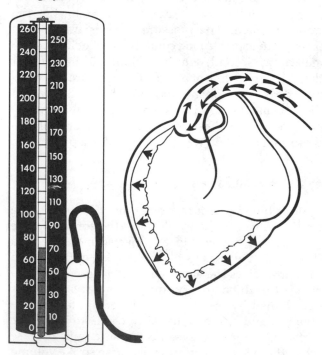

into a rigid aorta. This accounts, at least in part, for the systolic hypertension that is seen in elderly persons who have arteriosclerosis of the aorta.

Diastolic Blood Pressure

Diastolic blood pressure is determined largely by the *condition of the arteries* and their ability to accept the run-off of blood from the aorta. About two-thirds of the ventricular stroke volume remains in the aorta and in the large arteries at the end of systole, and it is this blood that maintains the blood pressure during diastole. The aorta is stretched during systole and as it recoils during diastole, it pushes the blood into the peripheral circulation. The forward movement of blood into the peripheral circulation is facilitated by the sudden closure of the aortic valve which occurs at the end of systole (Fig. 12-3). Because the heart is not contracting during this period of time, the diastolic pressure depends on the ability of the arteries to stretch and accept the run-off of blood from the aorta. In persons with atherosclerosis, the diastolic pressure becomes elevated because the arteries are rigid and cannot stretch during diastole.

Pulse Pressure

The pulse pressure, which is an important component of blood pressure, is simply the difference between the systolic and diastolic pressures (Fig. 12-4). Because diastolic pressure remains relatively constant, the pulse pressure is usually considered to be a good indicator of stroke volume. In hypovolemic shock, the pulse pressure is often decreased; this is because an increase in total peripheral resistance maintains the diastolic pressure, while systolic pressure declines because of a reduction in stroke volume.

Mean Arterial Blood Pressure

The mean arterial blood pressure represents the average blood pressure in the systemic circulation. It is the mean arterial pressure that determines tissue blood flow. In Figure 12-4 it can be observed that the mean arterial pressure is equal to the total area under the arterial pressure tracing. Mean arterial pressure can be calculated by using the formula:

$$\text{mean arterial pressure} = \text{diastolic pressure} + \frac{\text{pulse pressure}}{3}$$

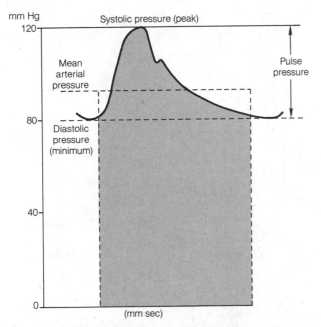

Figure 12–4. Intra-arterial pressure tracing made from the brachial artery. Pulse pressure is the difference between systolic and diastolic pressures. The shaded area under the pressure tracing represents the mean arterial pressure which can be calculated by using the formula: mean arterial pressure = diastolic pressure + $\frac{\text{pulse pressure}}{3}$.

Autonomic Control of Blood Pressure

The autonomic nervous system serves as the final common pathway for interpreting the effects of both physiologic and psychologic stress on blood pressure. The autonomic nervous system is divided into two parts—the parasympathetic and the sympathetic nervous systems. The parasympathetic nervous system exerts its main control on blood pressure through vagal slowing of heart rate. The effects of sympathetic control are more diffuse. This control utilizes three basic mechanisms: (1) controlling the diameter of the arterioles or resistance vessels, (2) increasing the heart rate and force of ventricular contraction, and (3) causing constriction of the large capacitance veins, which leads to an increase in venous return to the heart with a subsequent increase in cardiac output.

The Renin–Angiotensin–Aldosterone Mechanism

The renin–angiotensin–aldosterone mechanism regulates blood pressure through vasoconstriction and changes in body fluid volume (Fig. 12-5).

Renin is an enzyme produced by the kidney in response to a decrease in renal blood flow. Renin

Figure 12–5. Control of blood pressure by the renin–angiotensin–aldosterone mechanism.

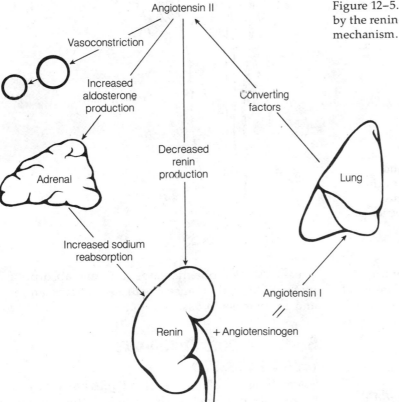

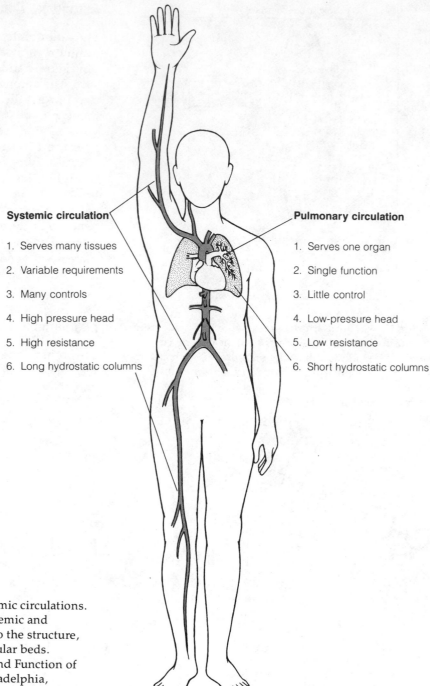

Systemic circulation

1. Serves many tissues

2. Variable requirements

3. Many controls

4. High pressure head

5. High resistance

6. Long hydrostatic columns

Pulmonary circulation

1. Serves one organ

2. Single function

3. Little control

4. Low-pressure head

5. Low resistance

6. Short hydrostatic columns

Figure 12–6. The pulmonary and systemic circulations. There are marked differences in the systemic and pulmonary circulations that are related to the structure, function, and location of these two vascular beds. (Adapted from Rushmer RF: Structure and Function of the Cardiovascular System, 2nd ed. Philadelphia, WB Saunders, 1976)

combines with a circulating plasma protein, angiotensinogen, to form angiotensin I. Angiotensin I is activated in the lung to form angiotensin II, which acts both as a vasoconstrictor and as a feedback regulator to decrease renin release. Although still speculative, recent evidence suggests that increased sodium levels may enhance the vascular action of angiotensin II.

Angiotensin II, or its breakdown products, stimulate the adrenal cortex to increase aldosterone release. Aldosterone increases sodium reabsorption by the kidney; this causes increased water retention and an increase in vascular volume.

:Systemic and Pulmonary Blood Pressure

Systemic and pulmonary blood pressures vary in magnitude and function (Fig. 12-6). To this point we have discussed blood pressure in the systemic circulation which reflects the action of the left heart. Systemic blood pressure is responsible for blood flow to all parts of the body except the lungs. The systemic circulation supplies the brain, the heart, the kidneys, skeletal muscles, and other organs.

The pulmonary circulation is controlled in much the same manner as the systemic circulation. In this system, the right heart serves to pump blood through the lungs. The pressure in the pulmonary circulation is much lower than in the systemic circulation (22/8 as compared with 120/70). The pulse pressure in the pulmonary circulation is maintained at two-thirds that of the systemic circulation. The low-resistance, low-pressure characteristics of the pulmonary circulation are consistent with the close proximity of the lungs to the heart and with the single gas exchange function of the lungs. Unlike the systemic circulation, sympathetic activity exerts little effect on blood pressures in the pulmonary vessels.

In summary, blood pressure is the force used to push blood through blood vessels in the systemic and pulmonary circulations. Because of the close proximity of the heart to the lungs, blood pressure in the pulmonary circulation is only about one-sixth that of the systemic circulation. Blood pressure is the product of cardiac output and peripheral resistance. The greatest determinant of systolic pressure is the stroke volume, whereas diastolic pressure is determined largely by the condition of the arteries.

:Study Guide

After you have studied this chapter, you should be able to meet the following objectives:

: : Compare systolic and diastolic pressure.

: : Compare blood pressure measurement in the adult and in the child.

: : State the determinants of systolic and diastolic pressure.

: : Define *pulse pressure*.

: : Give the formula for calculating mean arterial blood pressure.

: : State the influence of the autonomic nervous system on blood pressure.

: : Trace the physiology of the renin–angiotensin–aldosterone mechanism.

: : Distinguish pulmonary blood pressure from systemic blood pressure.

:References

1. Kirkendall WM, Burton AC, Epstein FH et al: Recommendations for Human Blood Pressure Determination by Sphygmomanometers, p 14. New York, American Heart Association, 1967
2. Smith JJ, Kampine JP: Circulatory Physiology, pp 56-57. Baltimore, Williams and Wilkins, 1980

:Suggested Readings

Cohn J: Blood pressure measurements in shock. JAMA 199, No. 13:118, 1967

Corns R: Maintenance of blood pressure equipment. Am J Nurs 76, No. 5:771, 1976

Federspiel B: Renin and blood pressure. Am J Nurs 75, No. 9:1462, 1975

Feinbeib M, Darwin D, Kuller L: Criteria for evaluation of automated blood pressure measuring devices for use in hypertensive screening programs. Circulation 49, No. 3:6, 1974

Lieberman E: Hypertension in childhood and adolescence. Clin Symp 30, No. 3:3, 1978

Lancour J: How to avoid pitfalls in measuring blood pressure. Am J Nurs 76, No. 5:773, 1976

Keeping your sphygmomanometer in accurate and good repair: An equipment evaluation report. Patient Care 8, No. 1:146, 1974

13

Hypertension

Hypertension is a chronic elevation in arterial blood pressure. Although there seems to be general agreement as to the normal physiologic range for arterial blood pressure, there are still divergent views on the exact level above which these pressures become clinically abnormal. Criteria established by the World Health Organization (WHO) define hypertension as pressures that exceed 160 mm Hg systolic and 95 mm Hg diastolic. These figures are, however, somewhat arbitrary and fail to account for changes that occur with age and other variables that tend to affect blood pressure.* It has become rather common practice to expand the WHO definition to include a category for borderline hypertension—pressures in the range of 140 to 160 mm Hg systolic and 90 to 95 mm Hg diastolic.

Regardless of the definition used, hypertension remains a major health problem with an accompanying threat of complications and a decrease in life expectancy. Studies indicate that over 34 million people, or 15% to 20% of the American population, are afflicted with hypertension.[1] Tragically, only about half of these persons are aware that they have hypertension. As indicated in Figure 13-1, the incidence of hypertension increases with age and is seen more frequently among blacks. This disorder occurs in all geographic areas of the country and affects individuals from low-, middle- and upper-income groups.

Hypertension is usually divided into two categories, primary and secondary. In primary or essential hypertension, the chronic elevation of blood pressure itself is descriptive of the disorder. On the other hand, in secondary hypertension, the elevation in blood pressure accompanies some other disorder, such as kidney disease. Malignant hypertension, as the name implies, is an accelerated form of hypertension. This chapter discusses each of these forms of hypertension.

:Primary or Essential Hypertension

In 90% to 95% of all cases of hypertension, no specific cause can be found—hence the term primary or essential hypertension. The term benign hypertension has been used to describe the disorder, but

---

*The criteria used for hypertension screening by the Milwaukee Blood Pressure Program were: 18 to 49 years, ≥ 140/90 mm Hg; 50 to 59 years ≥ 150/95; and over age 60 ≥ 180/100. (Kochar, Mahendr S, Daniels, Lynda M: Hypertension Control for Nurses and Other Health Professionals, p 2. St. Louis, CV Mosby Company, 1978)

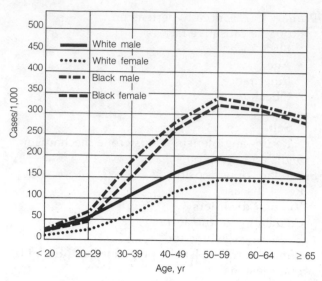

Figure 13–1.   Prevalence of elevated blood pressure at screening (diastolic ≥ 95 mm Hg) according to age and race. (Stamler J et al: Hypertension Screening in 1 Million Americans. JAMA 235, No. 21:2301. Copyright 1976, American Medical Association)

considering the effects of long-term elevations in blood pressure, such a description seems rather inappropriate.

Probable Causative Factors

Although the cause or causes of essential hypertension are largely unknown, various factors have been implicated as contributing to its development. These contributing (or risk) factors include (1) old age, (2) black race, (3) genetic predisposition, (4) environmental factors such as obesity and emotional stress, (5) increased levels or exaggerated responses to sodium, and (6) alterations in renin, angiotensin, and aldosterone regulation (Table 13-1). As with

Table 13-1 Contributing Factors to Development of Essential Hypertension

Old age

Black race

Family history of hypertension

Environmental factors
    Obesity
    Stress
    Drugs (amphetamines, alcohol, nicotine, others)

Increased salt/sodium intake or exaggerated response to sodium

Alterations in renin–angiotensin–aldosterone regulation

other disease conditions, it is probable that there is not a single cause which is responsible for the development of essential hypertension, or for that matter, that the condition is in fact a single disease. Because of the widespread implications for primary prevention, early detection, and proper management of diagnosed hypertension, each of the contributing factors is discussed separately.

Before we continue the discussion of causative factors, it should be pointed out that essentially all of the risk factors contribute to the development of hypertension by either (1) increasing body fluid levels or, (2) increasing the total peripheral resistance. Some of the contributing factors may involve both mechanisms.

Black race

Hypertension is not only more prevalent in blacks than in whites, it is also more severe. The mortality risk for hypertensive blacks is approximately two to three times that of the white population. There is a greater prevalence of diastolic hypertension among young black men than among young white men.[2,3] The reasons for this are largely unknown. It has been proposed that many blacks have a diet that is high in salt and low in potassium and that they may have difficulty excreting sodium.[4] It may also be that stress associated with social and economic problems contributes to the development of hypertension in blacks.

Age

Maturation and growth are known to cause predictable increases in blood pressure. For example, in the newborn, arterial blood pressure is normally only about 50 mm Hg systolic and 40 mm Hg diastolic. Sequentially, blood pressure increases with physical growth from a value of 78 mm Hg systolic at 10 days of age to 120 mm Hg at the end of adolescence. Blood pressure usually continues to undergo a slow rate of increase during the adult years (Fig. 13-1). The relationship between the aging process and hypertension is commonly accepted. The author can recall many older persons describing the normal range of blood pressure as being "one hundred plus your age." While this definition is not entirely correct, it is quite possible that the cardiovascular and autonomic nervous system changes that are part of the normal aging process do, in fact, contribute to the increased blood pressures observed in older persons. It must be remembered, however, that individuals tend to age differently; this factor undoubtedly accounts for some of the great variations in blood pressure among elderly persons.

Inheritance

The inclusion of inheritance as a contributing factor in the development of hypertension is supported by the fact that hypertension is seen most frequently among members of the same family. Current studies suggest that in persons with a positive family history the risk for developing essential hypertension is approximately twice that of persons with a negative family history. The inherited predisposition does not seem to rely on other risk factors, but when they are present the risk seems to be additive. This is particularly true of obesity. When overweight and a genetic predisposition are both present the risk of developing hypertension becomes three to four times as high.[5] The pattern of inheritance is unclear, i.e., it is not known whether a single gene or multiple genes are involved. Whatever the explanation, the high incidence of hypertension among close family members seems significant enough to be presented as a case for recommending that persons from so-called high risk families be encouraged to participate in hypertensive screening programs. This recommendation should include children from such families. It is recommended that all children three years and older, particularly those with a family history of hypertension, should have their blood pressure checked annually.[6]

Obesity

Excessive weight is commonly observed in association with hypertension. In a large nationwide screening program of over a million persons, it was found that the frequency of hypertension in overweight persons ages 20 to 39 was double that of persons of normal weight and triple that of underweight persons.[7] The exact manner in which obesity contributes to the development of hypertension is largely unknown, though it may be that mechanisms responsible for elevating blood pressure in the overweight person are related to the metabolic needs of excess adipose tissue, along with the increased demands on the cardiovascular system to provide adequate blood flow through the enlarged body mass. It is also quite possible that the dietary habits of the overweight person include the ingestion of excess salt along with an increased caloric intake. Whatever the cause, it is known that weight loss is effective in reducing blood pressure in a sizable number of obese hypertensive individuals. It is important to stress, however, that any beneficial effects of weight loss will probably be determined by the duration and severity of the hypertension and its residual damaging effects on the circulatory system.

Stress

Physical and emotional stress undoubtedly contributes to transient alterations in blood pressure. Studies in which arterial blood pressure was continually monitored on a 24-hour basis as individuals performed their normal activities showed marked fluctuations in pressure associated with normal life stresses—increasing during periods of physical discomfort and family crisis and declining during rest and sleep.[8] As with other risk factors, the role of stress-related episodes of transient hypertension in producing the chronically elevated pressures seen in essential hypertension is still speculative. It may be that vascular smooth muscle hypertrophies with increased activity in a manner similar to that of skeletal muscle, or that the central integrative pathways in the brain become adapted to the frequent stress-related input.

Psychologic techniques involving biofeedback, relaxation, and transcendental meditation have recently emerged as methods to control stress-related alterations in blood pressure. It is still too early to tell whether these techniques will offer information about the role of stress in the production of hypertension or will prove useful in its treatment.

Salt

Increased salt intake has long been suspected as an etiologic factor in the development of hypertension. The relationship between body levels of sodium and hypertension is based, at least partially, on the finding of a decreased incidence of hypertension among primitive, unacculturated people from widely different parts of the world. For example, among the Yanomamo Indians of northern Brazil, who excrete only about 1 mEq of sodium per day, the average blood pressure in men ages 40 to 49 is 107/67 mm Hg and in women of the same age, 98/62 mm Hg.[9]

Just how increased salt intake contributes to the development of hypertension is still largely unclear. It may be that it causes an elevation in blood volume, increases resistance in the resistance vessels, or that it exerts its effects through some other mechanism such as the renin–angiotensin–aldosterone mechanism. Interestingly, it has been observed that excess salt does not cause hypertension in all persons, nor does reduction in salt intake reduce blood pressure in all hypertensives. This probably means that some people are more susceptible, and others less so, to the effects of increased sodium intake. Evidence to support individual and group susceptibility to the hypertensive effects of sodium comes from observations made from the development of a strain of spon-

taneously hypertensive rats. These rats develop hypertension earlier than do other strains and the hypertension is more severe when extra salt is added to their diet.

More recently, it has been proposed that it may be the ratio of sodium to potassium intake, rather than sodium intake alone, that influences blood pressure.[10] It has been suggested that food preparation today involves not only the addition of salt but the leaching out of potassium as a result of modern preparation methods in which the cooking water is discarded.

Renin–angiotensin–aldosterone mechanism

The renin–angiotensin–aldosterone feedback mechanism and its contribution to blood pressure control was mentioned in Chapter 12. Secondary hypertension occurs in renal disease due to increased renin levels and in primary aldosteronism due to increased production of aldosterone by the adrenal gland. Although plasma renin levels are usually normal in essential hypertension, about 25% of such persons have what has been determined to be low renin levels. Interestingly, patients with low-renin hypertension have normal aldosterone levels, suggesting that there is a defect in the renin–angiotensin–aldosterone feedback mechanism. Low-renin hypertensives tend to have fewer vascular complications and have a better response to diuretic therapy.[11]

Signs and Symptoms

Essential hypertension frequently is asymptomatic, and diagnosis is often made by chance during screening procedures or when an individual seeks medical care for other purposes. Although headache is often considered to be an early symptom of hypertension, it is present only in a small number of hypertensives at the time of diagnosis. When present, the headache associated with hypertension is believed to be due to intense vasodilatation. It occurs most frequently on awakening and is usually felt in the back of the neck. A common early symptom of long-term hypertension is nocturia, which indicates that the kidney is losing its ability to concentrate urine. Epistaxis (nosebleeds), tinnitus (ringing in the ears), and vertigo (dizziness), although often claimed to be characteristic of hypertension, have been found to be no more frequent among persons with recognized hypertension than among those with normal blood pressures.

Other commonly associated signs and symptoms are probably related to the complications of hypertension—the long-term effects of blood pressure elevation on other organ systems in the body, such as the kidneys, eyes, heart, and blood vessels.

Aside from elevated blood pressure measurements, there are few diagnostic tests that are useful in detecting and diagnosing essential hypertension. In this respect, the increased availability of hypertensive screening clinics provides a means for early detection. The reader is reminded that blood pressure varies in response to stress, time of day, and other factors. For this reason a diagnosis of essential hypertension is never based on a single blood pressure reading. Contributing factors such as a family history of hypertension or the presence of obesity often assist in confirming the diagnosis. Laboratory tests, x-ray films, and other diagnostic tests are usually done for the purpose of ruling out secondary hypertension or for detecting associated complications.

:Secondary Hypertension

Only 5% to 10% of hypertensive cases are currently classified as secondary hypertension—that is, hypertension due to another disease condition. In secondary hypertension, as with other alterations in physiologic function, the presence of an elevation in blood pressure may be a homeostatic response that is recruited in an effort to maintain body function at least partially; or the elevated pressure may be due to an actual alteration in body structures that control or affect blood pressure. Disease states that most frequently give rise to secondary hypertension are (1) kidney disease, (2) vascular disorders, (3) alterations in endocrine function and hormone levels, (4) acute brain lesions, and (5) more recently, some epidemiologic evidence that links alcohol consumption with blood pressure elevation. To avoid duplication in descriptions, the mechanisms associated with elevations of blood pressure in the disorders already mentioned are discussed briefly, and a more detailed discussion of specific disease disorders is reserved for other sections of the book.

Renal Disease

With the dominant role that the kidney assumes in blood pressure regulation, it is not surprising that the largest single cause of secondary hypertension is renal disease (for further discussion of hypertension in renal disease see Chapter 26). By controlling salt and water levels, the kidney is probably involved in virtually all types of hypertension. In renal disease,

salt and water retention undoubtedly plays a major role in elevated blood pressure. Also implicated in the development of renal hypertension is an imbalance between the vasoconstrictor and vasodepressor substances produced by the kidney.

The classic Goldblatt kidney experiments of the 1930s showed that renal ischemia contributes to the development of hypertension through the renin–angiotensin mechanism. In these experiments hypertension occurred regularly in animals in which one renal artery was constricted to produce renal ischemia. These experiments revealed that the ischemic kidney secretes large amounts of renin; this secretion leads to formation of angiotensin II and an aldosterone-mediated increase in salt and water retention by the nonischemic kidney. There is also evidence that the kidneys produce one or more vasodepressor substances. The most likely candidate for this action is a member of the prostaglandin family, although other substances such as kallikrein, a neutral lipid from the renomedullary tissue, and bradykinin have also been suggested. The data are inconclusive, but continuing research will probably bring further insight.

Vascular Disorders

As mentioned in the earlier part of this chapter, hypertension itself predisposes to vascular disorders and vascular pathology tends to produce or perpetuate hypertension. The effects of arteriosclerosis on blood pressure are generally interpreted as changes in total peripheral resistance. In arteriosclerosis of the aorta and large arteries, the rigid vessel walls resist the run-off of blood ejected from the heart during systole, so the blood pressure rises and remains elevated during diastole. When renal blood vessels are affected, additional renal mechanisms contribute to the blood pressure elevation. The exaggerated vascular changes seen in malignant hypertension are discussed toward the end of this chapter.

Coarctation of the Aorta

An unusual form of hypertension occurs in coarctation of the aorta (adult form) in which there is a narrowing of that vessel as it exits from the heart, most commonly beyond the subclavian arteries (see Chapter 16). In the infantile form, the narrowing occurs proximal to the ductus arteriosus, in which case heart failure and other problems are present. As a result, many affected babies die within their first year of life. In the adult form of coarctation there is often an increase in cardiac output that results from renal compensatory mechanisms; the ejection of a large stroke volume into a narrowed aorta with limited ability to accept the run-off results in an increase in systolic blood pressure and blood flow to the upper part of the body. Blood pressure in the lower extremities may be normal, although it is frequently low. The pulse pressure in the legs is almost always narrowed and the femoral pulses are weak. Because the aortic capacity is diminished, there is usually a marked increase in systolic pressure (measured in the arms) during exercise when both stroke volume and heart rate are exaggerated.

Endocrine Dysfunction

Secondary hypertension due to endocrine disorders is rare; when it does occur it is usually of adrenal origin. It involves either the adrenal medullary or cortical tissue.

A *pheochromocytoma* is a tumor of chromaffin tissue usually found in the adrenal medulla, but it may also arise in other sites where there is chromaffin tissue, such as the sympathetic ganglia. Like adrenal medullary cells, the tumor cells of a pheochromocytoma produce and secrete the catecholamines epinephrine and norepinephrine. Thus the hypertension results from the massive release of these catecholamines. Often their release is paroxysmal rather than continuous, causing periodic episodes of hypertension, tachycardia, sweating, anxiety, and other signs of excessive sympathetic activity. Several tests are available to differentiate this type of hypertension from other types. Provocative tests which use a drug such as histamine, glucagon, or tyramine cause release of catecholamines with a resultant elevation in blood pressure; this confirms that the hypertension is of sympathetic origin. In another test, an alpha adrenergic blocking drug, such as phentolamine, is administered; it blocks the vasoconstrictor action of the catecholamines, and the blood pressure falls. A third less hazardous diagnostic measure is the determination of urinary catecholamines and their metabolites, including vanillylmandelic acid (VMA).

Increased levels of *adrenal cortical hormones* can also give rise to hypertension. Both primary hyperaldosteronism (excess production of aldosterone by the adrenal cortex), and excess levels of glucocorticoids (Cushing's disease or syndrome) tend to raise blood pressure (see Chapter 33). These hormones facilitate salt and water retention by the kidney; the hypertension that accompanies excessive levels of either hormone is probably related to this factor. It

has been observed that in primary hyperaldosteronism a salt-restricted diet often brings the blood pressure down. Because aldosterone acts on the distal renal tubule to promote sodium exchange for the potassium lost in the urine, persons with hyperaldosteronism usually have decreased potassium levels. The drug spironolactone is an aldosterone antagonist, and is therefore used in the medical management of patients with an excess of this hormone; the drug increases sodium excretion and potassium retention.

Female Hormone Levels; Pregnancy and the Pill

About one out of every fifteen pregnancies is accompanied by hypertension, resulting from preeclampsia, eclampsia, or other forms of hypertension. The triad of hypertension (blood pressures above 140/90 on at least two occasions, six or more hours apart), or a rise in systolic pressure of at least 30 mm Hg, or a rise in diastolic pressure of at least 15 mm Hg over previously known blood pressures; proteinuria (300 mg/liter in 24 hours); and edema (weight gain in excess of two pounds/week) developing after the twentieth week of pregnancy are classic findings in preeclampsia. Eclampsia is an exaggerated form of preeclampsia that has progressed to include convulsions and possibly coma.

Preeclampsia, or toxemia of pregnancy, is seen most frequently in young teenage primigravida (first pregnancy), in diabetics, in pregnant women with multiple fetuses, and in women with hydatidiform moles. Preeclampsia disappears spontaneously within about 48 hours after the pregnancy is terminated. No specific causes of preeclampsia or the hypertension that symbolizes its presence have been established. It is known that renin levels are reduced in preeclampsia and that plasma levels of aldosterone and desoxycorticosterone fall considerably, although not back to the prepregnant state. The observed decrease in both renin and aldosterone has prompted questions about the advisability of routine salt restriction and frequent use of diuretics during pregnancy. For a more thorough discussion of toxemias of pregnancy, the reader is referred to an appropriate text.

Oral contraceptives are known to cause hypertension. Why this is true is largely unknown, although it has been suggested that increased sodium retention, plasma volume, and weight gain, along with changes in the level and action of renin, angiotensin, and aldosterone may play a part. The fact that the various contraceptive drugs contain different amounts and combinations of estrogen and progestational agents may contribute to the varying incidence of hypertension among pill users. Fortunately, the hypertension associated with contraceptives usually disappears once the drugs have been discontinued. Reduction to normal may require as much as six months. However, in some women the blood pressure may not return to normal, and it may be that they are among that portion of the population that was at risk for developing hypertension.

Brain Lesions

The hypertension associated with brain lesions is usually of short duration and should be considered a protective homeostatic mechanism. It is mentioned here because it tells us quite a bit about intracranial pressure and cerebral blood flow. The brain and other cerebral structures being located within the rigid confines of the skull with no room for expansion, any increase in intracranial pressure tends to compress the blood vessels that supply the brain. Because adequate blood flow is essential to life, it is not surprising that brain lesions which increase intracranial pressure and impede cerebral blood flow trigger a vasoconstrictor response (the Cushing reaction) designed to elevate blood pressure as a way to restore blood flow to the brain. This flow is re-established when the arterial pressure increases to a level higher than the increase in the intracranial pressure that caused compression of the vessels. Should the intracranial pressure rise to the point where the blood supply to the vasomotor center becomes inadequate, vasoconstrictor tone is lost, and the blood pressure begins to fall.

Alcohol Consumption

A study of close to 84,000 persons with known drinking habits at the Oakland–San Francisco Kaiser–Permanente Medical Care Program revealed an interesting relationship between alcohol consumption and blood pressure[12] in that regular consumption of three or more alcoholic drinks per day increases the risk of hypertension. Systolic blood pressures were more markedly affected in persons with increased alcohol consumption than were the diastolic pressures. Only recently has the link between alcohol consumption and hypertension come to light, and it is expected that further studies will shed more light on this relationship.

:Malignant Hypertension

Five to ten percent of persons with essential and secondary hypertension develop an accelerated and potentially fatal form of the disease—malignant hypertension. It is usually a disease of younger persons, particularly young black men, women with toxemias of pregnancy, and persons with renal and collagen diseases.

Malignant hypertension is characterized by marked elevations in blood pressure with diastolic values above 120 mm Hg, encephalopathy, renal disorders, vascular changes, and retinopathy. There may be intense arterial spasm of the cerebral arteries with hypertensive encephalopathy. Cerebral vasoconstriction is probably an exaggerated homeostatic response designed to protect the brain from excesses of blood pressure and flow. The regulatory mechanisms are often insufficient to protect the capillaries and cerebral edema frequently develops. As it advances, papilledema (swelling of the optic nerve at its point of entrance into the eye) ensues, giving evidence of the effects of pressure on the optic nerve and retinal vessels. There may be headache, restlessness, confusion, stupor, motor and sensory deficits, and visual disturbances. In severe cases convulsions and coma follow.

Prolonged and severe exposure to exaggerated levels of blood pressure in malignant hypertension injures the walls of the arterioles, and there may be intravascular coagulation and fragmentation of red blood cells. The renal blood vessels are particularly vulnerable to hypertensive damage. In fact, renal damage due to vascular changes is probably the most important prognostic determinant in malignant hypertension. Elevated levels of blood urea nitrogen and serum creatinine, metabolic acidosis, hypocalcemia, and proteinuria provide evidence of renal impairment.

The complications associated with hypertensive crisis demand immediate and rigorous medical treatment. With proper therapy, the death rate from this cause can be markedly reduced, as can further episodes. Two drugs to treat hypertensive emergencies are mentioned here, although others also may be required to bring the blood pressure down to a safe level. These two drugs—diazoxide, which causes arteriolar dilatation, and sodium nitroprusside, a vasodilator that also affects the venous system—are administered intravenously. Sodium nitroprusside is mixed with 5% glucose in water and administered as a continuous intravenous drip. The drug must be freshly prepared at the time of administration and its action and rate of administration must be carefully monitored by intra-arterial blood pressure methods.

:Effects of Hypertension

The complications and mortality associated with primary and secondary hypertension can be explained as the "increased wear and tear" on the heart and blood vessels.

The increased work load on the left ventricle to pump against the elevated pressures in the systemic circulation is directly related to the degree and duration of the hypertension. This increased work is the stimulus for ventricular muscle hypertrophy and it increases the heart's need for oxygen. If the increased work demands exceed the heart's compensatory efforts, heart failure occurs. The individual who develops coronary artery disease along with hypertension is at particularly high risk, since the heart's oxygen transport facilities are impaired in the presence of increased oxygen needs. Surprisingly, many individuals seem to tolerate elevated levels of blood pressure for many years before its detrimental effects on cardiac function are detected. The hypertrophied left ventricle is usually visible on an x-ray film, and on the electrocardiogram shows a characteristic left axis deviation.

Arteries and arterioles throughout the body experience the effects of the mechanical stress associated with hypertension. Again, it is the severity and duration of the increase that largely determine the

extent of vascular changes. In general, hypertension has been implicated in accelerating the development of atherosclerosis, which causes a narrowing of the vessel lumen, and in weakening the vessels. Also, there is greater risk of aortic aneurysm, coronary heart disease, renal complications, retinopathy, and cerebral vascular disease.

:Hypertension in Children

The incidence of hypertension in children is not known. Part of the reason for this uncertainty is that blood pressure measurements in children have been a neglected part of the physical examination. According to one survey, only 5% of children in three large outpatient clinics had their blood pressures measured during a physical examination.[13] Although there has been some change in these figures, the extent of change is not known. Lauer (1975) found a 1.2% incidence of hypertension in children ages six to nine and a 12.2% incidence in adolescents of 14 to 18 years.[14] Secondary hypertension is more common in children and is usually related to some other health problem such as kidney disease. There is a greater incidence of essential hypertension among adolescents; probably as much as 25% of adolescent hypertension can be labeled essential.[15] The risk factors associated with essential hypertension are similar to those in the adult—a family history of hypertension, increased salt intake, and obesity.

Figure 13–2.   Percentiles of blood pressure measurement in boys and girls (right arm, seated). (High Blood Pressure Information Center, 120/80, NIH, Bethesda)

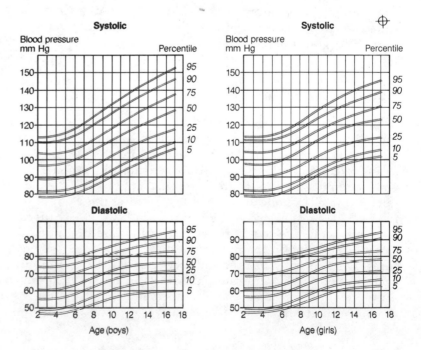

The National Heart, Lung, and Blood Institute (NHLBI) convened a Task Force to review the situation, consult with experts in the field, and develop recommendations for evaluation and treatment of childhood hypertension. The Task Force developed a grid of blood pressures for chidren ages 2 to 18 years (Fig. 13-2), based on readings obtained from more than 11,000 normal children. The Task Force recommended that the term "high normal blood pressure" be used to describe an otherwise healthy child with a single systolic or diastolic pressure reading above the 95th percentile; it was also recommended that these children be re-examined. The term "sustained elevated blood pressure" was suggested to describe those children whose reading is above the 95th percentile on four separate consecutive occasions. "Report of the Task Force on Blood Pressure Control in Children" was published in 1977.[16] The reader is referred to this report and to other readings for further discussion.

:Treatment of Hypertension

In *secondary hypertension*, efforts are made to correct or control the disease condition that is the cause of the hypertension. Antihypertensive medications and other treatment measures supplement the treatment of the underlying disease.

For some individuals, restriction of dietary sodium, weight loss, and efforts to reduce stress factors may be sufficient to control the blood pressure in *essential hypertension*. When changes in life style are ineffective or inappropriate, antihypertensive medications are often prescribed. The medications fall into three categories: (1) diuretics, (2) sympathetic inhibitors, and (3) vasodilators (Table 13-2).

Diuretics, such as the thiazides, spironolactone, and triamterene produce a decrease in vascular volume which helps reduce blood pressure. Of the three, the thiazides appear to have a direct blood pressure lowering effect that is separate from their diuretic action.

Sympathetic inhibitors act at various levels of the sympathetic nervous system. They decrease sympathetic outflow from the brain; they decrease the level of sympathetic neuromediators that are available; or they block transmission of impulses at the sympathetic ganglia or peripheral nerve endings. Inhibition of sympathetic activity often affects functions other than those related to blood pressure; it also tends to enhance parasympathetic nervous system activity. Thus a number of the side effects of these drugs are related to the altered autonomic responses

they induce—either decreased sympathetic or increased parasympathetic function.

Vasodilator drugs promote a decrease in total peripheral resistance by causing relaxation of vascular smooth muscle, particularly the arterioles. These drugs often stimulate tachycardia as a result of the decreased filling of the vascular compartment.

Several drugs are under investigation for use in the treatment of hypertension. Some new adrenergic beta-blocking drugs and enzyme inhibitors prevent conversion of angiotensin I to angiotensin II. Captopril is one of the converting enzyme inhibitors that has recently been released for use.

There are at least three factors that the physician usually considers when prescribing drugs to control hypertension: (1) the drug is not highly toxic and causes minimal side effects, (2) the cost of the drug is not prohibitive, and (3) the procedure for taking the medication is compatible with the patient's life style, i.e., he may take antihypertensive drugs once a day, but may refuse (or forget) to comply with a plan that requires more frequent taking of medications. More than one drug may be prescribed to take advantage of drug synergism; i.e., each of the drugs enhances the action of the others so that none needs to be prescribed in high doses.

The Joint National Committee on Detection, Evaluation and Treatment of High Blood Pressure[17] has recommended a step-wise approach to the treatment of hypertension. This plan involves the addition of antihypertensive drugs in four steps. Step one involves initiation of treatment with the use of a diuretic alone; an additional drug selected from the step two category is added when control is not effected by the diuretic alone. Step three requires the addition of a vasodilator. In the fourth step, guanethidine sulfate is added if control has not yet been achieved. The specific drugs recommended at each step are not cited in this discussion because newer drugs undoubtedly will become available which may or may not fit the step-wise method.

In summary, hypertension is a chronic health problem that presently affects about one out of every five Americans. It may present as a primary disorder or may be a symptom of some other disease. The incidence of hypertension increases with age, is seen more frequently in men than women, and is more prevalent among blacks. It is also linked to a family history of the disorder, obesity, and increased salt intake. Because hypertension is often "silent," hypertension screening programs provide an effective means of early detection. The importance of screening lies in the fact that hypertension can usually be controlled and its complications prevented or minimized with appropriate treatment measures.

Table 13–2 Actions and Side Effects of Antihypertensive Drugs*

Drug	Actions	Frequent Side-Effects (greater than 5%)
Sympathetic Inhibitors		
Rauwolfia alkaloids (reserpine)	Acts centrally and peripherally; causes depletion of catecholamines	Nasal congestion, drowsiness, sedation, *depression*, increased appetite, and weight gain
Methyldopa (Aldomet)	Reduces the level of neurotransmitter in the central and peripheral nervous system	Fatigue, drowsiness, and sedation; postural and exercise dizziness; dry mouth and headache; may cause abnormal liver function tests and positive direct Coombs' test
Clonidine (Catapres)	Diminishes sympathetic outflow from the brain	Dry mouth, drowsiness, sedation, fatigue, dizziness, and vertigo; dry mouth and constipation; *sudden discontinuance of the drug may result in hypertensive crisis*
Propranolol (Inderal)	Adrenergic beta receptor blocking drug (central and peripheral); reduces cardiac output and renin release	Nausea, anorexia, fatigue, dizziness, lightheadedness, bradycardia; blocks beta receptors in bronchioles and can cause bronchospasm in predisposed persons; may intensify hypoglycemia in diabetics on insulin or oral agents
Guanethidine (Ismelin)	Postganglionic sympathetic blocking agent	Orthostatic hypotension, bradycardia, diarrhea, muscular weakness and fatigue, nasal stuffiness, edema, weight gain, headaches, inhibition of ejaculation, impotence, elevation of BUN and creatinine
Vasodilators		
Hydralazine hydrochloride (Apresoline)	Reduces the total peripheral resistance by relaxing smooth muscle in the arterioles	Headache, nausea, vomiting, tachycardia, palpitations, dizziness, weakness, lethargy, and postural hypotension
Prazosin hydrochloride (Minipres)	Smooth muscle relaxant; acts directly on peripheral arterioles	Dizziness, postural hypotension, syncope, weakness, palpitations, nausea, drowsiness, lack of energy, weakness, nausea, and vomiting; patients usually started on low initial dose to avoid severe syncope
Minoxidil (Loniten)	Smooth muscle relaxant; action most pronounced at level of the arterioles	Fluid retention, angina, tachycardia, hair growth (hypertrichosis) of face and extremities

(Based on data from McMahon FG: Management of Essential Hypertension. Mount Kisco, Futura Publishing, 1978)
*The actions of diuretic drugs are given in Chapter 25, Table 25-1.

:Study Guide

After you have studied this chapter, you should be able to meet the following objectives:

: : Describe the possible influence of age, race, heredity, and environment on essential hypertension.

: : State the postulated roles of obesity, stress, and salt intake in hypertension.

: : Differentiate essential or primary hypertension from secondary hypertension.

: : Relate renal disease to the occurrence of hypertension.

: : Describe the relationship between arteriosclerosis and blood pressure.

: : State the role of aortic coarctation in the development of hypertension.

: : Explain the role of catecholamines in the development of hypertension.

: : State the parameters used to determine the presence of preeclampsia.

: : Explain why the vasoconstrictor response is protective in brain lesions.

: : Describe the effects of malignant hypertension on the vascular system.

: : List the three categories of drugs used to treat hypertension and the chief characteristics of each.

:References

1. American Heart Association: Heart Facts, p 10. Dallas, 1980
2. Itskovitz HD et al: Patterns of blood pressure in Milwaukee. JAMA 238, No. 8:864, 1977
3. Stamler J et al: Hypertension screening of 1 million Americans. JAMA 235, No. 21:2299, 1976
4. Langford HG: Hypertension in blacks. Cardiovasc Clin 9, No. 1:323, 1978
5. Stamler J et al: Hypertension screening of 1 million Americans. JAMA 235, No. 21:2299, 1976
6. Recommendations of the Task Force on Blood Pressure Control in Children. Pediatrics 59, No. 5 (Suppl):797, 1977
7. Stamler R et al: Weight and blood pressure. JAMA 240, No. 15:1607, 1978
8. Bevan AT, Hanour AJ, Stott FH: Direct arterial pressure recording in unrestricted man. Clin Sci Molec Med 36:329, 1969
9. Oliver WJ, Cohen EL, Neel JV: Blood pressure, sodium intake, and sodium related hormones in the Yanomamo Indians, a "no-salt" culture. Circulation 52, No. 1:146, 1975
10. Meneely GR, Battarbee HD: High sodium-low potassium environment and hypertension. Am J Cardiol 38:768, 1976
11. Kaplan NM: Clinical Hypertension, 2nd ed, p 299. Baltimore, Williams & Wilkins, 1978
12. Klatsky AL et al: Alcohol consumption and blood pressure. N Eng J Med 296, No. 21:1194, 1977
13. Pazdral PT et al: Awareness of pediatric hypertension: Measuring blood pressure. JAMA 235, No. 21:2320, 1976
14. Lauer RM et al: Coronary heart disease risk factors in school children: The Muskatine Study. J Pediatr 86:696, 1975
15. Adelman RD: Elevated blood pressures in infants and children. J Fam Pract 6, No. 2:360, 1978
16. National Heart, Lung and Blood Institute: Report of the Task Force on Blood Pressure Control in Children. Pediatrics 59:797, 1977
17. Moser M (chairman): Report of the National Committee on Detection, Evaluation, and Treatment of High Blood Pressure. JAMA 237, No. 3:255, 1977

:Suggested Readings

Bear RA, Erenrich N: Essential hypertension and pregnancy. Can Med Assoc J 118, No. 8:936, 1978

Daniels L, Kochar MS: Monitoring and facilitating adherence to hypertension therapeutic regimens. Cardio-Vasc Nurs 16, No. 2:7, 1980

Federspiel B: Renin and blood pressure. Am J Nurs 75, No. 9:1462, 1975

Harburg E et al: Skin color, ethnicity, and blood pressure I: Detroit blacks. Am J Public Health 68, No. 12:1177, 1978

Hartshorn JC: What to do when the patient's in hypertensive crisis. Nursing '80 10, No. 7:37, 1980

Jones MB: Hypertensive disorders of pregnancy. J Obstet Gynecol Neonatal Nurs 8, No. 2:92, 1979

Kannel WB, Sorlie P, Gordon T: Labile hypertension: A faulty concept: The Framingham study. Circulation 61, No. 6:1183, 1980

Lees MM: Central circulatory responses in normotensive and hypertensive pregnancy. Postgrad Med J 55, No. 5:311, 1979

Lieberman E: Hypertension in childhood and adolescence. Clin Symp 30, No. 3:3, 1978

Lindheimer MS, Katz AI: Sodium and diuretics in pregnancy. N Eng J Med 288, No. 17:891, 1973

Londe S, Goldring D: High blood pressure in children: Problems and guidelines for evaluation and treatment. Am J Cardiol 37, No. 3:650, 1976

Marcinek MB: Hypertension: What it does to the body. Am J Nurs 80, No. 2:928, 1980

Moser M: Hypertension: How therapy works. Am J Nurs 80, No. 2:937, 1980

Niarchos AP, Laragh JH: Hypertension in the elderly. Mod Concepts Cardiovasc Dis 44, No. 8:43, 1980

Reisin E et al: Effect of weight loss without salt restriction on the reduction of blood pressure in overweight hypertensive patients. N Eng J Med 298, No. 1:1, 1978

Stamler R et al: Family (parental) history and prevalence of hypertension. JAMA 241, No. 1:43, 1979

Tobian L: Hypertension and obesity. N Eng J Med 298, No. 1:46, 1978

Tobian L: What we now know about the mechanisms of essential hypertension. Med Times 106, No. 5:79, 1978

Ward GW, Bandy P, Fink JW: Treating and counseling the hypertensive patient. Am J Nurs 78, No. 5:824, 1978

Welt SI, Crenshaw MC: Concurrent hypertension and pregnancy. Clin Obstet Gynecol 21:619, 1978

Wyka C et al: Group education for the hypertensive. Cardio-Vasc Nurs 16, No. 1:1, 1980

14

Hypotension and Shock

Cardiac output is closely related to blood pressure. In health, blood pressure is maintained within a range that provides adequate cardiac output and blood flow to meet the metabolic demands of all body cells. This chapter focuses on two clinical conditions in which hypotension occurs. The first of these is the life-threatening condition called circulatory shock and the second is orthostatic hypotension.

:Shock

In 1895 a Harvard surgeon published what has come to be recognized as the classic manifestations of irreversible shock.

> A patient is brought into the hospital with a compound comminuted fracture . . ., where the bleeding has been slight. As the litter is gently deposited on the floor he makes no effort to move or look about him. He lies staring at the surgeon with an expression of complete indifference as to his condition. There is no movement of the muscles of the face; the eyes, which are deeply sunken in their sockets, have a weird, uncanny look. The features are pinched and the face shrunken. A cold, clammy sweat

Table 14-1 Classification of Shock

1. Hypovolemic
  Loss of whole blood
  Loss of plasma
  Loss of extracellular fluid

2. Cardiogenic
  Failure of the heart as a pump (myocardial damage)
  Severe alterations in rhythm (heart block or severe bradycardia)
  Inability to fill properly (cardiac tamponade)
  Obstruction to outflow (pulmonary embolus or thoracic aortic aneurysm)

3. Peripheral Pooling
  Loss of sympathetic vasomotor tone
  Presence of vasodilator substances in the blood (anaphylactic shock)

4. Septic Shock
  Vasodilatation
  Arteriovenous shunting
  Failure of body cells to utilize oxygen

Based on data from MacLean LD: Shock: Causes and management of circulatory collapse. In Davis–Christopher Textbook of Surgery. 11th ed, p 67. Sabiston, DC (ed): Philadelphia, WB Saunders, 1977

exudes from the pores of the skin, which has an appearance of profound anaemia. The lips are bloodless and the fingers and nails are blue. The pulse is almost imperceptible; a weak, thread-like stream may, however, be detected in the radial artery. The thermometer, placed in the rectum, registers 96° or 97° F. The muscles are not paralyzed anywhere, but the patient seems disinclined to make any muscular effort. Even respiratory movements seem for the time to be reduced to a minimum. Occasionally the patient may feebly throw about one of his limbs and give vent to a hoarse, weak groan. There is no insensibility . . ., but he is strangely apathetic, and seems to realize but imperfectly the full meaning of the questions put to him. There is no use to attempt an operation until appropriate remedies have brought about a reaction. The pulse, however, does not respond; it grows feebler and finally disappears, and "this momentary pause in the act of death" is soon followed by the grim reality. A post-mortem examination reveals no visible changes in the internal organs.[1]

Definition

Shock is not a specific disease; it can occur in the course of many life-threatening traumatic or disease states. Shock can be due to trauma, blood loss, myocardial infarction, hypersensitivity reactions, infections, and other injuries. Neither is shock a simple state of hypotension. Rather, shock is a clinical condition characterized by "*an inadequate blood flow to vital organs or the inability of the body cell mass to metabolize nutrients normally.*"[2]

Although blood flow relies on blood pressure, the two are not synonymous. Blood flow relies not only on pressure, but on a vessel diameter that is large enough to facilitate flow and on sufficient blood volume to fill the vascular compartment. In shock, vasoconstriction often serves to maintain blood pressure while compromising blood flow.

Types of Shock

Adequate perfusion of body tissues depends upon the pumping ability of the heart; a vascular circuit that transports blood to the cell and back to the heart; a sufficient amount of blood to fill the circulatory system; and tissues that are able to use and extract oxygen and nutrients from the blood delivered to the capillaries of the microcirculation. There are several ways to classify shock. For our purposes the following classification is useful: (1) hypovolemic, (2) cardiogenic, (3) peripheral pooling, and (4) septic shock. The four types of shock are summarized in Table 14-1.

Hypovolemic shock

Hypovolemic shock occurs when there is an acute loss of 15% to 20% of the circulating blood volume. The decrease may be due to a loss of whole blood (hemorrhage), plasma (severe burns), or extracellular fluid (gastrointestinal fluids lost in vomiting or diarrhea). Hypovolemic shock can also occur with third space losses, when extracellular fluid is trapped outside the vascular compartment. Often blood and fluid losses are concealed. One source cites the case of an elderly man who suffered severe crushing injuries of both legs. The patient had no external evidence of bleeding yet required eight liters of blood over a period of seven hours for stabilization of vital signs.[3]

Of the four types of shock, hypovolemic shock has been the most widely studied, and usually serves as a prototype in discussions of the manifestations of shock. The severity and clinical findings associated with hypovolemic shock are summarized in Table 14-2.

The progression of hypovolemic shock can be divided into four stages. There is an *initial stage* during which the circulatory blood volume is decreased but not enough to cause serious effects. The second stage is the *compensatory stage*; although the circulating blood volume is reduced compensatory mechanisms are able to maintain blood pressure and tissue perfusion at a level sufficient to prevent cell damage. The third stage is the *progressive stage* or *stage of decompensated shock*. At this point unfavorable signs begin to appear: blood pressure begins to fall; blood flow to the heart and brain is impaired; capillary permeability is increased; fluid begins to leave the capillary; blood flow becomes sluggish; and there is damage to body cells and their enzyme systems. The fourth and final stage of shock is the *irreversible stage*. In irreversible shock, even though the blood volume may have been temporarily re-

Table 14-2   Correlation of Clinical Findings and the Magnitude of Volume Deficit in Hemorrhagic Shock

Severity of Shock	Clinical Findings	Reduction in Blood Volume* (percent)
None	None; normal blood donation	Up to 10% (500 ml)†
Mild	Minimal tachycardia	15%–25% (750 ml to 1250 ml)
	Slight decrease in blood pressure	
	Mild evidence of peripheral vasoconstriction with cool hands and feet	
Moderate	Tachycardia 100–120	25%–35% (1250 ml to 1750 ml)
	Decrease in pulse pressure	
	Systolic pressure 90–100 mm Hg	
	Restlessness	
	Increased sweating	
	Pallor	
	Oliguria	
Severe	Tachycardia, over 120	Up to 50% (2500 ml)
	Blood pressure below 60 mm Hg systolic and frequently unobtainable by cuff	
	Mental stupor	
	Extreme pallor, cold extremities	
	Anuria	

*Blood volume changes based on the clinical observations of Beecher et al.
†Based on blood volume of 7% in a 70-kg male of medium build.
(Weil M, Shubin H: Diagnosis and Treatment of Shock, p 118. Baltimore, Williams & Wilkins, 1967)

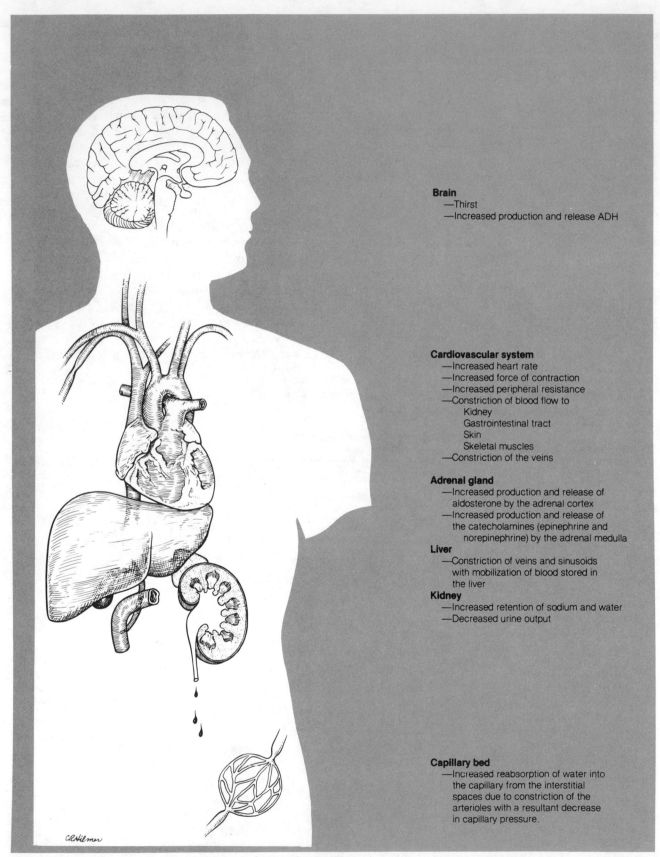

Brain
—Thirst
—Increased production and release ADH

Cardiovascular system
—Increased heart rate
—Increased force of contraction
—Increased peripheral resistance
—Constriction of blood flow to
  Kidney
  Gastrointestinal tract
  Skin
  Skeletal muscles
—Constriction of the veins

Adrenal gland
—Increased production and release of
  aldosterone by the adrenal cortex
—Increased production and release of
  the catecholamines (epinephrine and
    norepinephrine) by the adrenal medulla

Liver
—Constriction of veins and sinusoids
  with mobilization of blood stored in
  the liver

Kidney
—Increased retention of sodium and water
—Decreased urine output

Capillary bed
—Increased reabsorption of water into
  the capillary from the interstitial
  spaces due to constriction of the
  arterioles with a resultant decrease
  in capillary pressure.

Figure 14–1.   Compensatory mechanisms in hypovolemic shock.

stored and vital signs stabilized, death ensues in a matter of time. Although the factors that determine recovery from severe shock have not been clearly identified, it appears that they are related to blood flow at the level of the microcirculation.

Compensatory mechanisms in hypovolemic shock.

Three major compensatory mechanisms are activated in hypovolemic shock: (1) vasoconstrictor response, (2) shift of fluid from the interstitial to the intravascular compartment, and (3) increased pumping efficiency of the heart. The compensatory mechanisms in hypovolemic shock are summarized in Figure 14-1.

Within seconds after the onset of hemorrhage or loss of blood volume there are signs of *sympathetic* and *adrenal medullary activity*. During the early stages, vasoconstriction causes reduction in the size of the vascular compartment and increase in peripheral vascular resistance. This response is usually all that is needed when the injury is slight, and blood loss is arrested at this point. Ten percent of a person's total volume of blood can be removed without significantly affecting blood pressure—the reader is reminded that the average blood donor loses a pint of blood without suffering adverse effects. Figure 14-2 shows how blood loss influences cardiac output and blood pressure. It can be seen that the changes in blood pressure lag behind the drop in cardiac output. This is due to the vasoconstriction and increase in heart rate occurring as blood leaves the circulatory system. It is also apparent that cardiac output and tissue blood flow will decrease before signs of hypotension occur.

As shock progresses, heart rate and cardiac contractility increase and vasoconstriction becomes more intense. Blood flow to the skin, skeletal muscles, kidneys, and abdominal organs decreases. The sympathetic vasoconstrictor response affects both the arterioles and veins. Arteriolar constriction helps to maintain blood pressure by increasing the total peripheral resistance, while venous constriction mobilizes blood that has been stored in the capacitance side of the circulation. There is considerable capacity for blood storage in the large veins of the abdomen and the liver. About 350 ml of blood that can be mobilized in shock is stored in the liver.

The compensatory changes in heart rate, cardiac contractility, and vascular tone developing in shock are mediated through the sympathetic nervous system. In the absence of sympathetic reflexes only about 15% to 20% of the blood can be removed over a period of 30 minutes before death occurs as compared to the 30% to 40% that can be removed over a

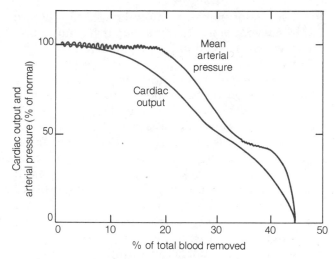

Figure 14-2.   Effect of hemorrhage on cardiac output and arterial pressure. (Guyton AC: Textbook of Medical Physiology, 5th ed. Philadelphia, WB Saunders, 1976)

similar time period with intact sympathetic innervation.[4] Sympathetic stimulation does not cause constriction of the cerebral and coronary vessels, and blood flow through the heart and brain is maintained at essentially normal levels as long as the mean arterial pressure remains above 70 mm Hg.

As has been stated, vasoconstriction causes a reduction in the size of the vascular compartment, so that it can be adequately filled by a smaller blood volume. There are also compensatory mechanisms designed to replace fluid lost from the vascular compartment. During shock, a decline in capillary pressure causes water to be drawn into the vascular compartment from the interstitial spaces. The maintenance of vascular volume is further enhanced by renal mechanisms that conserve fluid. The previously described decrease in renal blood flow resulting from sympathetic vasoconstriction causes both a decrease in glomerular filtration rate and an increase in reabsorption of sodium and water, due to activation of the renin–angiotensin–aldosterone mechanism. The decrease in blood volume also stimulates centers in the hypothalamus that regulate ADH and thirst; a decrease in blood volume of 10% is sufficient to activate both these mechanisms.[5]

Cardiogenic shock

Cardiogenic shock implies failure of the heart to adequately pump blood. Cardiogenic shock can occur because of myocardial damage, ineffective pumping due to cardiac arrhythmias, failure to fill properly, obstruction to outflow from the heart, and problems associated with open-heart surgery.

Cardiogenic shock is frequently encountered

both because of an increase in coronary heart disease and because of better treatment of arrhythmias that in earlier times would have been fatal. It develops in 10% to 24% of persons admitted to hospital with a diagnosis of myocardial infarction, and its severity and progression appear to be related to the amount of myocardium involved. Patients dying of cardiogenic shock generally have lost at least 40% of the contracting muscle in the left ventricle due to either recent or old infarcts.

Cardiogenic shock can follow other types of shock associated with inadequate coronary blood flow; or it can develop because substances released from ischemic tissues impair cardiac function. One such substance, myocardial toxic factor (MTF), is released into the circulation during severe shock. The MTF has a severe depressant effect on myocardial contractility, frequently reducing cardiac contractile efficiency by as much as 50%. The MTF is thought to originate in the pancreas as the result of cellular ischemia in that organ.[6]

Peripheral pooling

With loss of blood vessel tone, the capacity of the vascular compartment expands to the extent that a normal volume of blood does not fill the circulatory system. Loss of vessel tone has two main causes: (1) a decrease in sympathetic control of vasomotor tone, and (2) the presence of vasodilator substances in the blood. There is a decrease in venous return in peripheral pooling which leads to a diminished cardiac output, but no decrease in total blood volume, hence this type of shock is often referred to as *normovolemic shock*.

The term *neurogenic shock* describes shock due to decreased sympathetic control of blood vessel tone; there may be a defect in vasomotor center function in the brain stem, or in sympathetic outflow to the blood vessels. Output from the vasomotor center can be interrupted by brain injury, the depressant action of drugs, hypoxia, or lack of glucose (e.g., insulin reaction). Fainting due to emotional causes is a transient form of neurogenic shock. General anesthetic agents can depress the vasomotor center, and spinal anesthesia or spinal cord injury can interrupt transmission of outflow from the vasomotor center. In contrast to hypovolemic shock, the heart rate is often slower than normal in neurogenic shock, and the skin is dry and warm.

Vasodilator substances in the blood can produce massive vasodilatation with peripheral blood pooling. This in fact is what happens in *anaphylactic shock*. This type of shock is due to a hypersensitivity reaction in which histamine and histamine-like substances are released into the blood. These substances cause dilatation of both arterioles and venules along with a marked increase in capillary permeability. The vascular response in anaphylactic shock is accompanied by contraction of other nonvascular smooth muscle such as the bronchioles. Penicillin, shellfish, insect stings, animal sera, and plant pollens are antigens that are frequent causes of anaphylactic shock.

Anaphylactic shock is usually *of sudden origin; death can occur within a matter of minutes unless appropriate medical intervention is promptly instituted.* Signs and symptoms associated with impending anaphylactic shock include abdominal cramps, apprehension, burning and warm sensation of the skin, itching, urticaria (hives), coughing, choking, wheezing, tightness of the chest, and difficult breathing. Once blood begins to pool peripherally, there is a precipitous drop in blood pressure and the pulse becomes so weak as to be detected with difficulty. Airway obstruction may ensue due to laryngeal edema.

Prevention of anaphylactic shock is always preferable to treatment. Once a patient has been sensitized to an antigen there is always risk of a fatal outcome. All persons with known hypersensitivities should carry some form of warning to alert medical personnel should they become unconscious or unable to relate this information. Information about Medic Alert bracelets and tags is available through most pharmacies. Patients should be carefully questioned about any earlier drug reactions and should be told what medications they are to receive before the medications are administered. It is also recommended that persons being treated as outpatients remain in the facility for thirty minutes following any injection of medication known to produce anaphylaxis, as most serious reactions occur within this period of time.

Unfortunately, it is not always possible to prevent anaphylactic shock. Therefore, all health care personnel should be aware of the characteristic signs and symptoms so that appropriate care can be promptly instituted. Epinephrine constricts blood vessels and relaxes the smooth muscle in the bronchioles; it is usually the first drug to be given to a patient believed to be experiencing an anaphylactic reaction. Other treatment measures include the administration of oxygen, antihistamine drugs, and hydrocortisone. Resuscitation measures may be required. It is often helpful to institute measures to decrease absorption when the antigenic agent has been injected into the tissues. This can be accomplished by application of ice, which constricts blood vessels. Measures to reduce absorption should not be used to replace other treatment measures, but they may be particularly helpful in situations in which medical treatment is not immediately available; for example, application of ice may delay absorption of the antigen from a bee sting so that there is time to secure medical attention.

Septic shock

It has been only in the past 30 years that septic shock has come to be recognized as a clinical entity. There has been a noted increase in its incidence in recent years. At present it has a mortality rate of about 50%. Septic shock is most frequently associated with gram-negative bacteremia, although it can be caused by gram-positive bacilli and other micro-organisms. Unlike other types of shock, septic shock is often associated with other pathologic complications, such as pulmonary insufficiency (shock lung) and disseminated intravascular clotting (DIC).

There are two major predisposing factors involved in the development of septic shock: access to the vascular compartment by an infectious agent, and a susceptible host. The elderly and those with extensive trauma and burns, neoplastic disease, and diabetes are particularly susceptible to infection and the development of septic shock. Another cause is the presence of an indwelling urinary or intravenous catheter. It has been proposed that the rising incidence of septic shock is related to (1) the widespread use of antibiotics, with development of a reservoir of virulent and resistant organisms, (2) concentration in hospitals of larger numbers of infections, (3) more extensive operations on elderly and poor-risk patients, (4) an increase in the number of patients suffering from severe trauma, and (5) use of steroids and immunosuppressant and anticancer drugs.[7]

Unlike other forms of shock, septic shock often presents with fever and vasodilatation, and the skin is usually flushed and warm. There appear to be several hemodynamic patterns associated with septic shock, dependent upon the patient's vascular volume at the onset of shock.[8] The first pattern is a hyperdynamic circulatory response in patients with a normal blood volume at the onset of sepsis. These patients have a high cardiac output, normal or increased central venous pressure, increased pulse pressure, and warm and flushed skin. This response is seen most frequently in young healthy persons, for example, young women who have had a septic abortion. The second response pattern is seen in patients who have a decreased blood volume at the onset of sepsis. They present with a low cardiac output, low central venous pressure, and cold, cyanotic extremities.

Although the pathophysiology of septic shock is not clearly understood, many investigators believe that it is due to a primary defect in cellular uptake and utilization of oxygen. Mild hyperventilation, respiratory alkalosis, and an altered sensorium may be the earliest signs of septic shock. These signs, which are thought to be a primary response to the bacteremia, often precede the usual signs and symptoms of sepsis by several hours or days.

Pathophysiologic Changes

The compensatory mechanisms that the body recruits in shock are not intended for long-term use. When injury is severe or its effects are prolonged, the compensatory mechanisms begin to have detrimental effects. The intense vasoconstriction causes a decrease in tissue perfusion, impaired cellular metabolism, liberation of lactic acid, and cell death. Once circulatory function has been re-established at the onset of shock, whether the shock will be irreversible or the patient will survive is determined largely at the cellular level.

Flow in the microcirculation

Delivery of oxygen and nutrients to body cells and removal of metabolic waste products is dependent upon adequate blood flow throughout the capillaries of the microcirculation. There are two types of capillary flow—one is called *nutrient flow* and the other *nonnutrient flow* (see Figure 14-3). Nutrient flow describes flow in the true capillary pathways that supply cells with oxygen and nutrients. In nonnutrient flow, blood is shunted directly from the arterial to the venous side of the circulation without passing through the true capillary pathways. Nonnutrient flow provides warmth, but not oxygen and nutrients, to the tissues. In septic shock, nonnutrient flow is increased and the skin is warm and flushed. On the other hand, both nutrient and nonnutrient flow are decreased in hypovolemic shock and the skin is cool and clammy.

In severe and prolonged shock, there is failure of the vascular system. When this occurs, there is relaxation of the arterioles and venules, a fall in arterial pressure, and venous pooling of blood. At the capillary level, hypoxia and products of cell deterioration cause increased capillary permeability, stagnation of blood flow, and formation of small blood clots.

Cellular changes. At the cellular level, oxygen and nutrients supply the energy needed to maintain cellular function. Within the cell, oxygen and fuel substrates are converted to adenosine triphosphate (ATP), the cell's energy source. The cell uses ATP for a number of purposes including protein synthesis and

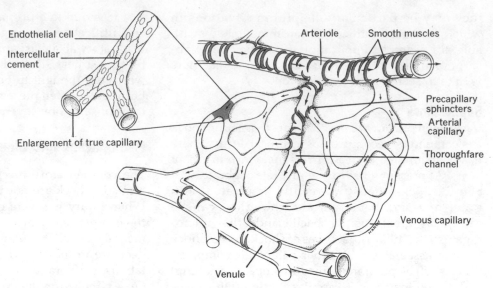

Figure 14–3. Diagram of a capillary bed. When the precapillary sphincters are relaxed, blood flows through the true capillary pathways that supply cells with oxygen and nutrients. Non-nutrient flow occurs when the sphincters constrict, causing blood to be shunted directly from the arteriole to the venule. (Chaffee EE, Lytle IM: Basic Physiology and Anatomy, 4th ed. Philadelphia, JB Lippincott, 1980)

operation of the sodium and potassium membrane pump which extrudes sodium from the cell while returning potassium to its interior.

The cell utilizes two pathways to convert nutrients to energy. The first is the *anaerobic* (nonoxygen) *glycolytic* pathway which is located in the cytoplasm (Fig. 14-4). Glycolysis converts glucose to pyruvate. The second pathway is the *aerobic citric acid cycle* (Krebs cycle) which is located in the mitochondria. When oxygen is available, pyruvate from the glycolytic pathway moves into the mito-

Figure 14–4. Aerobic and anaerobic metabolic pathways in the cells. Lactic acid is formed during anaerobic metabolism, whereas, carbon dioxide and water are the byproducts of aerobic metabolism.

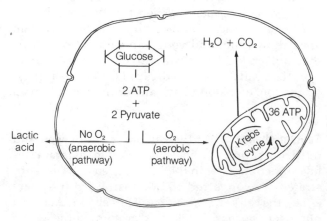

chondria and enters the citric acid cycle where it is transformed into ATP. Breakdown products of fatty acids and proteins can also be metabolized in the mitochondrial pathway. Carbon dioxide and water are formed as byproducts of aerobic metabolism. When there is a lack of oxygen, pyruvate does not enter the citric acid cycle; instead, it is converted to *lactic acid*. In severe shock, cellular metabolic processes are essentially anaerobic which means that excess amounts of lactic acid accumulate in both the cellular and extracellular compartments.

The anaerobic pathway, while allowing energy production to continue in the absence of oxygen, is relatively inefficient—it produces only two ATP units, whereas the citric acid cycle produces 36 ATP units. Without sufficient energy production, normal cell function cannot be maintained (Fig. 14-5). The activity of the cell membrane pump is impaired— potassium leaves the cell and there is an influx of sodium and water. The cell swells and the membrane becomes more permeable. The mitochondria swell and the lysosomal membranes rupture. This is followed by cell death and release of intracellular contents into the serum. Lastly, there is reason to believe that the release of lysosomal enzymes and vasoactive peptides leads to changes in the microcirculation that adversely affect recovery from shock. The lysosomal enzymes from the pancreas have been implicated in the release of MTF from the pancreas.

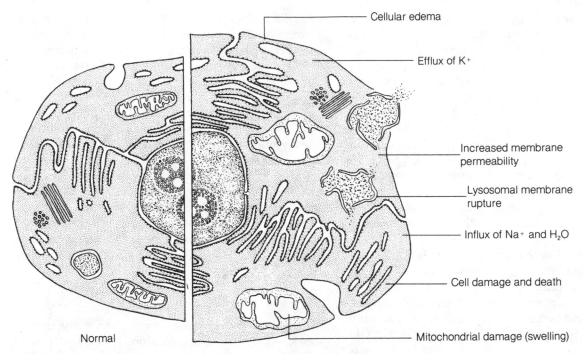

Figure 14–5.   Cellular effects of shock.

Signs and Symptoms

The signs and symptoms of shock are closely related to low peripheral blood flow and excessive sympathetic stimulation. For purposes of discussion, the manifestations of shock have been divided into the following categories: (1) thirst, (2) skin and body temperature changes, (3) arterial and venous pressure, (4) pulse, (5) urine output, and (6) changes in sensorium.

Thirst

Thirst is an early symptom in hypovolemic shock, easily overlooked in situations where there is concealed bleeding. Explanations regarding the causes of thirst are many, although the underlying cause is probably related to changes in blood volume and osmolarity. Patients with trauma frequently have a decreased renal blood flow due to an intense adrenal medullary response along with an increase in ADH levels. Water should, therefore, be given cautiously because water intoxication can occur in a patient who continues to drink water in the face of altered renal function.

Skin and body temperature

The skin reflects the fact that there are two different peripheral responses to shock. In one, sympathetic stimulation leads to intense vasoconstriction of the skin vessels with activation of the sweat glands—the

skin is cool and moist. In the other, there is vasodilatation—the skin is warm and flushed. The former can be observed in hypovolemic and cardiogenic shock, the latter, in hyperdynamic septic shock. In cardiogenic shock, the lips, nailbeds, and skin are cyanotic due to stagnation of blood flow and increased extraction of oxygen from the hemoglobin as it passes through the capillary bed. In hemorrhagic shock the loss of red blood cells leaves the skin and mucous membranes pale.

The decrease in body temperature, often observed in shock, reflects a decrease in the body's metabolic rate. There is a reported correlation between the temperature in the great toe (great toe temperature minus environmental temperature) and the survival rate in shock, in that patients who had increases in toe temperature during dopamine treatment for shock had the highest survival rate. These differences were not accounted for by a simultaneous increase in rectal temperature and were therefore thought to reflect differences in peripheral blood flow to the distal extremities.[9] In septic shock, body temperature may be elevated due to infection and the skin may be warm due to nonnutrient shunting of blood flow in the capillary beds of the skin and peripheral tissues.

Arterial and venous pressures

There has been considerable controversy over the value of blood pressure measurements in diagnosis and management of shock. *This is because compensatory mechanisms tend to preserve blood pressure until shock is relatively far advanced.* Furthermore, *an adequate arterial pressure does not ensure adequate perfusion of vital structures such as the liver and kidney.* This is not to imply that blood pressure should not be measured in patients at risk for developing shock, but it does indicate the need for other assessment measures by which shock may be detected at an earlier stage.

In shock, blood pressure is often measured intra-arterially, as the sphygmomanometer may not always provide an accurate means; systolic pressures measured by the cuff method are consistently lower than those measured intra-arterially. This is because, in shock, the increased vascular resistance in the upper extremities prevents the hemodynamic events that normally produce Korotkoff sounds. Thus, the first tapping sounds detectable with the stethoscope will be heard at a pressure considerably lower than that measured from the artery. The *Doppler method*, in which blood pressure is measured noninvasively by ultrasound, often provides a more accurate estimate of Korotkoff's sounds when they are no longer audible through the stethoscope. In some instances, this method may be used as an alternative to continuous intra-arterial monitoring.

Peripheral venous pressures are decreased in hypovolemic shock. Sympathetic stimulation causes intense venoconstriction such that the veins collapse and it becomes difficult to start an intravenous infusion. *Central venous pressure* reflects the amount of blood returning to the heart and the ability of the heart to pump the blood forward into the arterial system. Measurements of central venous pressure can be obtained by means of a catheter inserted into the superior vena cava through a peripheral vein. This pressure is decreased in hypovolemia and increased in heart failure. The changes that occur in central venous pressure over time are usually more significant than the absolute numerical values obtained during a single reading.

Pulmonary capillary wedge pressure (PCWP) is obtained by means of a flow-directed, balloon-tipped Swan–Ganz catheter. This catheter is introduced through a peripheral vein and is then advanced into the superior vena cava. The balloon is inflated with air once the catheter is in the thorax; it then floats through the right heart and pulmonary artery until it becomes wedged in one of the small pulmonary arteries. Once the catheter is in place, the balloon is inflated *only* when the PCWP is being measured, to prevent necrosis of pulmonary tissue.

With the balloon inflated, the catheter monitors pulmonary capillary pressures in direct communication with pressures from the left atrium. The pulmonary capillary pressures provide a means of assessing the pumping ability of the left heart.

One type of Swan–Ganz catheter is equipped with a thermistor probe to obtain *thermodilution measurements of cardiac output.* In this method, a known amount of iced solution of a known temperature is injected into the right atrium through an opening in the catheter, and the temperature of the blood is measured downstream in the pulmonary artery by means of a thermistor probe located at the end of that catheter. A microcomputer calculates blood flow (and cardiac output) by the difference between the temperatures recorded from the two sites.

Pulse

An increase in heart rate is often an early sign of shock. As with vasoconstriction, the tachycardia of early shock is a sign of sympathetic nervous system response to injury. Tachycardia may also reflect emotional aspects surrounding the injury or the pain associated with the trauma. Blood volume and vessel tone are reflected in the quality of the pulse. *A weak and thready pulse indicates vasoconstriction and a reduction in filling of the vascular compartment.*

Urine output

Urine output decreases in the initial stages of shock, as discussed earlier. Compensatory mechanisms decrease renal blood flow as a means of diverting blood flow to the heart and brain. *Oliguria of 20 ml per hour or less is indicative of severe shock and inadequate renal perfusion. Continuous measurement of urine output is essential for assessing the circulatory status of the patient in shock.*

Sensorium

Restlessness and apprehension are common behaviors in early hypovolemic shock. As the shock progresses, the restlessness of an earlier stage is replaced by apathy and stupor. During this latter stage, there is no longer an expression of concern about the outcome of the injury, and complaints of pain and discomfort cease. If shock is unchecked, the apathy will progress to coma. Coma due to blood loss alone and not related to head injury or other factors is usually an unfavorable sign; it usually means that the patient has sustained a lethal blood loss.[10]

Complications of Shock

Wiggers, a noted circulatory physiologist, has aptly stated, "Shock not only stops the machine, but it wrecks the machinery."[11] Indeed, many body systems are "wrecked" by severe shock. Four major complications of severe shock are (1) shock lung, (2) acute renal failure, (3) gastrointestinal ulceration, and (4) disseminated intravascular clotting. Thus, the complications of shock are serious, often fatal.

Shock lung

Shock lung or the *adult respiratory distress syndrome* is a potentially lethal form of respiratory failure that can follow severe shock. The term "shock lung" was introduced during the Vietnam War to describe the progressive pulmonary failure seen in soldiers who suffered major trauma. The symptoms do not usually develop until 24 to 48 hours after the initial trauma, in some instances longer. Characteristically there is a decrease in pulmonary compliance; more pressure (effort) is needed to inflate the lung, so that there is an increase in the rate and effort of breathing. Alveolar capillary permeability is increased and interstitial edema develops; the lung becomes engorged and gas exchange is impaired. Hypoxia usually is severe despite oxygen therapy. Some patients develop a hyaline membrane similar to that seen in respiratory distress syndrome of the newborn.

The exact cause of the adult respiratory syndrome is unknown. It has been suggested that the problem results from (1) a decrease in lung perfusion and ischemia of the type II alveolar cells which produce surfactant; (2) oxygen toxicity; (3) neurogenic factors that cause pulmonary venoconstriction and pulmonary edema due to sympathetic nervous factors; (4) fluid overload with stretching and disruption of the pulmonary capillaries; or (5) damage to the lung by endotoxins and substances released as the result of sepsis. One very widely accepted cause of the adult respiratory syndrome is disseminated intravascular clotting—the presence of thromboemboli in the pulmonary microcirculation. It is possible that multiple mechanisms operate to cause a similar pattern of injury or to trigger a common response (e.g., intravascular clotting) which, in turn, produces the pulmonary damage.

Acute renal failure

The renal tubules are particularly vulnerable to ischemia, and *renal failure* is one important late cause of death in severe shock. The degree of renal damage is related to the severity and duration of shock; the normal kidney is able to tolerate severe ischemia for a period of fifteen to twenty minutes. The renal lesion most frequently seen after severe shock is *acute tubular necrosis*. Acute tubular necrosis is reversible, although return to normal renal function may require weeks or months (see Chap. 27 for further discussion). *Continuous monitoring of urine output during shock provides a means for assessing renal blood flow.*

Gastrointestinal ulceration

The gastrointestinal tract is particularly vulnerable to ischemia due to the circulatory pattern of its mucosal surface. In shock there is widespread constriction of blood vessels supplying the gastrointestinal tract; this causes a redistribution of blood flow such that mucosal perfusion is severely diminished. Superficial mucosal lesions of the stomach and duodenum can develop within hours of severe trauma, sepsis, or burn. (Stress ulcers associated with burns are called Curling's ulcers.) Bleeding is a frequent sign of gastrointestinal ulceration due to shock. Hemorrhage has its onset usually within two to ten days following the original insult, and often it gives no warning.

Disseminated intravascular clotting (DIC)

Disseminated intravascular clotting, a complication of septic shock, is characterized by the formation of small clots in the microcirculation. There is consumption and depletion of platelets, fibrinogen, and other clotting factors, leading to disruption of the normal clotting process with abnormal bleeding or hemorrhage.

Treatment Measures

The treatment of shock is directed toward *correcting* or *controlling the underlying cause* and *improving tissue perfusion*. This chapter presents an overview of commonly employed treatments.

In *hypovolemic shock*, the goal of treatment is to *restore vascular volume*. This can be accomplished through *intravenous administration of fluids and blood*. The plasma expanders (*dextrans* and *colloidal albumin solutions*) have a high molecular weight, do not necessitate blood typing, and remain in the circulation for longer periods of time than the crystalloids such as glucose and saline. The *dextrans must be used with caution, however, as they may induce serious or fatal reactions, including anaphylaxis.*

In *cardiogenic shock*, treatment measures are directed toward reducing the work of the heart while improving its pumping efficiency. An intra-aortic balloon may be used to supplement cardiac pumping in situations of severe cardiogenic shock. The balloon pump is inserted retrograde into the thoracic aorta through a peripheral artery. The balloon, filled with helium, is synchronized to inflate during diastole and deflate during systole. Diastolic inflation creates a diastolic pressure wave that results in increased perfusion to all the organs including the myocardium. The sudden release of pressure at the onset of systole lowers resistance to ejection of blood from the left ventricle, thereby increasing the heart's pumping efficiency.

Vasoactive drugs

Vasoactive drugs are agents capable of either constricting or dilating blood vessels. Currently, there is considerable controversy about the advantages or disadvantages related to use of these drugs. The major vasoactive drugs used to treat shock are summarized in Table 14-3.

There are two types of receptors for the sympathetic nervous system—alpha and beta. Beta receptors are further subdivided into beta-1 and beta-2. In the cardiorespiratory system stimulation of the alpha receptors causes vasoconstriction; stimulation of beta-1 receptors causes an increase in heart rate and the force of myocardial contraction; and stim-

ulation of beta-2 receptors produces vasodilatation of the skeletal muscle beds and relaxation of the bronchioles. Currently, dopamine is prescribed to treat shock because it induces a more favorable array of alpha and beta receptor actions than many of the adrenergic drugs. Dopamine is thought to increase blood flow to the kidneys, liver, and other abdominal organs while maintaining vasoconstriction of less vital structures such as the skin and skeletal muscles. *Nitroprusside* (Nipride), a vasodilator drug, is used to treat cardiogenic shock. It causes both arterial and venous dilatation, thus a decrease in venous return to the heart with a reduction in arterial resistance against which the left heart must pump. The arterial pressure is maintained by an increased ventricular stroke volume that is ejected against a lowered resistance; this allows blood to be redistributed from the pulmonary vascular bed to the systemic circulation.

In summary, shock is an acute emergency situation in which body tissues are either deprived of oxygen or cellular nutrients or are unable to use these materials in their metabolic processes. Shock may develop because there is not enough blood in the circulatory system (hypovolemic shock); because the heart fails as a pump (cardiogenic shock); because blood is pooled in the periphery (vasogenic or neurogenic shock); or because the tissues are unable to utilize oxygen and nutrients (septic shock).

Table 14–3   Vasoactive Drugs Used in Treatment of Shock

Drug	Mechanism	Action*
Epinephrine (Adrenalin)	alpha beta 1 and 2	Vasoconstriction (specific for anaphylactic shock) Increase in heart rate and cardiac contractility Causes a decrease in renal and splanchnic blood flow while increasing skeletal muscle flow
Norepinephrine (Levophed)	alpha beta 1	Vasoconstriction Increase in heart rate and cardiac contractility
Isoproterenol (Isuprel)	beta 1 beta 2	Increase in heart rate and cardiac contractility Vasodilatation and perfusion of cerebral and renal tissue
Metaraminol (Aramine)	alpha beta 1	Vasoconstriction Increase in heart rate and cardiac contractility.
Dopamine (Intropin)	alpha beta 1 dopaminergic	Vasoconstriction with large doses Increased heart rate and cardiac contractility Vasodilatation of splanchnic and renal vessels
Dobutamine	beta 1	Increases cardiac contractility with minimal increase in heart rate (specific in cardiogenic shock)
Nitroprusside (Nipride)	dilator of venous and arterial smooth muscle	Decreases venous return to the heart causing a decrease in end-diastolic volume and pressure Decreases systemic vascular resistance with a resultant decrease in left ventricular stroke work (specific for cardiogenic shock)

*This list is not intended to be inclusive; it encompasses the drug actions related only to treatment of shock.

:Orthostatic Hypotension

By orthostatic hypotension is meant a fall in both systolic and diastolic blood pressure upon standing. In the absence of normal baroreflex function, blood pools in the lower part of the body when the standing position is assumed, cardiac output falls, and blood flow to the brain is inadequate. Dizziness, fainting, or both may then occur.

On assumption of the upright position, there is usually a momentary shift in blood to the lower part of the body with an accompanying fall in central blood volume and arterial pressure. Normally, this fall in blood pressure is transient, lasting through several cardiac cycles. This is because the baroreceptors located in the thorax and carotid sinus area sense the fall in blood pressure and initiate reflex constriction of the veins and arterioles as well as an increase in heart rate that brings blood pressure back to normal. Within a few minutes of standing, blood levels of ADH and sympathetic neuromediators increase as a secondary means of ensuring maintenance of normal blood pressure in the standing position. Muscle movement in the lower extremities also aids venous return to the heart by pumping blood out of the legs.

In persons with healthy blood vessels and normal autonomic function, cerebral blood flow is usually not reduced in the upright position unless arterial pressure falls below 70 mm Hg. The strategic location of the arterial baroreceptors, between the heart and brain, is designed to ensure that the arterial pressure is maintained within a range sufficient to prevent a reduction in cerebral blood flow.

Causes

In orthostatic hypotension, mean arterial and pulse pressure are decreased by at least 30 to 35 mm Hg after 10 minutes of standing.[12] It has been reported to occur with (1) increased age, (2) decreased blood volume, (3) defective autonomic function, (4) severe varicose veins, and (5) immobility or impaired function of the skeletal muscle pumps.

The elderly
Weakness and dizziness on standing are common complaints of the elderly. It has been reported that about 10% of persons over the age of 65 have a fall in systolic pressure of 20 mm Hg or more on assumption of the upright position,[13] since cerebral blood flow is primarily dependent upon systolic pressure. Patients with impaired cerebral circulation may experience symptoms of weakness, ataxia, dizziness,

and syncope when their arterial pressure falls even slightly. This may happen in older persons who are immobilized for brief periods of time, or whose blood volume is decreased due to inadequate fluid intake or over zealous use of diuretics.

Fluid deficit
Orthostatic hypotension is often an early sign of fluid deficit. When blood volume is decreased the vascular compartment is only partially filled; although when a person is in the recumbent position cardiac output may be adequate, it often decreases to the point of causing weakness and fainting when the person assumes the standing position. Common causes of orthostatic hypotension related to hypovolemia are (1) excessive use of diuretics, (2) excessive diaphoresis, (3) loss of gastrointestinal fluids through vomiting and diarrhea, and (4) loss of fluid volume associated with prolonged bed rest.

Autonomic dysfunction
The sympathetic nervous system plays an essential role in adjustment to the upright position. Sympathetic stimulation increases heart rate and cardiac contractility, and causes constriction of peripheral veins and arterioles. Orthostatic hypotension due to altered autonomic function is common in peripheral neuropathies associated with diabetes mellitus, following injury or disease of the spinal cord, or as the result of a cerebral vascular accident in which sympathetic outflow from the brain stem is disrupted. Another cause of autonomically mediated orthostatic hypotension is the use of drugs that interfere with sympathetic activity (Table 14-4).

Prolonged bedrest
With prolonged bedrest there is a reduction in plasma volume, a decrease in venous tone, failure of peripheral vasoconstriction and weakness of the skeletal muscles of the veins, which help return blood to the heart. Orthostatic intolerance is a recognized problem of space flight—a potential risk upon reentry into the earth's gravitational field. Physical deconditioning follows even short periods of bedrest. After three to four days, blood volume is decreased. Loss of vascular and skeletal muscle tone is less predictable, but probably becomes maximal after about two weeks of bedrest.

Idiopathic orthostatic hypotension
Idiopathic orthostatic hypotension is unrelated to drug therapy or other pathologic conditions. It may be of two types: (1) idiopathic orthostatic hypotension not accompanied by other signs of neurologic

Table 14–4 Drugs Known to Cause Orthostatic Hypotension*

Drug Groups	Specific Drugs	Mechanism of Action
Antihypertensive drugs	Pentolinium (Ansolysen) Trimetaphan (Arfonad)	Blocks transmission of sympathetic impulses at the autonomic ganglia
	Guanethidine (Ismelin)	Blocks sympathetic impulses at the postganglionic sites
	Methyldopa (Aldomet) Clonidine (Catapres)	Decreases sympathetic outflow from the central nervous system
	Hydralazine (Apresoline) Prazosin (Minipres) Minoxidil (Loniten)	Direct vasodilator action
Antiparkinson drugs	Levodopa preparations Amantadine (Symmetrel)	Vasodilatation due to beta adrenergic stimulation or alpha blockade of the peripheral vascular system
Antipsychotic drugs	Chlorpromazine (Thorazine) Thiethylperazine (Torecan) Thioridazine (Mellaril)	Loss of reflex vasoconstriction due to blocking of alpha receptors; these drugs also impair sympathetic outflow from the brain
Vasodilator drugs	Nitrates (nitroglycerin and long-acting nitrates)	Direct vasodilator action

*This list is not intended to be inclusive; it encompasses some of the widely prescribed drugs.

deficits, and (2) idiopathic hypotension accompanied by multiple neurologic deficits (Shy–Drager syndrome). The Shy–Drager syndrome is characterized by upper motor neuron damage with uncoordinated movements, urinary incontinence, constipation, and other signs of neurologic pathology.

Assessment

Orthostatic hypotension can be assessed with the blood pressure cuff. A reading should be made when the patient is supine, immediately upon assumption of the seated or upright position, and at two to three minute intervals for a period of ten to fifteen minutes. It is strongly recommended that a second person be available when blood pressure is measured in the standing position, to prevent injury should the patient become faint. A tilt table can also be used for the purpose. With a tilt table, the patient is recumbent, while the table is tilted so that the patient is in a head-up position.

Treatment

Treatment of orthostatic hypotension is usually directed toward alleviating the cause or if this is not possible, toward helping the patient cope. Correction of fluid deficit, and trying a different antihypertensive medication, are examples of measures designed to correct the cause. Measures designed to

help the patients cope are (1) gradual ambulation, i.e., sitting on the edge of the bed for several minutes before standing to allow the circulatory system to adjust, (2) avoidance of situations that encourage excessive vasodilatation (such as drinking alcohol or exercising vigorously in a warm environment), and (3) avoidance of excess diuresis (use of diuretics), diaphoresis, or loss of body fluids. Tight-fitting elastic support hose or an abdominal support garment may help prevent pooling of blood in the lower extremities and abdomen.

In summary, orthostatic hypotension refers to an abnormal fall in both systolic and diastolic blood pressures that occurs on assumption of the upright position. Among the factors that contribute to its occurrence are (1) advanced age, (2) decreased blood volume, (3) defective function of the autonomic nervous system, (4) severe varicose veins, and (5) the effects of immobility.

:Study Guide

After you have studied this chapter, you should be able to meet the following objectives:

: : State a clinical definition of *shock*.

: : List the chief characteristics of hypovolemic shock, cardiogenic shock, peripheral pooling, and septic shock.

: : List and describe the four stages of hypovolemic shock.

: : Trace the compensatory mechanisms that are activated in hypovolemic shock.

: : State the basis of cardiogenic shock.

: : State the common features of normovolemic shock, neurogenic shock and anaphylactic shock.

: : List immediate treatment measures that health care professionals should take in anaphylactic shock.

: : Differentiate nutrient flow from nonnutrient flow.

: : Trace the conversion of oxygen and fuel substrates to ATP.

: : State the physiologic basis of thirst in shock.

: : State the manifestations of shock revealed in the skin and the body temperature.

: : Describe the central problem involved in measuring blood pressure in shock.

: : Describe changes in pulse rate, urinary output, and sensorium that are indicative of shock.

: : Describe the pathology seen in shock lung.

: : Describe the damage to the renal system and the gastrointestinal system associated with shock.

: : State the rationale for treatment measures to correct and reverse shock.

: : Describe the pathologic changes that culminate in orthostatic hypotension.

: : State why older persons are more likely than younger ones to experience orthostatic hypotension.

: : State the relationship between orthostatic hypotension and fluid deficit.

: : Describe the mechanisms of drug action that may induce orthostatic hypotension.

: : Describe treatment measures in orthostatic hypotension.

:References

1. MacLean LD: Shock: Causes and management of circulatory shock. In Sabiston DC (ed): Davis–Christopher's Textbook of Surgery, 11th ed, p 65. Philadelphia, WB Saunders, 1977
2. MacLean LD: Shock: Causes and management of circulatory shock. In Sabiston DC (ed): Davis–Christopher's Textbook of Surgery, 11th ed, p 67. Philadelphia, WB Saunders, 1977
3. MacLean LD: Shock: Causes and management of circulatory shock. In Sabiston DC (ed): Davis–Christopher's Textbook of Surgery, 11th ed, p 69. Philadelphia, WB Saunders, 1977
4. Guyton AC: Textbook of Medical Physiology, 6th ed, p 333. Philadelphia, WB Saunders, 1981
5. Guyton AC: Textbook of Medical Physiology, 6th ed, p 441. Philadelphia, WB Saunders, 1981
6. Guyton AC: Textbook of Medical Physiology, 6th ed, p 336. Philadelphia, WB Saunders, 1981
7. Altemeier WA, Todd JC, Inge WW: Gram-negative septicemia: A growing threat. Ann Surg 166:530, 1967
8. MacLean LD: Shock: Causes and Management of circulatory shock. In Sabiston DC (ed): Davis–Christopher's Textbook of Surgery, 11th ed, p 82, 1977
9. Ruiz CE, Weil MH, Carlson RW: Treatment of circulatory shock with dopamine. JAMA 242, No. 2:167, 1979
10. Shires et al: In Schwartz SI et al (ed): Principles of Surgery, p 136. New York, McGraw-Hill, 1980
11. As cited in Smith JJ, Kampine JP: Circulatory Physiology, p 298. Baltimore, Williams & Wilkins, 1980
12. Ziegler MG, Lake CR, Kopin IJ: The sympathetic-nervous-system deficit in primary orthostatic hypotension. N Engl J Med 296, No. 6:293, 1977
13. Johnson RH et al: Effect of posture on blood-pressure in elderly patients. Lancet 731, 1965

:Suggested Readings
Shock

Foster SB, Canty KA: Pump failure following myocardial infarction: An overview. Heart Lung 9, No. 2:293, 1979
McCaffree RD: Shock: How to recognize its early stages and what to do about it. Med Times 107, No. 9:25, 1979
Mohr JA, Coussons T: Septic shock. Med Times 107, No. 9:39, 1979
Pepine CJ, Nichols WW, Alexander JA: Guidelines to evaluation and management of shock. Hosp Med 15, No. 3:88, 1979
Rackley CE et al: Cardiogenic shock. Med Times 107, No. 9:33, 1979
Schumer W: Metabolism during shock and sepsis. Heart Lung 5, No. 3:416, 1975
Weil M: Current understanding of mechanisms and treatment of circulatory shock caused by bacterial infections. Ann Clin Res 9:181, 1977
Whitsett TL: Medical management of shock: Drugs of choice and their choice. Med Times 107, No. 9:59, 1979
Wilson RF: The diagnosis and management of severe sepsis and septic shock. Heart Lung 5, No. 3:422, 1976
Wilson RF: The pathophysiology of shock. Intens Care Med 6:89, 1980
Zamora B: Management of hemorrhagic shock. Hosp Med 15, No. 7:6, 1979

Orthostatic hypotension

Adelman EM: When the patient's blood pressure falls: What does it mean? What do you do? Nursing '80 10, No. 2:26, 1980

Hickler RB: Orthostatic hypotension and syncope. N Engl J Med 296, No. 6:336, 1977

Johnson RH, Smith AC, Spalding JMK et al: Effect of posture on blood pressure in elderly patients. Lancet:731, 1965

Melada GA, Goldman RH, Luetscher JA et al: Hemodynamics, renal function, plasma renin, and aldosterone in man after 5 to 14 days of bedrest. Aviation, Space and Environmental Medicine. 1049, 1975

Mooss AN, Sketch MH: Orthostatic hypotension: Evaluation and therapy. Hosp Med 15, No. 12:16, 1979

Moss AJ, Glaser W, Topol E: Atrial tachypacing in the treatment of a patient with primary orthostatic hypotension. N Engl J Med 302, No. 26:1456, 1980

Myers MG, Kearns P, Shedletsky R et al: Postural hypotension and mental function in the elderly. Can Med Assoc J 119:1061, 1978

15

Control
of Cardiac
Function

The heart is a four-chambered pump that beats on the average of seventy times a minute, twenty-four hours a day, three hundred and sixty-five days a year for a lifetime. In one day this pump moves over 1800 gallons of blood throughout the body, and during a lifetime, the work performed by the heart would lift thirty tons to a height of thirty thousand feet. This chapter discusses the overall structure and function of the heart in preparation for the understanding of the chapters that follow.

The heart is located between the lungs, in the mediastinal space of the intrathoracic cavity, within a tough fibrous sac called the pericardium. The wall of the heart is composed of three layers: an outer layer called the epicardium which is adjacent to the pericardium, the myocardium or muscle layer, and the smooth endocardial layer that lines the heart.

Figure 15–1. Diagram of the pulmonary and systemic circulations. (Chaffee EE, Lytle IM: Basic Physiology and Anatomy, 4th ed. Philadelphia, JB Lippincott, 1980)

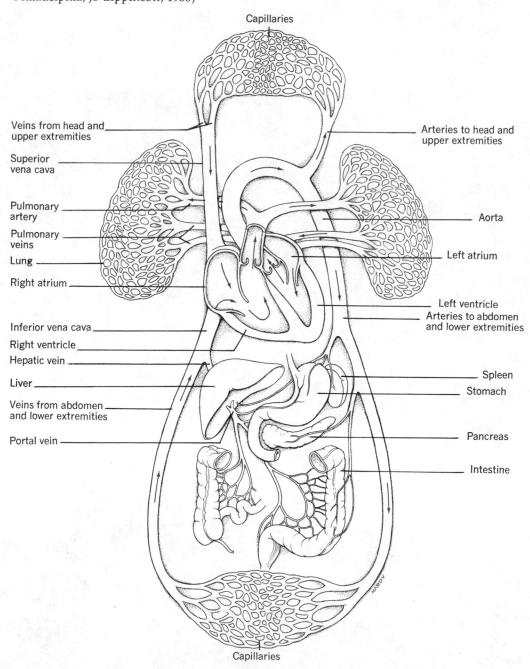

:The Heart as a Pump

The heart is actually two two-chambered pumps—a right and left pump (Fig. 15-1). The lower chambers, or ventricles, provide the heart's pumping action. The upper chambers, or atria, serve mainly as primer pumps which gain importance during increased activity when the filling time of the heart is decreased, or in situations where heart disease impairs ventricular filling. In these two situations, cardiac output would fall drastically, were it not for the action of the atria. It has been estimated that atrial contraction can contribute as much as 30% to cardiac reserve during periods of stress, while having little or no effect on cardiac output during rest.

The right heart delivers blood to the lungs for renewal of its oxygen supply and for removal of carbon dioxide. Because of the close proximity of the lungs to the heart and the low resistance to flow in the pulmonary circulation, the right heart operates as a low-pressure pump (pulmonary artery pressure is about 22/8 mm Hg). The left heart, on the other hand, must pump blood throughout the entire systemic circulation, where the distance and resistance to blood flow demands that this side operate as a high-pressure system (systemic arterial blood pressure is approximately 120/70 mm Hg). The increased thickness of the left ventricular wall results from the additional work this ventricle is required to perform. As an additional point of emphasis, the reader is reminded that both sides of the heart must pump the same amount of blood over a period of time. This will become clearer when the effects of heart failure are discussed.

The Cardiac Cycle

The cardiac cycle consists of a period of contraction (*systole*) during which blood is ejected from the heart, and a period of relaxation (*diastole*) during which the heart fills with blood. The amount of blood that is ejected from the heart with each beat is called the *stroke volume*. During diastole the ventricles normally increase their volume to about 120 ml (called the end-diastolic volume), and at the end of systole about 50 ml of blood remain in the ventricles (end-systolic volume). The difference between the end-diastolic and end-systolic volumes (about 70 ml) is the stroke volume.

Valvular Structures

Effective pumping action requires directional control so that blood moves in a forward direction through the chambers of the heart. This control is provided by the heart's four valvular structures— the two atrioventricular valves (tricuspid and mitral), and the two semilunar (aortic and pulmonic) valves. Figure 15-2 shows the valvular structures of the heart. The valves are formed of fibrous tissue that is covered with endocardium. The edges of the valves form thin leaflets pointing in the direction of blood flow.

The edges of the atrioventricular (A–V) valves form cusps, two on the left (bicuspid) and three on the right (tricuspid). The atrioventricular valves are supported by the *papillary muscles* and the *chordae tendineae*. Contraction of the papillary muscles at the onset of systole causes the A–V valves to complete their closure. The chordae tendineae prevent the valves from turning inside out and everting into the atria during systole.

Because of their shape, the aortic and pulmonic valves are often referred to as the *semilunar* valves. Actually the semilunar valves are shaped more like "tea cups" which collect the retrograde, or backward, flow of blood that occurs toward the end of systole, as a means of enhancing closure.

There are no valves at the atrial sites where

Figure 15–2.   Diagram showing the valvular structures of the heart. The atrioventricular valves are in an open position and the semilunar valves are closed. There are no valves to control the flow of blood at the inflow channels (vena cava and pulmonary veins) to the heart.

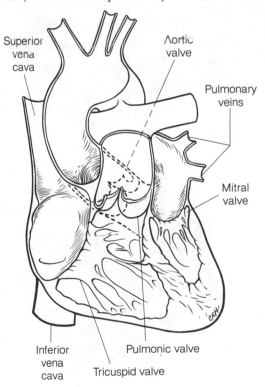

blood enters the heart, i.e., the vena cava and the pulmonary veins. This means that the flow of blood into the heart is almost continuous depending upon the intrathoracic pressure. For example, there are times during forced expiration that intrathoracic pressure rises above the pressure in the right atria and, at this time, venous return to the heart is temporarily impeded. The absence of valves at the inflow channels of the heart means that excess blood will be pushed back into the veins when the atria become distended. In severe right-sided failure, for example, the jugular veins often become prominent in the standing position when they normally should be collapsed.

The Conduction System

Heart muscle differs from skeletal muscle in its ability to generate its own action potentials or electrical impulses. This unique rhythmic property allows the heart to continue beating independently of the nervous system.

In certain areas of the heart, the tissue has been modified to form the specialized cells of the con-

Figure 15–3. The conduction system of the heart showing the intra-atrial conduction pathways and the left anterior and posterior fascicles of the ventricular conduction system. (Goldman MJ: Principles of Clinical Electro-Cardiography. Copyright 1976 by Lange Medical Publications, Los Altos, CA)

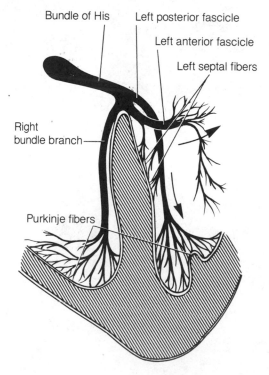

duction system. Although most myocardial cells are capable of initiating and conducting impulses, it is the heart's conduction system that maintains its pumping efficiency. Specialized pacemaker cells are able to generate impulses at a faster rate and the conduction tissue transmits impulses more rapidly than other types of heart tissue. It is these properties that allow the conduction system to control the cardiac rhythm.

Each cardiac contraction is initiated by an impulse that originates in the *sinoatrial (S–A) node*, which is called the pacemaker. The S–A node is located in the posterior wall of the right atrium near the entrance to the vena cava. The S–A node is able to act as the pacemaker of the heart because it has the fastest inherent rate of firing in relation to other parts of the conduction system. The impulse from the S–A node travels through the atria to the *atrioventricular (A–V)* node. The conduction pathways of the heart are illustrated in Figure 15-3. There are at least four intra-atrial pathways, including Bachmann's bundle that connects the S–A and A–V nodes. Junctional fibers in the A–V node connect with the *bundle of His* of the ventricular conduction system. The bundle of His separates into right and *left bundle branches* as it reaches the intraventricular septum. The right and left bundle branches move through the subendocardial tissues toward the papillary muscles and then divide into the *Purkinje* branches that supply the outer walls of the ventricle. The left bundle branch fans out and divides into two segments, the *left posterior* and the *left anterior fascicle*, as it enters the septal area. The Purkinje system has large fibers that allow for rapid conduction and almost simultaneous excitation of the entire right and left ventricles. This rapid rate of conduction through the Purkinje system is necessary for rapid and efficient ejection of blood from the heart.

Essentially the heart has two separate conduction systems: one controls atrial activity, the other, ventricular activity. The two systems are connected by junctional fibers in the A–V node. Because the A–V node is the only connection between the atrial and ventricular conduction systems, the atria and the ventricles beat independently of each other when there is a complete block in transmission at the A–V node.

Autonomic control of heart rate

The activity of the conduction system and the contractile properties of the heart can be modified by the autonomic nervous system. The *vagus* nerve carries impulses from the parasympathetic nervous system to the heart, mainly to the S–A and A–V nodes. The sympathetic nervous system supplies these structures as well as the ventricles.

The *parasympathetic nervous* system has two effects on the heart: it slows the rate of impulse formation in the S–A node, and slows transmission of the impulse through the A–V node. This system is tonically active and has a constraining effect on heart rate. Strong vagal stimulation can actually stop impulse formation in the S–A node or block transmission in the A–V node. When this happens, there is a delay of about 10 to 15 seconds after which a ventricular pacemaker takes over, causing the ventricles to begin beating at a rate of 15 to 40 beats-per-minute. On the other hand, the drug atropine blocks vagal stimulation to the heart and causes its rate to increase.

The *sympathetic nervous system* increases both the heart rate and the force of cardiac contraction. The sympathetic receptors in the heart are beta receptors. This will become more meaningful when the effects of sympathetic drugs on cardiac function are discussed. The beta receptors in the heart respond to both direct neural stimulation and to sympathetic neuromediators in the blood.

:Coronary Circulation

Myocardial contraction requires constant utilization of oxygen and other nutrients (carbohydrates, ketones, and fatty acids). While other nutrients can be stored in muscle cells, oxygen must be supplied continuously. The oxygen supply for the heart is derived from the blood that flows through the coronary arteries (see Fig. 16-2). Under normal conditions the heart extracts and uses about 60% to 80% of the oxygen from the blood flowing through the coronary arteries, as compared with the 25% to 35% that is extracted from the blood by the skeletal muscles. The heart's metabolic requirements may easily exceed the amount of oxygen available when blood flow through the coronary arteries is reduced.

The Work of the Heart and Oxygen Consumption

Oxygen consumption and the need for oxygen delivery by the coronary arteries is determined largely by the tension that the heart must produce during contraction in order for ejection of blood to occur and by the time that this tension must be maintained (tension × time). Oxygen consumption is further determined by the myocardial wall tension, the stroke

work, the contractile state of the myocardium, and the heart rate.

The *myocardial wall tension* is determined by the *amount of blood* that is present in the heart at the end of *diastole*. When the diameter of the ventricle is greatly increased the heart must use additional energy just to decrease its size and to create the tension and pressure needed to eject blood.

The *stroke work* is the effort the heart expends to pump blood. The reader will probably recall that work is generally defined as force multiplied by distance. The main (external) work of the heart is related to the *amount of blood* that is pumped (force) with each beat and the *pressure* (distance) that the ventricle must develop to move that blood into the aorta or pulmonary artery.

stroke work =
stroke volume × mean arterial blood pressure

This means that the stroke work of the left ventricle pumping against a mean systemic pressure of 85 mm Hg is going to be greater than the stroke work of the right ventricle pumping against a mean pulmonary artery pressure of only 15 mm Hg. Stroke work is increased in the presence of hypertension and valvular disorders, which reduce the size of the opening through which the blood must be ejected.

The *contractile state* of the heart refers to its ability to change its force of contraction, without a change in end-diastolic volume, the heart rate, or arterial pressure. Oxygen consumed to maintain the contractile state is used to produce the interactions between the actin and myosin filaments of the myocardial fibers.

Heart rate increases myocardial oxygen requirements by increasing the frequency with which the heart goes through all the processes that require oxygen consumption.

Sometimes the factors that influence cardiac performance are spoken of as preload and afterload stresses. Changes in diastolic filling are called *preload* factors because they are applied *before* the contraction begins. A decrease in venous return to the right heart is often referred to as a decrease in preload. The *afterload*, on the other hand, is the force the heart must pump against *after* the contraction has commenced. The mean arterial blood pressure is an afterload stress.

Coronary Blood Flow

Contraction of the myocardial muscle fibers affects the flow of blood through the coronary arteries. During systole, contraction of myocardial muscle compresses the coronary arteries and causes a reduction in blood flow. Because of the high pressure that the left ventricle must generate, the decrease in flow is greatest in the arteries that supply this chamber. It has been estimated that about 70% of blood flow through the coronaries occurs during diastole. This is particularly significant in situations of tachycardia in which the increase in heart rate causes an increase in oxygen consumption, while the time spent in diastole is markedly reduced. An increase in heart rate probably has little effect on oxygen delivery in the normal heart because the process of autoregulation causes the coronary arteries to dilate. On the other hand, rigid atherosclerotic vessels probably have limited capacity for dilatation, in which case an increase in heart rate may impair oxygen delivery to the myocardium.

Cardiac Output

The efficiency of the heart as a pump is often measured in terms of cardiac output. *Cardiac output* is the product of the stroke volume and the heart rate.

cardiac output = stroke volume × heart rate

Output varies with body size and with the metabolic needs of the tissues. It increases during physical activity and decreases during rest and sleep. The normal average cardiac output in an adult ranges from 3.5 to 8.0 liters-per-minute. In the trained athlete this value can increase to levels as high as 35 liters-per-minute. The *cardiac reserve* refers to the maximum percentage that the cardiac output can increase above the normal resting level. The normal young adult has a cardiac reserve of slightly more than 300%.

Regulation of cardiac output

The heart's capacity to increase its output according to body needs is dependent upon three factors: diastolic filling, cardiac contractility, and heart rate.

Diastolic filling. The heart muscle, or myocardium, is composed of myofibrils made up of *actin* and *myosin* filaments (Fig. 15-4). During systole they interact to shorten muscle and during diastole the interaction is broken so that the muscle relaxes.

The anatomic arrangement of the myocardial fibers is such that the tension or force of contraction is greatest if the muscle is stretched just before it begins to contract. The maximum force of contraction is achieved when an increase in diastolic filling causes the muscle fibers to be stretched to about two and one-half times beyond their normal resting length. When the muscle fibers are thus stretched, the actin and myosin filaments are op-

Figure 15–4.   Structure of the myofibrils showing the actin and myosin filaments. During contraction the cross bridges form linkages, causing the filaments to slide across each other. This results in shortened myofibrils. (Rushmir RF: Structure and Function of the Cardiovascular System. Philadelphia, WB Saunders, 1976)

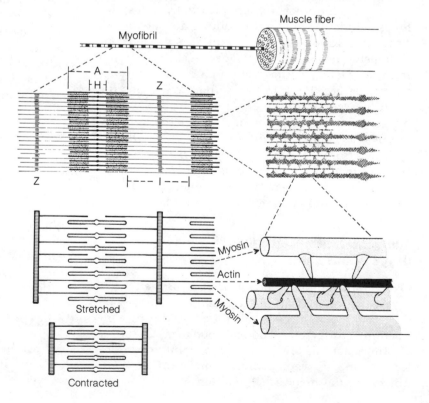

timally approximated. The increased force of cardiac contraction that accompanies an increase in diastolic filling is referred to as the *Frank–Starling mechanism* or *Starling's law of the heart*. The Frank–Starling mechanism allows the heart to adjust its pumping ability to accommodate various levels of venous return.

Cardiac contractility. Cardiac contractility refers to the ability of the heart to change its force of contraction without changing its resting (diastolic) length. The contractile state of the myocardial muscle is determined by the biochemical and biophysical properties that govern the actin and myosin interactions within the myocardial cells. An *inotropic* influence is one that modifies the contractile state of the myocardium. For instance, hypoxia exerts a negative inotropic effect by decreasing cardiac contractility, while sympathetic stimulation produces a positive inotropic effect by increasing cardiac contractility.

Heart rate. Heart rate increases cardiac output by increasing the frequency with which blood is ejected from the heart. As heart rate increases, however, the time spent in diastole is reduced, and there is less time for filling of the ventricles prior to the onset of systole. This leads to a decrease in stroke volume and at high heart rates it may actually lead to a decrease in cardiac output. In fact, one of the dangers of ventricular tachycardia is reduction in cardiac output because the heart does not have time to fill.

In summary, the heart is a two-sided electrically driven pump that derives oxygen for its energy needs from blood flow delivered by the coronary arteries. The heart, like other body structures, is able to adapt to the metabolic needs of the various tissues, and when disease threatens its integrity the heart responds in a manner that strives to maintain this function.

:Study Guide

After you have studied this chapter, you should be able to meet the following objectives:

: : Describe the pumping action of the heart.

: : State the significance of the cardiac cycle.

: : Describe the regulation of cardiac pumping action by the atrioventricular valves and the semilunar valves.

: : Describe the control of atrial activity and the control of ventricular activity by the cardiac conduction system.

: : Describe the relationship between the autonomic nervous system and the cardiac conduction system.

: : State the determinants of oxygen consumption.

: : State the formula for measuring stroke work.

: : State the formula for measuring cardiac output.

: : Describe the role of diastolic filling, cardiac contractility, and heart rate in regulation of cardiac output.

:Suggested Readings

Berne RM: Cardiovascular Physiology, 3rd ed. St Louis, CV Mosby, 1977

Chaffee EE, Lytle IM: Basic Physiology and Anatomy, 4th ed., pp 312-328. Philadelphia, JB Lippincott, 1980

Guyton AC: Textbook of Medical Physiology, 6th ed., pp 150-202. Philadelphia, WB Saunders, 1981

Honig CR: Modern Cardiovascular Physiology. Boston, Little, Brown & Co., 1981

Smith JJ, Kampine JP: Circulatory Physiology. Baltimore, Williams & Wilkins, 1980

16

Alterations in Cardiac Function

There are many ways to classify heart disease. In this book they are divided into acquired and congenital diseases.

:Acquired Heart Disease

Acquired types of heart disease are conditions that develop following birth and that can occur as the result of ischemia, inflammation, immune responses, and malnutrition. They can affect any of the cardiac structures. In this section of the chapter, the focus is on the structural layers of the heart—the pericardium, myocardium, and endocardium. A discussion of conduction disturbances is included with disorders of the myocardium, valvular dysfunction with disorders of the endocardium.

:The Pericardium

The heart is located in the thorax, behind and largely to the left of the lower two-thirds of the sternum. It is anchored at the top, or base, by the great vessels, and it is encased in a double-layered sac, the *pericardium* (Fig. 16-1). The pericardium isolates the heart from the other thoracic structures, maintains its position in the thorax, and prevents overfilling. The two layers of the pericardium are separated by a thin layer of serous fluid, which serves to prevent frictional forces from developing as the visceral layer, adherent to the pericardium, comes in contact with the outer fibrous layer, the parietal pericardium.

Figure 16–1. Diagram of the layers of the heart that shows the visceral pericardium, the pericardial cavity, and the parietal pericardium.

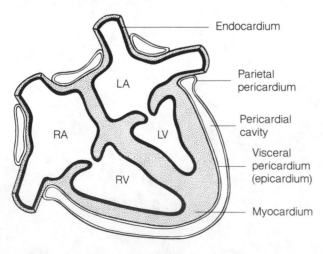

The pericardium is subject to many of the pathologic processes that affect structures elsewhere in the body, including infection and immune responses, ischemia and necrosis, metabolic disorders, injury, and neoplastic infiltrations. For the most part, these pathologic processes serve as stimuli for the inflammatory response. The pericarditis resulting from these pathologic processes can be acute; it can be chronic with formation of exudate (pericardial effusion); or it can cause extensive fibrosis and fusion between the layers of the pericardial sac (constrictive pericarditis).

Acute Pericarditis

Although acute pericarditis can be caused by a number of organisms, its most likely cause is a viral infection. This form of pericarditis is seen most commonly in men aged 20 to 30. Nearly all patients with acute pericarditis have pain. It is usually abrupt in onset, occupies the precordial area, and is frequently described as being sharp. It may radiate to the arm, shoulder, back, or epigastric area. Unlike the constant pain associated with myocardial infarction, pericardial pain is worse with breathing, coughing, swallowing, or positional changes. Often the patient will seek relief of pain by sitting up and leaning forward. The pain may mimic angina in quality and location, but, unlike angina, it is not relieved by rest or taking nitroglycerin.

A rubbing, called friction rub, develops between the inflamed surfaces of the pericardium and it can be heard through a stethoscope placed on the chest. The sound associated with friction rub is often described as having a "leathery" or "close to the ear" sound. It is usually heard best when the patient is in the seated position and is leaning forward, with the stethoscope placed along the left sternal border, over the xiphoid process, or near the lower border of the sternum. The friction rub associated with acute pericarditis usually lasts from 7 to 10 days.

As with other acute infections, acute pericarditis is usually accompanied by systemic signs of inflammation—fever, leukocytosis, and elevated sedimentation rate. Involvement of the adjacent myocardial tissue produces characteristic changes in the S–T segment of the electrocardiogram.

Pericardial Effusion

As the inflammatory process progresses, the pericardium reacts by producing an exudate. The exudate varies in amount and type depending on the causative agent; it can be serous, purulent, hemorrhagic, fibrinous, or any combination of these types. Acute fibrinous pericarditis usually heals by resolution; whereas other forms of exudative pericarditis may lead to deposition of scar tissue and formation of adhesions between the layers of the pericardium. When excessive exudate is formed it is called *pericardial effusion*.

Chronic Pericarditis with Effusion

Chronic pericarditis with effusion is characterized by an increase in inflammatory exudate which continues beyond the anticipated period of time. In some cases, the exudate will persist for several years. In the majority of cases of chronic pericarditis, no specific pathogen can be identified. The process is commonly associated with other forms of heart disease, such as rheumatic fever, congenital heart lesions, or hypertensive heart disease. Systemic diseases such as lupus erythematosus, rheumatoid arthritis, scleroderma, and myxedema are also causes of chronic pericarditis, as are metabolic disturbances associated with acute and chronic renal failure. Unlike the situation in acute pericarditis, the signs and symptoms of the chronic form are often minimal; many times the disease is detected for the first time on a routine chest film. As the condition progresses, the fluid may accumulate and compress the adjacent cardiac structures and impair cardiac filling.

Constrictive Pericarditis

In constrictive pericarditis, scar tissue develops on the epicardium, pericardium, or on both structures. In time, the scar tissue contracts and interferes with cardiac filling, at which point, cardiac output and cardiac reserve become fixed. Additionally, venous congestion causes portal hypertension and ascites. Ascites is a prominent early finding, often occurring without signs of accompanying peripheral edema. There is also distention of the jugular veins. *Kussmaul's sign* is an *inspiratory distention* of the cervical veins due to inability of the right atrium, encased in its rigid pericardium, to accommodate the increase in venous return which occurs with inspiration.

Cardiac Tamponade

Cardiac tamponade is a compression due to excess fluid or blood in the pericardial sac. It can occur as the result of trauma, effusion, cardiac rupture, or dissecting aneurysm. The signs and symptoms are related to restriction of venous return to the heart and a reduction in cardiac output. The obstruction to venous return usually causes distention of the jugu-

lar veins and an elevation in central venous pressure; the reduction in cardiac output produces signs and symptoms of circulatory shock.

Pulsus paradoxus is a decrease in pulse volume and systolic blood pressure during inspiration. It is most often observed when the blood pressure is measured, although changes in the quality of the peripheral pulse may be obvious in some patients, i.e., the peripheral pulse may decrease and almost disappear during inspiration. To observe for pulsus paradoxus, the sphygmomanometer cuff is inflated and then slowly deflated to the point where the Korotkoff sounds can be heard throughout the respiratory cycle. Normally, the systolic pressure fluctuates about 5 to 10 mm Hg during respiration, but in pulsus paradoxus, fluctuation is increased by 20 to 30 mm Hg. This extreme decrease in systolic pressure during inspiration is thought to be caused by a greater than normal decrease in stroke volume during this phase of respiration.

Diagnosis and Treatment

Various diagnostic tests confirm the presence of pericardial disease. These measures include chest x-ray studies, electrocardiography, echocardiography, and cardiac catheterization with angiographic studies. Aspiration and laboratory analysis of the pericardial fluid may be used to identify the causative agent.

Treatment is dependent upon the etiology. Antibiotics that are specific for the causative agent are usually prescribed. Anti-inflammatory drugs may minimize the inflammatory response and the accompanying undesirable effects. Pericardiocentesis, the removal of fluid from the pericardial sac, may be a life-saving measure in severe cardiac tamponade. Surgical treatment may be required in traumatic lesions of the heart, or in constrictive pericarditis in which cardiac filling is severely impaired.

In summary, pericarditis is an inflammation of the pericardial sac due to one of a number of agents. It may be acute or chronic. It is significant because of its potential for restricting cardiac filling.

:The Myocardium

Although the myocardium is subject to pathologic conditions arising from a variety of agents—inflammation, immune responses, trauma, and metabolic disturbances—by far the most common cause is ischemia and infarction. The coronary arteries supply blood to the myocardium, and it is these arteries that are prone to develop atherosclerosis with resultant myocardial ischemia and infarction.

There are two main coronary arteries, the right and left, which arise from the coronary sinus just above the aortic valve (Fig. 16-2). The *left coronary artery* divides almost immediately into the anterior descending and circumflex branches. The *left anterior descending artery* passes down through the groove between the two ventricles, giving off *diagonal branches* that supply the left ventricle and *perforating branches* that supply the anterior portion of the intraventricular septum and the anterior papillary muscle of the left ventricle. The *circumflex branch* of the left coronary artery passes to the left and moves posteriorly in the groove that separates the left atrium and ventricle, giving off branches that supply the left lateral wall of the left ventricle. The *right coronary* lies in the right atrioventricular groove, and its branches supply the right ventricle. The right coronary artery usually moves to the back of the heart where it forms the *posterior descending artery* that supplies the posterior portion of the heart (the intraventricular septum, atrioventricular node, and posterior papillary muscle). The sinoatrial node is also usually supplied by the right coronary artery. In about 10% of the population, the left circumflex rather than the right coronary artery moves posteri-

orly to form the posterior descending artery. The term *dominant* designates the main coronary artery that extends to form the posterior descending artery. Dominant left circulation tells us that the posterior descending artery is a branch of the left circumflex, and dominant right circulation tells us that the posterior descending artery is a branch of the right coronary artery.

The larger coronary arteries lie on the surface of the heart, with smaller intramuscular branches coming off and penetrating the myocardium. Although there are no connections between the large coronary arteries, there are anastomotic channels that join the small arteries (Fig. 16-3). With gradual occlusion of the larger vessels, the smaller collateral vessels increase in size and provide alternate channels for blood flow. One of the reasons that coronary disease does not produce symptoms until it is far advanced is that the collateral channels develop at the same time that the atherosclerotic changes are occurring.

Coronary Heart Disease

In 99% of cases, coronary heart disease is due to atherosclerosis. Most men and women in the United States over age fifty probably have moderately far advanced coronary atherosclerosis even though

Figure 16–2. Diagram of the coronary arteries that arise from the aorta and some of the coronary veins.

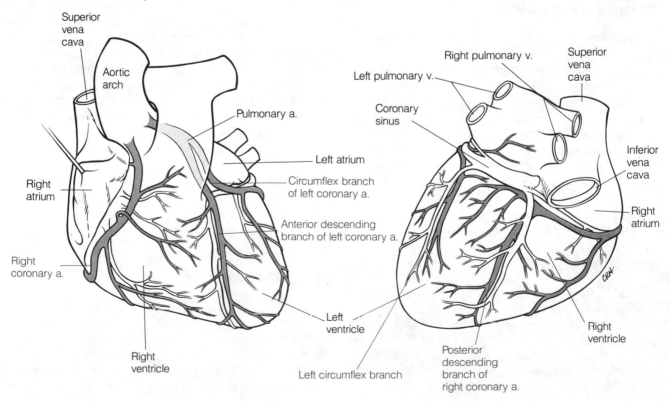

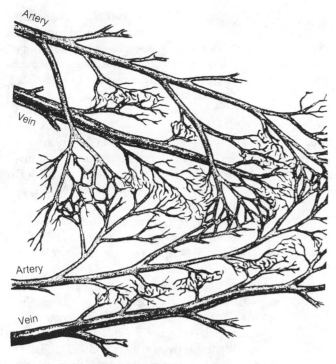

Figure 16–3.   Anastomoses of the smaller coronary arterial vessels. (Guyton AC: Textbook of Medical Physiology, 6th ed. Philadelphia, WB Saunders, 1981)

most of them have no symptoms of heart disease.[1] Risk factors and the pathogenesis of atherosclerosis are discussed in Chapter 9. Coronary heart disease can affect one or all of the coronary arteries (1, 2, or 3 vessel disease), and it can be diffuse or localized to one area of a single vessel. Usually 75% or more of the vessel lumen must be occluded before there is significant reduction in coronary blood flow. Disease of the coronary vessels can cause angina, myocardial infarction, cardiac arrhythmias, conduction defects, heart failure, or sudden death. Each of these conditions is characterized by a disparity between oxygen needs of the myocardium and the ability of the coronary arteries to supply the blood to meet these needs.

Methods of Diagnosis

Coronary heart disease is often a silent disorder; at the time that symptoms such as angina occur the disease is usually far advanced. At present, there are no simple screening tests to detect coronary artery disease. Diagnostic tests are usually done when symptoms are present and are often used to determine the severity and localize the areas of involvement. Noninvasive diagnostic methods include electrocardiography, exercise stress testing, and

echocardiography. Cardiac catheterization is an invasive procedure that permits localization of heart defects and lesions in the coronary arteries.

The *electrocardiogram* (ECG) provides a recording of the electrical events in the cardiac cycle. The depolarization and repolarization of the heart tissue may be altered. A *vectorcardiogram* is a three-dimensional ECG; it displays a vector loop of impulses on the frontal (right to left and head to toe), sagittal (front to back and head to toe), and horizontal (front to back and left to right) planes of the body.

The *echocardiogram* uses an ultrasonic beam to scan and construct a picture of the heart in motion. It is useful for determining ventricular dimensions and valve movements and to obtain data on the movement of the left ventricular wall and septum, estimates of diastolic and systolic volumes, and motion of individual segments of the left ventricular wall during systole and diastole. It can be used for studying valvular disease and detecting pericardial effusion.

Nuclear imaging involves the use of radionuclides to detect the presence of myocardial ischemia and infarction. When injected intravenously, these agents (for example, thallium-201), are distributed to the myocardium in proportion to the magnitude of blood flow. Following injection, an external detection device describes the distribution of the radioactive material. An ischemic or necrotic area appears as a "cold spot" which lacks radioactive uptake. Technetium-99m, tagged to pyrophosphate is another radioactive imaging agent that demonstrates the general location and extent of suspected myocardial infarction within 24 to 48 hours after the event has occurred.

Cardiac catheterization involves the passage of flexible catheters into the great vessels and chambers of the heart. In right heart catheterization, the catheters are inserted into a peripheral vein and then advanced into the right heart. The left heart catheter is inserted into a peripheral artery and then passed retrograde into the aorta and left heart. The cardiac catheterization laboratory, where the procedure is done, is equipped for viewing and recording fluoroscopic images of the heart and vessels in the chest and for measuring pressures within the heart and great vessels. There is also equipment for cardiac output studies and for obtaining samples of blood for blood gas analysis. Angiographic studies are made by injecting a contrast medium into the heart so that an outline of the moving structures can be visualized and filmed. Coronary arteriography involves the injection of a contrast medium into the coronary arteries; this permits visualization of lesions within these vessels.

Exercise stress testing is a means of observing cardiac function under stress. Three types of tests are utilized: the step test, the bicycle ergometer, and the treadmill, with the treadmill being used most frequently in the United States. Many Americans are not accustomed to riding bicycles, and the step test requires considerable motivation on the part of the patient. During treadmill testing, the person walks or runs on a moving belt. The level of physical activity, or workload, that the person performs can be gradually increased by changing the speed and incline of the belt; this is usually done in stages. The ECG is monitored continuously during the test and blood pressure is taken at predetermined intervals. It is also possible to monitor oxygen consumption, although a person is assumed to have reached the limit for oxygen uptake at the point of exhaustion.* Usually the person being tested continues to exercise, completing successive stages of the test, until reaching the point of exhaustion, or until a predetermined target heart rate is reached. The target heart rate is determined by age (Table 16-1). The person may be asked to continue until the maximal heart rate is achieved or until a percentage (i.e., 85% to 90%) of the maximal rate is reached. The presence of chest pain, severe shortness of breath, arrhythmias, S–T segment changes on the ECG, or a decrease in blood pressure is suggestive of coronary heart disease, and the test is usually terminated when these signs appear.

Angina Pectoris

Angina pectoris is a choking paroxysmal pain associated with transient myocardial ischemia. The pain of angina is assumed to occur when myocardial need for oxygen exceeds the ability of the coronary vessels to supply adequate blood flow to meet these needs. Stressful states, such as cold, physical exertion, and emotional stress, are known to produce angina. Angina is usually associated with coronary atherosclerosis, although only a small number of persons with coronary atherosclerosis experience angina. In many instances, myocardial infarction occurs without a prior history of angina. And in rare instances, other factors that increase the work of the heart, such as severe aortic stenosis or anemia, may cause angina. Recently, it has been shown that angina can result from spasms of the coronary arteries.

Pain is a classic manifestation of angina. Typically, the pain is described as "constricting, squeezing, or suffocating." The pain is usually steady, increasing in intensity only at the onset and end of the attack. The pain of angina is usually located in the precordial or substernal area; it is similar to myocardial infarction in that it may radiate to the left shoulder, jaw, arm, or other areas of the chest. In some persons, the arm or shoulder pain may be confused with arthritis; in others, the epigastric pain is thought to result from indigestion. The duration of anginal pain is brief—seldom does it last more than 5 minutes. Of particular diagnostic significance is the fact that the pain is relieved by rest or administration of nitroglycerin; this is not true of other forms of chest pain.

Electrocardiographic changes are not always present in angina, particularly if the recording is made while the person is resting or at a time when pain is not present. Exercise and pain may cause S–T segment displacement. Exercise stress testing is useful in differentiating angina from other forms of chest pain.

---

*Tables have been developed which convert workload of the exercise tests to levels of oxygen consumption.

Table 16–1 Predicted Maximal Heart Rates by Age, and Recommended Target Heart Rates for Submaximal Exercise Testing

	Maximal and Submaximal Heart Rates Predicted by Age												
Ages (yrs)	20	25	30	35	40	45	50	55	60	65	70	75	80
Maximal heart rate (untrained)	197	195	193	191	189	187	184	182	180	178	176	174	172
90% of maximal heart rate	177	175	173	172	170	168	166	164	162	160	158	157	155

From American Heart Association. Exercise Testing and Training of Apparently Healthy Individuals: A Handbook for Physicians. The Committee on Exercise. Kattus, Albert A, Chairman, 1972, p 14. Reprinted with permission.

Unstable angina

Unstable angina is an accelerated form of angina in which the pain begins to appear more frequently and is more severe. The pain lasts longer and there is less relief with nitroglycerin. The pain may appear at rest. Unstable angina is sometimes called preinfarction angina because of its propensity for accelerating to myocardial infarction.

Variant angina

While classical angina is associated with exercise, a variant form of nonexertional angina exists. Variant (Prinzmetal's) angina is caused by spasms of the coronary arteries. In most instances, the spasms occur in the presence of coronary artery stenosis; however, it has been shown to occur in the absence of visible disease. Unlike the classical forms of angina, the varient form often occurs during rest and frequently follows a cyclic or regular pattern or occurrence (e.g., it happens at the same time each night). Arrhythmias are often present when the pain is severe and the individual suffering the attack is often aware of their presence. Electrocardiographic changes are significant if recorded during an attack. Typically the S–T segment is elevated on the same lead during each attack. As with classical angina, nitroglycerin is usually effective in relieving the attack of variant angina.

Diagnosis and Treatment

The diagnosis of angina is usually based on history, electrocardiographic findings, response to administration of nitroglycerin, and results of exercise stress testing.

Measures for treatment of angina are usually directed toward reducing the work demands of the heart, since the diseased coronary vessels are probably maximally dilated and carrying as much blood as they are capable of carrying. Treatment measures directed at decreasing preload and afterload stress include the selective pacing of physical activities, stress reduction, avoidance of cold, weight reduction if obesity is present, use of nitroglycerin and long-acting nitrates, the beta-blocking drug propranolol, and a new group of drugs called calcium antagonists. At this writing, the calcium antagonists are not available in the United States. Immediate cessation of activity is often sufficient to abort an anginal attack. Sitting down or standing quietly is often preferable to lying down, since these positions tend to promote pooling of blood in the lower extremities. Sudden exposure to cold tends to increase vasoconstriction; thus, patients with angina are usually cautioned against drinking cold liquids and breathing extremely cold air. Anxiety often precipitates angina because it causes an increase in both heart rate and blood pressure.

Nitroglycerin (glycerol trinitrate) provides prompt relief from anginal pain. It is a vasodilating drug which causes relaxation of both venous and arterial vessels. Venous dilatation reduces venous return to the heart, thereby emptying the heart and decreasing the amount of blood that the heart must pump. With this decrease there is less tension on the wall of the ventricle and less pressure is needed to pump blood. Nitroglycerin also relaxes the arterioles, reducing the pressure against which the left heart must pump. Nitroglycerin must be given *sublingually*, since it is rapidly destroyed in the liver once it has been absorbed. Absorption is rapid, and relief of pain usually begins in 30 seconds. Nitroglycerin is also available in ointment form, for topical application. This form has a longer duration of action, usually 4 to 6 hours. The beta adrenergic blocking drug *propranolol* (Inderal) blocks sympathetic stimulation to the heart, and has a direct effect on the myocardium. It depresses diastolic depolarization, decreases conduction velocity, and exerts a negative inotropic effect on the heart. The reader is referred to a pharmacology text for a more complete discussion of drugs used to treat angina.

The surgical treatment of angina—aortocoronary bypass surgery—has gained popularity particularly in patients who have significant coronary disease. Although it cannot be documented that this surgery significantly alters disease progress, it does relieve pain, so that patients may have a more productive life. In one study, 60% of patients who had bypass surgery for angina showed marked improvement or were pain-free 1 year later as compared with 16% who had corresponding relief when treated medically.[2] In another study, which viewed patients' employment pattern following bypass surgery, 90% of those under age 55 were still employed 4 years later; 68% of men 55 to 59 remained employed after 4 years; and 44% of men over age 60.[3]

Myocardial Infarction

Myocardial infarction is ischemic death of myocardial tissue associated with obstruction of a coronary vessel. Thrombosis is ultimately linked with vessel occlusion during myocardial infarction, although the time sequence of thrombus development is controversial. Recently, it has been suggested that thrombosis follows, rather than precedes, the ischemic event. This opinion is supported by nec-

Figure 16–4.   Anatomy and distribution of the coronary arteries and the topography of infarction. (James TN: Arrhythmias and conduction disturbances in acute myocardial infarction. Am Heart J 64:3,416-426, 1962)

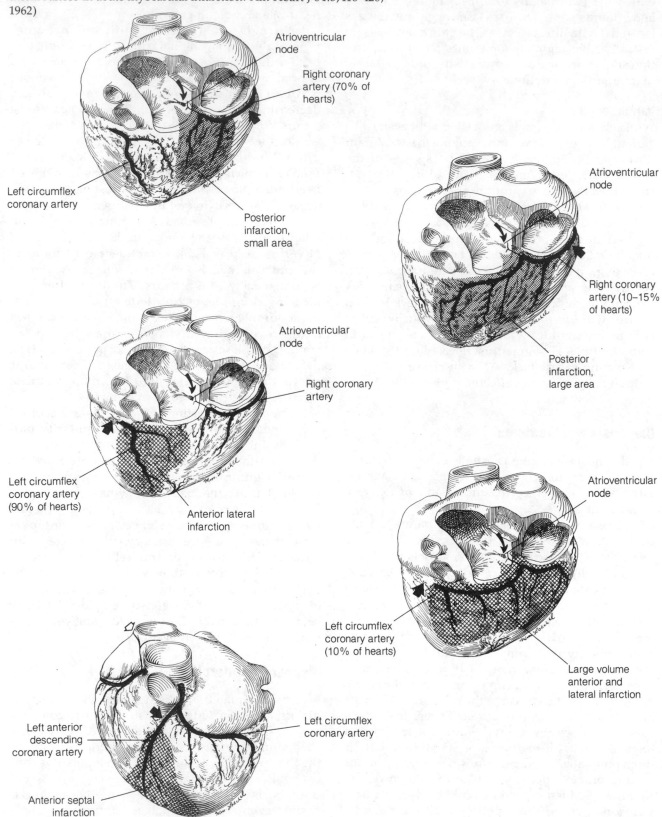

ropsy data in which complete occlusion with thrombosis was not demonstrated in a large percentage of patients dying with myocardial infarction.[4] The frequency of thrombosis increases with the duration of survival and the size of the infarct. It is quite possible that the event responsible for the infarct—vessel spasm or excess myocardial oxygen requirements—may also predispose to thrombus formation in the vessel supplying the area. Even though thrombosis may not be the initiating event in myocardial infarction, almost all patients dying of myocardial infarction have been found to have severe coronary atherosclerosis.[5]

An infarct may involve the endocardium, myocardium, epicardium, or a combination of these. An *intramural* infarct is one that is contained within the myocardium whereas a *transmural* infarct involves all three layers. Most infarcts are transmural, involving the free wall of the left ventricle and the intraventricular septum. The increased vulnerability of the left ventricle is probably related to its increased work demands. According to Robbins,[6] about 30% to 40% of infarcts affect the right coronary, 40% to 50% the left anterior descending artery, and the remaining 15% to 20% the left circumflex artery. This distribution is depicted in Figure 16-4.

Although gross tissue changes are not apparent for hours following myocardial infarction (Table 16-2), it has been reported that the ischemic area ceases to function within a matter of minutes and

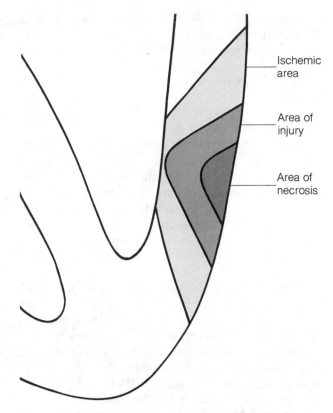

Figure 16–5.   Tissue damage after myocardial infarction.

that irreversible damage to cells occurs in about 40 minutes. There is also evidence to suggest that an area of injury and ischemic zone borders the necrotic area (Fig. 16-5). There is reason to believe that the fate of the remaining viable cells in the area of injury and ischemic zone is not determined until sometime after the onset of infarction.[7] Recently, there has been considerable concern for salvaging the ischemic area and thereby reducing the size of the infarct. Measures said to reduce infarct size are (1) decreasing myocardial oxygen consumption, and (2) increasing oxygen availability. Since *sympathetic activity* increases the *metabolic activity of the myocardium* and myocardial oxygen consumption, the sympathetic beta-blocking drug propranolol may be used to reduce sympathetic stimulation of the heart following infarction. A second means to decrease oxygen consumption is by vasodilator drugs, such as nitroglycerin, nitroprusside, and hydralazine, because they decrease venous return (reduce preload) and the arterial pressure against which the left ventricle must pump (afterload). The intra-aortic balloon pump augments left ventricular pumping and aids perfusion (Chap. 14). Oxygen is administered to make it readily available to the ischemic myocardium. Of interest is the possibility of aug-

Table 16–2   Tissue Changes Following Myocardial Infarction

Time Following Onset	Gross Tissue Changes
6 to 12 hours	No gross changes
18 to 24 hours	Pale to gray–brown Slight pallor of area
2 to 4 days	Necrosis of area is apparent. Area is yellow–brown in center and hyperemic around the edges.
4 to 10 days	Area becomes soft; fatty changes in the center are well developed. Hemorrhagic areas are present in the infarcted area. Rupture of the heart, when it occurs, happens during this period.
10 days and on	Fibrotic (scar) tissue replacement and revascularization commences.
6 weeks	Scar tissue replacement of necrotic tissue is usually complete, depends on size of infarct.

Developed from data in Robbins SL, Cotran R: Pathologic Basis of Disease, ed. 2, Philadelphia: W. B. Saunders, 1979, p. 656.

menting the production of ATP by the myocardial cells through the anaerobic pathway in an effort to supply needed energy. Efforts in this area have focused on the use of glucose-insulin-potassium infusions, antilipolytic agents, and lipid-free albumin solutions.

Signs and symptoms

The signs and symptoms of myocardial infarction can be categorized into four groups: (1) pain and autonomic responses associated with the ischemic event; (2) weakness and signs related to impaired myocardial function; (3) arrhythmias and electrocardiographic changes associated with ischemia and death of myocardial cells; and (4) signs of inflammation and elevated serum enzyme levels indicative of tissue death.

The onset of infarction is usually abrupt, with pain as the significant symptom. Typically, the pain is severe and crushing, often described as being constrictive, suffocating, or like "someone sitting on my chest." The pain is usually retrosternal with radiation to the left arm, neck, or jaw, although it may be experienced in other areas of the chest. Unlike angina, the pain associated with infarction is more prolonged and is not relieved by rest or nitroglycerin and frequently, narcotics are required. There may be a sensation of *epigastric distress*; nausea and vomiting may occur. These symptoms are thought to be related to the severity of the pain and to vagal stimulation. This epigastric distress may be mistaken for indigestion and the patient may seek relief with use of antacids or other home remedies, which only delays getting medical attention. Frequently, he complains of *fatigue and weakness*, especially of the arms and legs. Pain and sympathetic stimulation combine to give rise to *tachycardia, anxiety, restlessness*, and *feelings of impending doom*. The *skin* is often *pale, cool*, and *moist*. The impaired myocardial function may lead to hypotension and shock.

Electrocardiographic changes are not always present immediately following the onset of symptoms, except as arrhythmias. Typical changes associated with death of myocardial tissue include prolongation of the Q wave, S–T segment elevation, and T wave inversion. The ECG changes are variable and complex, and interested readers and those intending to work in the coronary care unit are referred to specialty texts for full discussion.

Cell death causes inflammation and release of intracellular enzymes. Fever and leukocytosis usually develop within about 24 hours and continue for 3 to 7 days. The sedimentation rate rises on the second and third days and remains elevated for 1 to 3 weeks. Enzymes released include creatine phosphokinase (CPK), lactic dehydrogenase (LDH), and glutamic-oxaloacetic transaminase (GOT). As indicated in Table 16-3, these enzymes become elevated at different times postinfarction and provide useful diagnostic information. The enzyme CPK (MB band), which is one of three isoenzymes of CPK, has been found to be a more reliable indicator of myocardial infarction than other enzymes (singly or in combination) or the electrocardiogram.[9]

Complications

The stages of recovery are closely related to the size of the infarct and changes that have taken place within the infarcted area. Fibrous tissue lacks the contractile, elastic, and conductive properties of normal myocardial cells; hence, the residual effects as well as complications are determined essentially by the extent and location of injury.

Sudden death

Sudden death is death occurring within an hour after onset of symptoms, and it is usually attributed to fatal arrhythmias, which may occur without evidence of infarction. Sulfinpyrazone, a drug that inhibits platelet aggregation, has been reported to decrease the incidence of sudden death.[10] At this

Table 16–3   Elevation of Serum Enzymes Postmyocardial Infarction

| | Time Postinfarction | | |
Enzyme	Exceeds Normal Value	Reaches Peak Value	Returns to Normal
CPK (Creatine phosphokinase)*	4 to 8 hours	24 hours	3 to 4 days
LDH (Lactic dehydrogenase)†	12 to 24 hours	3 to 6 days	8 to 14 days
GOT (Glutamic oxaloacetic transaminase)	8 to 12 hours	24 to 48 hours	4 to 7 days

*There are three isoenzymes of CPK; myocardial cells possess the isoenzyme MB.

†There are five isoenzymes of LDH; myocardial cells have both LDH_1 and LDH_2. Normally the ratio of LDH_1 to LDH_2 is less than one; following myocardial infarction, this ratio is reversed.

writing, the benefits of the drug are investigational. Should its effectiveness be established, it will then be necessary to develop a means of identifying persons at risk, since many of those who die suddenly have had no history of heart disease.

Heart failure and cardiogenic shock

Both heart failure and cardiogenic shock are dreaded complications of myocardial infarction. They are discussed in Chapters 17 and 14.

Pericarditis and Dressler's syndrome

Pericarditis may complicate the course of acute myocardial infarction. It usually appears on the second or third day postinfarction. At this time, the patient experiences a new type of pain which is aggravated with deep inspiration and positional changes. A pericardial rub may or may not be heard in all patients who have postinfarction pericarditis, and often it is transitory, usually resolving uneventfully. Dressler's syndrome describes signs and symptoms associated with pericarditis, pleurisy, and pneumonitis: fever, chest pain, dyspnea, and abnormal laboratory (elevated white blood cell count and sedimentation rate) and ECG findings. The symptoms may arise between one day and several weeks following infarction, and are thought to represent a hypersensitivity response to tissue necrosis.

Thromboemboli

Thromboemboli are a potential complication, arising either as venous thrombi or, occasionally, as a clot from the wall of the ventricle. Immobility and impaired cardiac function contribute to stasis of blood in the venous system. Elastic stockings, along with active and passive leg exercises, are usually included in the postinfarction treatment plan as a means of preventing thrombus formation.

Rupture of the heart, septum, or papillary muscle

The acute postmyocardial infarction period can be complicated by rupture of the myocardium, the intraventricular septum, or a papillary muscle. Myocardial rupture is usually fatal, occurring at the time when the injured ventricular tissue is soft and weak, about the seventh to the tenth day. Necrosis of the septal wall or papillary muscle may also lead to rupture of either of these structures with a worsening of ventricular performance. Surgical repair is usually indicated, but whenever possible, it is delayed until the heart has had time to recover from the initial infarction. Vasodilator therapy and the aortic balloon counterpulsation pump may provide supportive assistance during this period.

Ventricular aneurysm

Scar tissue does not have the characteristics of normal myocardial tissue. When a large section of ventricular muscle is replaced by scar tissue, that section does not contract with the rest of the ventricle; instead there is outpouching—aneurysm—of the ventricle during systole, which diminishes myocardial pumping efficiency (Fig. 16-6). This increases the work of the left ventricle and predisposes to heart failure. The ischemia in the surrounding area predisposes to development of arrhythmias, and within the aneurysm stasis of blood can lead to thrombus formation. Surgical resection is often corrective.

Treatment

The treatment of myocardial infarction has changed drastically during the past decade. Patients are ambulated earlier, leave the hospital sooner, and are encouraged to return to an active and productive life; this is in contrast to the prolonged restriction of activity and limited return to work that were imposed in past years.

Figure 16–6. Paradoxical movement of a ventricular aneurysm during systole.

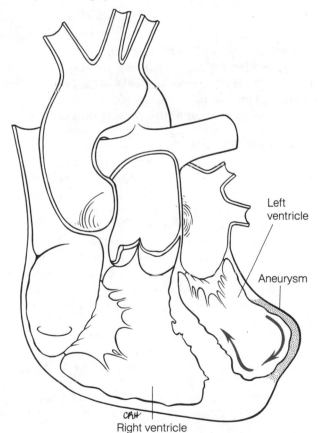

Left ventricle

Aneurysm

Right ventricle

Surveillance during the immediate postinfarction period

Immediate postinfarction care focuses on early detection and treatment of arrhythmias and on the impaired cardiac pumping ability. The danger of potentially fatal arrhythmias early postinfarction usually warrants continual electrocardiographic monitoring. The coronary care unit ensures access to constant supervision, monitoring, and emergency treatment if required. Currently there is interest in identifying patients at low risk for developing arrhythmias and other complications, with the intent that these patients could be managed in less acute hospital units or even in the home-care setting.

Relieving pain and decreasing oxygen needs

Protecting the oxygen supply to the heart and decreasing myocardial oxygen consumption as much as possible are additional concerns in treatment. The severe pain of myocardial infarction gives rise to anxiety, with recruitment of autonomic responses, and these increase the work demands on the heart. Morphine and meperidine (Demerol) are often given intravenously because they have a rapid onset of action, and the intravenous route does not elevate cardiac enzyme levels. A second early treatment measure involves the use of low-flow oxygen to augment oxygen content of the inspired air. Arterial oxygen levels may fall precipitously following myocardial infarction, and oxygen administration maintains the oxygen content of the blood perfusing the coronary circulation. Modifying the diet to include foods that are low in salt and easy to digest is another treatment measure. Laxatives are often prescribed to prevent constipation and straining on defecation.

Activity and exercise

It has been suggested that patients with severe coronary heart disease avoid activities that may involve the *Valsalva maneuver*. The Valsalva maneuver is the act of exhaling against a closed glottis as occurs in straining at stool or lifting while holding the breath. The resultant increase in intrathoracic pressure impedes venous return to the heart, so stroke volume and pulse pressure are decreased; this causes a reflex-mediated increase in heart rate and total peripheral resistance. Then, when the strain is released, the blood quickly returns to the right heart, with a sudden increase in blood pressure (arterial pressure overshoot); this causes a reflex bradycardia. The hemodynamic changes during the Valsalva maneuver are rapid and of short duration, usually lasting only seconds. The maneuver has been safely used as a test of autonomic function in patients with coronary heart disease.[11] It has been reported that some patients obtain relief of angina through self-prescribed use of the maneuver.[12] Probably the pain relief is due to temporary decrease in venous return occurring during the maneuver. Patients with congestive heart failure do not have a decrease in stroke volume or pulse pressure with the maneuver, because their increase in central blood volume does not impede the sudden venous return to the heart. The Valsalva maneuver causes an abrupt translocation of blood from the chest to the veins of the legs; probably one of the greatest dangers associated with the maneuver is that thromboemboli may be mobilized from these veins. The benefits of the Valsalva maneuver are controversial, and it may be wise to instruct patients to avoid holding their breath in any activity in which the maneuver may be involved.

Static or isometric exercise involves the development of tension without a change in muscle length. Static exercise causes an increase in heart rate and blood pressure, increasing the pressure load against which the left ventricle must pump and therefore myocardial oxygen consumption. Lifting, carrying, and pushing are examples of activities that involve the use of isometric exercises.

Dynamic exercise has become an integral part of the rehabilitation program of most cardiac patients. It includes such activities as walking, swimming, and jogging; these exercises cause changes in muscle length and rhythmic contractions of muscle groups. The exercise program is usually individually designed to meet the patient's physical and psychological needs. The goal of the exercise program is to increase maximal oxygen uptake by the tissues, so that the patient will be enabled to perform more work at a lower heart rate and blood pressure.

:The Conduction System

The conduction system controls the rhythm and the pumping action of the heart. The process of impulse generation in the heart and other excitable tissue involves the movement or flow of electrical charges at the level of the cell membrane. There are three phases in impulse generation: the nonexcited state, depolarization, and repolarization (Fig. 16-7). In the resting or nonexcited state, positive and negative charges are separated by the cell membrane, which is impermeable to the flow of electrical charges. Depolarization can be likened to the flipping of a light switch; during this phase the characteristics of the cell membrane are changed and there is flow of charge (current) along the membrane. Repolariza-

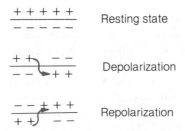

Resting state

Depolarization

Repolarization

Figure 16–7. The flow of charge during impulse generation in excitable tissue. During the resting state, opposite charges are separated by the cell membrane. Depolarization represents the flow of charge across the membrane and repolarization of the return of the membrane potential to its resting state.

tion is similar to recharging a battery; this phase involves the movement of charges back across the membrane and the return of the membrane to its nonexcited state. A cell must be sufficiently recovered before it can be depolarized again.

Impulses from the heart are transmitted to the surface of the body where they are sensed and recorded on an electrocardiogram (ECG) (Fig. 16-8).

The horizontal axis of the ECG tracing measures time, and the vertical axis measures the amplitude of the impulse (in millivolts). The P wave represents depolarization of the S–A node and the atria, the QRS complex records the events that occur during ventricular depolarization, and the T wave occurs with ventricular repolarization. Atrial repolarization occurs during the period of the QRS complex and is not visible on the ECG.

Arrhythmias and Conduction Defects

The specialized cells in the conduction system manifest four inherent characteristics: (1) automaticity, (2) excitability, (3) conductivity, and (4) refractoriness. *Automaticity* is the ability of certain cells of the conduction system to initiate an impulse or action potential. The S–A node has an inherent discharge rate of 60 to 100 times per minute; normally it acts as the pacemaker of the heart, because it reaches the threshold for excitation before other parts of the conduction system have recovered sufficiently to be depolarized. If the sinus node fires more slowly, or if S–A conduction is blocked, another site of impulse generation will take over as pacemaker. These pacemakers have a slower rate of discharge; the A–V node has an inherent firing rate of 40–60 times per

Figure 16–8. Diagram of the electrocardiogram (lead II) and representative depolarization and repolarization of the atria and ventricle. The P wave represents atrial depolarization; the QRS complex ventricular depolarization; and the T wave ventricular repolarization. Atrial repolarization occurs during ventricular depolarization and is hidden under the QRS complex.

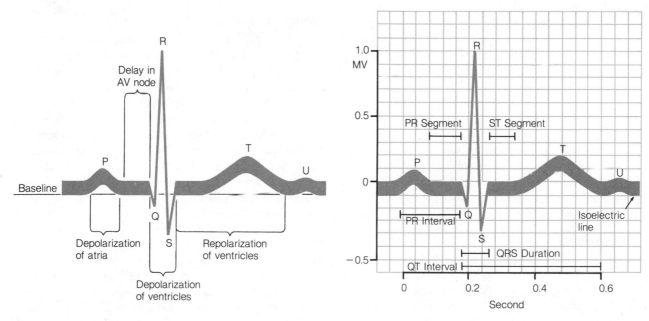

minute, and the Purkinje system 30–40 times per minute. Even when the S–A node is functioning properly, other cardiac cells can assume the properties of *automaticity* and begin to initiate impulses when injured, deprived of oxygen, or exposed to certain chemicals or drugs.

An *ectopic pacemaker* is an excitable focus outside the normally functioning S–A node. These pacemakers can reside in other parts of the conduction system or in muscle cells of the atria or ventricles. A premature contraction occurs when an ectopic pacemaker initiates a beat. In general, premature contractions do not follow the normal conductive pathways; they are not coupled with normal mechanical events; and they often render the heart refractory, or incapable of responding to the next normal impulse that arises from the S–A node. Premature contractions occur without incident in persons with healthy hearts in response to sympathetic stimulation or to stimulants such as caffeine. In the diseased heart, the premature contraction may lead to more serious arrhythmias. *Excitability* describes the ability of a cell to respond to an impulse and generate an action potential. Myocardial cells that have been injured and replaced by scar tissue do not possess the properties of excitability; neither do they possess the property of *conductivity* or the ability to conduct the flow of electrical charge. *Refractoriness* is the inability to respond to an incoming stimulus; the refractory period of cardiac impulse is the interval in the repolarization period during which an excitable cell has not recovered sufficiently so that it can be reexcited. Each of the four characteristics of the cells in the conduction system can be altered to the extent that it contributes to the development of arrhythmias.

Disorders of heart beat arise as the result of disturbances in impulse generation or automaticity and conduction of impulses in the heart. There are many causes of altered cardiac rhythms, including congenital defects of the conduction system, degenerative changes, ischemia and myocardial infarction, fluid and electrolyte imbalances, and effects of drug ingestion. Arrhythmias are not necessarily pathologic; they can occur in the healthy as well as the diseased heart. Disturbances in cardiac rhythms exert their harmful effects by interfering with the heart's pumping ability.

Sinus arrhythmias

The normal rhythm of the heart with the sinus node in command is regular and ranges from 60 to 100 beats per minute. On the electrocardiogram a P wave may be observed to precede every QRS complex.

Alterations in the function of the S–A node lead to a change in the rate and regularity of the heart beat. *Sinus bradycardia* describes a rate less than 60 beats per minute. In sinus bradycardia, a P wave precedes each QRS; this confirms that the impulse is originating in the S–A node rather than in a part of the conduction system that has a slower heart rate. Vagal stimulation decreases the firing rate of the S–A node and conduction through the A–V node to cause a decrease in heart rate. A slow resting rate of 50 to 60 beats per minute may be normal in a well-trained athlete who maintains a large stroke volume. *Sinus tachycardia* refers to an increase in heart rate, to 100 to 160 beats per minute, that has its origin in the S–A node. Sympathetic stimulation or withdrawal of vagal tone incites an increase in heart rate. Sinus tachycardia is normal during exercise and in situations that incite sympathetic stimulation. *Sinus arrhythmia* is a condition in which the heart rate speeds up and then slows down in an irregular, but cyclic, pattern; it is often associated with respiration and alterations in autonomic control. *Sinus arrest* refers to failure of the S–A node to discharge and results in an irregular pulse. An escape rhythm develops as another pacemaker takes over. Sinus arrest may result in prolonged periods of asystole and often predisposes to other arrhythmias. Causes of sinus arrest include disease of the S–A node, digitalis toxicity, and excess vagal tone. The *sick sinus syndrome* is a term that describes a condition of periods of bradycardia alternating with tachycardia. The bradycardia is caused by disease of the sinus node (or other intraatrial conduction pathways) and the tachycardia, by paroxysmal atrial or junctional arrhythmias.

Arrhythmias originating in the atria

The impulse from the S–A node passes through the conductive pathways in the atria to the A–V node. An *atrial premature contraction* can originate in the atrial conduction pathways or in atrial muscle cells. This contraction is transmitted to the ventricle as well as back to the S–A node. The retrograde transmission to the S–A node often interrupts the timing of the next sinus beat so there is a pause between the two normally conducted beats. *Atrial flutter* describes an atrial rate of 160 to 350. There is a delay in conduction through the A–V node, and the ventricles respond to every second, third or fourth beat (for example, when conduction from the atria to the ventricles is 3:1, an atrial flutter rate of 225 will result in a ventricular rate of only 75). *Atrial fibrillation* describes an atrial rate in excess of 350, usually 450 to 600 beats per minute. Here, conduction through the A–V node is totally disorganized, the peripheral pulse is grossly irregular, and a pulse deficit can be observed. The pulse deficit is the difference between the apical and peripheral pulses. In atrial fibrillation, the rate may be such that there is not sufficient stroke output to be felt at the wrist, causing a difference between the apical heartbeat and peripheral pulses. Atrial fibrillation can occur as the result of left atrial distention due to mitral stenosis. It is the most common atrial arrhythmia in the elderly.[13] Atrial fibrillation predisposes to thrombus formation in the atria, with subsequent risk of formation of systemic emboli.

During rest and moderate activity ventricular filling is not dependent upon atrial contraction. Atrial contraction contributes only about 25% to 30% of cardiac reserve; therefore, atrial arrhythmias may go unnoticed unless they are transmitted to the ventricle. These arrhythmias are usually diagnosed electrocardiographically.

Alterations in A-V conduction

The A–V node is the only relay station between the atrial and ventricular conduction systems. Junctional fibers in the A–V node have high resistance characteristics, which cause a delay in transmission of impulses from the atria to the ventricles; this allows for filling of the ventricles and protects them from abnormally rapid rates that arise in the atria. Conduction defects are most commonly due to fibrosis or scar tissue in fibers of the conduction system. Conduction defects of the A–V node can also occur as the result of digitalis toxicity.

Heart block occurs when conduction through the A–V node is delayed or interrupted. It may occur in the A–V nodal fibers or in the A–V bundle (bundle of His), which is continuous with the Purkinje conduction system that supplies the ventricles. The P–R interval on the ECG corresponds with the time that it takes for the cardiac impulse to travel from the S–A node to the ventricular pathways; the normal range is 0.12 to 0.20 second. *A first-degree heart block* is the situation in which conduction through the A–V pathway is delayed and the P–R interval is longer than 0.20 second. In *second-degree block*, one or more of the atrial impulses are blocked. There are two types of second-degree block: the *Mobitz type I*, or *Wenckebach phenomenon*, describes a progressive increase in the P–R interval until the point where one P wave is totally blocked; the *Mobitz type II block* describes the situation in which there is a sudden block in one or more atrial impulses without an antecedent prolongation of the P–R interval. In a Mobitz type II block, the ventricular rate is irregular and reflects the degree of block; this type of block is significant because it often precedes complete heart block. *Third-degree* or *complete* heart block occurs

when the conduction link between the atria and ventricles is completely lost; the atria continue to beat at a normal rate and the ventricles develop their own rate, which is normally slow (30 to 40 beats per minute). Complete heart block causes a decrease in cardiac output with possible periods of syncope (called a Stokes–Adams attack). Patients with complete heart block usually require a pacemaker.

The A–V node can act as a pacemaker in the event the S–A node fails to initiate an impulse. Junctional fibers in the A–V node or bundle can also serve as ectopic pacemakers, producing *premature junctional contractions*.

Disorders of ventricular conduction

The junctional fibers in the A–V node join with the Purkinje conduction system of the ventricles. On leaving the junctional fibers, the cardiac impulse travels through the A–V bundle, moves down the right and left bundle branches that lie beneath the endocardium on either side of the septum, and then spreads out through the walls of the ventricles. Interruption of impulse conduction through the bundle branches does not usually cause alterations in the rhythm of the heart beat; this is because the impulse is usually conducted along an alternate or detour pathway. It does, however, take longer for the impulse to be transmitted through the Purkinje system when there is a conduction defect; this produces changes in the QRS complex of the ECG and causes the QRS complex to be wider than the normal 0.08 to 0.12 second. The left bundle branch is divided into two parts called fascicles (see Fig. 15-3). A hemiblock refers to involvement of one of the fascicles of the left bundle branch.

Ventricular arrhythmias

Arrhythmias arising in the ventricles are usually considered to be more serious than those arising in the atria; this is because they afford the potential for interfering with the pumping action of the heart. *A premature ventricular contraction* is caused by a ventricular ectopic pacemaker. Following a premature contraction, the ventricle is usually not able to repolarize sufficiently to respond to the next impulse that arises in the S–A node; this causes the "compensatory pause," which occurs while the ventricle waits to reestablish its previous rhythm. With a premature contraction, the diastolic volume is usually insufficient for ejection of blood into the arterial system; this causes a skipped beat. In the absence of heart disease, premature ventricular contractions are usually not of great clinical significance. They can occur in digitalis toxicity and in myocardial ischemia and infarction. The occurrence of frequent premature ventricular contractions in the diseased heart predisposes to other more serious arrhythmias, including ventricular tachycardia and fibrillation. *Ventricular tachycardia* describes a ventricular rate of 160 to 250; it is dangerous because it causes a reduction in the diastolic filling time to the point where the cardiac output is severely diminished or nonexistent. Ventricular tachycardia leads to compromised coronary perfusion and predisposes to fibrillation. *Ventricular fibrillation* is a fatal arrhythmia, unless interrupted by cardioversion. During ventricular fibrillation, the ventricle quivers but does not contract, with cessation of cardiac output.

Diagnosis and Treatment

Diagnosis of conduction defects and cardiac arrhythmias is usually made on the basis of the electrocardiograph tracing.

The treatment of arrhythmias is directed toward controlling the arrhythmia and correcting the cause, and preventing more serious or fatal arrhythmias. Correction may involve simply adjustment of an electrolyte disturbance or withholding a medication such as digitalis. Preventing more serious arrhythmias often involves drug therapy (Table 16-4). Correction of the conduction defect can involve use of an electronic pacemaker or cardioversion in ventricular fibrillation. A *pacemaker* is an electronic device that delivers an electrical stimulus to the heart, and it may be a temporary or a permanent measure.

Temporary pacing involves the passage of a venous catheter with electrodes at its tip. The catheter is advanced under fluoroscopic or electrocardiographic control into the right atrium or ventricle, where it is wedged against the endocardium. Permanent pacing requires insertion of pacemaker electrodes attached directly into the epicardium, or transvenous insertion into the apex of the right ventricle, where the electrode comes in contact with the endocardium. Defibrillation or DC cardioversion (400 watt-seconds) is the only reliable method for treating ventricular fibrillation. The current from the defibrillator interrupts the disorganized impulses allowing the S-A node to regain control of the heart beat.

:The Endocardium and Valvular Structures

The endocardium has a smooth surface which interfaces with blood moving through the heart. The endocardium covers the septum, the papillary muscles, the latticework of muscular columns called the trabeculae carneae, and the valvular structures. The smoothness of this layer is an essential characteristic in preventing platelet aggregation and clot formation. This section discusses two diseases of the endocardium, rheumatic fever and endocarditis. The final part of the discussion focuses on valvular defects of the aortic and mitral valves.

Table 16–4 Antiarrhythmic Drugs*.

Drug	Indication for Use	Action
Quinidine	Atrial fibrillation	Prolongs the refractory time Decreases myocardial excitability Prolongs conduction Decreases automaticity
Digitalis	Atrial tachycardia, flutter and fibrillation A–V junctional tachycardia	Causes vagal slowing Increases the refractory period in the A–V node to block some of the atrial impulses
Phenytoin (Dilantin)	Ventricular arrhythmias and digitalis toxicity	Depresses automaticity
Lidocaine (Xylocaine)	Ventricular arrhythmias	Depresses automaticity of Purkinje fibers (to suppress ectopic pacemakers)
Procainamide (Pronestyl)	Ventricular arrhythmias	Prolongs the refractory period Depresses excitability of the atrium and ventricles Prolongs conduction time Decreases automaticity of pacemaker cells
Disopyramide (Norpace)	Ventricular arrhythmias	Same as quinidine and procainamide

*The reader is referred to another source of drug information for a more complete discussion of these drugs.

Rheumatic Fever

Rheumatic fever is an important disease because of its potential for causing chronic heart problems. It currently affects 100,000 children and 1,750,000 adults in the United States. Although generally a preventable disease, the death rate from rheumatic fever in 1977 was 12,770.[14] Rheumatic fever is more prevalent in groups subjected to poor nutrition, crowded living conditions, and inadequate health care.

Age plays an important role in the epidemiology of rheumatic fever. It is most prevalent in school-age children. Ninety percent of all patients had their initial attack between ages five and fifteen,[15] and it is seldom seen in children under age four or in persons over age fifty.

Rheumatic fever is associated with infection due to group A beta-hemolytic streptococcus and usually follows an inciting pharyngeal infection by 1 to 4 weeks. It is of particular significance that rheumatic fever and its cardiac complications can be prevented by antibiotic treatment of the initial streptococcal infection.

The pathogenesis of the disease is unclear, and the question why only 3% of persons with uncomplicated streptococcal infections develop rheumatic fever remains to be answered. The time frame for development of symptoms in relation to the sore throat, as well as the presence of antibodies to the streptococcus organism, strongly suggests an immunologic origin. Like other immunologic phenomena, rheumatic fever requires an initial sensitizing exposure to the offending (streptococcus) agent, and the risk of recurrence is high following each subsequent exposure. Rheumatic fever can present as an acute, recurrent, or chronic disorder.

The acute stage includes a history of an initiating streptococcal infection and subsequent involvement of the mesenchymal connective tissue of the heart, blood vessels, joints, and subcutaneous tissues. Common to all is the presence of a lesion called the *Aschoff body*. The Aschoff body is a localized area of tissue necrosis containing fibrinoid material. The recurrent phase usually involves extension of the cardiac effects of the disease. The chronic problems are associated with valvular defects due to the disease.

The child with rheumatic fever usually has had a history of sore throat, headache, fever, abdominal pain, nausea and vomiting, swollen glands (usually at the angle of the jaw), and other signs of a streptococcal infection. Throat cultures taken at the time of the acute infection are positive for streptococcus.

The sedimentation rate, C-reactive protein, and white blood cell count are usually elevated at the time that heart or joint manifestations begin to appear. A high or rising antistreptolysin O titer is also suggestive of rheumatic fever. Streptolysin O is a hemolytic factor produced by most strains of group A beta-hemolytic streptococci; antistreptolysin O (ASO) is an antibody against the hemolytic factor produced by the streptococci. Other signs and symptoms associated with an acute episode of rheumatic fever are related to the structures involved in the disease process.

Rheumatic fever can affect any of the three layers of the heart: pericardium, myocardium, and endocardium. Usually all three layers are involved. Rheumatic pericarditis causes the production of a fibrinous or serofibrinous exudate. Myocardial changes are for the most part reversible, and produce minimal changes in cardiac function. It is the involvement of the endocardium and valvular structures that produces the permanent and disabling effects of the disease. Although any of the four valves can be involved, it is the mitral and aortic valves that are affected most often. During the acute inflammatory stage of the disease, the valvular structures become reddened and swollen; small vegetative lesions develop on the valve leaflets. Gradually, the acute inflammatory changes proceed to fibrous scar tissue development, which tends to contract and cause deformity of the valve leaflets and shortening of the chordae tendineae. In some cases, the edges or commissures of the leaflets fuse together as healing occurs.

Joint involvement, while not a cause of permanent disability, is a frequent finding in rheumatic fever. The inflammatory process affects the synovial membrane of the joint, causing swelling and discomfort. Often the arthritis is migratory in nature, affecting one joint and then moving to another. The transitory nature of the joint pains has at times caused the disorder to be mistaken for "growing pains."

The *skin lesions* seen in rheumatic fever are of two types, subcutaneous nodules and erythema marginatum. The *subcutaneous nodules* range in size from 1 to 4 cm; they are hard, painless, and freely movable, and usually overlie the extensor muscles of the wrist, elbow, ankle, and knee joints. *Erythema marginatum* lesions are maplike macular areas, seen most commonly on the trunk or inner aspects of the upper arm and thigh. Skin lesions are present only in about 10% of patients who have rheumatic fever; they are transitory and disappear during the course of the disease.

Chorea (Sydenham's chorea), sometimes called St. Vitus' dance, is the major central nervous system manifestation. It is seen most frequently in girls. Typically, there is an insidious onset of irritability and other behavior problems. The child is often fidgety, cries easily, begins to walk clumsily, and tends to drop things. The choreic movements are spontaneous, rapid, purposeless jerking movements, which tend to interfere with voluntary activities. Facial grimaces are common, and even speech may be affected. Fortunately, the chorea is self-limiting, usually running its course within a matter of weeks or months.

Recurrent nosebleeds (epistaxis) are thought to be a subclinical manifestation of rheumatic fever.

Treatment

Treatment is designed to control the acute inflammatory process and to prevent cardiac complications and recurrence of the disease. During the acute phase, prevention of residual cardiac effects becomes of primary concern. Administration of antibiotics and anti-inflammatory drugs, and selective restriction of physical activities are usually carried out during the acute stage of illness. Secondary prevention involves the prophylactic use of penicillin (or another antibiotic in penicillin-sensitive patients) for a period of at least 5 years to prevent recurrence. Penicillin is also the antibiotic of choice for treating the acute illness. Salicylates and corticosteroids are also widely used.

Secondary prevention and compliance with a plan for prophylactic administration of penicillin requires that the patient and the family understand the rationale for such measures as well as the measures themselves. Patients also need to be instructed to report possible streptococcal infections to their physician. They should be instructed to inform their dentist about them so that they can be adequately protected during dental procedures that might traumatize the oral mucosa.

Bacterial Endocarditis

The significance of bacterial endocarditis lies in the tendency for it to develop in persons with a damaged heart. It can be caused by almost any pathogen, the most common being *Streptococcus viridans*. Staphylococci, gram-negative bacteria, and fungi have also been isolated as causes of endocarditis.

Two predisposing factors contribute to the development of endocarditis. One is a *damaged endocardial surface*, the other a *portal of entry* by which the organism gains access to the blood stream. The presence of valvular disease, rheumatic heart disease, or congenital heart defects provides an environment conducive to bacterial growth. The second factor, bacteremia, may emerge in the course of seemingly minor health problems, such as an upper respiratory tract infection, a skin lesion, or a dental procedure. Simple gum massage or an innocuous oral lesion may afford the pathogenic bacteria access to the blood stream. Bacterial endocarditis is reported to be a significant potential disease in narcotic addicts who "mainline." And it is a potential complication in patients with intravascular catheters that remain in place for long periods of time.

The vegetative lesion characteristic of bacterial endocarditis consists of a collection of pathogens and cellular debris, enmeshed in the fibrin strands of clotted blood. These lesions may be singular or multiple, may reach a size of several centimeters, and are usually found loosely attached to the free edges of the valve surface. The loose organization of the lesion permits the organisms to disseminate, and fragments are carried by the blood to give rise to small hemorrhages, abscesses, and infarcted areas in other parts of the body—kidneys, spleen, brain, and joints.

Bacterial endocarditis may occur in an acute or subacute form. *Acute bacterial endocarditis* is thought to affect primarily persons with normal hearts, whereas *subacute bacterial endocarditis* (SBE) is seen most frequently in patients with damaged hearts. The signs and symptoms include fever, change in the character of an existing heart murmur, and evidence of embolic distribution of the vegetative lesions. In the acute form, the fever is usually spiking and accompanied by chills. In the subacute form, the fever is usually low grade and of gradual onset, and is frequently accompanied by other systemic signs of inflammation such as anorexia, malaise, and lethargy. Small petechial hemorrhages frequently result when emboli lodge in the small vessels of the skin, nailbeds, and mucous membranes.

The blood culture is the most significant diagnostic aid in bacterial endocarditis. Usually a series of three to six cultures are obtained during a 36- to 48-hour period to ensure adequate sampling.

The focus of treatment is toward identifying and destroying the causative organism, minimizing the residual cardiac effects, and treating the pathology induced by the emboli. The blood cultures usually identify the organism so its sensitivity to antibiotics can be assessed. An appropriate antibiotic is prescribed to eradicate the pathogen. This active treatment stands in contrast to preantibiotic days when bacterial endocarditis often was fatal. Of even

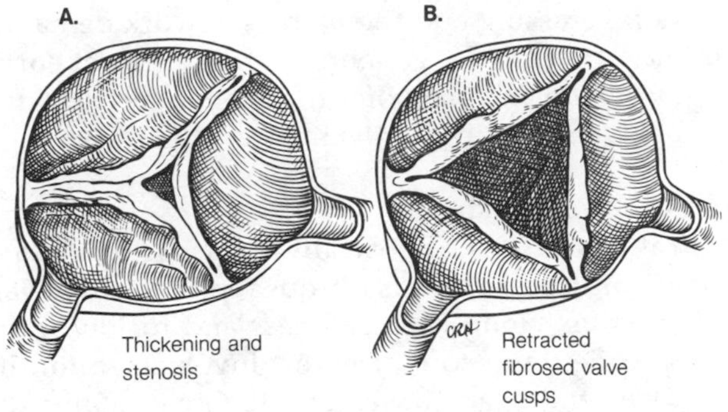

Figure 16–9. Disease of the arotic valve as viewed from the aorta: (*A*) depicts stenosis of the valve opening, and (*B*) an incompetent or regurgitant valve that is unable to close completely.

greater importance is prevention in persons known to be at risk. Prevention can be largely accomplished through prophylactic administration of an antibiotic prior to dental procedures and others that may cause bacteremia.

Valvular Disease

Dysfunction of the heart valves can result from a number of disorders, including congenital defects, trauma, ischemic damage, degenerative changes, and inflammation. Rheumatic endocarditis is the most common cause. Its inflammatory changes cause scar tissue to form on the valve leaflets and the chordae tendineae with a subsequent shortening of the chordae and deformation of the valve structure. In valvular disease there may be two types of mechanical disruptions (1) narrowing or stenosis of the valve opening; or (2) a valve that fails to close completely (Fig. 16-9).

Valvular disease can be either stenotic (failure to open completely) or regurgitant (failure to close completely), but often there is a combination of both stenotic and regurgitant effects. The influence of valvular disease on cardiac function is related to alterations in blood flow and increased work demands on the heart. Any of the four heart valves can become diseased; this discussion is limited to defects of the aortic and mitral valves.

Stenosis causes a decrease in flow through the valve, with an increased work demand on the heart chamber in front of the diseased valve. In mitral stenosis, for example, the left atrium becomes distended and the work output required of this chamber is increased. As the condition advances, blood return from the lungs is impeded, and the pulmonary circulation becomes congested. Blood flow through a normal valve can increase to five to seven times the resting value; consequently, valvular stenosis must be severe before it causes life-threatening problems.[16] The first evidence of symptoms usually is noted during exercise.

An incompetent (regurgitant) valve permits blood flow to continue while the valve is closed, flowing into the left ventricle during diastole when the aortic valve is affected, and into the left atrium during systole when the mitral valve is diseased. With an incompetent valve, the work demands of both the heart chamber in front and that in back of the affected valve are increased. In mitral regurgitation, the left atrium is presented with an increased volume and the left ventricle with a bidirectional flow pattern such that blood is propelled into both the left atrium and the aorta during systole.

Aortic valvular defects

The orifices of the coronary arteries are strategically located in the aorta, just distal to the aortic valve leaflets (Fig. 16-10). In aortic stenosis, the velocity of flow through the narrowed valve orifice is increased at the expense of the lateral pressure needed to perfuse the coronary arteries. In aortic regurgitation, failure of aortic valve closure during diastole causes diastolic pressure to fall; this decreases the pressure needed to perfuse the coronary arteries.

Aortic stenosis causes resistance to ejection of blood into the aorta, so the work demands on the left ventricle are increased and the volume of blood ejected into the systemic circulation decreases. The most common causes of aortic stenosis are rheumatic fever and congenital heart defects. In the elderly, it may be related to degenerative atherosclerotic changes of the valve leaflets.

Figure 16–10. Location of the orifices for the coronary arteries and the direction of flow during systole and diastole.

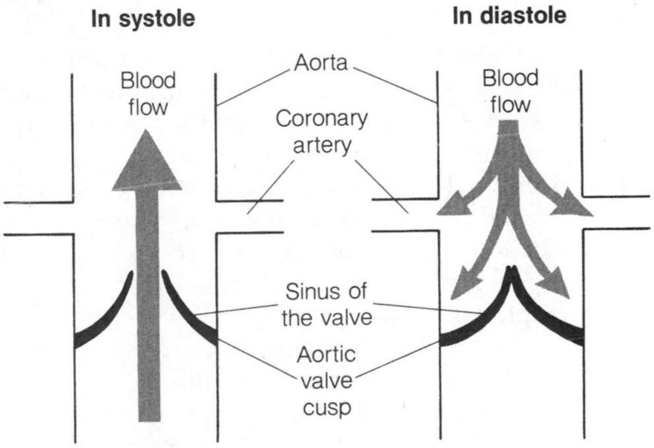

Obstruction to aortic outflow causes a decrease in stroke volume, in which blood pressure is low and pulse pressure narrow. Thus it takes a longer time for the heart to eject blood; the heart rate is often slow and the pulse of low amplitude. Resistance to flow through the aortic valve gives rise to an auscultatory murmur in systole.

• The onset of signs and symptoms is dependent to a large extent on the person's activity level; in one who leads a sedentary life, the disease may be far advanced before symptoms are noted. Exertional dyspnea is a common presenting symptom. It is characterized by vertigo and syncope when the stroke volume falls to levels insufficient for cerebral needs. Also, the combination of increased work demands on the hypertrophied left ventricle and decreased perfusion of the coronary vessels may cause angina.

An *incompetent aortic valve* allows blood to return to the left ventricle during diastole. This defect may result from conditions that cause scarring of the valve leaflets or from enlargement of the valve orifice to the extent that the valve leaflets no longer meet. Rheumatic fever ranks first on the list of causes of aortic regurgitation.

A widening of the pulse pressure is characteristic of aortic regurgitation, so that the systolic pressure is frequently increased and the diastolic pressure decreased. Widening of the pulse pressure has two underlying mechanisms: first, there is an increase in the stroke volume as the left ventricle must eject blood entering from the lungs, as well as the blood that has leaked back across the aortic valve into the ventricle during diastole; secondly, because the aortic valve fails to close completely, diastolic pressure cannot be maintained. The left ventricle hypertrophies due to the increased volume load on this chamber. Turbulence of flow across the aortic valve during diastole produces a high-pitched or blowing type of murmur.

The large stroke volume and rapid runoff of blood from the aorta produce characteristic changes in the peripheral pulses: prominent carotid pulsations in the neck, throbbing peripheral pulses, and a left ventricular impulse that causes the chest to move with each beat. The term "waterhammer" pulse is often used to describe the hyperkinetic peripheral pulse found in persons with aortic regurgitation. The pulsations in the carotid can become so intense that the person's head may nod with each heart beat.

Symptoms of aortic regurgitation are those associated with heart failure: exertional dyspnea, dizziness, pulmonary edema, and orthopnea. Angina follows the impaired coronary perfusion due to a low diastolic pressure and the increased work demands on the left ventricle. Patients with significant aortic regurgitation complain of throbbing of the chest due to the hyperdynamic left ventricle.

Mitral valve defects

Mitral stenosis is almost always associated with rheumatic fever. There is fibrous replacement of valvular tissue, along with stiffness and fusion of the valve leaflets and commissures. Involvement of the chordae tendineae causes shortening, pulling the valvular structures more deeply into the ventricles.

The clinical findings are due to obstruction to blood flow between the left atrium and ventricle. Initially, the impediment to flow causes an increase in left atrial volume and pressure. As the disease progresses, the increased pressure is transmitted back to the pulmonary circulation, resulting in pulmonary congestion and hypertension, and this increases work demands on the right ventricle and finally failure of this side of the heart. Also, there is inadequate filling of the left ventricle with clinical manifestations due to low cardiac output. The murmur of mitral stenosis is found during diastole when blood is flowing through the constricted valve orifice; it is usually a low-pitched rumbling murmur, best heard at the apex of the heart.

Signs and symptoms depend on the severity of the obstruction and are generally related to (1) right heart failure, (2) left atrial distention and mural thrombus formation, and (3) decreased cardiac output due to impaired left ventricular filling. Symptoms are those of pulmonary congestion, including nocturnal paroxysmal dyspnea and orthopnea. Atrial fibrillation may occur, the result of distention of the left atrium. Together, the fibrillation and distention predispose to mural thrombus formation, from which systemic emboli may form. Palpitations are a frequent symptom, and chest pain, weakness, and fatigue are other complaints.

Diagnosis and Treatment

Valvular defects are usually detected through cardiac auscultation. Diagnosis is aided by the use of the phonocardiogram, echocardiogram, and catheterization. The phonocardiogram, obtained by placing a microphone on the chest wall, provides a graphic recording of heart sounds. Simultaneous ECG recordings are usually made to provide reference points for use in interpreting the phonocardiogram.

Treatment of valvular defects consists of (1) medical management of heart failure and associated problems and (2) surgical intervention to either repair or replace the defective valve. Mitral commissurotomy is the surgical enlargement of a stenotic valve. It may be performed as either an open or a closed procedure. The open procedure requires extracorporeal circulation (cardiopulmonary bypass), but has the advantage of affording the surgeon direct visualization of the operative site. Valvular replacement, either with a prosthetic device or a homograft, is usually reserved for severe disease. Unfortunately, the ideal substitute valve has not yet been invented, consequently, valve replacement is usually reserved for patients with severe disease.

:Congenital Heart Disease

Approximately eight babies out of every thousand are born with a congenital heart defect. About one-third of them have a severe defect that would cause death within the first year if it were not corrected. This section of the chapter is designed to provide an overview of congenital heart defects, including a discussion of the embryonic development of the heart, the hemodynamic changes that accompany congenital heart disorders, and the more common defects. Depending on the type of defect that is present, children with congenital heart disease will experience varying signs and symptoms associated with altered heart action, heart failure, and difficulty in supplying the peripheral tissues with oxygen and other nutrients.

Embryonic Development of the Heart

When one considers the rapid sequential changes required to transform the embryonic tubular heart into a functioning four-chambered directional pump, it is not difficult to imagine the variability and extent of developmental errors that could occur.

During the third week following conception the heart of the developing embryo begins its first pulsatile movements—the heart is the first functioning organ of the body. This early development is essential for the rapidly growing embryo as it outgrows its ability to meet its nutritional and elimination needs through diffusion alone.

The developing heart begins its function as a single tubular structure and rapidly undergoes a series of synchronized folding and positional changes as both it and the embryo continue to grow and develop (Fig. 16-11). Besides these changes, the embryonic tubular heart undergoes internal changes by which it becomes partitioned both vertically and

horizontally; in such manner the tubular heart is transformed into a four-chambered version of the adult heart.

Vertically, the atrial and ventricular septa develop to form a separate left and right heart. De-

Figure 16–11.   Ventral views of the developing heart (20–25 days). (Adapted from Moore KL: The Developing Human, 2nd ed. Philadelphia, WB Saunders, 1977)

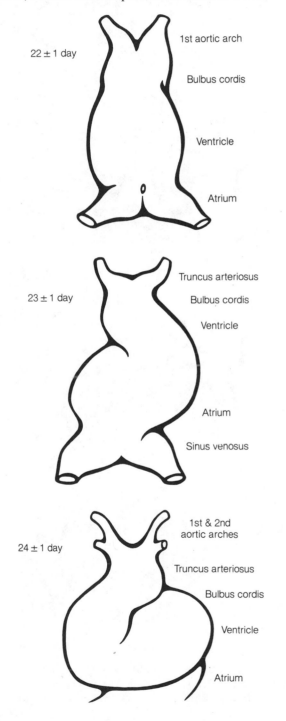

velopment of a closed ventricular septum is usually completed by the end of the seventh week. Development of the atrial septum is more complex and closure does not occur until after birth. During formation of the atrial septum, an opening called the *foramen ovale* develops to establish a communicating channel between the two upper chambers of the heart. This opening allows blood from the umbilical vein to pass directly into the left heart, bypassing the lungs (Fig. 16-12). As the lungs expand following birth, the pulmonary and systemic circulations separate into two systems, and the foramen ovale closes.

Horizontal separation of the heart accompanies vertical positioning. The atria and the ventricles separate as the tissue bundles, called the endocardial cushions, begin to form in the midportion of the dorsal and ventral walls, and grow inward. As the endocardial cushions enlarge, they meet and fuse, forming a right and a left atrioventricular channel (Fig. 16-13). It is in these channels that the mitral and tricuspid valves develop.

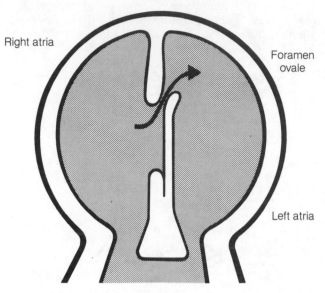

Figure 16–12.   Illustration of the foramen ovale. (Adapted from Moore KL: The Developing Human, 2nd ed. Philadelphia, WB Saunders, 1977)

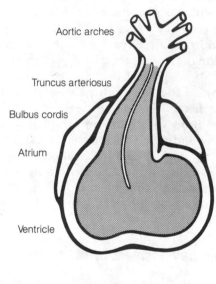

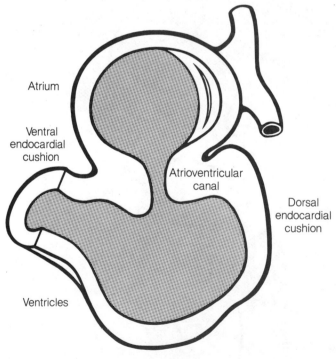

Figure 16–13.   Development of the endocardial cushions. (Adapted from Moore KL: The Developing Human, 2nd ed. Philadelphia, WB Saunders, 1977)

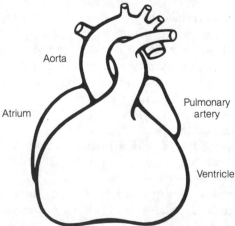

Figure 16–14.   Separation and twisting of the truncus arteriosus to form the pulmonary artery and aorta. (Adapted from Moore KL: The Developing Human, 2nd ed. Philadelphia, WB Saunders, 1977)

To complete the developmental process, provision must be made for separating blood pumped from the right heart, so it can be diverted into the pulmonary circulation while blood from the left heart is pumped into the systemic circulation. This separation of blood flow is accomplished by the outlet channels of the tubular heart, the *bulbus cordis* and the *truncus arteriosus*, which undergo spiral twisting and vertical partitioning (Fig. 16-14). In the process of forming a separate pulmonary trunk and aorta, the *ductus arteriosus* arises to allow blood entering the pulmonary trunk to be shunted into the aorta as a means of bypassing the lungs. Like the foramen ovale, the ductus arteriosus usually closes shortly after birth.

Normal development of the heart requires a precise and orderly sequence of differentiation and growth. Congenital heart defects can arise at any stage of development, with structural abnormalities reflecting growth that was occurring at the time the disturbance arose. Table 16-5 is designed to assist the reader in understanding the embryonic origin of specific defects.

Table 16-5   Classification of Congenital Heart Defects According to Site of Embryonic Origin

Stage of Embryonic Development	Defect
Development of the atrial septum	Atrial septal defect of septum secondum
	Atrial septal defect of septum primum
Development of the ventricular septum	Ventricular septal defect of muscular septum
	Ventricular septal defect of membranous septum
Development of the endocardial cushions	Ebstein's anomaly of the tricuspid valve
	Abnormalities of the tricuspid and mitral valve
	Defect in ostium primum
	Defect in membranous portion of the ventricular septum
Spiraling and partitioning of the truncus arteriosus and bulbus cordis	Transposition of the great vessels
	Persistent truncus
	Tetralogy of Fallot
	Pulmonary stenosis
	Pulmonary outflow obstruction
Development of the aortic arches	Coarctation of the aorta
	Patent ductus arteriosus

Causes of Congenital Heart Defects

Development of the heart and major blood vessels is usually completed by the end of the eighth week of gestation. Included in this brief span of time is the critical period between weeks three and eight with its complex changes in cardiac development. Causes of congenital heart defects have been attributed to environmental, genetic, and chromosomal influences.

Maternal rubella during this critical period of fetal development is associated with an increased incidence of heart defects; in one study, congenital heart disease was identified in 52% of babies who were born with congenital rubella during the 1964-65 New York City epidemic.[17] Also, it appears that other viruses, some drugs, and radiation are causes of congenital heart defects.

Chromosomal and genetic factors are thought to account for about 5% of congenital heart defects. Characteristic of these influences is the number of cardiac lesions observed in children born with Down's syndrome (trisomy of chromosome 21). The familial clustering of a number of congenital heart defects suggests that these defects are polygenic in origin. The 3% risk of polygenic recurrence that occurs with the presence of one affected child increases substantially as a second and third child are found to have similar defects.

Although both environmental and genetic influences have been cited as causes of congenital heart disease, often the cause is unknown, and it has been postulated that perhaps both genetic and environmental factors interact and contribute to the defect.

Hemodynamic changes accompanying congenital heart defects

Congenital heart defects produce their major effects through (1) shunting or mixing of arterial and venous blood, and (2) alterations in pulmonary blood flow and production of pulmonary hypertension.

Shunting.   Shunting of blood refers to the diverting of blood flow from one system to the other—from the arterial to the venous or the venous to the arterial system. The shunting of blood in congenital heart defects usually originates with the presence of an *abnormal opening* between the right and left circulations and the presence of a *pressure difference* that facilitates flow.

In atrial defects, blood usually moves from the left atria into the right atria because of the higher pressure in the left heart. In a more complicated pressure-flow situation, such as a ventricular septal defect accompanied by obstruction of the pulmonary outflow channel, pressure builds up in the right ventricle to the extent that it may exceed left ventricular pressure; in this case, blood is pushed from the right side of the heart to the left side. The presence of a left-to-right shunt results in unoxygenated blood being ejected into the systemic circulation, causing cyanosis. In the left-to-right shunt, blood intended for ejection into the systemic circulation is recirculated through the right heart and back through the lungs; the increased volume distends the right heart and pulmonary circulation and increases the workload placed on the right ventricle. Children with a septal defect that causes left-to-right shunting usually have an enlarged right heart and pulmonary blood vessels.

Alterations in Pulmonary Blood Flow and Pressure

The complications of congenital heart disorders are due to their effect on the pulmonary circulation, which may be exposed to either an increase or a decrease in blood flow.

In contrast to the arterioles in the systemic circulation, the mature pulmonary arterioles are thin-walled vessels, so they can accommodate various levels of stroke volume from the right heart. The maturation process that produces thinning of the smooth muscle layer in these vessels is delayed until after birth. But in congenital heart disease, the increase in pulmonary blood flow during the early neonatal period results in delay or impairment of maturation. When this happens, there is increased resistance to flow in the pulmonary circulation, and pulmonary hypertension develops. How damaging this blood flow will be to the maturing pulmonary vessels depends on the time of onset and the extent of increased flow. In many instances, the volume overload occurs after the pulmonary vessels have already developed their low-resistance properties.

In situations in which the shunting of systemic blood flow into the pulmonary circulation threatens permanent injury to the pulmonary vessels, a surgical procedure may be done in an attempt to reduce the flow by increasing resistance to outflow from the right ventricle. This procedure, called pulmonary banding, consists of placing a constrictive band around the main pulmonary artery. The banding technique is often used as a temporary measure to alleviate the symptoms and protect the pulmonary vessels in anticipation of later surgical repair of the defect.

There are also defects that decrease flow, producing inadequate oxygenation of blood. The affected child often experiences fatigue, exertional dyspnea, impaired growth, and even syncope.

Septal Defects
Atrial septal defects
Atrial septal defects are more common in girls than in boys. Embryologically, division of the atria is facilitated by the development of two separate septa, which lie side-by-side; septum primum is formed first and septum secondum develops later. Neither septum completely separates the atria, and an oblique opening, the foramen ovale, allows blood to flow from the right atria into the left heart as a means of bypassing the uninflated lungs. As you will note in Figure 16-12, septum primum acts as a one-way valve to prevent the backward flow of blood. At birth, the lungs expand, umbilical blood flow is interrupted, and left atrial pressure rises, pushing septum primum against septum secondum. The continued contact of septum primum with septum secondum induces permanent closure of the foramen ovale, and the foramen ovale is usually completely closed by the second or third month of extrauterine life.

In atrial septal defect, there is aberrant development of septum primum or septum secondum or, more frequently, it comes about because the foramen ovale fails to close. The affected child often is asymptomatic because the defect is so small. In the case of an isolated septal defect that is large enough to allow shunting, the flow of blood will usually be from the left to the right side of the heart (remember that the pressure in the left heart is greater than that in the right); when this happens, there is an increase in the volume of the right heart and pulmonary artery (Fig. 16-15). This increased blood volume that must be ejected from the right heart prolongs closure of the pulmonic valve and produces a separation, or fixed splitting, of the aortic and pulmonic components of the second heart sound.

Ventricular septal defects
Ventricular septal defects are the most common form of congenital heart defect; 20% of all patients with congenital heart disease have a ventricular defect as the only abnormality, and males are affected more frequently than females. These defects vary in size, and can be located in almost any part of the structure, the site being determined by the embryological event that was occurring at the time that growth was interrupted. The ventricular septum originates from

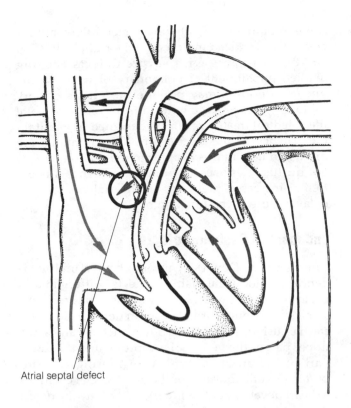

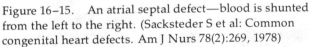

Atrial septal defect

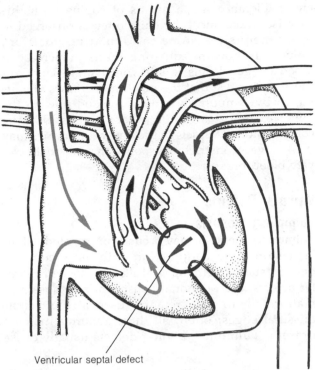

Ventricular septal defect

Figure 16–15.   An atrial septal defect—blood is shunted from the left to the right. (Sacksteder S et al: Common congenital heart defects. Am J Nurs 78(2):269, 1978)

Figure 16–16.   A ventricular septal defect—blood is usually shunted from the left to the right. (Am J Nurs 78(2):269, 1978)

two sources: the intraventricular groove of the folded tubular heart gives rise to the muscular part of the septum, and the endocardial cushions fuse to separate the atria and extend to form the membranous portion of the septum. The upper membranous portion of the septum is the last area to close and it is here that most defects occur.

A ventricular septal defect may be the only cardiac defect or may be one of multiple cardiac anomalies. Many defects of medium or small size in the muscular septum close spontaneously.

As with atrial septal defects, the alterations in cardiac function related to openings in the ventricular septum depend on the presence of other heart defects and their size and location. The shunting of blood across the defect is determined largely by the pressures within the two ventricles. Flow is usually left to right because of the higher pressure in the left ventricle (Fig. 16-16). In situations where an obstruction to pulmonary outflow accompanies a ventricular defect, right ventricular pressure may exceed left ventricular pressure, and then flow will be from right to left. Depending on the size of the opening, the signs and symptoms may range from the presence of an asymptomatic systolic murmur to frank congestive heart failure. Often, ventricular

septal defects are a component of a defect of greater complexity, such as tetralogy of Fallot.

Tetralogy of Fallot

As the name implies, tetralogy of Fallot consists of four associated congenital heart defects: (1) ventricular septal defects involving the membranous septum and the anterior portion of the muscular septum; (2) dextroposition of shifting to the right of the aorta, so that it overrides the right ventricle and is in communication with the septal defect; (3) obstruction or narrowing of the pulmonary outflow channel, including a pulmonic valve stenosis, a decrease in the size of the pulmonary trunk, or both; and (4) hypertrophy of the right ventricle due to the increased work required to pump blood through the obstructed pulmonary channels (Fig. 16-17).

Most children with tetralogy of Fallot display varying degrees of cyanosis—hence the term "blue babies." The cyanosis develops as the result of decreased pulmonary blood flow and because the right-to-left shunt causes mixing of unoxygenated blood with the oxygenated blood being ejected into the peripheral circulation. Because of the decreased oxygen availability, these children have limited exercise tolerance. As a means of coping with this exercise intolerance, the child often is observed to spontaneously assume the squatting position, though just how the squatting effects an increase in blood oxygen levels is still conjectural. Some authorities suggest that the position increases venous return by temporarily reducing blood flow to the lower extremities, while others suggest that the compression of vessels in the lower extremities may incite a vasoconstrictor response that serves to elevate blood pressure.

Valvular Defects

Pulmonary stenosis

Pulmonary stenosis may occur as an isolated valvular lesion or in conjunction with more complex defects, such as tetralogy of Fallot. In isolated valvular defects, the pulmonary cusps may be absent or malformed, or may remain fused at their commissural edges; often, all three abnormalities are present. Pulmonic valvular defects usually cause

Figure 16–17. Tetralogy of Fallot, which involves a ventricular septal defect, dextroposition of the aorta, right ventricular outflow obstruction, and hypertrophy of the right ventricle. (Am J Nurs 78(2):267, 1978)

some impairment of pulmonary blood flow and increase the workload imposed on the right heart (Fig. 16-18). In infants with severe defects causing marked impairment of pulmonary blood flow, the ductus arteriosus may provide the vital accessory route for perfusing the lungs during early postnatal life. Medical treatment efforts designed to maintain the patency of the ductus in affected infants are discussed later in this chapter in the section on patent ductus arteriosus. If pulmonary stenosis is extreme, increased pressures in the right heart may delay closure of the foramen ovale.

Endocardial Cushion Defects

Children with Down's syndrome have a high incidence of endocardial cushion defects, with estimates indicating that as many as 50% of such children have some form of endocardial cushion defect. The endocardial cushions form the atrioventricular canals, the upper part of the ventricular septum, and the lower part of the atrial septum. Considering the embryologic contributions of the endocardial cushions to heart development, it is easy to see why the defect

Figure 16–18. Pulmonary stenosis causes obstruction of flow into the pulmonary artery and a decrease in pulmonary flow. (Am J Nurs 78(2):272, 1978)

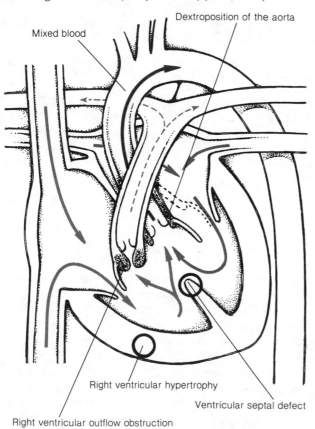

Mixed blood

Dextroposition of the aorta

Right ventricular hypertrophy

Ventricular septal defect

Right ventricular outflow obstruction

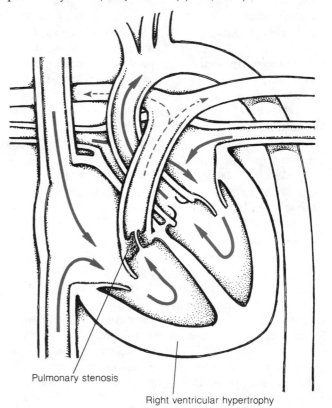

Pulmonary stenosis

Right ventricular hypertrophy

can cause so many different types of defects. In its most severe form, the defect involves both the atrial and ventricular septa and the tricuspid and mitral valves. When growth is halted at a later stage of development, there may be an ostium primum defect and a cleft in the mitral valve. Any single defect or combination of endocardial defects is possible (Fig. 16-19).

Ebstein's anomaly is a defect in endocardial cushion development characterized by displacement of tricuspid valvular tissue into the ventricle. The displaced tricuspid leaflets are either attached directly to the right ventricular endocardial surface or to shortened or malformed chordae tendineae.

Defects in Partitioning of the Truncus Arteriosus

Transposition of the great vessels

In transposition of the great vessels, the aorta originates in the right ventricle and the pulmonary trunk in the left. The structural defect present in this anomaly suggests that during embryonic partitioning of the aorta and pulmonary trunk there was failure in the spiral movement of the bulbus cordis and truncus arteriosus (Fig. 16-20). In infants born with this defect, survival is dependent upon com-

munication between the right and left heart, either in the form of a septal defect or as a patent ductus arteriosus. A procedure called a balloon atrial septostomy may be done to increase blood flow between the two sides of the heart. It is done by inserting a balloon-tipped catheter into the heart through the vena cava, then passing the catheter through the foramen ovale into the left atrium. The balloon is then inflated and as it is brought back through the foramen ovale, the opening is enlarged.

A surgical procedure, the Mustard operation, in which the atrial septum is removed and a new wall is created so that blood is directed into the proper outflow channels, corrects the defect.

Aortic Arch Defects

Patent ductus arteriosus

In fetal life, the ductus arteriosus is the vital link by which blood from the right heart bypasses the lungs and enters the systemic circulation (Fig. 16-21). Following birth this passage is no longer needed, and it usually closes during the first 24 to 72 hours. The

Figure 16–19. Endocardial cushion defect—blood flows between the chambers of the heart. (Am J Nurs 78(2):272, 1978)

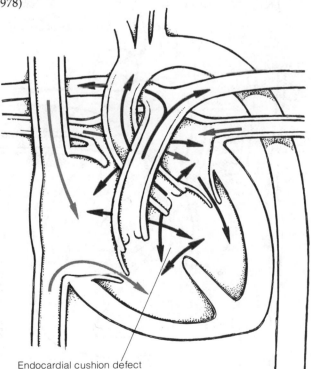

Endocardial cushion defect

Figure 16–20. Transposition of the great vessels, in which the pulmonary artery is attached to the left side of the heart and the aorta to the right side of the heart. The survival of an infant born with this defect depends on an opening between the two sides of the heart (patent ductus arteriosus or patent foramen ovale). (Am J Nurs 78(2):267, 1978)

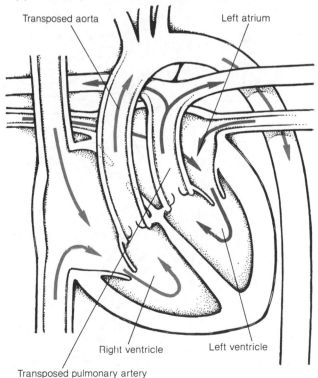

Transposed aorta Left atrium

Right ventricle Left ventricle

Transposed pulmonary artery

physiologic stimulus and mechanisms associated with permanent closure of the ductus are not entirely known, although maternal rubella and infant hypoxia during or shortly after birth are found in many cases. As is true of other heart and circulatory defects, patency of the ductus arteriosus may be present in various forms; the opening may be of small, medium, or large size.

The function of the ductus arteriosus in providing a right-to-left shunt in prenatal life has prompted the surgical creation of an aortic–pulmonary shunt as a means of improving pulmonary blood flow in children with severe pulmonary outflow disorders. Recent research has focused on the role of type E prostaglandins in maintaining patency of the ductus; several researchers have found by injecting prostaglandin E into the umbilical vein of infants who require a ductal shunt, closure has been delayed or prevented.[18] Other research suggests that inhibiting prostaglandin activity with drugs such as aspirin and indomethacin has prompted closure of the ductus.[19,20]

Coarctation of the aorta

Coarctation of the aorta can be described as a localized narrowing of the aorta, either proximal to the ductus (preductal) or distal to the ductus (postductal). (See Fig. 16-22.)

Figure 16–21.   Patent ductus arteriosus—the high pressure in the aorta causes blood to be shunted back into the pulmonary artery. (Am J Nurs 78(2):267, 1978)

In *preductal* coarctation, the ductus remains open and shunts blood from the pulmonary artery, through the ductus arteriosus, into the aorta. It is frequently seen with other cardiac anomalies, and carries a high mortality. Because of the position of the defect, there is reduction in blood flow throughout the systemic circulation, and the affected infant develops heart failure at an early age due to the increased workload imposed on the left ventricle.

In *postductal* coarctation, symptoms often do not arise until late adolescence or adult life. In these persons, the narrowing of the aorta distal to the subclavian artery and proximal to the descending aorta creates disparity between the pulses and blood pressure of the upper and lower extremities (Chap. 13).

Manifestations and Treatment

Congenital heart defects present with numerous signs and symptoms. Some defects, such as patent ductus arteriosus and small ventricular septal defects, often close spontaneously, and in other less severe defects, there are no signs and symptoms. Often, the disorder is discovered during a routine health examination. Pulmonary congestion, cardiac failure, and decreased peripheral perfusion are the chief concerns in children with more severe defects. Such defects often cause problems shortly after birth

Figure 16–22.   Postductal coarctation of the aorta. (Am J Nurs 78(2):270, 1978)

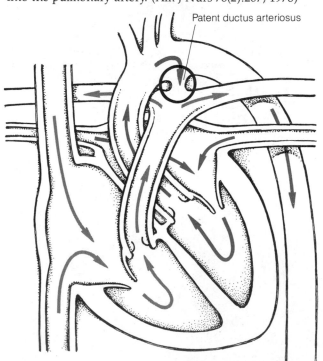

Patent ductus arteriosus

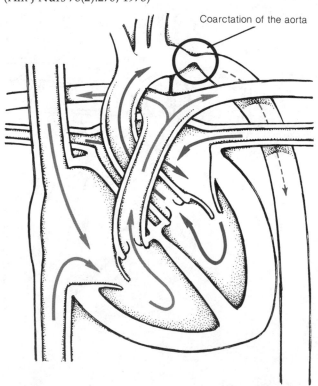

Coarctation of the aorta

or in early infancy. The child often exhibits cyanosis, respiratory difficulty, and fatigability, and is likely to have difficulty with feeding and failure to thrive. A generalized cyanosis that persists more than 3 hours following birth is suggestive of congenital heart disease.

One technique of evaluating the infant consists of administering 100% oxygen for 10 minutes. If the infant "pinks up," the cyanosis is probably due to respiratory problems. Because infant cyanosis may appear as a duskiness, it is important to assess the color of the mucous membranes, fingernails, toenails, tongue, and lips. Pulmonary congestion in the infant causes an increase in respiratory rate, orthopnea, grunting, wheezing, coughing, and rales. The baby whose peripheral perfusion is markedly decreased may appear to be in a shock-like state. The manifestations and treatment of heart failure in the infant and small child are similar in many ways to those in the adult (Chapter 17), but the infant's small size and limited physical reserve give them added seriousness and make treatment more difficult. The treatment plan usually includes supportive therapy designed to help the infant compensate for the limitations in cardiac reserve and to prevent complications. Surgical intervention is often required in severe defects, and it may be done in the early weeks of life, or conditions permitting, may be delayed until the child is older. The reader is referred to a pediatric textbook for a complete description of treatment.

In summary, congenital heart defects affect about eight out of every thousand neonates. The fetal heart develops during weeks three to eight following conception, and it is during this period that defects in its development arise. The defect reflects the stage of development at the time when the causative event occurred. There are a number of factors that are thought to contribute to the development of congenital heart defects, including genetic and chromosomal influences, viruses, and environmental agents such as drugs and radiation. Often the cause of the defect is unknown. The defect may produce no effects or it may markedly affect cardiac function. Infants with severe congenital heart defects often suffer from pulmonary congestion, heart failure, and decreased peripheral perfusion.

:Study Guide

After you have studied this chapter, you should be able to meet the following objectives:

: : Compare the manifestations of acute pericarditis with those of chronic pericarditis with effusion.

: : State the characteristics of constrictive pericarditis.

: : Relate the term *tamponade* to its manifestations in cardiac tamponade.

: : Describe the anatomy of the right and the left coronary arteries.

: : State the significance of atherosclerosis in the occurrence of coronary heart disease.

: : Describe the purpose of electrocardiogram, echocardiogram, and nuclear imaging in diagnosis of coronary heart disease.

: : Describe the use of exercise stress testing.

: : Distinguish unstable angina from variant angina.

: : State the overall goal in treatment of angina, and its rationale.

: : State the relationship between thrombosis and myocardial infarction.

: : List the chief signs and symptoms by which the health professional can recognize myocardial infarction.

: : State four or more possible complications of myocardial infarction and the manifestations of each.

: : Describe the immediate postinfarction and later postinfarction treatment measures that the professional health care team should follow.

: : Describe the sequence of events by which the conduction system controls cardiac rhythm and pumping action.

: : Compare sinus arrhythmia with atrial arrhythmia.

: : Describe the characteristics of first, second, and third degree heart block.

: : State the potential complications associated with premature ventricular contractions.

: : State the probable sequence of events in rheumatic fever.

: : State the predisposing factors in bacterial endocarditis and the significance of each.

: : Relate the presence of valvular disease to cardiac function.

: : Describe the pathophysiology of aortic stenosis and aortic regurgitation.

: : Describe the clinical findings in mitral valve defects.

: : Describe the sequence of events in embryonic development of the heart.

: : Relate the occurrence of Down's syndrome to congenital heart defects.

: : State the effect of altered pulmonary blood flow on congenital heart disease.

: : Compare the features of atrial septal defects with those of ventricular septal defects.

: : Explain why the phrase "blue baby" is used to describe a baby with tetralogy of Fallot.

: : State the effect of congenital pulmonary stenosis on pulmonary blood flow.

: : Explain the significance of endocardial cushion defects.

: : Describe the anatomical situation in transposition of the great vessels.

: : Explain the function of the ductus arteriosus in fetal life.

: : Describe the effect on blood flow of preductal and postductal coarctation of the aorta.

:References

1. Arteriosclerosis. Report of the 1977 Working Group to Review the Report of the National Heart and Lung Institute Task Force on Arteriosclerosis. U.S. Department of Health, Education and Welfare, p 14, Dec, 1977

2. Peduzzi P, Hultgren H: Effect of medical vs. surgical treatment on symptoms of stable angina pectoris. Circulation 60, No. 4:888, 1979

3. Anderson AJ, Barboriak JJ, Hoffmann RG, Mullen DC: Retention or resumption of employment after aortocoronary bypass operation. JAMA 243, No. 6:543, Feb, 1980

4. Robbins SL: Cardiac pathology—a look at the last five years. Human Pathology 5:9, 1974

5. Robbins SL, Cotran RS: Pathologic Basis of Disease, ed. 2, WB Saunders, Philadelphia, p 652, 1979

6. Robbins SL, Cotran RS: Pathologic Basis of Disease, ed. 2, WB Saunders, Philadelphia, p 655, 1979

7. Hillis LD, Braunwald E: Myocardial ischemia. N Engl J Med 296, No. 18:1034, 1977

8. Hillis LD, Braunwald E: Myocardial ischemia. N Engl J Med 296, No. 18:1034, 1977

9. Grande P et al: Optimal diagnosis in acute myocardial infarction. Circulation 61, No. 4:723, 1980

10. The Anturane Reinfarction Trial Research Group: Sulfinpyrazone in the prevention of sudden death after myocardial infarction. N Engl J Med 302, No. 5:250, 1980

11. Porth CJ et al: Stroke volume and blood pressure changes in coronary heart disease patients during graded Valsalva. Fed Proc 39, No. 3:1169, 1980

12. Pepine CV, Wiener L: Effects of Valsalva maneuver on myocardial ischemia in patients with coronary heart disease. Circulation 59, No. 6:1304, 1978

13. Sokolow M, McIlroy MB: Clinical Cardiology. Los Altos, California, Lange Medical Publications, p 470, 1977

14. Heart Facts: American Heart Association, p 10, 1980

15. Robbins SL, Cotran RS: Pathologic Basis of Disease, ed. 2, Philadelphia, WB Saunders, p 666, 1979

16. Sokolow M, McIlroy MB: Clinical Cardiology. Los Altos, California: Lange Medical Publications, p 351, 1977

17. Engle MA, Adams F, Betson C, DuShande J, Elliott L, McNamara DG, Rashkind WJ, Talner NS: Primary prevention of congenital heart disease. Circulation 41: A26, June, 1970

18. Rudolph AM, Heymann MA: Medical treatment of ductus arteriosus. Hosp Pract 12, No. 2:57, 1977

19. Heymann MA, Rudolph AM, Silverman NH: Closure of the ductus arteriosus in premature infants by inhibition of prostaglandin synthesis. N Engl J Med 295, No. 10:530, 1976

20. Smith, ME: Nonsurgical closure of patent ductus arteriosus in preterm infants. Heart Lung 8, No. 2:308, 1979

:Suggested Readings

Bacterial endocarditis and rheumatic fever

DiSciascio G, Taranta A: Rheumatic fever in children. Am Heart J 99, No. 5:635, 1980

Kaplan EL et al: Prevention of bacterial endocarditis. Circulation 56, A139, 1977

Pankey GA: The prevention and treatment of bacterial endocarditis. Am Heart J 98, No. 1:102, 1979

Conduction defects

Atkinson AJ, Nevin MJ: Antiarrhythmic therapy with procainamide. Cardio-Vasc Nurs 13, No. 5:17, 1977

Heger JJ, Fisch C: Axioms on cardiac arrhythmias. Hosp Med 15, No. 1:20, 1979

Roffman JA, Fieldman A: Ventricular conduction defects: significance and prognosis. Heart Lung 9, No. 1:111, 1980

Standford JL, Felmer JM, Arenberg D: Antiarrhythmic drug therapy. Am J Nurs 80, No. 7:1288, 1980

Congenital heart defects

Argarwala B, Baffes B: Congestive heart failure in the infant. Heart Lung 5, No. 1:63, 1976

Engle MA et al: Primary prevention of congenital heart disease. Circulation 41:A25-28, 1970

Modrcin MA, Schott J: An update of congestive heart failure in infants. Issues Comp Pediat Nurs 3:5, 1979

Nadas AS: Heart disease in children. Hosp Prac 12, No. 1:103, 1977

Nadas A, Fyler D: Pediatric Cardiology. WB Saunders, Philadelphia, 1972

Rudolph AM, Heymann MA: Medical treatment of ductus arteriosus. Hosp Prac 12, No. 2:57, 1977

Sacksteder S: Embryology and fetal circulation. Am J Nurs 78, No. 2:262, 1978

Sacksteder S, Gildea H, Dassy C: Common congenital cardiac defects. Am J Nurs 78, No. 2:266, 1978

Shor VZ: Congenital cardiac defects. Am J Nurs 78, No. 2:256, 1978

Smith ME: Nonsurgical closure of patent ductus arteriosus in preterm infants. Heart Lung 8, No. 2:308, 1979

Exercise testing and rehabilitation

Dehn M: Rehabilitation of the cardiac patient: The effects of exercise. Am J Nurs 80, No. 3:435, 1980

Merril S, Froelicher VF: Exercise testing. Cardio-Vasc Nurs 13, No. 6:23, 1977

Sivarajan ES, Halpenny CJ: Exercise testing. Am J Nurs 79, No. 12:1262, 1979

Winslow EH, Weber TM: Rehabilitation of the cardiac patient. Progressive exercise to combat the hazards of bed rest. Am J Nurs 80, No. 3:440, 1980

Diseases of the myocardium

Abrams J: Nitroglycerin and long-acting nitrates. N Engl J Med 302, No. 22:1234, 1980

Alexander JK, Fred HL, Wright KE, Turell DJ, Jackson RA, Jackson D: Exercise and coronary artery disease. Heart Lung 7, No. 1, 1978

Arcebal AG, Lemberg L: Angina pectoris in the absence of coronary artery disease. Heart Lung 9, No. 4:728, 1980

Braunwald E: Treatment of the patient after myocardial infarction. N Engl J Med 302, No. 5:290, 1980

Cain RS, Ferguson R, Tillisch JH: Variant angina: A nursing approach. Heart Lung 8, No. 6:1122, 1979

Devny AM: Rehabilitation of the cardiac patient: bridging the gap between in-hospital and outpatient care. Am J Nurs 80, No. 3:446, 1980

Foster SB, Canty KA: Pump failure following myocardial infarction: An overview. Heart Lung 9, No. 2:293, 1980

Fuller EO: The effect of antianginal drugs on myocardial oxygen consumption. Am J Nurs 80, No. 2:250, 1980

Gronim SS: Helping the client with unstable angina. Am J Nurs 78, No. 10:1677, 1978

Hirsh AT: Postmyocardial infarction syndrome. Am J Nurs 79, No. 7:1240, 1979

Kannel WB, Sorlie P, McNamara, PM: Prognosis after initial myocardial infarction: the Framingham study. Am J Cardiol No. 44:53, 1979

McIntosh H, Entman ML, Evans RI, Martin RR, Jackson D: Smoking as a risk factor. Heart Lung 7, No. 1:445, 1978

McIntosh HD, Stamler J, Jackson DJ: Introduction to risk factors in coronary artery disease. Heart Lung 7, No. 1:126, 1978

Norris RM: Prognosis in myocardial infarction. Heart Lung 4, No. 1:75, 1975

Oliver MF: The metabolic response to a heart attack. Heart Lung 4, No. 1:57, 1975

Scheer E: Enzymatic changes and myocardial infarction: A nursing update. Cardio-Vasc Nurs 14, No. 2:5, 1978

Schroeder JS, Lamb I, Hu M: Do patients in whom myocardial infarction has been ruled out have a better prognosis after hospitalization than those surviving infarction? N Engl J Med 303, No. 1:1, 1980

Tanner G: Heart failure in the MI patient. Am J Nurs 77, No. 2:230, 1977

Westfall UE: Electrical and mechanical events in the cardiac cycle. Am J Nurs 76, No. 2:231, 1976

Diseases of the pericardium

Buselmeier TJ, Davin TD, Simmons RL, Najarian JS, Kjellstrand CM: Treatment of intractable uremic pericardial effusion. J Am Med A 240:1358, 1978

Domby WR, Whitcomb MF: Pleural effusion as a manifestation of Dressler's syndrome in the distant post-infarction period. Am Heart J 96, No. 2:243, 1978

Hirschmann JV: Pericardial constriction. Am Heart J 96, No. 1:110, 1978

Spodick DH: Acute pericarditis and pericardial effusion: Guide to diagnosis and management. Hosp Med 15:72, May, 1979

Zeluff GW, Eknoyan G, Jackson D: Pericarditis in renal failure. Heart Lung 8, No. 6:1139, 1979

17

Heart Failure

Heart failure is not a specific disease. It is failure of the heart as a pump which can occur in the course of many heart diseases—any condition that places an excessive work load on the heart. Two such problems—congestive heart failure and acute pulmonary edema—are the subject of this chapter.

:Cardiac Reserve and Recruitment of Compensatory Mechanisms

The heart has the amazing capacity to adjust its activity to meet the varying needs of the body—during sleep, its output declines, and during exercise it is markedly increased. This ability to increase output during increased activity is called the *cardiac reserve*. For example, competitive swimmers and long-distance runners have a large cardiac reserve as evidenced by the fact that during exercise their cardiac output rapidly increases by as much as five to six times its normal resting level. In sharp contrast to the healthy athlete, persons with heart failure even at rest are often using their cardiac reserve. For them, even such simple activities as climbing a flight of stairs may cause shortness of breath because they have exceeded their cardiac reserve.

Cardiac reserve is maintained through *compensatory mechanisms*. In many forms of heart disease, early decreases in cardiac function are unnoticed because these compensatory mechanisms serve to maintain cardiac output. In persons with heart failure there are three main compensatory mechanisms that help maintain cardiac output: (1) increased sympathetic activity, (2) fluid retention, and (3) myocardial hypertrophy. It seems, however, that these adaptive mechanisms were not intended for long-term use, because in severe and prolonged heart failure, the compensatory mechanisms, themselves, begin to cause problems.

Increased Sympathetic Stimulation

Cardiac output is the product of heart rate and stroke volume. Increases in sympathetic activity produce increase in both heart rate and cardiac contractility. In severe heart failure, the sympathetic receptors may remain functional, but the failing heart may be unable to synthesize the neuromediator norepinephrine, and must depend on neuromediators carried in the blood stream.[1] The heart's metabolic needs increase with sympathetic stimulation and in situations where coronary blood flow may not be adequate to meet these needs, myocardial ischemia and angina may develop.

Fluid Retention

Fluid retention is an important early compensatory mechanism in heart failure. Initially, there is a renin-angiotensin-aldosterone-mediated increase in sodium and water retention by the kidney as cardiac output falls to the point where renal blood flow is decreased. The fluid retained by the kidneys causes a progressive increase in vascular volume with an accompanying increase in venous return to the heart. This leads to increased filling and stretching of the myocardial fibers during diastole and a resultant increase in the force of cardiac contraction (the Frank–Starling mechanism, discussed in Chapter 15). The Frank–Starling mechanism becomes ineffective when the heart becomes overfilled and the muscle fibers are overstretched. The increase in vascular volume also leads to edema.

Muscle Hypertrophy

Muscle hypertrophy is a long-term compensatory mechanism. Cardiac muscle, like skeletal muscle, responds to an increase in work demands by undergoing hypertrophy. Heart disease, by increasing resistance to ejection of blood from the ventricles, is the greatest stimulus for hypertrophy; for example, the left ventricle may increase in size to six times normal in severe aortic stenosis. If portions of the heart muscle are damaged and replaced with scar tissue, the undamaged part of the myocardium often hypertrophies as a means of improving the pumping capacity of the ventricle. However, myocardial hypertrophy is no longer beneficial when the oxygen requirements of the increased muscle mass exceed the ability of the coronary vessels to bring blood to the area.

:Congestive Heart Failure

Heart failure occurs when the heart fails to pump sufficient blood to meet the metabolic needs of body tissues. In congestive heart failure, fluid accumulates in body tissues along with a decrease in cardiac output. Table 17-1 lists the causes of heart failure.

When the heart fails as a pump, there may be two direct effects on the circulation. First, *backward failure* allows blood to accumulate in the vessels or heart chambers located behind the failing ventricles, resulting in congestion of the pulmonary and venous systemic circulations. Second, *forward failure* impairs the forward movement of blood into the vessels emerging from the heart. Although the initial event that leads to heart failure may be primarily right-sided or left-sided in origin, long-term heart

Table 17–1   Causes of Heart Failure

Impaired Cardiac Function	Excess Work Demands
Myocardial disease	**Increased pressure work**
Cardiomyopathies	Systemic hypertension
Myocarditis	Pulmonary hypertension
Coronary insufficiency	Coarctation of the aorta
Myocardial infarction	
Valvular heart disease	**Increased volume work**
Stenotic valvular disease	Arteriovenous shunt
Regurgitant valvular disease	Excess administration of intravenous fluids
Congenital heart defects	**Increased perfusion work**
	Thyrotoxicosis
	Anemia
Constrictive pericarditis	

failure usually involves both sides. It is easier, however, to understand the physiologic mechanisms associated with heart failure when right- and left-sided failure are discussed separately.

Right-sided Failure

Right-sided heart failure is characterized by an accumulation or "damming back" of blood in the systemic venous system. This causes an increase in right atrial and peripheral venous pressures, with subsequent development of edema in the peripheral tissues, and congestion of the abdominal organs. The peripheral edema is most pronounced in the lower extremities and in the area over the sacrum. As venous distention advances, blood backs up in the hepatic veins that drain into the inferior vena cava, and the liver becomes engorged. In severe and prolonged right-sided failure, liver function is frequently impaired, and liver cells may die. Congestion of the portal circulation may also lead to enlargement of the spleen with transudation of fluid into the peritoneal cavity (ascites). Congestion of the gut may cause gastrointestinal disturbances, including anorexia, abdominal pain, and loss of weight. The jugular veins are above the level of the heart and normally collapsed in the standing position. In severe right-sided failure, the external jugular veins become distended and can be visualized when the person is standing. The manifestations of right-sided heart failure are depicted in Figure 17-1.

Left-sided Failure

With impairment of left heart function, blood tends to accumulate in the pulmonary circulation. An increase in pulmonary capillary pressure reflects the

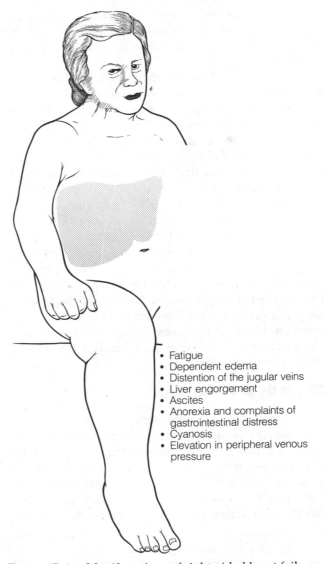

- Fatigue
- Dependent edema
- Distention of the jugular veins
- Liver engorgement
- Ascites
- Anorexia and complaints of gastrointestinal distress
- Cyanosis
- Elevation in peripheral venous pressure

Figure 17–1.   Manifestations of right-sided heart failure.

increased left atrial pressure and leads to pulmonary edema. In severe pulmonary edema, capillary fluid moves into the alveoli. The accumulated fluid causes shortness of breath and interferes with the ability of the lungs to oxygenate blood, and causes fluid to collect in the alveoli and respiratory passages.

One of the major manifestations of left-sided heart failure is shortness of breath. A perceived shortness of breath is called *dyspnea*. Dyspnea related to an increase in activity is called *exertional dyspnea*. *Orthopnea* is shortness of breath that occurs when a person is supine or lying down. The gravitational forces which caused fluid to become sequestered in the lower legs and feet when the person was sitting, are no longer operational when the person is supine, and these fluids are then mobilized and redistributed to an already distended pulmonary circulation. *Paroxysmal nocturnal dyspnea* is a sudden attack of dyspnea during sleep. It disrupts sleep, and the waking person may recall having had a bad dream.

Fatigue and limb weakness often accompany diminished output from the left ventricle. Cardiac fatigue is different from emotional fatigue in that it is usually not present in the morning, but progresses as activity increases during the day. In acute or severe left-sided failure, cardiac output may fall to levels that are insufficient for providing the brain with adequate oxygen, and there are indications of mental confusion and disturbed behavior.

Cyanosis may occur in either right- or left-sided heart failure. In left-sided failure, impairment of the gas-exchange function of the lung interferes with oxygenation of the blood, and the hemoglobin leaves the pulmonary circulation without being fully oxygenated. In right-sided failure, blood flow is sluggish, and there is increased extraction of oxygen from the blood as it passes through the capillaries; the quantity of deoxygenated hemoglobin in the blood then increases.*

Diagnosis and Treatment

As was stated earlier, heart failure is a manifestation of a number of heart diseases or other systemic pathology. Consequently, treatment measures are usually directed toward determining the cause of the primary disorder. The functional classification of the New York Heart Association is one guide to classifying the underlying problems (Table 17-2).

---

*The blue discoloration associated with cyanosis requires the presence of 5 g of deoxygenated hemoglobin. A severely anemic person may not have sufficient hemoglobin to permit 5 g to become deoxygenated. Some of the success credited to the bloodletting practices of the 18th and 19th centuries probably resulted from treating cyanosis by causing anemia.

Table 17–2 Classification of Patients with Diseases of the Heart

Cardiac status
1. Uncompromised
2. Slightly compromised
3. Moderately compromised
4. Severely compromised

Prognosis
1. Good
2. Good with therapy
3. Fair with therapy
4. Guarded despite therapy

The treatment of heart failure is directed toward (1) correcting the cause, (2) improving cardiac function, (3) maintaining fluid volume within a compensatory range, and (4) arriving at an activity pattern consistent with individual limitations in cardiac reserve.

Surgical correction of a ventricular defect and replacement of a defective valve are examples of measures directed at correcting the cause of heart failure. Digitalis is often prescribed to increase the heart's pumping efficiency. Restriction of salt intake and diuretic therapy facilitate excretion of edema fluid. Counseling, health teaching, and other assistive measures help persons with heart failure to manage their activity patterns appropriately.

Digitalis has been a recognized treatment for congestive heart failure for the past 200 years. The various forms of digitalis are called *cardiac glycosides*. They improve cardiac function by increasing the force and strength of ventricular contraction. Also, they slow the heart rate by decreasing S-A node activity and decreasing conduction through the A-V node, thus increasing diastolic filling time. Although not a diuretic, digitalis promotes urine output by improving renal blood flow. The margin between therapeutic and toxic doses of digitalis is very narrow. Low potassium levels predispose patients to digitalis toxicity, an important consideration in patients who are on digitalis, since many of them are also taking diuretics which promote potassium losses.

Digitalis toxicity can be described by its effect on three body systems—the heart, gastrointestinal tract, and central nervous system. The most serious is digitalis-induced arrhythmias. These arrhythmias can take many forms and can mimic most disturbances of cardiac rhythm. Anorexia, nausea, and vomiting are common gastrointestinal indications of toxicity. They may occur in patients receiving parenteral digitalis which suggests that they are due to disturbances in the central nervous system, rather than to direct irritation of the gastrointestinal tract. Psychic and visual problems are signs of toxicity to the central nervous system. Some patients have described the visual disturbance as "looking through yellow-green glasses." A recent advance in laboratory methods allows for monitoring of serum digitalis levels.

:Acute Pulmonary Edema

Acute pulmonary edema is a life-threatening situation. Although pulmonary edema is often associated with left heart failure, it can also result from increased permeability of the pulmonary capillary membrane, which in turn may be due to an infectious process, exposure to toxic gases, drug reactions, or other conditions. Hypervolemia due to rapid infusion of intravenous fluids or a blood transfusion in an elderly person or in a person with limited cardiac reserve may precipitate an episode of pulmonary edema. The following discussion centers on pulmonary edema due to heart failure.

In left-sided heart failure, an episode of pulmonary edema usually happens at night when the person has been reclining for a period of time; gravitational forces are not exerted on the circulatory system, so that edema fluid that had been sequestered in the lower extremities is redistributed to the pulmonary circulation (as was discussed). Or the acute episode may be a complication of impaired cardiac pumping ability in myocardial infarction.

A person with pulmonary edema is usually seen sitting and gasping for air (Fig. 17-2). The apprehension is obvious. The pulse is rapid; the skin is moist and cool, and the lips and nailbeds are cyanotic. As the edema worsens and oxygen supply to the brain falls off, confusion and stupor appear. Dyspnea and air hunger are accompanied by a cough productive of a frothy and often blood-tinged sputum—the effect of air mixing with the plasma and blood cells that have exuded into the alveoli. The movement of air through the alveolar fluid produces a fine crepitant sound, called *rales*, which can be heard through a stethoscope placed on the chest. As fluid moves into the larger airways, the breathing is louder. In the terminal stage it is called the *death rattle*. In severe pulmonary edema, persons literally drown in their own secretions.

Treatment Measures

The goals of treatment are directed toward reducing the fluid volume in the pulmonary circulation. This can be accomplished by reducing the amount of blood that the right heart delivers to the lungs or by improving the work performance of the left heart.

A number of measures are available that decrease the blood volume in the pulmonary circulation, and the seriousness of the pulmonary edema will determine which are to be used. One of the simplest measures to relieve orthopnea is assumption of the seated position. For many persons, sitting up or standing is almost reflex in nature and may be sufficient to relieve the symptoms associated with mild accumulation of fluid.

Diuretics

Diuretics promote excretion of edema fluid, and in emergencies, they are often administered intravenously. The diuretic furosemide (Lasix) appears to

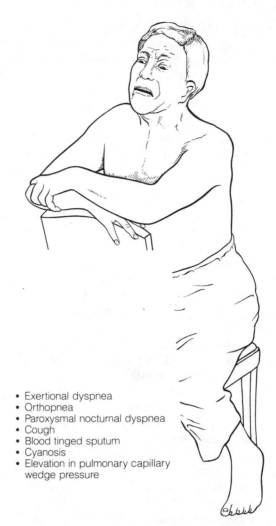

- Exertional dyspnea
- Orthopnea
- Paroxysmal nocturnal dyspnea
- Cough
- Blood tinged sputum
- Cyanosis
- Elevation in pulmonary capillary wedge pressure

Figure 17–2.   Manifestations of acute left-sided heart failure.

have a biphasic effect on pulmonary congestion. When given intravenously, it appears to produce venous dilatation almost immediately with increased venous pooling of blood and a decrease in venous return to the right heart. The decrease in venous tone that occurs when furosemide is administered intravenously precedes its diuretic action by about 30 to 60 minutes.[2]

Vasodilator drugs

Vasodilator drugs cause relaxation of smooth muscle. These drugs induce venous pooling of blood, produce relaxation of the pulmonary arterial and venous vessels, and reduce resistance in the systemic arterial vessels. With pooling of blood in the peripheral veins, there is less blood available to the right heart for delivery to the pulmonary circulation. Relaxation of the pulmonary vessels diminishes pressure in the pulmonary capillaries and allows fluid to be reabsorbed from the interstitium of the lung and from the alveoli. (The reader is referred to

Chapter 24 for a discussion of edema formation.) With a decrease in the resistance of the systemic arterial vessels, there is less pressure against which the left heart must pump and thus the work of the left venticle is decreased. Table 17-3 lists some vasodilator drugs used to treat acute pulmonary edema. Note that some of them exert their major action on the arterial system, some on the venous system, and some on both the arterial and venous systems.

General measures

Measures to *improve left heart performance* focus on (1) reducing the filling pressure of the left ventricle and (2) reducing the afterload against which the left heart must pump. This can be accomplished through use of *vasodilator drugs*, *treatment of arrhythmias* that impair cardiac function, and by improving the contractile properties of the left ventricle with digitalis. *Rapid digitalization* may be accomplished with intravenous digitalis.

   Oxygen therapy affords oxygenation of the blood and helps relieve anxiety. *Positive-pressure breathing* increases the intra-alveolar pressure which opposes the capillary filtration pressure in the pulmonary capillaries, and is a temporary measure to decrease the amount of fluid moving into the alveoli.

   Although its mechanisms of action are unclear, *morphine sulfate* is usually a drug of choice in acute pulmonary edema. Morphine relieves anxiety and depresses the pulmonary reflexes that cause spasm of the pulmonary vessels. Aminophylline is another drug, administered intravenously, that may be useful. It reduces bronchospasm, increases glomerular filtration rate, and promotes urinary excretion of sodium and water. This drug relieves Cheyne–Stokes respirations which sometimes occur in severe heart failure. Relief is due not to the theophylline itself, but to the ethylenediamine in which the theophylline is solubilized.

   Another way to reduce pulmonary blood vol-

ume in severe life-threatening situations is by venesection or alternating tourniquets. Fortunately, with modern pharmacologic treatments, there is less need for these treatment methods. Venesection consists of removing 300 to 500 ml of blood from the body. (It seems likely that the success of the barbershop surgeon with his bloodletting practices was due at least partly to the temporary relief of symptoms of pulmonary congestion.) Alternating tourniquets afford a means of trapping venous blood in the extremities. The tourniquets are inflated to levels between the arterial and venous pressures; this permits some inflow of arterial blood while preventing outflow of venous blood. Four cuffs are used: one cuff is alternately deflated every 15 to 20 minutes so that venous flow from any one extremity is occluded only for a period of 45 to 60 minutes. Alternating tourniquets are an interim measure, while other forms of treatment are being initiated. Care must be taken when discontinuing the use of the tourniquets, so that the heart is not suddenly confronted with increase in venous return.

In summary, heart failure is characterized by impaired pumping ability of the heart and represents the outcome of many forms of heart disease and other conditions which place excess demands on the heart. Heart failure may be either right-sided or left-sided. In right-sided failure there is congestion of the systemic venous system, and in left-sided failure there is pulmonary congestion. Usually heart failure affects both sides of the circulation.

:Study Guide

After you have studied this chapter, you should be able to meet the following objectives:

: : Explain the phrase *cardiac reserve*.

: : Explain how the compensatory mechanisms of increased sympathetic stimulation, fluid retention, and muscle hypertrophy maintain cardiac reserve.

: : Describe the effects of backward failure and forward failure on the circulation.

: : Explain the gastrointestinal disturbances due to right-sided heart failure.

: : Explain the respiratory disturbances due to left-sided heart failure.

: : Describe the effects of digitalis on cardiac function.

: : Describe the clinical picture seen in pulmonary edema.

Table 17–3   Vasodilator Drugs Used in Pulmonary Edema

Drugs	Site of Action Arteries	Veins
Hydralazine	X	
Phentolamine	X	
Nitrates		X
Nitroprusside	X	X
Prazosin	X	X
Trimethaphan	X	X
Hexamethonium	X	X

From: Giles, Thomas D. Principles of vasodilator therapy in left ventricular congestive heart failure. Heart Lung 9(2):274, 1980

: : Explain why diuretics are prescribed to treat pulmonary edema.

: : Describe the action of vasodilator drugs on the respiratory system.

: : Describe the use of alternating tourniquets in treatment of pulmonary edema.

:References

1. Braunwald E: The sympathetic nervous system in heart failure. Hosp Pract 5, No. 12:31-38, 1970
2. Dikshit K et al: Renal and extrarenal effects of furosemide in congestive heart failure after acute myocardial infarction. N Engl J Med 288(21):1087-1090, 1973

:Suggested Readings

Heart failure

Arbeit S, Fiedler J, Landau T, Rubin I: Recognizing digitalis toxicity. Am J Nurs 77(12):1936-45, 1977

Atkins FL: New therapies in the management of congestive heart failure. J Kansas Med Soc 81(2):83-85, 1980

Brigham KL: Pulmonary edema: cardiac and noncardiac. Am J Surg 138:361-367, 1979

Brigham KL: Lung vascular permeability and primary pulmonary edema. Western J Med 130(3):222-226, 1979

Carlet J, Francoual M, Lhoste F, Regnier B, Lemaire F: Pharmacological treatment of pulmonary edema. Intens Care Med 6:113-122, 1980

Dack S: Acute pulmonary edema. Hosp Med 14, No. 3·112, 1978

DeSanctis RW, Atkinson AJ, Mullins CB: Congestive heart failure: diagnosis and treatment today. Emerg Med 11:108-114+, 1979

Dickenson CJ, Marks J: Heart failure: Pathophysiological considerations. Developments in Cardiovascular Medicine. MTP Press, Lancaster, England, 1978, pp. 213-232

Hildner FJ: Pulmonary edema associated with low left ventricular filling pressures. Am J Card 44:1410-1411, 1979

Isacson LM, Schulz K: Treating pulmonary edema. Nursing '78, 8:42-46, 1978

Jodice J: Management of acute pulmonary edema. J Emerg Nurs 4:19-22, 1978

Moore SJ: Digitalis toxicity and treatment with phenytoin: a neurological mechanism of action. Heart Lung 6(6):1035-1040, 1977

Segal BL: New approaches to therapy of acute heart failure. Am Fam Phys 21(2):131-135, 1980

Sibbald WJ, Anderson RR, Holliday RL: Pathogenesis of pulmonary edema associated with the adult respiratory distress syndrome. Can Med Assoc J 120(4): 445-450, 1979

Sidd J: Congestive heart failure. Orth Clin N Am 9(3): 745-760, 1978

Snashall PD: Pulmonary edema. Brit J Dis Chest 74(2):2-22, 1980

Sochocky S: Pulmonary edema. Brit J Clin Prac 33(5):127, 1979

Spooner B, Cross BW, Hasko BA: Diverse implications of laboratory values in congestive heart failure. Crit Care Quart 2:37-45, 1979

Spragg R: Adult respiratory distress syndrome. Hosp Med 15, No. 3:31, 1979

An update of congestive heart failure in infants. Issues Comp Pediat Nurs 3:5-22, 1979

Weber KT, Janicki JS: The heart as a muscle-pump system and the concept of heart failure. Am Heart J 98(3): 371-384, 1979

18

Control of Respiratory Function

Respiration provides the body with a means for gas exchange. Although respiration also includes gas exchange at the cellular level (internal respiration), this chapter is mainly concerned with external respiration, or the exchange of gases between the internal and external environments. Respiration can be divided into three parts: (1) ventilation, (2) perfusion, or flow of blood in the pulmonary circulation, and (3) diffusion of gases between the alveoli and the blood in the pulmonary circulation. The discussion in this chapter focuses on the structure and function of the respiratory system as it relates to these three aspects of respiration. Included in the chapter is a discussion of breathing and cough which is needed for an understanding of the content in subsequent chapters. Blood gases are discussed in Chapter 20.

:Structure and Function of the Respiratory System

The respiratory system can be divided into two parts: the conducting airways and the respiratory tissues, where gas exchange takes place. The conducting portion of the respiratory tract consists of the nose, nasopharynx, larynx, trachea, bronchi, and bronchioles (Fig. 18-1). The true respiratory portion of the lung consists of the alveolar structures and the pulmonary capillaries.

The Conducting Airways

The conducting airways are lined with a pseudostratified ciliated columnar epithelium, which contains serous glands and mucus-secreting goblet cells (Fig. 18-2). The mucus produced by these cells forms a blanket-like layer, the *mucociliary blanket*, which protects the respiratory system and entraps dust and other foreign particles as they move through the conducting airways. Cilia, the hair-like projections lining the mucous membrane of the respiratory tract, which are in constant motion, move the mucous blanket with its entrapped particles conveyor-belt fashion toward the pharynx whence it is either expectorated or swallowed. Figure 18-2 shows the secreting goblet cells and the cilia that line the conducting airways.

Cigarette smoking tends to inhibit the cilia to the extent that the movement of the mucociliary blanket may be slowed down or stopped. This slowing allows the residue from tobacco smoke, dust, and other particles to accumulate in the lungs. There is also evidence that smoking causes hyperplasia of the goblet cells, which results in an increase in respiratory tract secretions. As is discussed in Chapter 19, these changes are thought to contribute to the development of chronic bronchitis and emphysema.

Nasal cavities

The nose is the preferred airway for entrance of air into the respiratory tract during normal breathing.

Figure 18–1. The respiratory system. (Chaffee EE, Lytle IM: Basic Physiology and Anatomy, 4th ed. Philadelphia, JB Lippincott, 1980)

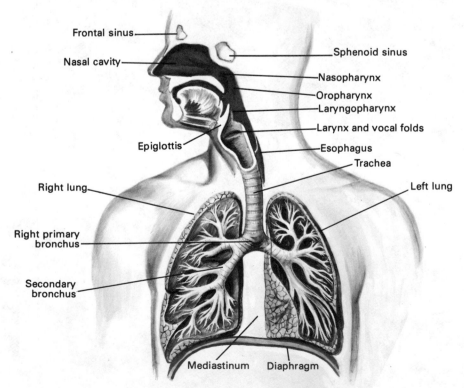

Frontal sinus
Nasal cavity
Sphenoid sinus
Nasopharynx
Oropharynx
Laryngopharynx
Larynx and vocal folds
Epiglottis
Esophagus
Trachea
Right lung
Left lung
Right primary bronchus
Secondary bronchus
Mediastinum   Diaphragm

As air passes through the nasal passages, it is filtered, warmed, and humidified. The outer part of the nasal passages is lined with coarse hair, which aids in filtering dust and large particles from the air. The upper portion of the nasal cavity is lined with mucous membrane supplied with a rich network of small blood vessels, and it is this portion of the nasal cavity that supplies the warmth and moisture to the air breathed.

The *relative humidity* is the percentage of water vapor in the air at a specific temperature in relation to the maximum capacity of the air at that same temperature. The capacity of the air to contain water vapor without condensation occurring increases as the temperature rises. The *air in the alveoli*, which is maintained at body temperature, is *completely satu-*

rated with water vapor (relative humidity 100 percent), and usually contains considerably more water than is present in the air breathed. The difference between the water vapor contained in the air breathed and that found in the alveoli is drawn from the moist surface of the mucous membranes that line the respiratory passages. Under normal conditions, the nasal mucosal surfaces produce about a pint of water per day in the process of humidifying the air breathed.[1] This amount is increased when a person breathes dry air or has a fever. During such periods, the respiratory secretions often become thick and the protective function of the mucociliary blanket may become impaired. This is particularly true of persons in whom water intake is inadequate. With mouth breathing or breathing through a tracheot-

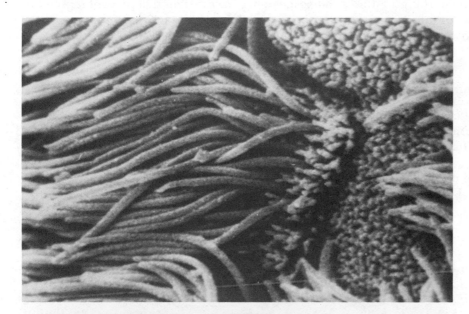

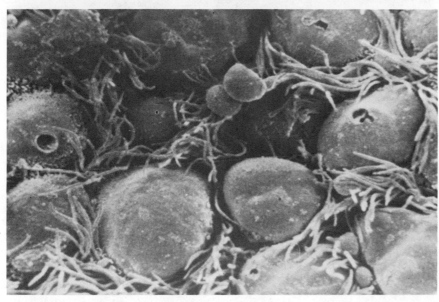

Figure 18–2. (Top) Scanning electron micrograph showing cilia (longer projections) which are in constant motion moving the mucociliary blanket upward in a conveyor-belt fashion toward the pharynx. The small flat clusters are the microvilli which transport fluid across the bronchial lining. (Bottom) Scanning electron micrograph of the small round goblet cells that secrete mucus. (Courtesy of Janice Nowell of the University of California, Santa Cruz, California)

omy (opening in the throat), air entering the lungs is not warmed, filtered, or humidified as it would be when breathing through the nose.

The mouth and the pharynx

The mouth serves as an alternative airway when the nasal passages are plugged or when there is need for exchange of large amounts of air, such as occurs during exercise. The pharynx is the only opening between the nasal and mouth openings and the lungs. Consequently, obstruction of the pharynx leads to immediate cessation of ventilation. Control of the tongue and pharyngeal muscles is impaired in coma and in certain types of neurologic diseases. In these conditions, the tongue tends to fall back into the pharynx and obstructs the airway, particularly if the person is lying on the back. Swelling of the pharyngeal structures due to injury or infection also predisposes a person to airway obstruction, as does the presence of a foreign body.

The larynx

The larynx connects the pharynx with the trachea. The epiglottis is a thin leaf-shaped structure that aids in covering the larynx during the act of swallowing to prevent food and fluids from entering the larynx. The walls of the larynx are supported by cartilaginous structures that prevent collapse during inspiration. The functions of the larynx can be divided into two categories: (1) those functions associated with speech, and (2) those associated with

protecting the lung by preventing the entrance of substances other than air. The larynx is located in a strategic position between the upper airways and the lungs, and is sometimes referred to as the "watchdog" of the lungs. When confronted with a substance other than air, the laryngeal muscles contract and close off the airway. At the same time, the cough reflex is initiated as a means of removing the foreign substance from the airway. Paralysis of the laryngeal muscles predisposes to aspiration of foreign materials into the lungs.

The tracheobronchial tree

The trachea, or windpipe, is a continuous tube that connects the larynx and the major bronchi of the lungs. The walls of the trachea are supported by horseshoe-shaped cartilages that prevent it from collapsing during inspiration, when the pressure in the thorax is negative.

The trachea divides to form the right and left *primary* bronchi, which enter the lung through a slit called the *hilus*. The point at which the trachea divides is called the *carina*. The carina is heavily innervated, and coughing and bronchospasm may result when this area is stimulated. The right primary bronchus is shorter and wider, and continues at a more vertical angle with the trachea than the left primary bronchus. This makes it easier for foreign bodies to enter the right main bronchus rather than the left.

Each primary bronchus divides into *secondary*

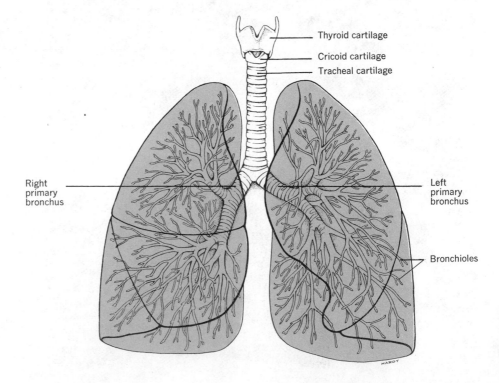

Figure 18–3.   Diagram of the larynx, trachea, and bronchial tree (anterior view). (Chaffee EE, Lytle IM: Basic Physiology and Anatomy, 4th ed. Philadelphia, JB Lippincott, 1980)

Thyroid cartilage

Cricoid cartilage

Tracheal cartilage

Right primary bronchus

Left primary bronchus

Bronchioles

bronchi, which supply each of the lobes of the lungs—*three in the right lung* and *two in the left* (Fig. 18-3). The bronchi continue to branch, forming *smaller bronchi*, until they become the *terminal bronchioles*, the smallest of the conducting airways. The structure of the primary bronchi is similar to that of the trachea in that both of these airways are supported by *cartilaginous rings*. As the bronchi become smaller, however, the cartilaginous support thins out until it disappears at the level of the bronchioles. Instead, the bronchioles are encircled with a *spiraling layer of smooth muscle fibers* (Fig. 18-4). Bronchospasm, or contraction, of these muscles causes narrowing of the bronchioles and impairs air flow. Bronchial smooth muscle is innervated by the autonomic nervous system. Stimulation of the *parasympathetic fibers*, derived from the *vagus*, results in *bronchoconstriction*. *Sympathetic stimulation*, on the other hand, causes *relaxation* of the bronchial smooth muscle.

The Respiratory Tissues

The lobules are the functional units of the lung where gas exchange takes place. Each lobule is supplied with structures that provide for both gas ex-

Figure 18–4.   Arrangement of smooth muscle fibers that surround the bronchioles.

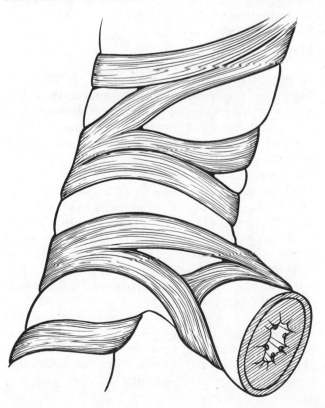

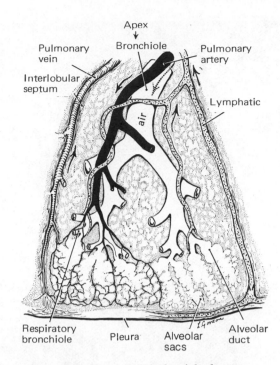

Figure 18–5.   Diagram of a lobule of the lung. (Chaffee EE, Lytle IM: Basic Physiology and Anatomy, 4th ed. Philadelphia, JB Lippincott, 1980)

change and circulation of blood (Fig. 18-5). The gas exchange structures consist of a bronchiole and the alveolar ducts and sacs. In circulation, blood enters the lobule through a pulmonary artery and then exits through a pulmonary vein. Lymphatic structures surround the lobule and aid in removal of plasma proteins and other particles from the interstitial spaces.

The alveolar sacs are cup-shaped, thin-walled structures separated from each other by thin alveolar septa. Most of the septa are occupied by a single network of capillaries, so that the blood is exposed to air on both sides. It has been estimated that there are about 300 million alveoli in an adult lung with a surface area of about 50 to 100 square meters.[2] Unlike the bronchioles, which are tubes with their own separate walls, the alveoli are interconnecting spaces that have no separate walls (Fig. 18-6). As a result of this arrangement, there is a continual mixing of air between the alveolar structures. Small discontinuities in the alveolar wall, the "pores of Kohn," probably contribute to the mixing of air under certain conditions.

The alveolar structures are composed of three types of cells—the type I alveolar cells, the type II alveolar cells, and the alveolar macrophages. The type I alveolar cells are flat squamous epithelial cells, across which gas exchange takes place. The alveolar macrophages are responsible for removal of offend-

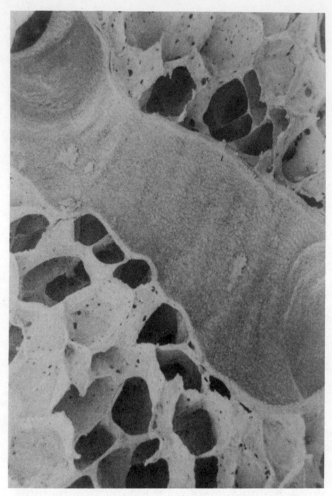

Figure 18–6.   A closeup of a cross section of a small bronchus and surrounding alveoli. (Courtesy of Janice A. Nowell of the University of California, Santa Cruz, California)

ing matter from the alveolar epithelium. Evidence is available suggesting that smoking impairs the function of the macrophages. The type II alveolar cells produce surfactant, a lipoprotein substance that decreases the surface tension within the alveoli. This action allows for greater ease of lung inflation and helps to prevent collapse of the smaller airways. Without surfactant, lung inflation would be extremely difficult, requiring intrapleural pressures as low as -20 to -30 mm Hg.[3] The intrapleural pressure during normal breathing ranges from about -4 to -12 mm Hg. Respiratory pressures are often expressed in cm H_2O, which can be converted to mm Hg by multiplying by 1.35. (The specific gravity of mercury is 13.546.)

The type II alveolar cells do not begin to mature until weeks 26 to 28 of gestation and, consequently, many premature babies are born with poorly func-

tioning type II alveolar cells and have difficulty producing sufficient amounts of surfactant. In these babies, the collapse of the lungs due to lack of surfactant is called respiratory distress syndrome (RDS), or hyaline membrane disease. The production of surfactant also requires adequate amounts of oxygen and blood flow for delivery of substrates such as fatty acids. Among infants predisposed to develop RDS are premature infants, infants of diabetic mothers, infants born by cesarean section (when performed prior to the 38th week of gestation), and those suffering from hypoxia, acidosis, and hypothermia.

When there is need to consider the early delivery of an infant, it is possible to obtain an estimate of the maturity of the type II alveolar cells by measuring the *lecithin* to *sphingomyelin* (L/S) ratio in the amniotic fluid through amniocentesis. In this way, it is often possible to delay the delivery of an infant until the type II alveolar cells are sufficiently mature to permit its survival. Under special circumstances, the administration of corticosteroid drugs to the mother may speed lung maturation in the fetus and thereby prevent RDS. There appears to be a lesser incidence of RDS among premature babies born through vaginal delivery compared with those born by cesarean section, and it has been speculated that the stress of vaginal delivery may increase the infant's corticosteroid levels.

Surfactant production is also impaired in adult respiratory distress syndrome (ARDS), or shock lung, discussed in Chapter 14.

Pleura

A thin, transparent, double-layered serous membrane lines the thoracic cavity and encases the lungs. The outer parietal layer lies adjacent to the wall of the chest, and the inner visceral layer adheres to the surface of the lung. There is a thin film of serous fluid separating the two pleural layers, and this allows the two layers to glide over each other and yet hold together, so there is no separation between the lungs and thorax. This adherence is similar to what occurs when a glassful of water is placed on a thin film of water that has been spilled on a table top. The pleural cavity is a potential space in which serous fluid or inflammatory exudate can accumulate. *Pleural effusion* is an abnormal collection of excess fluid or exudate in the pleural cavity.

During normal breathing, the pressure within the pleural cavity is always negative (-4 mm Hg when the alveolar spaces are open to the atmosphere, *i.e.*, between breaths when the mouth and glottis are open). Without this negative pressure, which holds the lungs against the chest wall, the elastic recoil properties of the lung would cause it to collapse. Collapse of the lung due to air in the pleural cavity is called *pneumothorax*.

Ventilation

There is nothing mystical about ventilation; it is purely a mechanical event that obeys the laws of physics as they relate to the behavior of gases. Some of these principles are summarized for the reader's review.

Atmospheric pressure
At sea level, the atmospheric pressure is 760 mm Hg, or 14.7 pounds per square inch. In measuring respiratory pressure, atmospheric pressure is assigned a value of zero. A pressure of +15 mm Hg means that the pressure is 15 mm Hg above atmospheric pressure, and a pressure of −15 mm Hg is 15 mm Hg less than atmospheric.

Pressure–volume relationship
Boyle's law states that the pressure of a gas will vary inversely with the volume of the container, provided the temperature is kept constant. This means that if equal amounts of a gas are placed into two containers, one with a smaller volume than the other, the pressure of the gas in the container with the smaller volume will be greater than the pressure of the gas in that with the larger volume. The movement of gases is always from an area of greater pressure to one of lesser pressure. In the example just given, if a connection were placed between the two containers, air would move from the smaller volume to the larger volume.

The law of partial pressures
The law of partial pressures states that the total pressure of a mixture of gases is equal to the sum of the partial pressures of the separate gases in the mixture. If the concentration of oxygen at 760 mm Hg is 20%, then its partial pressure is 152 mm Hg (760 × 0.20).

Water vapor pressure
The amount of water vapor that is contained in a gas mixture is determined by the temperature of the gas and is unrelated to atmospheric pressure. Air in the lungs is completely saturated (100% humidity) with water vapor. At a normal body temperature of 98.6°F., the pressure of water vapor in the lungs is 47 mm Hg. The water vapor pressure must be in-cluded in the sum of the total pressure of the gases in the alveoli (*i.e.*, the total pressure of other gases in the alveoli is 760 − 47 = 713 mm Hg).

Inspiration and Expiration

Ventilation is concerned with the movement of gases into and out of the lung. Ventilation is dependent upon a system of open airways and movement of the respiratory muscles—the diaphragm and the intercostals.

Inspiration
During inspiration, the diaphragm moves downward and the external intercostal muscles move outward so that both size and volume of the lungs are increased, thus causing the pressure within the airways of the lungs to decrease below that of atmospheric air. As a result, air moves into the lungs.

Expiration
During expiration, the elastic components of the chest wall and lung structures that were stretched in inspiration recoil passively, causing lung volume to decrease so that the pressure within the lungs is now greater than atmospheric (i.e., air then moves out of the lungs). Expiration is a passive event, contributing little to the work of breathing. Instead, energy is expended in the work of enlarging the chest during inspiration.

Lung Compliance

Lung compliance describes the ease with which the lungs can be inflated. Specifically, it refers to the change in lung volume that occurs with a given change in respiratory pressures.

$$\text{compliance} = \frac{\text{change in volume}}{\text{change in pressure}}$$

It takes less inspiratory effort, for example, to create the pressure needed to inflate a compliant lung than it does to inflate a stiff and noncompliant lung.

Respiratory Volumes

The amount of air that is inhaled and exhaled can be measured with a *spirometer* (Fig. 18-7). The bell of the spirometer moves down during inspiration and up during exhalation, causing the pen to move up and down and mark the chart paper. The tidal volume, about 500 ml, is the amount of air that moves into and out of the lungs during normal breathing. The maximum amount of air that can be inspired in

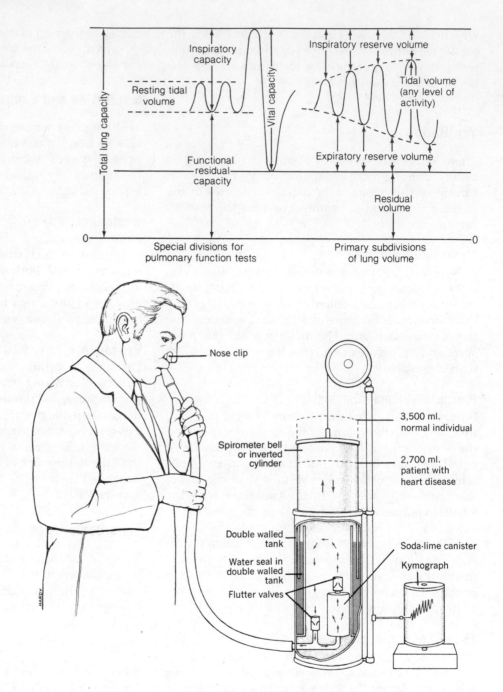

Figure 18–7. Measurement of vital capacity using a spirometer. (Chaffee EE, Lytle IM: Basic Physiology and Anatomy, 4th ed. Philadelphia, JB Lippincott, 1980)

excess of normal tidal volume is called the *inspiratory reserve* (about 3000 ml), and the maximum amount that can be exhaled in excess of the normal tidal volume is the *expiratory reserve* (1200 ml). The *vital capacity* is a measure of respiratory reserve, and is the amount of air that can be inhaled and forcibly exhaled in a single breath (usually about 4700 ml). There is always some air remaining in the lungs following forced expiration (1200 ml); this air is the *residual volume*. The residual volume tends to increase with age because there is more trapping of air in the lungs at the end of expiration.

The Efficiency and Work of Breathing

The *minute volume* is the amount of air that is exchanged in 1 minute; it is determined by the metabolic needs of the body. The minute volume is equal to the tidal volume multiplied by the respiratory rate, which is about 6000 ml (500 ml tidal volume × respiratory rate of 15 breaths per minute) during normal activity. The pattern of breathing—the tidal volume and the rate of breathing—is usually determined by the ease of lung expansion (compliance) and the effort needed to move air through the conducting airways. For example, *in persons with stiff and noncompliant lungs, expansion of the lungs is difficult*, and these persons usually find it easier to breathe if they keep their tidal volume low and breathe at a more rapid rate (*i.e.*, 300 × 20 = 6000 ml) to achieve their minute volume and meet their oxygen needs.

minute volume = tidal volume × respiratory rate

On the other hand, persons with *airway disease* usually find it less difficult to inflate the lungs, but *expend more energy in moving air through the airways*. As a result, these persons tend to take deeper breaths and to breathe at a slower rate (*i.e.*, 600 × 10 = 6000 ml) to achieve their oxygen needs.

Dead Air Space

Dead air space refers to the air that must be moved with each breath but *does not participate in gas exchange*. Movement of air through dead air space contributes to the work of breathing, but not to gas exchange. There are two types of dead air space: that contained in the *conducting airways (anatomic)*, and that contained in the *respiratory portion of the lung (physiologic dead space)*. The volume of airway dead space is fixed and is approximately 150 to 200 ml, depending on body size. It constitutes air contained in the nose, pharynx, trachea, bronchi, and so on. If the alveoli are ventilated but deprived of blood flow, they do not contribute to gas exchange and thus constitute alveolar, or physiologic, dead space. The total dead space is equal to the airway and alveolar dead air space. The effective minute volume is equal to the minute ventilation minus the physiologic dead air space. Creation of a tracheotomy decreases the dead space of the airways and can have the effect of decreasing the work of breathing.

Diffusion

Gas exchange takes place in the alveoli. Here gases *diffuse across the alveolar–capillary membrane, moving from an area of higher concentration to one of lower concentration*. Oxygen moves from the alveoli into the capillary, and carbon dioxide moves from the capillary network into the alveoli. There is rapid equilibration between the gases in the alveoli and those in the blood, so that the partial pressure of the blood gas at the venous end of the pulmonary capillary is approximately the same as that in the alveoli. Because of its greater solubility, the diffusion of carbon dioxide across the respiratory membrane is 20 times more rapid than that of oxygen.

The diffusion of gases in the lung is influenced by four factors: (1) the surface area available for diffusion, (2) the thickness of the alveolar–capillary membrane through which the gases diffuse, (3) the difference between the partial pressure of the gas on either side of the membrane, and (4) the characteristics of the gas. Diseases that destroy lung tissue or increase the thickness of the alveolar–capillary membrane influence the diffusing capacity of the lung. Removal of one lung, for example, reduces the diffusing surface by one-half. The thickness of the alveolar capillary membrane and the distance for diffusion are increased in pulmonary edema and pneumonia. Administration of high concentrations of oxygen increases the pressure difference between the two sides of the alveolar–capillary membrane and increases the diffusion of the gas. The characteristics of the gas and its molecular weight and solubility determine how rapidly it diffuses through the respiratory membranes. Carbon dioxide diffuses 20 times more rapidly than oxygen, because of its greater solubility in the respiratory membranes.

Blood Flow

The lungs have a dual blood supply, the bronchial and the pulmonary circulations. The *pulmonary circulation* provides for the *gas exchange function* of the lungs, while the *bronchial circulation* provides the *lung with blood to meet its nutritional needs*.

The *bronchial arteries* arise from the thoracic aorta and enter the lungs with the major bronchi, dividing and subdividing along with the bronchial tubes as it supplies them and the other lung structures with oxygen. The capillaries of the bronchial circulation drain into the *bronchial veins*, the larger of which empties into the vena cava and returns blood to the right heart. The smaller of the bronchial veins empties into the pulmonary veins. This blood is unoxygenated, since the bronchial circulation does not participate in gas exchange. As a result, this blood dilutes the oxygenated blood returning to the left heart from the lungs and reduces the saturation of hemoglobin so that it is less than 100% saturated as it leaves the left heart and moves into the systemic circulation.

The function of the *pulmonary circulation* is to *facilitate gas exchange*. In order to accomplish this, there must be a continuous flow of blood through the respiratory portion of the lungs. Unoxygenated blood enters the lung through the pulmonary artery, which has its origin in the right heart and enters the lung at the hilus, along with the primary bronchus. The pulmonary arteries branch in a manner similar

Normal

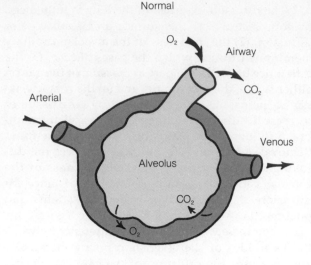

Perfusion without ventilation

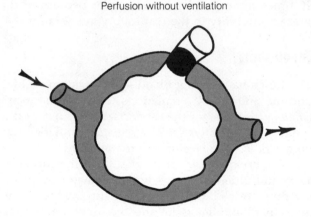

Ventilation without perfusion

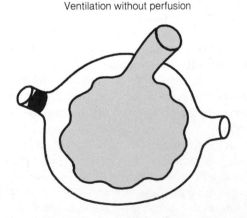

Figure 18–8. Diagram showing matching of ventilation and perfusion.

to that of the airways. The small pulmonary arteries accompany the bronchi as they move down the lobules and branch to supply the capillary network that surrounds the alveoli (see Fig. 18-5).

The meshwork of capillaries in the respiratory portion of the lung is so dense that the flow in these vessels is often described as being similar to a sheet of flowing blood. The oxygenated capillary blood is collected in the small pulmonary veins of the lobules, and from there it moves to the larger veins, to be collected finally in the four large pulmonary veins that empty into the left atrium.

The pulmonary vessels are thinner and more compliant than those in the systemic circulation, and the pressures in the pulmonary system are much lower (22/8 mm Hg vs 120/70 mm Hg). The low-pressure, low-resistance characteristics of this system serve to accommodate the delivery of varying amounts of blood from the systemic circulation without producing signs and symptoms of congestion. The movement of blood through the pulmonary capillary bed requires that the mean pulmonary arterial pressure be greater than the mean pulmonary venous pressure. Pulmonary venous pressure increases in left-sided heart failure, and this causes pressure in the capillary network to increase, with the result that there is transudation of capillary fluid into the alveoli. Acute pulmonary edema is discussed in Chapter 17.

Ventilation–Perfusion Relationships

The gas exchange properties of the lung are dependent upon the matching of ventilation and perfusion, so that there are equal amounts of air and blood entering the respiratory portion of the lungs. Two factors may interfere with the matching of ventilation and perfusion—hypoventilation and "shunt." Shunt refers to blood that moves from the venous to the arterial system without going through the ventilated portion of the lung. Intracardiac shunting of blood due to congenital heart defects is discussed in Chapter 16. Respiratory shunting of blood usually results from destructive lung disease, which impairs ventilation, or from heart failure in which there is interference with the movement of blood through sections of the lungs.

There are many causes of mismatched ventilation and perfusion, of which the most obvious are illustrated in Figure 18-8. Diagram A illustrates the desired ventilation and perfusion pattern in which there is normal ventilation of the alveoli and normal blood flow through the pulmonary capillary that surrounds it. Diagram B illustrates a situation of hypoventilation in which perfusion is normal while there is lack of ventilation due to airway obstruction. This is the type of situation that occurs in atelectasis (Chap. 19). In diagram C ventilation is normal, but there is obstruction of the pulmonary artery supplying the lobule. An example of this situation is pulmonary embolism. Most of the situations in which there is mismatching of ventilation and perfusion are less obvious. In lung disease, for example, there may be altered ventilation in one area of the lung and altered perfusion in another area.

Control of Respiration

Unlike the heart, which has inherent rhythmic properties and can beat independently of the nervous system, the movement of the muscles controlling respiration requires continuous input from the nervous system. Movement of the diaphragm, the intercostal muscles, the sternocleidomastoid and other accessory muscles controlling respiration is integrated by neurons in the respiratory center, located in the brain stem. One group of these neurons controls inspiration, and this section of the respiratory center is designated the inspiratory center. Another group, located in the expiratory portion, is responsible for the control of expiration. The cycling of impulses between the inspiratory and expiratory portions of the respiratory center provides for the regular pattern of breathing.

Activity of the respiratory center is regulated by input from other neural centers and by blood gases and blood pH. The influence of higher brain centers on the control of respiration is evidenced by the fact that one can consciously adjust the depth and rate of respiration. Fever, pain, and anxiety exert their influence through lower levels of brain function. The need for changes in respiration varies with metabolism. Tissue needs for oxygen delivery and removal of carbon dioxide are monitored by chemoreceptors that respond to changes in these blood gases and pH.

The most important chemoreceptors for monitoring changes in *carbon dioxide are located in the medulla*, near the respiratory center. These receptors are bathed in cerebral spinal fluid. Carbon dioxide diffuses from the blood into the cerebral spinal fluid; in the process, it combines with water to form carbonic acid, which dissociates to form *hydrogen ions*, and these have a *direct stimulating effect on the chemoreceptors*. Thus, the carbon dioxide content in the blood regulates ventilation through its effect on the pH of the cerebral spinal fluid. These chemoreceptors are extremely sensitive to *short-term changes* in carbon dioxide. The effect of an increase in carbon dioxide on ventilation reaches its peak within a minute or so and then declines within the next few hours to a day if the carbon dioxide level of the blood remains elevated. With *long-term elevations in carbon dioxide*, there occurs a *compensatory increase in the bicarbonate level* of the cerebral spinal fluid, which acts as a buffer for the hydrogen ions. Thus, *persons with chronically elevated levels of carbon dioxide no longer respond to this stimulus for increased ventilation*, but rely on the *stimulus provided by a decrease in blood oxygen*.

Arterial oxygen levels are monitored by *peripheral chemoreceptors* located in the *carotid and aortic bodies*. Although these chemoreceptors also monitor carbon dioxide, they play a much more important role in monitoring arterial blood oxygen levels. These receptors exert little control over ventilation until the PaO_2 has dropped to below 60 mm Hg. Hypoxia is the main stimulus for ventilation in persons with chronic hypercarbia. If these persons are given oxygen therapy at a level sufficient to increase the PaO_2 above that needed to stimulate the peripheral chemoreceptors, their ventilation may become severely depressed.

Breathing

The act of breathing is normally effortless and does not require conscious thought. In an adult, the normal rate of respiration is about 16 to 18 per minute, with about one breath for every four heart beats. This rate increases with exercise and other activities that increase body metabolism. In normal breathing, expiration is largely passive and is accomplished within 4 to 6 seconds.

Respiratory movements are normally smooth, with equal expansion of both sides of the chest. In men, respiratory movements tend to be primarily diaphragmatic, whereas in women, there tends to be greater movement of the intercostal muscles. When breathing becomes labored, the accessory muscles of the neck come into play, and there may be flaring of the nares.

The suffix *pnea* denotes a relationship to breathing. *Tachypnea* is rapid breathing, and *hyperpnea* is an increase in both the rate and depth of respiration (Fig. 18-9). Hyperpnea is normal during exercise. *Bradypnea* is an abnormally slow respiratory rate. *Hyperventilation* is ventilation in excess of

Normal

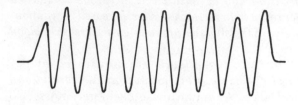

Bradypnea

Tachypnea

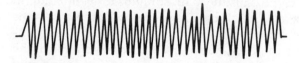

Hyperventilation

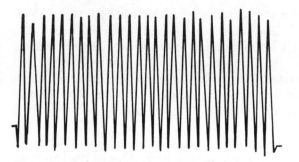

Periodic

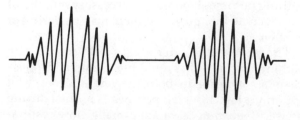

Figure 18–9.   Diagram of breathing patterns.

that needed to maintain a normal level of arterial PCO_2. Hyperventilation causes a decrease in PCO_2 and tends to lead to respiratory alkalosis (Chap. 23).

Breath Sounds

The sound produced as air moves through the airways during respiration can be heard with a stethoscope and is called breath sounds. *Vesicular breath sounds* result from air moving through the bronchioles and the alveoli. Normally these sounds are heard over most of the lung area. Breath sounds are absent when an area of the lung is not inflated during respiration, as occurs in pneumothorax and in atelectasis. Breath sounds are decreased in emphysema because of decreased air velocity and sound conduction due to air trapping. *Rales* and *rhonchi* are abnormal sounds that result from passage of air through secretions in the lung or passage of air moving through narrowed air passages. The reader is referred to a text on physical assessment for a complete description of breath sounds and respiratory assessment measures.

Periodic Breathing

Periodic breathing describes a breathing pattern in which there are episodes of apnea, or absence of breathing. *Cheyne–Stokes breathing* is a type of periodic breathing characterized by periods of slowly waxing and waning respirations, separated by a period of apnea that lasts up to 30 seconds (see Fig. 18-9). Cheyne–Stokes breathing is thought to be caused by impaired function of central feedback mechanisms which buffer the respiratory center's response to carbon dioxide. In order for Cheyne–Stokes respirations to occur, the hyperpneic and apneic phases of the breathing pattern must be long enough for sufficient changes in the carbon dioxide content of the blood to occur. During the hyperpneic phase of Cheyne–Stokes breathing, carbon dioxide levels fall, leading to a decreased stimulus for ventilation and finally to apnea. The period of apnea, in turn, causes the carbon dioxide content of the blood to accumulate, and this leads to the hyperpneic phase of the respiratory pattern. There are two types of disease conditions that cause predisposition to Cheyne–Stokes breathing. One is congestive heart failure, in which there is a great delay in moving blood with its altered carbon dioxide content from the lungs to the chemoreceptors in the brain that control ventilation. The other is impaired function of the brain centers regulating the feedback mechanisms that control respiration; that is, Cheyne–Stokes respirations may be seen in persons who have brain lesions that affect the area of the brain stem controlling the feedback gain of the respiratory center in response to changes in carbon dioxide level. This type of breathing is also seen in healthy individuals at high altitudes, especially during sleep.

Dyspnea

Dyspnea is a *subjective sensation of difficulty in breathing*, and seems to be related to the *work or effort of breathing*. Although dyspnea is often associated with respiratory or heart disease, its presence does not necessarily imply pathology; dyspnea occurs normally during exercise, particularly in untrained individuals. It also has an emotional component. Like other subjective symptoms, such as fatigue and pain, dyspnea is difficult to quantify because it relies on a person's perception of the problem. In an assessment of dyspnea, at times it is useful to observe the number of words that a person can utter between breaths. A person who is not having trouble breathing can often utter a full sentence or more before taking another breath. On the other hand, someone who is having great difficulty in breathing will often find it necessary to take a breath after every few words. Exertional dyspnea occurs with exercise and with an increase in activity. Dyspnea should not be confused with tachypnea, hyperpnea, or hyperventilation.

Dyspnea can be either inspiratory or expiratory. *Inspiratory dyspnea* occurs primarily when there is *obstruction of the trachea or large airways*, such as occurs in the presence of a foreign body, tumor, or infection of the large airways. Inspiratory dyspnea is often accompanied by a low-pitched crowing sound, called *stridor*, and *retraction of the chest structures*. Airflow into the chest is decreased with airway obstruction, even though the inspiratory effort and negative pressure in the chest is increased, resulting in retraction of the intercostal spaces. In infants and small children, there is often retraction of the entire sternum as well as the intercostal spaces. *Expiratory dyspnea* is primarily associated with *obstruction of the bronchioles and smaller bronchi*. *Expiratory dyspnea* causes *prolongation of the expiratory phase of respiration*, and this phase may be accompanied by a *wheezing* or whistling sound and bulging of the intercostal spaces due to air trapping.

Cough

The cough reflex protects the lung from accumulation of secretions and from entry of irritating and destructive substances; it is one of the primary defense mechanisms of the respiratory tract.

The cough reflex is initiated by receptors located in the tracheobronchial wall; they are extremely sensitive to irritating substances and to the presence of excess secretions. Afferent impulses from these receptors are transmitted through the vagus to the medullary center, which integrates the cough response.

Cough itself requires the rapid inspiration of a large volume of air (usually about 2.5 liters), followed by rapid closure of the glottis. This is followed by forceful contraction of the abdominal and expiratory muscles. As these muscles contract, there is a marked elevation of intrathoracic pressures to levels of 100 mm Hg or more. The rapid opening of the glottis, at this point, leads to an explosive expulsion of air.

There are many conditions that may interfere with the cough reflex and its protective function. The reflex is impaired in persons with *weakness of the abdominal or expiratory muscles*. This can be caused by disease conditions that lead to muscle weakness or paralysis, or by prolonged inactivity, or may be an outcome of surgery involving these muscles. Bedrest interferes with expansion of the chest and limits the amount of air that can be taken into the lungs in preparation for coughing, so the cough is weak and ineffective. Disease conditions that *prevent effective closure of the glottis and laryngeal muscles* interfere with accomplishment of the marked increase in intrathoracic pressure that is needed for effective coughing. The presence of a nasogastric tube, for example, may prevent closure of the upper airway structures. The presence of such a tube may also fatigue the receptors for the cough reflex that are located in the area. Lastly, the cough reflex is impaired when there is *depressed function of the medullary centers* in the brain which integrate the cough reflex. Interruption of the central integration aspect of the cough reflex can arise as the result of diseases of this part of the brain or the action of drugs that depress the cough center.

Although the cough reflex is basically a protective mechanism, frequent and prolonged coughing can be exhausting and painful, and can exert undesirable effects on the cardiovascular system and the elastic tissues of the lungs. This is particularly true in young children and the elderly.

Methods of cough relief fall into three categories. The *first is correction of the underlying cause*. When this fails or cannot be accomplished immediately, a *second method, administration of a drug with a cough suppressant action*, may be initiated, so long as the agent does not disrupt elimination of tracheobronchial secretions. The *third method relies on the use of expectorant drugs (or procedures)*, to increase the quantity of bronchial secretions or to liquefy them; this facilitates removal of secretions from the respiratory system and hence diminishes the need to cough. Table 18-1 lists various cough preparations and summarizes their mechanism of action.

Cough Suppressants (Antitussive Drugs)

Narcotics such as morphine, hydromorphone, and levorphanol cause *potent suppression of the cough reflex at the level of the medullary cough center*. These drugs also inhibit the *ciliary action of the respiratory mucous membrane, and depress respiration*. Therefore, persons receiving these drugs for control of pain need to be observed for development of respiratory complications, which can arise from depression of respiration and impairment of the cough reflex and respiratory defense mechanisms.

The *narcotics codeine and hydrocodone* also act as cough suppressants, but have fewer side effects and are therefore sometimes used as *antitussive drugs*. Some of the newer *non-narcotic agents such as dextromethorphan* are *effective in suppressing the cough* without creating drug dependence or other undesirable effects. It is these centrally acting non-narcotic antitussive drugs that are usually contained in the over-the-counter preparations.

Another group of drugs *act peripherally* to reduce stimulation of the afferent receptors of the cough reflex. One of these, benzonatate (Tessalon), is believed to have a local anesthetic effect. Another group of locally acting agents are the demulcents, such as glycerin and honey, which act by coating the irritated pharyngeal structures. Many cough syrups and lozenges contain a demulcent.

Expectorants

Expectorants are drugs or substances that increase the secretion of mucus in the bronchi and reduce its viscosity, making it easier to move the secretions toward the mouth, so they can be disposed of.

Water is probably one of the most effective and is certainly one of the best of the expectorants. In addition to its use to increase hydration, water is

Table 18-1 Medications Used in the Treatment of Cough

Classification of Preparations	Mechanism of Action
Antitussive Drugs	

Narcotics
  Codeine
  Hydrocodone
	Act centrally on the medullary cough center to suppress the cough

Non-narcotic Dextromethorphan	Acts centrally on the medullary cough center to suppress the cough
Antihistamine Diphenhydramine	Acts centrally on the cough center
Peripherally and centrally acting antitussive Benzonatate	Local anesthetic that acts peripherally on the stretch receptors in the lung and centrally to suppress the cough reflex

Peripherally acting demulcents
  Honey
  Glycerin
	Coat the irritated mucosal surface of the pharynx

Expectorants	

Gastric reflex stimulants
  Potassium iodide
  Syrup of ipecac
  Guaifenesin
  Ammonium chloride
	Increase the production of respiratory tract secretions by causing gastric irritation, which stimulates the gastric reflex

Bronchial secretory cell stimulant Elixir terpin hydrate	Acts on bronchial secretory glands to stimulate increased production of respiratory tract secretions
Mucolytic agent Acetylcysteine (Mucomyst)	Reduces the viscosity of mucus by depolymerizing (breaking down) mucopolysaccharides in mucus

also effective in the form of inhaled steam or moisture.

A number of expectorants are believed to act reflexly by causing gastric irritation, which in turn stimulates respiratory tract secretion. The reader is undoubtedly familiar with the increase in salivation and respiratory tract secretions that accompanies nausea and vomiting. Among the expectorants that act by causing gastric irritation are potassium iodide, ammonium chloride, syrup of ipecac, glyceryl guaiacolate (guaifenesin) (Table 18-1). Potassium iodide preparations leave a brassy taste in the mouth and lead to unpleasant hypersecretion from the eyes, nose, and mouth. It can also cause painful swelling of the parotid gland and an acneiform skin rash. Iodine preparations influence thyroid function and persons who use these medications over long periods may have changes in thyroid function. *Syrup of ipecac* is nauseating, and is a useful emetic in small children. It is included, in dilute forms, in some cough preparations. Glyceryl guaiacolate (guaifenesin) is incorporated into many over-the-counter cough medications, although its effectiveness as an expectorant is controversial. *Elixir of terpin hydrate* is thought to have a direct stimulatory effect on the bronchial secreting cells and is often combined with codeine in cough syrups. The mucolytic agent acetylcysteine is administered to liquefy the viscid mucus seen in cystic fibrosis.

Sputum

Sputum consists of respiratory secretions that are ejected from the mouth during coughing and expectoration. A cough is said to be productive or nonproductive, depending on the amount of sputum produced.

Sputum contains mucus produced by the epithelial cells that line the respiratory tract as well as any debris that has been inhaled. The normal adult produces about 100 ml of sputum per day, most of which is swallowed as it is propelled into the pharynx by the action of the mucociliary blanket. With infection of the respiratory tract, the sputum often contains infecting organisms and inflammatory debris, and becomes purulent. The color of the sputum is an important sign. Yellow sputum, for example, indicates infection. The presence of verdoperoxidase, liberated from the polymorphonuclear cells in the sputum, causes stagnant pus to turn green. Patients with lower respiratory tract infections may report having a green sputum upon arising in the morning, which turns yellow as the day progresses.

Pulmonary edema often causes exudation of red blood cells into the alveoli, thus producing frothy blood-tinged sputum. The coughing up of blood-tinged sputum is called hemoptysis.

In summary, the function of the respiratory system is to oxygenate the blood and to remove carbon dioxide from the blood. Respiration consists of ventilation, diffusion of oxygen and carbon dioxide across the alveolar–capillary membrane, and movement of blood through the respiratory portion of the lungs. For effective gas exchange to occur, ventilation and perfusion must be matched. The conducting airways of the respiratory tract are lined with a mucociliary blanket that protects the underlying respiratory structures and removes irritating substances from the lungs. The cough reflex is a protective mechanism to prevent accumulation of secretions in the lungs and to protect the respiratory tract from irritating substances.

:Study Guide

After you have studied this chapter, you should be able to meet the following objectives:

: : Describe the function of the mucociliary blanket.

: : Explain why nasal breathing is preferable to mouth breathing.

: : Trace the physiology of the mouth and pharynx, the larynx, and the tracheobronchial tree.

: : State the function of the three types of alveolar cells.

: : Relate Boyle's law to a clinical situation.

: : State the law of partial pressures.

: : Trace the sequence of events in inspiration and in expiration.

: : State the formula for determining lung compliance.

: : Define the terms *inspiratory reserve, expiratory reserve, vital capacity,* and *residual volume.*

: : State the formula for measuring minute volume.

: : Explain the use of the phrase *dead air space.*

: : Trace the exchange of gases in the alveoli.

: : Describe the role of the pulmonary circulation in gas exchange.

: : Explain why ventilation and perfusion must be matched.

: : Describe the physiology of respiration.

: :   Define four terms that denote alterations of normal breathing.

: :   Describe the type of periodic breathing known as Cheyne–Stokes breathing.

: :   Compare the conditions that give rise to inspiratory dyspnea with those that give rise to expiratory dyspnea.

: :   State the purpose of the cough reflex.

: :   Compare the physiologic basis for the use of cough suppressants with that for the use of expectorants.

:References

1. Ham AW: Histology ed. 7, Philadelphia: JB Lippincott Company, 1974, p 719
2. West JB: Respiratory Physiology. Baltimore, Williams and Wilkins, 1974, p 10
3. Guyton A: Textbook of Medical Physiology, ed 6. Philadelphia: WB Saunders, 1981, p 477

19

Alterations in Respiratory Function

Respiratory illnesses are one of the more common reasons for visits to physicians, for admission to hospital, and for forced inactivity among all age groups. Forty-seven million Americans—children and adults—suffer from one or more chronic respiratory diseases. Over 30,000 children under 5 years of age die each year of respiratory disease, more than 15,000 in the first year of life.[1] For purposes of discussion, respiratory diseases included in this chapter have been divided into four sections: (1) respiratory infections, (2) impaired expansion of the lungs, (3) chronic obstructive lung disease, and (4) cancer of the lung.

:Respiratory Infections

Respiratory infections are the leading cause of disability in the United States. The respiratory tract is susceptible to infectious processes caused by many types of microorganisms. For the most part, the signs and symptoms of respiratory tract infections depend on the function of structures involved, the severity of the infectious process, and the person's age and general health. This section discusses acute respiratory infections in children, pneumonias, and tuberculosis.

Acute Respiratory Infections in Children

In children, respiratory tract infections are frequent, and although they are troublesome, they are usually not serious. Frequent infections occur because in infants and small children the immune system has not been exposed to many common pathogens; consequently, they tend to develop infections with each new exposure. Although most such infections are not serious, the small size of an infant or child's airways tends to promote impaired airflow and obstruction. For example, an infection that causes only sore throat and hoarseness in an adult may result in serious airway obstruction in a small child.

Upper airway infections in childhood

Obstruction of the upper airways secondary to infection tends to exert its greatest effect during the inspiratory phase of respiration. Movement of air through an obstructed upper airway, particularly the vocal cords in the larynx, tends to produce a crowing sound called *stridor*. There can also be impairment of the expiratory phase of respiration; this causes a *wheezing* (whistling) sound as air moves through the obstructed area. With mild to moderate obstruction, inspiratory stridor is more prominent and expiratory wheezing is less noticeable because the airways tend to dilate with expiration. When the swelling and obstruction become severe, the airways can no longer dilate during expiration, and then there is both stridor and wheezing.

Cartilaginous support of the trachea and the larynx is poorly developed in infants and small children. As a result, these structures are soft and tend to collapse when a child cries and the inspiratory pressures become more negative. When this happens both the stridor and inspiratory effort are increased. The phenomenon of airway collapse in the small child is analogous to what happens when a thick beverage, such as a milkshake, is drunk through a soft paper straw. The straw will collapse when the negative pressure produced by the sucking effort exceeds the flow of liquid through the straw.

The marked decrease in intrathoracic pressure resulting from increased inspiratory effort in the presence of airway obstruction also tends to cause retraction (sucking in) of the softer chest structures, such as the supraclavicular spaces, the sternum, the epigastrium, and the intercostal spaces. The increased inspiratory effort also causes flaring of the nares.

There are two upper respiratory tract infections of early childhood that are serious—croup and epiglottitis. Croup is the more common one, and it is usually benign and self-limiting. Epiglottitis, on the other hand, is rapidly progressive and life-threatening. The characteristics of both infections are described in Table 19-1.

Croup. Croup is a *syndrome* characterized by an inspiratory stridor, hoarseness, and a barking cough. The British use the term *croup* to describe the cry of a crow or raven, and this is undoubtedly how the term originated. Croup is generally seen in children aged 3 months to 3 years and is usually of viral origin. The most common cause is an acute laryngotracheobronchitis, although acute laryngitis or laryngotracheitis may be implicated. One form of croup, spasmotic croup, characteristically occurs at night. The episode usually lasts for several hours, and may recur several nights in a row. Spasmotic croup tends to recur with subsequent respiratory infections.

Although the respiratory manifestations of croup often appear suddenly, they are usually preceded by upper respiratory infections which cause rhinorrhea (running nose), coryza (common cold), hoarseness, and a low-grade fever. The symptoms usually subside when the child is exposed to moist air. For example, letting the bathroom shower run

Table 19-1   Characteristics of Epiglottitis, Croup, and Bronchiolitis in Small Children

Characteristics	Epiglottitis	Croup	Bronchiolitis
Common causative agent	*Hemophilus influenzae,* type B bacterium	Parainfluenza virus	Respiratory syncytial virus
Most commonly affected age group	1 to 5 years	3 months to 3 years	Less than 18 months (most severe in infants under 6 months)
Onset and preceding history	Sudden onset	Usually follows symptoms of a cold	Preceded by stuffy nose and other signs
Prominent features	Child appears very sick and toxic	Stridor and a wet, barking cough	Breathlessness, rapid shallow breathing, wheezing, cough, and retractions of lower ribs and sternum during inspiration
	Sits with mouth open and chin thrust forward	Usually occurs at night	
	Stridor, difficulty swallowing, drooling, anxiety	Relieved by exposure to cold or moist air	
	Danger of airway obstruction and asphyxia		
Usual treatment	Intubation or tracheotomy	Mist tent or vaporizor	Supportive treatment and administration of oxygen
	Treatment with appropriate antibiotic		

and then taking the child into the bathroom often brings prompt and dramatic relief of symptoms. A mist tent or vaporizer is used for more continuous treatment. Exposure to cold air also seems to relieve the airway spasm; often, the severe symptoms will be relieved simply because the child is exposed to cold air on the way to the hospital emergency room.

Other treatments may be required when a mist tent is ineffective. One method is to administer a racemic mixture of epinephrine (L-epinephrine and D-epinephrine) by positive pressure breathing through a face mask. A second method involves administration of the anti-inflammatory adrenal corticosteroid hormones. Establishment of an artificial airway may become necessary in severe airway obstruction.

Epiglottitis.   Acute epiglottitis is caused by *Hemophilus influenzae,* type B bacterium. It is characterized by inflammatory edema of the supraglottic area, which includes the epiglottis and pharyngeal structures. It comes on suddenly, bringing danger of airway obstruction and asphyxia, and the child requires immediate hospitalization.

The child assumes a distinctive position—sitting up with the mouth open and the chin thrust forward. There is difficulty swallowing, a muffled voice, drooling, fever, and extreme anxiety.

The child usually needs immediate establishment of an airway, by either endotracheal tube or tracheotomy. If epiglottitis is suspected, the child should never be forced to lie down as this causes the epiglottis to fall backward and may lead to complete airway obstruction. Examination of the throat with a tongue blade or other instrument may cause fatal airway obstruction and should be done only by medical personnel experienced in intubation of small children. It is also unwise to attempt any procedure, such as drawing blood, that would heighten the child's anxiety because this, too, could precipitate airway spasm and cause death.

Recovery from epiglottitis is usually rapid and uneventful once an adequate airway has been established and appropriate antibiotic therapy has been initiated.

Lower airway infections in childhood

Lower airway obstruction produces air trapping with prolonged expiration. Wheezing results from bronchospasm, mucosal inflammation, and edema. The child presents with increased expiratory effort, increased respiratory rate, and wheezing. If the infection is severe, there will also be marked intercostal retractions and signs of impending respiratory failure.

Bronchiolitis.   Bronchiolitis is usually of viral origin. It is seen in toddlers under 18 months of age, with most serious cases occurring in babies under 6 months of age. They have a characteristic appearance—rapid respirations, wheezing, breathlessness, distressing cough, and retractions of the lower ribs and sternum. Treatment is supportive and usually includes oxygen administration.

Signs of Impending Respiratory Failure in Childhood

Respiratory problems of infants and small children are often of sudden origin, and recovery is usually rapid and complete. However, children are at risk for development of airway obstruction and respiratory failure due to obstructive disorders or lung infection. The child with epiglottitis is at risk for development of airway obstruction; the child with bronchiolitis, for development of respiratory failure due to impaired gas exchange. The signs and symptoms of impending respiratory failure are described in Table 19-2. Although respiratory failure is discussed in greater detail in Chapter 20, it seems appropriate to focus in this part of the text on its occurrence in small children.

Pneumonias

The term *pneumonia* describes inflammation of parenchymal structures of the lung, such as the alveoli and the bronchioles. Etiologic agents include both infections and noninfectious agents. For example,

Figure 19–1.   Diagram showing the distribution of lung involvement in lobar and bronchopneumonia.

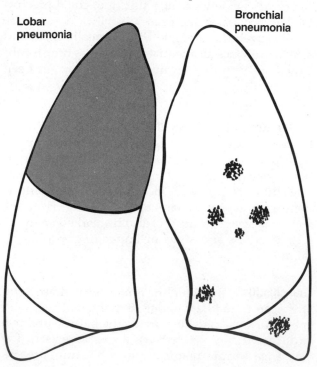

Lobar pneumonia

Bronchial pneumonia

Table 19-2   Signs of Respiratory Distress and Impending Respiratory Failure in the Infant and Small Child

Cyanosis that is not relieved by administration of oxygen (40%)
Heart rate of 150 per minute or greater and increasing
Bradycardia
Very rapid breathing (rate 60 per minute in the newborn to 6 months, or above 30 in children 6 months to 2 years)
Very depressed breathing (rate 20 per minute or below)
Retractions of the supraclavicular area, sternum, epigastrium, and intercostal spaces
Extreme anxiety and agitation
Fatigue
Decreased level of consciousness

inhalation of irritating fumes or aspiration of gastric contents can result in severe pneumonia.

Pneumonias are usually classified according to their etiologic agent and their anatomic distribution. The anatomic distribution can be considered under three general headings: (1) lobar, (2) bronchopneumonia, and (3) interstitial. In lobar pneumonia, there is involvement of a large portion or an entire lobe of a lung (Fig. 19-1). With bronchopneumonia, there is a patchy consolidation with involvement of multiple lobules. These lesions vary in size from 3 to 4 cm and, because of gravity, are more common in the lower and posterior portions of the lung. In interstitial pneumonia, the inflammatory process is more or less confined to the area within the wall that surrounds the alveoli and bronchioles. This type of pneumonia is generally caused by viral or mycoplasma infections.

Although antibiotics have significantly reduced mortality from the pneumonias, these diseases remain an important immediate cause of death in the elderly and in persons with debilitating diseases. In 1979 pneumonia was the sixth leading cause of death in the United States.[2]

The normal lung is sterile. Most of the agents that cause pneumonia are inhaled into the lung in air breathed. Depending upon the population being examined, pneumococci have been shown to be present in the nasopharynx in 5 to 59% of healthy persons;[3] normally, respiratory tract defense mechanisms would prevent these organisms from entering the lung. Loss of the cough reflex, damage to the ciliated endothelium that lines the respiratory tract, and lowered resistance to infection all increase susceptibility to pneumonia. Persons with immunologic deficiencies, congestive heart failure, or hypostatic pulmonary edema are particularly prone to develop pneumonia. Table 19-3 summarizes re-

Table 19-3 Respiratory Defense Mechanisms and Conditions That Impair Their Effectiveness

Defense Mechanism	Function	Factors That Impair Effectiveness
Nasopharyngeal defenses	Removes particles from the air; contact with surface lysosomes and immunoglobulins (IgA) protects against infection	IgA deficiency state, hayfever, "cold," trauma to the nose, others
Glottic and cough reflex	Protects against aspiration into tracheobronchial tree	Loss of cough reflex due to stroke or neural lesion; neuromuscular disease; abdominal or chest surgery; depression of the cough reflex due to sedation or anesthesia; presence of a nasogastric tube (tends to cause adaptation of afferent receptors)
Mucociliary blanket	Removes particles from the respiratory tract	Smoking; viral diseases; chilling; inhalation of irritating gases
Pulmonary macrophages	Remove microorganisms and foreign particles from the lung	Chilling; alcohol intoxication; tobacco; anoxia

spiratory tract defense mechanisms and factors that impair their effectiveness and thereby are predisposing factors to pneumonia.

Lobar pneumonia

Approximately 90 to 95% of cases of lobar pneumonia are caused by the pneumococcus *Streptococcus pneumoniae*.[4] Classically, lobar pneumonia occurs in otherwise healthy adults, and is relatively uncommon in infants and the elderly.

The tissue changes in lobar pneumonia are consistent with signs of acute inflammation. This acute inflammatory response can be divided into four stages: (1) the congestive stage, (2) red hepatization, (3) gray hepatization, and (4) resolution. Often its progress is modified by antibiotic therapy. The *congestive stage* represents the initial inflammatory response and is characterized by vascular engorgement of the alveolar vessels and transudation of serous fluid into the alveoli. The period of congestion lasts for about 24 hours and is followed by the stage of *red hepatization*. During this stage, there is extravasation of red blood cells and fibrin into the alveoli, and the lungs become firm and red with a liver-like appearance—hence the term red hepatization. The stage of *gray hepatization* is characterized by an accumulation of fibrin and beginning disintegration of the inflammatory white and red cells. Sometimes the infection extends into the pleural cavity causing *empyema*—pus in the pleural cavity. In untreated pneumonia, the stage of *resolution* occurs in about 8 to 10 days and represents the enzymatic digestion and removal of the inflammatory exudate from the infected lung area. The exudate is either coughed up or removed by macrophages.

The signs and symptoms of lobar pneumonia

coincide with the stage of the disease. The onset is usually sudden and is characterized by malaise, a severe shaking chill, and fever. The temperature may go as high as 106°F. During the congestive stage, coughing brings up a watery sputum, and breath sounds are limited, with fine crepitant rales. As the disease progresses, the character of the sputum changes; it may be blood-tinged (or rust-colored) to purulent. Pleuritic pain, a sharp pain that is more severe with respiratory movements, is common. With antibiotic therapy, fever usually subsides in about 48 to 72 hours and recovery is uneventful.

Bronchopneumonia

Bronchopneumonia is considered to be a disease of the very young, the very old, and the debilitated—the very young because their immunologic reserve and respiratory defense mechanisms have not as yet developed, and the very old because of a decline in immunity and because many have other diseases which predispose them to pneumonia.

Virtually any pathogenic organism can cause bronchopneumonia. Hospitalized patients are susceptible to bacteria present in the environment. These infections have been reported to occur in 0.5 to 5.0% of all hospitalized patients and in 12% of those sick enough to be admitted to intensive care units.[5] These nosocomial (hospital-acquired) infections are usually due to gram-negative microorganisms and are resistant to microbial therapy. Proper hand-washing and decontamination of inhalation equipment is important in preventing these infections.

In contrast to lobar pneumonia, which has a rapid onset, the early manifestations of bronchopneumonia are often insidious, in most cases including a low-grade fever, along with a cough and expiratory rales. Complications include formation of a lung abscess, empyema, and bacteremia.

Viral or mycoplasma pneumonias

Viral pneumonias can occur as a primary infection or as a complication of other diseases, such as chicken pox and measles. The influenza virus is the most common cause of viral pneumonia. In the adult, chicken pox is associated with pneumonia in 10 to 15% of cases, with a mortality rate of about 20%.[6] The mycoplasmas are the smallest free-living agents of disease, having characteristics of both viruses and bacteria. Pneumonias due to the mycoplasmas are sometimes called *primary atypical pneumonias*.

Viral or atypical pneumonias involve the interstitium of the lung and may masquerade as chest colds, with manifestations often confined to fever, headache, and muscle aches and pains. Viruses impair the respiratory tract defenses and are predisposing factors to secondary bacterial infections.

Immunization

Vaccines are available to protect against the pneumococcus and influenza virus. The pneumococcus vaccine is protective for 2 to 3 years against 80% of common types of pneumococcal bacteria.[7] The influenza vaccine contains inactivated A and B influenza viruses, and their antigenicity varies from year to year. Therefore, the formulation of the vaccine must be changed yearly in anticipation of changes that will be needed on the basis of current knowledge. Each year the Public Health Advisory Committee on Immunization Practices updates its recommendations about the composition of the vaccine. Because of variability in antigenicity and the frequency of adverse effects from the vaccine, influenza vaccine is not routinely administered to healthy persons. Both pneumococcal and viral vaccines are, however, recommended for persons in whom these infections represent a serious risk.

Tuberculosis

Tuberculosis is an infectious disease caused by *Mycobacterium tuberculosis*. The mycobacteria are slender rod-shaped, acid-fast, aerobic organisms. There are two forms of tuberculosis that pose a particular threat in humans—*Mycobacterium tuberculosis* and *Mycobacterium bovis*. Bovine tuberculosis is acquired by drinking milk from infected cows and has its initial effects on the gastrointestinal tract. This form of tuberculosis has been virtually eradicated in North America and other developed coun-

tries as a result of rigorous controls of dairy herds and pasteurization of milk. There has been a recent increase in the United States of atypical mycobacterial infections, including those caused by Group I, *Mycobacterium kansasii*, and Group III, *Mycobacterium intracellularis*.

There has been a marked decrease in the incidence of tuberculosis in the United States during the past several decades, with active cases falling from 76.7 per 100,000 in 1932 to 15.8 per 100,000 in 1974.[8] At present most infected persons are over age 30, and it has been suggested that most new cases will arise in persons already exposed to the disease. It has been estimated that 95% of children living in the U.S. will reach full maturity without ever having been exposed to the disease.[9]

Transmission

Tuberculosis is an airborne infection spread by *droplet nuclei*—minute, invisible particles harbored in the respiratory secretions of persons with active tuberculosis. Although the secretions often contain many larger particles, these larger particles tend to be filtered out of the air by gravity. If the larger particles are inhaled, they are usually trapped in the nasopharyngeal area and are removed by the action of the mucociliary blanket. Consequently, it is only the droplet nuclei that contribute to the transmission of the disease. These nuclei remain suspended in air and are circulated by air currents. They are so small that when inhaled they travel directly to the alveoli.

Pathogenesis

The destructiveness of tuberculosis is due not to the inherently destructive tubercle bacillus, but to the hypersensitivity response which it evokes. For purposes of discussion tuberculosis can be divided into primary and secondary infections, the initial infection being classified as primary tuberculosis and subsequent infections as secondary tuberculosis.

Primary tuberculosis is usually initiated in the alveolar wall as a result of inhaling tubercle bacilli. Primary tuberculosis has sometimes been called childhood tuberculosis, probably because contact with the disease occurred during childhood. The process begins as an acute inflammatory response and progresses to a chronic granulomatous inflammation (Chap. 4). Cell-mediated immunity and hypersensitivity reactions contribute to the evolution of the disease.

The initial response of the involved alveolar tissue is a local nonspecific pneumonitis. With initiation of the inflammatory response, polymorphonuclear leukocytes enter the area and phagocytize the bacilli but do not kill them. Within about 24 to 48 hours the polymorphonuclear cells are replaced by macrophages (histiocytes). Many of the bacilli engulfed by the macrophages remain viable, and proliferate. At some time, approximately days 10 to 20, the infiltrating macrophages begin to elongate and fuse together to form an epithelioid cell tubercle which becomes surrounded by lymphocytes. One or more tubercles may form. Following this period of time, the central portion of the lesion undergoes necrosis and forms a yellow cheesy mass called *caseous necrosis*. The tuberculin skin test becomes positive at about the time that the caseous necrosis occurs, suggesting that the necrosis results from the hypersensitivity response. Healing of the tubercular lesion occurs as collagenous scar tissue forms and encapsulates the lesion. In time most of these lesions become calcified, and are visible on a chest x-ray film. The primary lesion is known as a *Ghon focus*, and the combination of the tubercle lesion and the involved lymph nodes, the *Ghon complex*. The Ghon complex may contain viable organisms.

Occasionally, primary tuberculosis may progress, eroding into a bronchus and there discharging the contents of its necrotic center. An air-filled cavity forms, permitting bronchogenic spread of the disease. In rare instances, tuberculosis may erode into a blood vessel, giving rise to hematogenic dissemination. *Miliary tuberculosis* describes minute lesions resulting from this type of dissemination and may involve almost any organ, particularly the brain, meninges, liver, kidney, and bone marrow.

Secondary tuberculosis usually results from reactivation of a previously healed primary lesion. It often occurs in situations of impaired body defense mechanisms. The partial immunity that follows initial exposure affords protection against reinfection and to some extent aids in localizing the disease should secondary infection occur. The hypersensitivity reaction, on the other hand, is an aggravating factor in secondary tuberculosis, as evidenced by the frequency of cavitation and bronchial dissemination. The cavities may coalesce to a size of up to 10 to 15 centimeters in diameter. Pleural effusion and tuberculosis empyema are frequent as the disease progresses.

Clinical manifestations

Primary tuberculosis is usually asymptomatic, the only evidence of the disease being a positive tuberculin skin test and presence of calcified lesions on the chest x-ray film. Secondary tuberculosis may also be asymptomatic, particularly when the lesion is confined to the apices or upper portions of the lung. Often, however, there is an insidious onset of afternoon elevation of temperature, night sweats, weakness, fatigability, and loss of appetite and weight. As the disease advances, there may be dyspnea and orthopnea.

Diagnostic measures

The most frequently used screening methods for tuberculosis are the tuberculin skin tests and chest x-ray studies. Cultures of the sputum or gastric contents determine the presence of the organism. Gastric contents are aspirated after a fast of 8 to 10 hours, usually as the patient arises in the morning. These secretions contain tubercle bacilli swallowed during the night.

Skin testing.   The tuberculin skin test was introduced by Robert Koch in the late nineteenth century. The test measures delayed hypersensitivity (cell-mediated, type IV) that follows exposure to the tubercle bacillus. It is important to recognize that a positive reaction to the skin test does not mean that a person has tuberculosis, only that there has been exposure to the bacillus and that cell-mediated immunity to the organism has developed.

There are two skin tests, the multiple puncture technique and the intercutaneous technique. In the multiple puncture technique, purified protein derivative (PPD)—for example, Aplitest, SlavoTest PPD, Heaf test, or old tuberculin (Tine, MonoVacc) test—is the preferred method. A positive response is manifested by vesicle formation at the test site. The intercutaneous or Mantoux test (Aplisol or Tubersol) is the standard test for suspected tuberculosis. A positive reaction is evidenced by a discrete area of skin elevation of 10 mm or more. In tuberculosis, the areas of induration usually are between 15 and 20 mm or more.

Classification

The general classification of tuberculosis, published in 1974 by the American Thoracic Society, is as follows:

O. No tuberculosis exposure, not infected. No history of exposure, negative tuberculin test.

I. Tuberculosis exposure, no evidence of infection. History of exposure, negative tuberculin skin test.

II. Tuberculosis infection, without disease. Positive tuberculin skin test, negative bacteriologic studies (if done), no x-ray findings compatible with tuberculosis, no symptoms due to tuberculosis.

III. Tuberculosis: infected with disease. The current status of the patient's tuberculosis is described by three characteristics: location of the disease, bacteriologic status, and chemotherapy status.

In some cases, additional features—x-ray findings and the tuberculin skin test reaction—are included.

Treatment

Two groups of persons meet the criteria established for use of antimicrobial therapy: the first consists of those who have been in close contact with cases of active tuberculosis and who thus are at risk for developing an active form of the disease (classification I and/or II); the second includes persons with active tuberculosis (classification III).

Isoniazid (INH) is commonly given prophylactically to the first group, generally over a 12-month period. In clinically active cases, INH is given in conjunction with one or more other drugs, the most frequent first choice being *ethambutol* and *rifampin*. This treatment is followed for 6 to 12 months, after which ethambutol and INH are given for a total period of two years.

Isoniazid and rifampin are bactericidal—capable of killing the organisms. Isoniazid acts at the level of DNA synthesis, rifampin acts on RNA synthesis, and ethambutol is active in RNA synthesis. (It has been reported that rifampin may impair the effectiveness of oral contraceptives.) *Streptomycin*, the first drug found to be effective in tuberculosis, must be given parenterally, which limits its usefulness particularly in long-term therapy; it is of greatest value during the early weeks or months of therapy. *Aminosalicylic acid (PAS)* is a useful drug, often combined with INH for pediatric administration, ethambutol not being available for this use.

The reader is referred to a pharmacology text for a complete description of drugs used to treat tuberculosis.

Prevention

A vaccine containing an avirulent form of tubercle bacilli—bacille Calmette Guérin, or BCG—was introduced for human use in 1921. BCG incites both immunity and hypersensitivity to the tubercle bacillus. Many trials utilizing BCG have been carried out in efforts to reduce the incidence of tuberculosis in susceptible populations, and there is considerable controversy over its use. The reader probably will not see the vaccine used on a routine basis. While BCG increases resistance to infection, the hypersensitivity response which it provokes tends to heighten reaction to infection once it becomes established. The vaccine converts negative skin tests to positive ones, so it cannot be employed in screening for tuberculosis exposure.

In summary, this section has discussed three types of respiratory infections: acute respiratory tract infections in children, pneumonia, and tuberculosis. Respiratory tract infections are frequent in small children because their immune mechanisms are evolving and not fully developed. Among the serious respiratory infections in this age group are croup, epiglottitis, *and* bronchiolitis. *Epiglottitis is a life-threatening supraglottic infection carrying the danger of airway obstruction and asphyxia.* Pneumonia *describes an infection of the parenchymal tissues of the lung. Lobar pneumonia is most often caused by the pneumococcus, and involves a large portion or lobe of the lung. Bronchopneumonia is caused by numerous agents. It results in a patchy consolidation of multiple lobes of the lung and frequently affects persons with other debilitating diseases. Viral or atypical pneumonia can occur as a primary infection, such as that due to the influenza virus, or as a complication of other viral diseases such as measles. Viral or atypical pneumonias involve the interstitium of the lung and often masquerade as chest colds. Tuberculosis is a chronic respiratory infection caused by* Mycobacterium tuberculosis. *Tuberculosis, which is now being effectively treated by chemotherapeutic drugs, has decreased sharply in incidence during the past 4 to 5 decades.*

:Impaired Expansion of the Lung

Normal lung expansion requires the maintenance of a negative intrapleural pressure and unrestricted airflow in the conducting airways. Pneumothorax refers to collapse of the lung, which occurs when air gains entrance to the pleural space. Atelectasis is the incomplete expansion of a portion of the lung due to airway obstruction or lack of surfactant.

Pneumothorax

Pneumothorax can occur as a *spontaneous event* in which air leaks into the pleural space because of rupture of an air-filled bleb or blister on the lung surface or because air has entered the pleural space through a *wound or incision in the chest wall*. If the opening between the atmosphere and the pleural space remains patent, the pressure within the pleural space will become equal to that of the atmosphere, with consequent collapse of the lung and shift of the *mediastinum*, the *interpleural space* between the two lungs, in the direction of the collapsed lung. With a large or tension pneumothorax, the mediastinum may shift away from the involved side. The position of the trachea, normally located in the midline of the neck, deviates with the mediastinum, and thus is a means of assessing this portion of the chest.

A *tension pneumothorax* occurs when, because of a valve defect, air can enter but not leave the pleural space. It is a life-threatening situation, with a rapid increase in pressure within the chest which produces a *compression atelectasis of the lung*, a *shift of the mediastinum to the opposite side of the chest*, and *compression of the vena cava which interferes with venous return to the heart*. Emergency treatment of tension pneumothorax involves prompt insertion of a large-bore needle or chest tube into the affected side of the chest, along with water-seal drainage or continuous chest suction to aid in lung reexpansion.

Atelectasis

Atelectasis means collapse of the alveoli. It is due to a *lack of surfactant* (Chap. 18) or to *airway obstruction*. With complete obstruction of the airway there is absorption of oxygen from the dependent alveoli followed by collapse of that portion of the lung. A bronchus can be obstructed by a *mucus plug* that forms within the airway or by *external compression* due to fluid, tumor mass, exudate, or other cause in the area surrounding the airway. A small segment of lung or an entire lung lobe may be involved in atelectasis, and both chest expansion and breath sounds are decreased on the affected side. If the collapsed area is large, the trachea will deviate to the affected side. Signs of respiratory distress will be proportional to the extent of lung collapse.

There is increased danger of atelectasis following surgery. Anesthesia, pain, administration of narcotics, and immobility tend to promote retention of viscid bronchial secretions and hence airway obstruction. Encouraging a patient to cough and to take deep breaths along with frequent change of position, adequate hydration, and early ambulation decrease the likelihood of developing atelectasis.

In summary, adequate lung expansion is dependent upon a negative intrapleural pressure, patent airways, and adequate levels of surfactant. Pneumothorax occurs when air enters the pleural space, causing the lung to collapse. Atelectasis is partial collapse of a lung that results from airway obstruction or a deficiency in surfactant.

:Chronic Obstructive Lung Disease

In the United States, chronic lung disease ranks second to coronary heart disease as a cause of disability subject to Social Security payment. In 1979, chronic lung disease was the fifth leading cause of death in the United States.[10]

The terms chronic obstructive lung disease (COLD), chronic obstructive pulmonary disease (COPD), and chronic obstructive airway disease (COAD) denote a group of respiratory disorders characterized by obstruction to airflow in the lung. The most prevalent of these disorders are bronchial asthma, chronic bronchitis, and emphysema. Asthma is characterized by intermittent periods of reversible airway obstruction. In chronic bronchitis there is excessive mucus production by the mucosal cells of the bronchi and chronic productive cough (2 tablespoonsful of sputum a day or more) that has persisted for at least three months per year for two successive years or more. Pulmonary emphysema is an abnormal dilatation of the air spaces distal to the terminal bronchioles with destruction of the alveolar walls. In addition to these three causes of COLD, this section presents a brief description of two other causes of obstructive lung disease—bronchiectasis and cystic fibrosis.

Both the reversible (asthma) and persistent (chronic bronchitis and emphysema) disorders of the lung give rise to *hyperinflation, increased time needed for the expiratory phase of respiration*, and *impaired gas exchange* due to disproportion between ventilation and perfusion. The forced vital capacity (FVC) is the amount of air that can be forcibly exhaled following maximal inspiration. In a normal young adult, this should be achieved in 4 to 6 seconds.[11] The forced expiratory volume that can be achieved in one second is termed the $FEV_{1.0}$. In chronic lung disease the time required for FVC is increased, the $FEV_{1.0}$ is decreased, and the ratio of the $FEV_{1.0}$ to the FVC is decreased. These and other measurements of expiratory flow are determined by spirometry in diagnosis of COLD.

Bronchial Asthma

Conservative estimates indicate that between 8 and 10 million Americans suffer from bronchial asthma. The disease affects individuals of all ages and is the most common cause of chronic illness in children under age 17.

The disease is characterized by bronchial hyperreactivity to various stimuli, causing reversible bronchospasm, edema of the mucosal surface of the bronchioles, and increased production of mucus.

Wheezing and dyspnea occur due to airway obstruction. In severe cases there is hyperinflation of the lungs and an imbalance between ventilation and perfusion, with impairment of gas exchange. The attacks differ from person to person, and between attacks, many persons are symptom free. Both immune mechanisms (extrinsic asthma) and autonomic nervous system imbalances (intrinsic asthma) play a role in the associated bronchospasm, and they are described in the section titled "Types of asthma."

Immune response

Allergic asthma results primarily from a type I, IgE immune response (Chap. 5). The abundant mast cells of the bronchial tissues are rich in granules of chemical mediators—histamine, slow-reacting substance of anaphylaxis (SRS-A), eosinophil chemotactic factor, platelet-activating factor, and pros-

taglandins—which can provoke bronchospasm, vascular permeability, and increased mucus secretion, and in other ways may trigger an asthmatic attack. The granules from the sensitized mast cells are released on exposure to the offending allergen. Common allergens include house dust, pollen from trees, grass, and weeds, animal danders, and mold spores.

Autonomic nervous system (ANS) imbalance

The autonomic nervous system influences both bronchial smooth muscle and mediator release from the mast cells. The ANS parasympathetic component affects bronchoconstriction and promotes mediator release, while the sympathetic component affects bronchial relaxation and inhibits mediator release. Normally there are no chronically active bronchial relaxant (sympathetic) forces in operation, rather, a slight, vagally mediated bronchoconstrictor

Figure 19–2.　Diagram showing the site of action of drugs used in treatment of bronchial asthma. Cromolyn sodium prevents mast cell degranulation and mediator release. The sympathomimetic drugs (beta adrenergic agonists) and theophylline inhibit mediator production by the mast cells. The adrenal corticosteroid hormones, theophylline, sympathomimetic drugs and atropine decrease or prevent bronchospasm, edema, excess mucosal secretions, and inflammation. *Fair RS: Asthma in adults: The ambulatory patient. Hosp Pract 13(4): 113–123, 1978

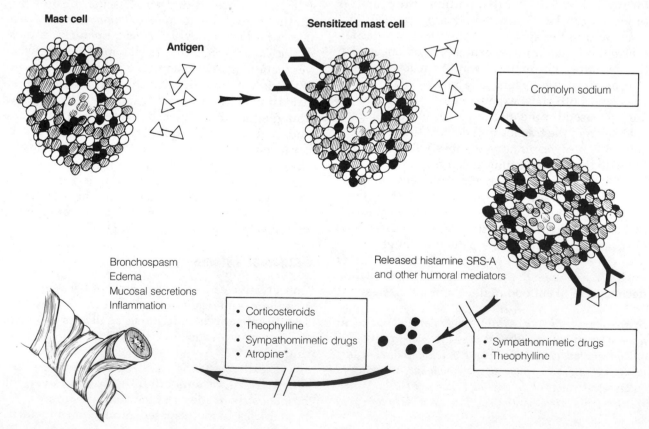

tone predominates. Hence a modest increase in sympathetic activity during periods of stress and increased oxygen need can bring about a marked decrease in airway resistance; this makes breathing easier and allows for increased ventilation.

The sympathetic nervous system has two types of receptors, alpha and beta receptors (Chap. 40). The beta type 2 receptors effect relaxation of the bronchioles. The smooth muscle tone and inflammatory mediator release from the mast cells are modulated by intercellular levels of the cyclic nucleotides, particularly adenosine monophosphate (cAMP). When the level of this second messenger (cAMP) falls, bronchial smooth muscle contracts. Beta adrenergic agonists such as adrenalin augment the cAMP levels in the mast cells so there is less mediator release from the mast cell granules. The interaction between autonomic nervous system influences, cAMP levels, and drugs used in asthma is depicted in Figure 19-2.

Types of asthma

There are two types of asthma, extrinsic and intrinsic. *Extrinsic* or allergic *asthma* is caused by release of inflammatory mediators from sensitized mast cells. Generally, this form of asthma is seen in persons with a family history of allergy and its onset occurs during childhood or adolescence. Persons with allergic asthma may also have other allergies such as hay fever. Attacks are related to exposure to specific allergens. Skin tests for the appropriate allergens are positive. *Intrinsic asthma* is characterized by an absence of clearly defined precipitating factors. Onset is usually after age 35. The attacks are frequently precipitated by factors such as infection, weather changes, exercise, emotion, and various drugs, including aspirin.

There is a small group of asthmatics in whom aspirin sensitivity is associated with severe asthmatic attacks, presence of nasal polyps, and recurrent episodes of rhinitis.[12] In addition, the yellow food dye tartrazine and nonsteroidal anti-inflammatory drugs, such as aminopyrine, phenylbutazone, ibuprofen, and indomethacin, may provoke attacks.

Exercise-induced asthma is seen in both intrinsic and extrinsic asthma, though the relationship between exercise and bronchial spasm is not understood. The response is often exaggerated when the person exercises in a cold environment; wearing a mask over the nose and mouth often minimizes the attack or prevents it. It appears that the proper selection of a mask could be important for persons subject to exercise-induced asthma, because it has been shown that increasing the humidity of the inhaled air is more important than simply heating the air.[13]

Clinical manifestations

Persons with asthma exhibit a wide range of signs and symptoms, from "chest tightness" to an acute immobilizing attack. Many sufferers are asymptomatic between attacks.

With progressive airway obstruction occurring during an attack, expiration becomes prolonged. The $FEV_{1.0}$ is decreased. Air becomes trapped in the lungs, increasing the residual volume (Chap. 18). The asthmatic must now breathe at a higher lung volume, and more energy is needed to overcome the tension already present in the lungs. Fatigue follows. Both inspiratory reserve capacity and vital capacity diminish. Because air is trapped in the alveoli and inspiration is occurring at higher lung volumes, the cough becomes less effective. As the condition progresses, the effectiveness of alveolar ventilation declines, with mismatching between ventilation and perfusion. Exchange of gases is impaired and cyanosis develops.

During an *acute attack*, the asthmatic generally prefers to sit up. There is visible use of the respiratory muscles. The skin is often moist, and anxiety and apprehension are obvious. The person wheezes during both inspiration and expiration, often audibly. Breath sounds may be coarse and loud. Vesicular breath sounds become quite distant due to trapping of air. Dyspnea may be severe, and often the person is able to speak only one or two words before taking a breath. A cough may accompany the wheezing. At the point where airflow is markedly decreased, the cough becomes ineffective despite being repetitive and hacking; this point often marks the onset of respiratory failure.

Treatment

Two treatment modalities are used in the management of bronchial asthma. One method focuses on prevention, the other on treatment. Figure 19-2 diagrams the action of various therapeutic drugs in relieving asthmatic bronchospasm.

Preventive measures include *avoidance of factors* such as allergens or breathing of cold air that are known to precipitate an attack. A careful history is often needed to identify all the contributory factors. When the offending agent cannot be avoided (for example, house dust), a *program of desensitization* may be undertaken (Chap. 5). The drug *cromolyn sodium* is sometimes effective in preventing allergic reactions. The drug is administered by inhalation. It *stabilizes the mast cells*, thereby preventing release of inflammatory mediators that cause the attack. This drug must be given prophylactically and is of no benefit when taken during an attack.

During the attack itself, bronchodilators are

used. These include the *beta adrenergic agonists* (such as epinephrine) and theophylline preparations. The adrenergic agents relax bronchial smooth muscle and relieve congestion of the bronchial mucosa. Certain forms of these drugs may be given by inhalation for rapid onset of action. *Theophylline* also acts by relaxing smooth muscle. Theophylline preparations can be administered by oral, rectal, or intravenous route. The adrenergic drugs and theophylline preparations have different mechanisms of action and are therefore complementary. The adrenergic drugs directly increase the levels of cyclic AMP in the bronchial smooth muscle, whereas theophylline decreases the metabolism of cyclic AMP. The *adrenocorticosteroid* drugs are also used to treat acute asthmatic attacks. It is thought that these drugs stabilize the lysosomes of the inflammatory cells, prevent the accumulation of histamine in mast cells, sensitize the beta adrenergic receptors, and exert other anti-inflammatory actions. The effects of these drugs are depicted in greater detail in Figure 19-2 and Table 19-4.

Relaxation techniques and *controlled breathing* help to allay the panic and anxiety that aggravate breathing difficulties. In a child, measures to encourage independence as it relates to symptom control, along with those directed at helping to develop a positive self-concept, are essential.

Chronic Bronchitis and Emphysema

Chronic bronchitis and pulmonary emphysema are closely related. Among persons with COLD, many will be found to have both chronic bronchitis and emphysema; some will have only chronic bronchitis; others will have emphysema.

For descriptive purposes, the euphemisms *"blue bloaters"* and *"pink puffers"* have been used to differentiate the clinical manifestations of chronic bronchitis and pulmonary emphysema. The reader will find that in actual practice, the distinction between them is not as vivid as presented here. This is because many individuals with COLD have combinations of both conditions. Characteristically, the secretions of chronic bronchitis obstruct airflow, causing an imbalance in ventilation and perfusion. For some unknown reason, persons with this form of COLD do not increase their total minute ventilation to compensate for the imbalance in ventilation and perfusion; consequently, they develop hypoxemia, cyanosis, and eventually cor pulmonale with systemic edema. These are the "blue bloaters." They are

Table 19–4 Characteristics of Chronic Bronchitis and Emphysematous Types of Chronic Lung Disease

Characteristic	Chronic Bronchitis ("Blue Bloaters")	Pulmonary Emphysema ("Pink Puffers")
Smoking history	Usual	Usual
Age of onset	Relatively younger	Relatively older
Clinical features		
Barrel chest (hyperinflation of the lungs)	May be present	Often dramatic
Weight loss	Infrequent	May be severe in advanced disease
Shortness of breath	Predominant early symptom, insidious in onset, exertional	May be absent early in disease
Decreased breath sounds	Variable	Characteristic
Wheezing	Variable	Usually absent
Rhonchi	Often prominent	Usually absent or minimal
Sputum	Frequent early manifestation, frequent infections, abundant purulent sputum	May be absent or may develop late in the course
Cyanosis	Often dramatic	Often absent, even late in the disease when there is low PO_2
Blood gases	Hypercapnia Hypoxia	Relatively normal
Cor pulmonale	Frequent Peripheral edema	Only in advanced cases
Polycythemia	Frequent	Only in advanced cases
Prognosis	Numerous life-threatening episodes due to acute exacerbations	Slowly progressive
	Death at relatively early age	Death usually at older age

also known as "nonfighters." With pulmonary emphysema there is a proportional loss of both ventilation and perfusion area in the lung. For whatever reason, these persons are "fighters"—able to struggle and overventilate, and thus to maintain relatively normal blood gas levels. They are the "pink puffers." The important features of these two forms of COLD are described in Table 19-4.

Chronic bronchitis

A chronic productive cough is the prominent feature in chronic bronchitis, and it is often present for many years before the onset of other symptoms. It is seen most commonly in middle-aged men and is associated with chronic irritation from inhaled substances and recurrent infections. In the United States, smoking is the most important cause of chronic bronchitis.

The disease involves both the major and the small airways, and is characterized by inflammation, edema, hyperplasia of the bronchial glands, and overproduction of mucus. Viral and bacterial infections are common and are thought to be a result of rather than a cause of the problem.

Shortness of breath on exertion and finally at rest is due to airway obstruction. Airway obstruction leads to imbalance between ventilation and perfusion, with *hypoxemia* and *cyanosis*. Then *pulmonary hypertension* ensues, associated with right heart failure, or *cor pulmonale*, and peripheral edema. The hypoxemia acts as a stimulus for red blood cell production with a resultant *polycythemia*. As the disease progresses, breathing is labored, even when the person is at rest. The expiratory phase of respiration is prolonged, and inspiratory and expiratory rales and rhonchi can be heard on auscultation. Another frequent finding in chronic bronchitis is *clubbing of the fingers*, a situation in which the tips of the fingers become bulbous, resembling drumsticks. Normally there is an obtuse angle of about 160° between the base of the nail and the adjacent dorsal surface of the finger; with clubbing, this angle exceeds 180°. In contrast to persons with emphysema, those with chronic bronchitis tend to maintain normal or elevated body weight.

Emphysema

In emphysema there is enlargement and destruction of the air spaces distal to the terminal bronchioles. Note loss of alveolar tissue demonstrated in Figure 19-3. The two principal types of emphysema are centrilobular and panlobular. The centrilobular type affects the respiratory bronchioles, with initial preservation of the alveolar ducts and sacs. In the panlobular form the peripheral alveoli are involved. Figure 19-4 depicts the alveolar involvement associated with centrilobular and panlobular emphysema.

There are several known or suspected causes of emphysema, the most important of which is cigarette smoking. The risk of emphysema increases with the number of cigarettes smoked.[14] A second cause of emphysema is a deficiency of alpha$_1$-antitrypsin. Alpha$_1$-antitrypsin is a proteinase inhibitor; it blocks the action of the proteolytic enzymes which are destructive to elastin and other substances in the alveolar wall. The deficiency is an inherited autosomal recessive disorder. Approximately 70 to 80% of persons with a homozygous pattern of inheritance for alpha$_1$-antitrypsin deficiency have COLD.[15] The severity of the condition and age of onset may vary from individual to individual. There is now evidence that cigarette smoking reduces the body stores of alpha$_1$-antitrypsin over time. Therefore, smoking and repeated respiratory tract infec-

Figure 19–3. Transmission electron micrograph of lung tissue. Top, normal tissue; bottom, emphysematous tissue (both at same magnification). Note enlargement of air spaces in the emphysematous lung. (Courtesy of Kenneth Siegesmund, Ph.D. Anatomy Department, The Medical College of Wisconsin)

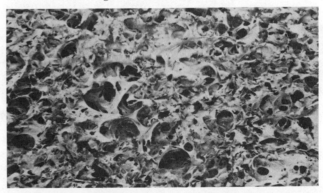

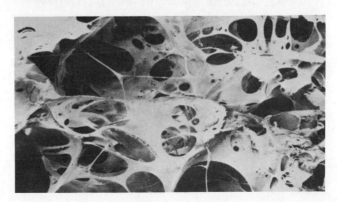

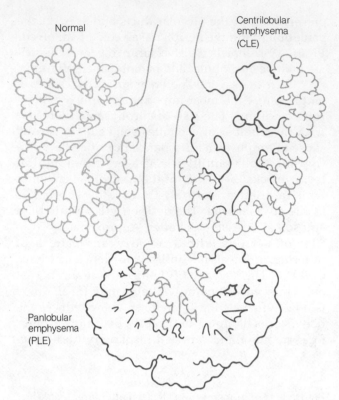

Normal

Centrilobular
emphysema
(CLE)

Panlobular
emphysema
(PLE)

Figure 19–4. Diagram showing the changes in alveolar structure associated with centrilobular and panlobular emphysema.

tions (which also impede normal secretion) tend to contribute to the development of emphysema in persons with an alpha$_1$-antitrypsin deficiency.

Emphysema causes trapping of air in the alveoli. Afflicted persons have marked *dyspnea, and struggle to maintain normal blood gas levels with increased ventilatory effort.* The work of breathing is greatly increased and eating is often difficult. As a result, there is often considerable *weight loss.* With hyperinflation of the lungs, there is an increase in the anterior-posterior dimensions of the chest—the so-called *barrel chest* typical of the person with emphysema. Usually *the seated position is preferred,* because it affords maximal use of the accessory muscles and serves to press the abdominal contents up against the diaphragm—a help in breathing. The *expiratory phase* of respiration is usually *prolonged* and generally accomplished through *pursed lips.* With hyperinflation of the lungs, there is a tendency toward airway collapse during expiration. The pursed-lip breathing serves to increase the airway pressure and thereby prevent such collapse. One popular test to assess the severity of obstructive airway disease which is employed in emphysema is the *match test.* In this test, a lit match is held 6 inches

from the mouth, and the patient is asked to extinguish it. Ability to extinguish the match indicates a maximum voluntary ventilation of 60 liters per minute and a forced expiratory volume at 1 second of 1.6 liters.[16]

Treatment of chronic bronchitis and emphysema

The treatment of COLD can be described under seven headings: (1) avoidance of smoking and environmental irritants; (2) prevention and control of respiratory infections; (3) maintenance of optimal nutritional status and fluid balance; (4) medications; (5) physical therapy and psychosocial rehabilitation; (6) control of shortness of breath; and (7) administration of oxygen or other methods of respiratory therapy. Obviously, not all persons with COLD have the same treatment needs.

Since COLD is a chronic disease, the outcomes of treatment are largely dependent upon self-care measures that involve both the afflicted person and the family members. These persons need to have a complete understanding of the disease process and the manner in which it affects respiratory function, as well as the purpose of the prescribed treatment measures.

Avoidance of environmental irritants. Avoidance of cigarette smoke and other environmental airway irritants is "a must." Vocational counseling may be needed if there is occupational exposure. Monitoring of air pollution levels and adjusting activities accordingly will aid in controlling shortness of breath. Wearing a cold weather mask often prevents bronchospasm due to breathing cold air.

Infection. Respiratory tract infections can prove fatal to persons with severe COLD. A person with COLD should avoid exposure to others with known respiratory tract infections, and should avoid attending large gatherings during periods of the year when influenza or respiratory tract infections are prevalent. Immunization for influenza and pneumococcal infections will decrease the likelihood of their occurrence. Persons with COLD should be taught to examine their sputum for signs of infection, so that antibiotics can be prescribed at the earliest sign of infection.

Maintenance of optimal nutrition and fluid balance. Because so much effort goes into breathing, many persons with COLD find it difficult to chew their food and to manage the effort of a large meal. This situation, combined with impaired diaphragm descent, air-swallowing, and medications that cause anorexia and nausea, impairs nutrition and promotes weight loss. Small, frequent, nutritious, and easily swallowed feedings aid in maintaining good nutrition and preventing weight loss. Vitamin supplements may be called for. Water is the most readily available expectorant for liquefying secretions, so fluid intake should be encouraged, particularly in persons who have thick, tenacious sputum. Fluid that is either too hot or too cold may aggravate breathing problems.

Medications. Several groups of medications are used in long-term management of COLD, including adrenergic (adrenalin-related) drugs, theophylline preparations, and expectorants. Adrenal corticosteroid hormones may be used in some cases. Expectorants are discussed in Chapter 18. Both *adrenergic* and *theophylline* preparations act by relaxing bronchiolar smooth muscle. Combination drugs, most often consisting of an adrenergic drug, a theophylline preparation, and a sedative to counteract CNS stimulation due to the adrenergic drug may be helpful. However, since sedative drugs depress the respiratory center, the combination drugs are used less frequently than in the past. Also, with the development of *adrenergic drugs* that act specifically on the *beta-2 receptors* of the lung and cause less central nervous system stimulation than the older adrenergics such as ephedrine and pseudoephedrine, there is less need for the combination drugs. The beta-2 agonists also have less effect on the cardiovascular system.

Theophylline preparations can be administered orally, rectally, or intravenously. They can be given intramuscularly, but cause much pain by this route. There is wide variability from case to case in the absorption and metabolism of these preparations; therefore, drug blood level serves as a guide in arriving at an effective dosage schedule. Although the adrenal corticosteroids are not usually prescribed in long-term treatment of COLD, a small number of persons do require them. The adrenal corticosteroids are available for local use in aerosol form, minimizing the undesirable effects that often accompany systemic use. Table 19-5 lists some of the common adrenergic drugs, their mechanisms of action, and their side-effects.

Many adrenergics are available in aerosol form for inhalation, and in this form they are particularly useful in controlling bronchospasm. Because they are convenient and effective, they can be abused by overuse. Of special concern is the potential for development of cardiac arrhythmias.

Physical therapy and psychosocial rehabilition. The maintenance or improvement of physical and psychosocial functioning is an essential component in the treatment plan for persons with COLD. During inspiration the diaphragm contracts and descends; during expiration it passively ascends, causing air to leave the lungs. In normal respiration, the diaphragm contributes 65% of the work of breathing, while the accessory muscles contribute about 35%.[17] In emphysema, the contribution of the diaphragm to the work of breathing is largely diminished due to loss of lung elasticity, with air trapping and lung distention. In order to compensate for this deficiency, persons with emphysema use their accessory muscles for breathing. Breathing is laborious, and the work of breathing increases. This labored breathing pattern may progress to the point where the diaphragm contributes only about 30% to the effort of breathing, while the accessory muscles carry 70% of the load.[18]

Breathing exercises and retraining focus on *improving gas exchange* and *restoring normal activity of the diaphragm*. *Physical conditioning*, with a gradual increase in activity, improves exercise tolerance. *Postural drainage* provides a means for removing excess secretions from the lungs. It is done by positioning the patient's body according to the distribution and configuration of the tracheobronchial tree so that gravity causes secretions to drain into the larger airways from which they can be effectively removed. The effectiveness of postural drainage may be enhanced by *percussion* or *vibration* of the chest wall, done by vibrating or tapping motions with the hands or by electronic vibrators or ultrasound generators. The reader is referred to other reference sources, some of which are listed at the end of the chapter, for a more complete description of these exercises and treatments.

Psychosocial rehabilitation must be individualized to meet the specific needs of persons with COLD and their families. These needs will vary with age, occupation, financial resources, social and recreational interest, and interpersonal and family relationships. Work simplification may be needed when impairment is severe.

Oxygen therapy. In advanced cases of COLD, the imbalance between ventilation and perfusion causes hypoxemia. Hypoxemia, with arterial PO_2 levels below 60 mm Hg, causes polycythemia and reflex vasoconstriction of the pulmonary vessels, with resultant pulmonary hypertension and further impairment of gas exchange in the lung. These patients are at risk for developing cor pulmonale.

Table 19-5   Bronchodilator Drugs Used in the Treatment of Chronic Obstructive Lung Diseases

Drug	Action	Route of Administration
Adrenergic Drugs	Drugs with a beta-2 action produce relaxation of the bronchial smooth muscle by acting at the level of adenyl cyclase to increase cyclic AMP; beta-1 agonists stimulate the heart, causing tachycardia and danger of arrhythmias; drugs with an alpha action cause vasoconstriction and raise blood pressure	
Epinephrine	Stimulates both alpha and beta receptors, producing tachycardia and blood pressure changes as well as bronchial dilatation	Usually given by inhalation or subcutaneous injection Intramuscular suspension preparations are available
Ephedrine (and related preparations such as pseudoephedrine)	Not a catecholamine; acts by inducing catecholamine release; has disadvantage of causing central nervous system stimulation and cardiovascular side-effects	Usually given orally, often in combinations of theophylline and a sedative
Isoproterenol	Both beta-1 and beta-2 actions	Usually given by inhalation Can be given sublingually
Metaproterenol	Mainly beta-2; can cause troublesome muscle tremors; may produce tachycardia and blood pressure changes	Oral and inhalation
Terbutaline	Beta-2 actions; may produce troublesome muscle tremors. May also produce tachycardia and blood pressure changes	Oral; subcutaneous
Isoetharine	Mainly beta-2	Inhalation
Albuterol	Mainly beta-2	Inhalation
Theophylline Preparations		
Theophylline Aminophylline (86 percent theophylline) Oxtriphylline (65 percent theophylline)	Produce bronchodilatation by inhibiting metabolism of cyclic AMP; can cause nausea and vomiting which is mediated through the central nervous system; may produce seizures at high levels, particularly in children	Usually given orally as a single agent, or occasionally as a combination preparation with an adrenergic drug and a sedative May be given intravenously or rectally

In such severe cases, administration of continuous low-flow (1–2 liters per min) oxygen by nasal cannula often improves arterial oxygen levels, decreases dyspnea, and improves exercise tolerance. Home oxygen administration is a recent development, and the criteria prescribing its use are evolving. It is generally agreed that the oxygen must be administered for at least 12 hours out of every 24 to be effective. However, cost alone—$300 or more a month—limits its use. At present, it is used mainly for persons who have severe dyspnea and an arterial PO_2 of 50 mm Hg or less.

There are some persons with COLD who experience *apnea* with severe hypoxemia *during sleep*. These periods of apnea are more apt to occur during rapid eye movement (REM) sleep. Most individuals who experience sleep apnea are unaware that it is occurring, although they may report having nightmares and restless sleep. Many will complain that they wake up feeling tired and are extremely tired throughout the day. These persons often complain of depression and nervousness when awake. Administration of tranquilizers and sedatives brings further depression of ventilation.

Oxygen administration in persons with COLD must be undertaken with a certain amount of caution. The saying, "A little bit is good, a whole lot is better," does not hold true for oxygen administration in COLD. The oxygen (liters per min) is usually titrated to provide an arterial PO_2 of about 60 mm Hg. Since the ventilatory drive associated with hypoxic stimulation of the peripheral chemoreceptors does not occur until the arterial PO_2 has been reduced to about 60 mm Hg or less, increasing the arterial oxygen above that level tends to depress stimulation for ventilation and often leads to hypoventilation and carbon dioxide retention.

Intermittent positive pressure breathing.   For those who need additional assistance in clearing secretions from the respiratory tract, mechanical devices that deliver medications in the form of a mist may be used. Hand-held nebulizers and, rarely, intermittent positive pressure breathing (IPPB) are employed. IPPB is accomplished by machines that deliver nebulized air to the lungs under increased pressure during inspiration. Bronchodilator drugs are often added to the nebulizer. IPPB should coincide with postural drainage.

Cystic Fibrosis

Cystic fibrosis is a hereditary disease transmitted as an *autosomal recessive trait*. It affects approximately 1 in 2000 children. It is an exocrine gland disorder involving both the mucus-secreting and the eccrine glands. Because cystic fibrosis involves production of a thick tenacious mucus, it is sometimes referred to as mucoviscidosis.

Clinically, cystic fibrosis is characterized by *elevation of sweat electrolytes*, *pancreatic insufficiency*, and *chronic lung disease*. There is excessive sodium and chloride in the sweat. Abnormalities in pancreatic function are present in about 80% of affected children. The pancreatic insufficiency gives rise to malabsorption and steatorrhea. In the newborn, meconium ileus may cause intestinal obstruction. Respiratory manifestations are due to an accumulation of viscid mucus in the bronchi which produces bronchial obstruction and dilatation. Mucus plugs can result in total obstruction of an airway, causing atelectasis.

Progress of the disease is variable. With improved medical management there has been an increased survival rate, which at present, is about 20 years of age.

Bronchiectasis

Bronchiectasis is an abnormal dilatation of the bronchioles associated with chronic necrotizing infection of the bronchi. There are a number of causes of bronchiectasis, including congenital abnormalities, cystic fibrosis, immunologic deficiencies, respiratory tract infections, and exposure to corrosive gases.

The disease is characterized by infection and obstruction of the bronchioles. The clinical manifestations are severe cough and recurrent bronchopulmonary infection with excessive production of purulent sputum. The quantity of sputum can often amount to cupfuls.

The basic therapy consists of early recognition and treatment of infection along with regular postural drainage. Prior to the advent of antibiotics, anaerobic infections were common, leading to malodorous sputum and breath—potentially a serious social handicap.

Cor Pulmonale

Cor pulmonale is a syndrome of *congestive failure of the right heart* occurring as a result of a long-standing *increase in pulmonary vascular resistance* due to chronic lung disease. The syndrome includes *hypertrophy of the right ventricle*. The pulmonary hypertension is thought to be caused by irreversible anatomic destruction of the pulmonary vessels and reversible spasm of the pulmonary arterioles resulting from hypoxemia. Cor pulmonale is usually accompanied by peripheral edema. Heart failure is discussed in Chapter 17.

In summary, chronic obstructive lung disease describes a group of conditions characterized by obstruction to airflow in the lungs. Among the conditions associated with COLD are bronchial asthma, chronic bronchitis, emphysema, cystic fibrosis, and bronchiectasis. The condition is manifested by hyperinflation of the lungs, increased time required for the expiratory phase of respiration, and mismatching of ventilation and perfusion. As the condition advances, signs of respiratory distress and impaired gas exchange are evident, with development of hypercapnia and hypoxemia.

:Cancer of the Lung

In the United States, lung cancer strikes more than 100,000 persons every year,[19] most commonly those between 40 and 70 years of age. Lung cancer is a leading cause of death among men, and a steadily increasing cause among women. These consistent increases over the past fifty years have coincided closely with the increase in cigarette smoking over the same span (Fig. 19-5). Many studies have shown that the risk of developing lung cancer increases with the number of cigarettes smoked, and that the average male smoker is 10 times more likely to develop lung cancer than is a nonsmoker.[20] Industrial

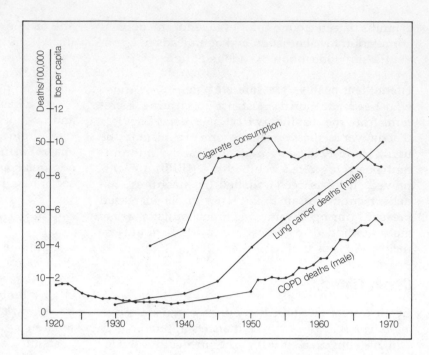

Figure 19–5. Increase in cigarette smoking and deaths due to lung cancer and COPD between 1920 and 1970. (Ayres SM: Cigarette Smoking and Lung Disease: An Update. Basics of RD 3(5):67, 1975)

hazards also contribute to the incidence of lung cancer. A commonly recognized hazard is exposure to asbestos, with the mean risk of lung cancer among asbestos workers significantly greater than in the general population. Tobacco smoke contributes heavily to the development of lung cancer in persons exposed to asbestos, the risk in this population group estimated to be 92 times greater than that for nonsmokers.[21]

Bronchogenic carcinoma is the cancer type seen in 90% to 95% of cases. These tumors can be further subdivided into epidermoid or squamous cell carcinoma (40% to 60%); adenocarcinoma (10% to 25%); small cell anaplastic (oat cell) carcinoma (7% to 25%); and bronchial carcinoid (5% to 10%).[22]

The tracheobronchial tree is lined with at least five types of epithelial cells which form the pseudostratified cell layer of these airways (Chap. 2). There are three types of columnar cells—the mucus-secreting goblet cells, the ciliated cells, and the brush cells. The basal cells are small, multiple, potential stem cells parallel to the basement membrane upon which the pseudostratified cell layer rests. One group of basal cells probably acts as reserve cells for the columnar cells, and the other, termed Kulchitsky (or K-type) cells, appears to be neuroendocrine in origin and is believed to have the capacity to secrete hormones. These cell characteristics would account for the paraneoplastic syndromes that occur in some forms of bronchogenic carcinoma. Squamous cell carcinoma probably arises from the basal reserve cells, adenocarcinoma from the mucin-secreting cells, and small cell and bronchial carcinoid cancers from the K-type cells.[23]

Manifestations

Cancer of the lungs develops insidiously, giving little if any warning of its presence. The earliest symptoms are cough, wheezing, slight shortness of breath, and an aching pain in the chest. Because these same symptoms are associated with chronic bronchitis and respiratory disorders associated with smoking, they are often disregarded.

The manifestations of lung cancer can be divided into four categories: (1) local respiratory disturbances, (2) the effects of metastatic lesions, (3) nonspecific effects such as weight loss, and (4) the paraneoplastic endocrine, neurologic, and connective tissue disorders.

Pleural effusion. Tumors adjacent to the visceral pleura often insidiously provoke pleural effusion (fluid in the pleural cavity). This effusion may cause dyspnea, but is less apt to cause fever, pleural friction rub, or pain as compared with pleural effusion due to other causes.

Paraneoplastic disorders. Paraneoplastic disorders are those that are unrelated to metastasis. No other type of cancer produces such disorders as frequently as lung cancer. Neurologic or muscular symptoms often develop 6 months to 4 years before the lung tumor is detected. One of the more common of these problems is weakness and wasting of the proximal muscles of the pelvic and shoulder girdles with decreased deep tendon reflexes, but without sensory changes.[24]

Certain bronchogenic carcinomas produce hormones. It has been estimated that approximately 10% of persons with bronchogenic cancer have evidence of ectopic hormone production.[25] The most frequently produced hormones are parathormone (causing hypercalcemia, Chap. 22), antidiuretic hormone (syndrome of inappropriate secretion of ADH, Chap. 22), and ACTH (clinical Cushing's syndrome, Chap. 33).

Prognosis

Because cancer of the lung is usually far advanced before it is discovered, the prognosis is generally poor, with a five-year survival rate of only 5% to 10%. The hope for the future rests with methods of earlier detection and with prevention.

In summary, cancer of the lung is a leading cause of death among men ages 40 to 70, and the death rate is increasing among women. In the United States this increased death rate has coincided with the increase in cigarette smoking. Industrial hazards, such as exposure to asbestos, increase the risk of developing lung cancer. Of all forms of lung cancer, bronchogenic carcinoma is the most common, accounting for 90% to 95% of cases. Because lung cancer develops insidiously, it is often far advanced before it is diagnosed, a fact that is used to explain the poor five-year survival rate for this cancer— only 5% to 10% of affected persons are alive and well five years after treatment.

:Study Guide

After you have studied this chapter, you should be able to meet the following objectives:

: : Explain why respiratory infections are common in young children.

: : Explain the pathophysiology underlying upper respiratory infections in children.

: : Describe the sequence of events associated with lobar pneumonia.

: : Explain why bronchopneumonia is often seen at the extremes of age.

: : Explain why the formulation of the influenza vaccine must be changed from time to time.

: : Describe the transmission of tuberculosis.

: : Differentiate between primary tuberculosis and secondary tuberculosis on the basis of their pathophysiology.

: : State the significance of a positive reaction to the skin test for tuberculosis.

: : State the American Thoracic Society classification of tuberculosis.

: : Describe the clinical condition known as spontaneous pneumothorax by comparing it with tension pneumothorax.

: : Explain why surgery increases the risk of atelectasis.

: : State the feature common to COLD, COPD, and COAD.

: : Describe the pathology seen in bronchial asthma.

: : Describe the clinical manifestations of bronchial asthma.

: : Explain the distinction between chronic bronchitis and emphysema.

: : State the usual sequence of events following airway obstruction in chronic bronchitis.

: : Explain why cigarette smoking may cause emphysema.

: : Describe the general guidelines that the health professional should be aware of in the treatment of chronic bronchitis and emphysema.

: : Describe the abnormalities characteristic of cystic fibrosis

: : State the chief manifestations of bronchiectasis.

: : Describe the features of the syndrome known as cor pulmonale.

: : State two environmental factors that may cause bronchogenic cancer.

:References

1. Facts About Lung Disease. American Lung Association, 1980
2. Vital Statistics Report: Annual Summary of the United States, 1979, Vol. 28(13). Washington, D.C., U.S. Department of Health and Human Services, 1980
3. Dowling JN, Sheehe PR, Feldman H: Pharyngeal pneumococcal acquisitions in "normal" families: A longitudinal study. J Infect Dis 124(1):9-19, 1971
4. Robbins SL, Cotran R: Pathologic Basis of Disease, 2nd ed, p. 847. Philadelphia, WB Saunders, 1979
5. National Nosocomial Infection Study, Fourth Quarter, 1972. U.S. Center for Disease Control, 1974

6. Jones DA: Viral infection of the respiratory system. Chest Heart Stroke J 3(5):48, 1979

7. Facts About Pneumococcal Pneumonia. American Lung Association

8. Tuberculosis Statistics—States and Cities, 1974. Washington, D.C., Public Health Service, U.S. Department of Health, Education and Welfare, Publication No. (CDC)76-8249, 1975

9. Youmans GP: Tuberculosis, p. 356. Philadelphia, WB Saunders, 1979

10. Vital Statistics Report: Annual Summary of the United States, 1979, Vol. 28, No. 13, U.S. Department of Health and Human Services

11. Chronic Obstructive Pulmonary Disease, 5th ed, inside front cover. American Lung Association and Medical Section, American Thoracic Association, 1977

12. Samter M, Beers RR: Intolerance to aspirin: Clinical studies and consideration of its pathogenesis. Ann Intern Med 68:975-983, 1968

13. McFadden ER, Ingram RH Jr.: Exercise-induced asthma. N Engl J Med 301(14):763-769, 1979

14. The Health Consequences of Smoking. Washington, D.C., U.S. Department of Health, Education and Welfare, 1971

15. Kueppers F, Black LP: Alpha-antitrypsin and its deficiency. Am Rev Respir Dis 110:176, 1974

16. Guenter CA, Welch MH: Pulmonary Medicine, p. 82. Philadelphia, JB Lippincott, 1977

17. Hodgkin JE et al: Chronic obstructive airway diseases: Current concepts in diagnosis and comprehensive care. JAMA 232(12):1253-1254, 1975

18. Hodgkin JE et al: Chronic obstructive airway diseases: Current concepts in diagnosis and comprehensive care. JAMA 232(12):1254, 1975

19. Facts on Lung Cancer. American Cancer Society, 1978

20. Progress Against Cancer of the Lung. Washington, D.C., U.S. Department of Health, Education and Welfare, Publication No. (NIH)76-526, 1974

21. Carr DT: Bronchogenic carcinoma. Basics of RD 5(5):54, 1977

22. Robbins SL, Cotran R: Pathologic Basis of Disease, 2nd ed, p. 866. Philadelphia, WB Saunders, 1979

23. Carr, DT, Rosenow EC: Bronchogenic carcinoma. Basics of RD 5(5):55, 1977

24. Rohwedder JJ: Neoplastic Disease. In Guenter CA, Welch MH: Pulmonary Medicine, p. 699. Philadelphia, JB Lippincott, 1977

25. Rohwedder JJ: Neoplastic Disease. In Guenter CA, Welch MH: Pulmonary Medicine, p. 702. Philadelphia, JB Lippincott, 1977

:Suggested Readings

Chronic obstructive lung disease

Benjamin SP, McCormick LJ: Structural abnormalities in COPD. Postgrad Med J 62(1):101-106, 1977

Bleich HL, Moore MJ (eds): Exercise-induced asthma: Observations on the initiating stimulus. Semin Med Beth Israel Hosp 301(14):763-769, 1979

Bode FR: Axioms on smoking and the respiratory tract. Hosp Med 14:35+, 1978

Buckley JM: The problem patient: Exercise-induced asthma. Hosp Pract 14, No. 5:119-120, 1979

Chakrin LW, Krell RD: Pathophysiology and pharmacotherapy of asthma: An overview. J Pharm Sci 69(2):236-238, 1980

Elpern EH: Asthma update: Pathophysiology and treatment. Heart Lung 9(4):665-670, 1980

Flenley DD, Calverly PMA, Douglas NJ et al: Nocturnal hypoxemia and long-term domiciliary oxygen therapy in "blue and bloated" bronchitis. Chest 77(2):305-307, 1980

Ghory AC, Patterson R: Treating asthma in the elderly. Geriatrics 35:32-38, 1980

Golish JA, Ahmad M: Management of COPD: A physiologic approach. Postgrad Med J 62(1):131-136, 1977

Harrison GN, Speir WA Jr: Drug therapy of chronic obstructive pulmonary disease. Hospital Formulary 13:869-872, 1978

Horton FO, Mackenthun AV, Anderson PS et al: Alpha, antitrypsin heterozygotes (Pi type mz): A longitudinal study of the risk of development of chronic air flow limitation. Chest 77(2):261-264, 1980

Huchinson DCS: The pathogenesis of pulmonary emphysema. Chest Heart Stroke J 3(5):18-25, 1979

Hudgel DW, Madsen LA: Acute and chronic asthma: A guide to intervention. Am J Nurs 80:1791-1795, 1980

Jacobs MM, Bowers B: Protocol: Chronic obstructive lung disease. Nurs Pract 4(6):11, 24-28, 1979

Kendig EL Jr: Chronic lung disease in children. Hosp Pract 12, No. 5:87-98, 1977

Massaro D: Clinical implications of the effect of breathing pattern on the lung. Respiratory Care 25(3):377-380, 1980

Mathews JJ: Chronic obstructive pulmonary disease. Topics Emerg Med 2:13-24, 1980

McCarthy DS: Chronic obstructive lung disease: Guide to diagnosis and management. Hosp Med 14, No. 12:40-41, 1978

Petty TL: Long-term outpatient oxygen therapy in advanced chronic obstructive pulmonary disease. Chest 77(2):304, 1980

Reed CE: Physiology and pharmacology of beta$_2$ adrenergic agents. Chest 73(6):914-926, 1978

Snider GL: Control of bronchospasm in patients with chronic obstructive pulmonary diseases. Chest 73(6):927-934, 1978

Tomashefski JF: Symposium: Definition, differentiation and classification of COPD. Postgrad Med J 62(1):88-97, 1977

Unger KM, Moser KM, Hansen P: Selection of an exercise program for patients with chronic obstructive pulmonary disease. Heart Lung 9(1):68-76, 1980

Webb-Johnson DC, Andrews JL: Drug therapy: Bronchodilator therapy (Part I). N Engl J Med 297(9):476-481, 1977

Weiss EB: Bronchial asthma. Clin Symp 27(1, 2), 1975

Pneumonia

Austrian R: Maxwell Finland lecture: Random gleanings from a life with the pneumococcus. J Infect Dis 131(4):474-484, 1975

Davidson M, Tempest B, Palmer D: Bacteriologic diagnosis of acute pneumonia: Comparison of sputum, transtracheal aspirates, and lung aspirates. JAMA 235(2):158-163, 1976

Finland M: Pneumonia and pneumococcal infections, with special reference to pneumococcal pneumonia. Am Rev Respir Dis 120:481-502, 1979

Hendley JO, Sande MA, Stewart PM, Zwaltney JM Jr: Spread of streptococcus pneumoniae in families: I. Carriage rates and distribution of types. J Infect Dis 132(1):55-61, 1975

Kesarwala HH: Pneumonia: A clinical review. J Med Soc NJ 77(1):43-46, 1980

Kilbourn JP: Bacterial flora of the respiratory tract. J Am Med Tech 42:218-226, 1980

Murray BE, Moellering RC: Antimicrobial agents in pulmonary infections. Med Clin North Am 64(3):319-320, 1980

Murray HW, Tuazon C: Atypical pneumonias. Med Clin North Am 64(3):507-527, 1980

Reichman RC, Dolin R: Viral pneumonias. Med Clin North Am 64(3):491-505, 1980

Tuazon C: Gram-positive pneumonias. Med Clin North Am 64(3):343-361, 1980

Weatherstone RM: The pneumonias. Chest Heart Stroke J 3(5):66-70, 1979

Respiratory infections in children

Barker GA: Current management of croup and epiglottitis. Pediatr Clin North Am 26(3):565-579, 1979

Cramblett HG: American Academy of Pediatrics Proceedings: Croup—present-day concept. Pediatrics 25(6):1071-1076, 1980

Cropp GJA: The problem of lung disease in children and adolescents. Am Lung Assoc Bull 62(10):10-14, 1976

Denny FW, Collier AM, Henderson FW, Clyde WA: The epidemiology of bronchitis. Pediatr Res 11:234-236, 1977

Evans HE: Lung Diseases of Children. American Lung Association, 1979

Glezen WP: Pathogenesis of bronchiolitis—epidemiologic considerations. Pediatr Res 11:239-243, 1977

Jones R, Santos JI, Overall JC Jr: Bacterial tracheitis. JAMA 242(8):721-726, 1979

Mendelsohn J: Pediatric respiratory emergencies. Topics Emerg Med 2:25-34, 1980

Organ AE: Lower respiratory tract infection in childhood. Issues Compr Pediatr Nurs 3(2):12-23, 1978

Page HS: Croup and epiglottitis: Sudden trouble for young children. American Lung Association Bulletin 67(2):9-11, 1981

Sims DG: Acute bronchiolitis in infancy. Nurs Times 75:1842-1844, 1979

Taussig LM: Pitfalls in pediatric pulmonary. Emerg Med 12:24-29, 1980

Tuberculosis

Ogasawara FR: A totally new classification of tuberculosis. American Lung Association Bulletin 25, 1975

Ogasawara FR, Popper H, Reichman LB, Zimmerman HJ: Preventive therapy of tuberculosis infection. Am Rev Respir Dis 110(3):59, 1974

Stead WW: Understanding Tuberculosis Today: A Handbook for Patients, 5th ed., 1980

Weg JC: Tuberculosis and Other Mycobacterial Diseases. American Lung Association, 1976

20

Respiratory Failure and Alterations in Oxygen Transport

Without oxygen, the cells soon die. It is a well-known fact that brain cells begin to die within four to six minutes of oxygen deprivation, and cells of other tissues soon after. Although the body is better able to tolerate an accumulation of carbon dioxide, this too can be lethal. Oxygenation of tissues and removal of carbon dioxide require not only an adequately functioning circulatory system, but also lungs capable of gas exchange and red blood cells capable of transporting oxygen to the tissues.

This chapter is divided into three parts: (1) regulation of blood gases, (2) respiratory failure, and (3) disorders of the red blood cells.

:Regulation of Blood Gases

The lungs enable inhaled air to come in close proximity to blood flowing through the pulmonary capillaries so that exchange of gases between the internal environment of the body and the external environment can take place. They thus restore the oxygen content of the arterial blood and remove the carbon dioxide from the venous blood. The red blood cells, in turn, facilitate transport of gases as they move between the lungs and the tissues.

Regulation of Blood Oxygen Levels

Oxygen is transported in two forms—in chemical combination with hemoglobin and physically dissolved in blood plasma. The *partial pressure (PO$_2$)*, or *oxygen tension*, is the level of the *dissolved gas,*[*] much like the dissolved carbon dioxide in a capped bottle of a carbonated soft drink. It is the dissolved form of oxygen that crosses the cell membrane and participates in cell metabolism. Hemoglobin in the red blood cell is the transport vehicle, binding oxygen in the pulmonary capillaries and releasing it into the tissue capillaries. The released oxygen becomes dissolved in the plasma as it moves between the red blood cell and the tissue cells.

Dissolved oxygen

Only about 1% of the oxygen carried in the blood is in the dissolved state, the remainder being carried with the hemoglobin. The amount of oxygen that will dissolve in plasma is determined by two factors: (1) the solubility of oxygen in plasma, and (2) the partial pressure of the gas in the alveoli. The solubility of oxygen in plasma is fixed and is very small. For every *1 mm Hg PO$_2$ present in the alveoli, 0.003 ml of oxygen becomes dissolved in 100 ml of plasma.* This means that at a normal alveolar PO$_2$ of 100 mm

Hg the blood carries only 0.3 ml of dissolved oxygen in every 100 ml of plasma. As will be discussed, this amount is very small when compared with the amount that can be carried in an equal amount of blood when oxygen is attached to hemoglobin.

Although the oxygen carried in plasma is insignificant, as just described, it may be a lifesaving mode of transport in carbon monoxide poisoning when most of the hemoglobin sites are occupied by carbon monoxide and are unavailable for transport of oxygen. The hyperbaric chamber, in which 100% oxygen at high atmospheric pressures is administered to treat certain disorders, increases the amount of oxygen that can be carried in the dissolved state, so that sufficient oxygen may be made available to prevent death of vital structures such as brain cells. The reader may want to calculate the amount of oxygen that can be carried in the plasma when a person breathes 100% oxygen at 3 atmospheres, the pressure frequently employed in hyperbaric chambers.[†]

Hemoglobin transport

In the lung, oxygen moves across the alveolar capillary membrane, through the plasma, and into the red blood cell where it forms a loose and reversible bond with the hemoglobin molecule (Fig. 20-1). In the normal lung, this process is rapid, so that even with a fast heart rate, the hemoglobin is almost completely saturated with oxygen during the short time that it spends in the pulmonary capillary bed. A small amount of unoxygenated blood from the bronchial circulation is mixed with the oxygenated blood in the pulmonary veins and as a result, the hemoglobin is only about 95 to 97% saturated as it moves into the arterial circulation.

Hemoglobin is a highly efficient carrier of oxygen, and approximately 98 to 99% of the oxygen used by body tissues is carried in this manner. *Each gram of hemoglobin is capable of carrying about 1.34 ml of oxygen when completely saturated.* This means that a person with a hemoglobin of 14 gm per 100 ml of

---

[*]The partial pressure of oxygen in arterial blood is usually designated by PaO$_2$, and the partial pressure in venous blood by PvO$_2$. The pressure of gas in the alveoli is designated by P$_A$O$_2$. In this discussion PO$_2$ is the designation for partial pressure.

[†]2280 (760 mm Hg × 3 atmospheres) × 0.003 (solubility of O$_2$ in plasma) = 6.8 ml/100 ml of plasma. The actual value would be slightly less than this, since the calculation does not take into account the partial pressure of carbon dioxide or water vapor pressure in the alveoli.

blood carries 18.8 ml of oxygen in each 100 ml of blood in the form of oxyhemoglobin.

The oxygenated hemoglobin is transported in the arterial blood to the peripheral capillaries where the oxygen is released and made available to the tissues for use in cell metabolism (Fig. 20-1). As the oxygen moves out of the capillaries in response to the needs of the tissues, the hemoglobin saturation, which was about 95 to 97% as the blood left the left heart, drops to about 75% as the mixed venous blood returns to the right heart.

Oxygen-hemoglobin dissociation

Oxygen that remains bound to hemoglobin cannot participate in tissue metabolism. The efficiency of the oxygen transport system is dependent upon the ability of the hemoglobin molecule to bind oxygen in the lung and release it on demand. The affinity of hemoglobin refers to its capacity to bind oxygen, thus, when affinity is increased, the hemoglobin binds oxygen readily, and when decreased, it releases oxygen.

Hemoglobin is made up of *four polypeptide chains* (the globin portion). Each of the polypeptide chains is covalently bonded with *heme* (a protoporphyrin molecule that contains iron). There are four binding sites for oxygen on a hemoglobin unit since each of the chains has one heme group. Each hemoglobin unit has two types of chains which are *genetically* determined. Normal "adult" hemoglobin has two α chains and two β chains ($\alpha_2\beta_2$). Fetal hemoglobin has two α chains and two v chains (α_2v_2). This increases oxygen affinity and facilitates transfer of oxygen across the placenta. The heme-heme interactions of the two types of chains ($\alpha_2\beta_2$) account for the normal oxygen-carrying capacity of hemoglobin. As will be discussed, sickle cell hemoglobin has a different amino acid substituted into the β chain and it is this that causes the deoxygenated hemoglobin molecule (hemoglobin with oxygen removed) to form a crescent or "sickle" shape.

Hemoglobin's affinity for oxygen is influenced by *p*H, in that it binds oxygen under alkaline conditions and releases it under acid conditions. Carbon dioxide moves out of the blood in the lungs, raising

Figure 20–1.   Transport of oxygen by the red blood cell. In (*A*) oxygen moves from the alveoli to the hemoglobin, and carbon dioxide moves from the red cell to the alveoli. In (*B*) oxygen moves from the red blood cell to the capillary fluid and then into the interstitial fluid where it becomes available to the cell, while carbon dioxide moves in the opposite direction.

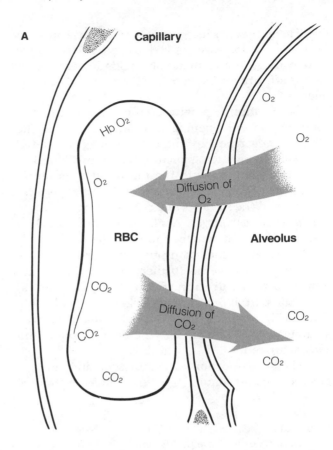

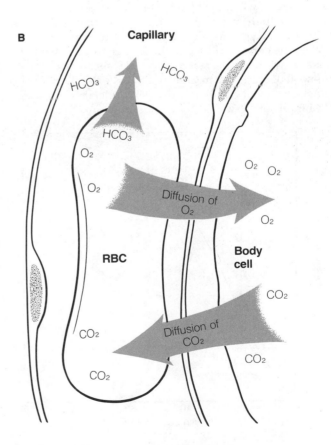

the pH and thereby increasing the oxygen affinity. In the tissues, a decrease in pH due to cellular release of carbon dioxide and metabolic acids lowers hemoglobin affinity for oxygen and thereby enhances its release.

The relationship between the oxygen carried in combination with hemoglobin and the PO_2 of the blood is described by the *oxygen-hemoglobin dissociation curve* which is pictured in Figure 20-2. The curve is S-shaped, with the top *flat portion* representing the binding of oxygen to the *hemoglobin in the lung* and the *steep portion* representing its *release into the tissue capillaries*. At about 100 mm Hg PO_2, a plateau occurs at which point the hemoglobin is 100% saturated. Increasing the alveolar PO_2 above this level will have no further effect in increasing hemoglobin saturation. Even at high altitudes, when the partial pressure of oxygen is considerably decreased, the hemoglobin remains relatively well saturated. At 60 mm Hg PO_2 the hemoglobin is still 89% saturated.

The steep portion of the dissociation curve—between 60 and 40 mm Hg—represents the removal

Figure 20–2.   Graph showing the oxygen hemoglobin dissociation curve. Note that when the carbon dioxide is increased or when the blood pH is decreased, the curve is shifted to the right, and therefore the hemoglobin binds less oxygen for any partial pressure of oxygen. When the curve is shifted to the left, as occurs when the carbon dioxide is decreased or the pH is increased, the opposite occurs. (From Chaffee EE, Lytle IM: Basic Physiology and Anatomy, 4th ed. Philadelphia, JB Lippincott, 1980)

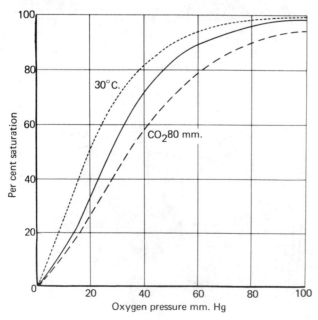

of oxygen from the hemoglobin as it moves through the tissue capillaries. This portion of the curve is of great importance for it permits considerable transfer of oxygen from hemoglobin to the tissues with only a small drop in oxygen tension. Normally the tissues remove about 5 ml of oxygen per 100 ml of blood, and the hemoglobin of mixed venous blood as it returns to the right heart is about 75% saturated (PO_2 40 mm Hg). In this portion of the dissociation curve, the rate at which oxygen is released from the hemoglobin is largely determined by tissue utilization. During heavy exercise, for example, the muscle cells may remove as much as 15 ml of oxygen per 100 ml of blood from the hemoglobin.

Hemoglobin can be regarded as an "oxygen buffer" system that regulates oxygen pressure in the tissues. Thus, hemoglobin affinity for oxygen must change with the metabolic needs of the tissues. This change is represented by a *shift* in the dissociation curve to the *right* or the *left*, as pictured in Figure 20-2.

As the curve shifts to the right, the tissue PO_2 is greater for any given level of hemoglobin saturation. A shift to the right is usually caused by conditions such as fever, acidosis, or an increase in PCO_2, which reflects increased tissue metabolism. Hypoxia also causes the dissociation curve to shift to the right. The red blood cells, unlike other tissues, contain high levels of the glycolytic intermediate 2,3-diphosphoglycerate (2,3-DPG), the levels of which increase during hypoxia; this reduces hemoglobin affinity for oxygen and favors its release to the tissues. A shift to the right due to an increase in 2,3-DPG occurs in various conditions of hypoxia, including those resulting from high altitude, pulmonary insufficiency, heart failure, and severe anemia.

A shift to the left of the dissociation curve represents an enhanced affinity of hemoglobin for oxygen and occurs in situations associated with a decrease in tissue metabolism, such as alkalosis, decreased body temperature, and decreased carbon dioxide levels. The degree of change in affinity is indicated by the P_{50}, or the *partial pressure of oxygen that is needed to achieve a 50% saturation of hemoglobin*. Returning to Figure 20-2, the reader will note that the dissociation curve on the left has a P_{50} of about 20 mm Hg; the normal curve, a P_{50} of 26; and the curve on the right, a P_{50} 35 mm Hg.

Cyanosis
Reduced hemoglobin—hemoglobin from which the oxygen has been removed—is purple. *Cyanosis* is the *purplish discoloration* of the skin, nailbeds, and

mucous membranes due to the presence of excessive reduced hemoglobin in the superficial capillaries. Cyanosis does not occur until there is at least *5 gm of reduced hemoglobin per 100 ml of blood* in these capillaries. The appearance of cyanosis depends on the thickness and pigment of the skin, the peripheral blood flow, and the amount of hemoglobin present. Consequently, cyanosis is not always a sensitive index of hypoxia. It is difficult to detect in persons with dark skin. Cyanosis is deceiving; it can occur when there is a local decrease in blood flow and does not necessarily reflect the oxygen content of blood flow in other parts of the body. For example, it is common for the fingers to turn blue during cold exposure. This is because of sluggish blood flow with increased extraction of oxygen from the blood as it flows through the superficial vessels. Since cyanosis appears when there is 5 gm of reduced hemoglobin in 100 ml of blood, a person with polycythemia, an excess of red blood cells, may easily carry 5 gm reduced hemoglobin per 100 ml of blood without evidence of hypoxemia. A person with anemia, on the other hand, may not have sufficient hemoglobin so that 5 gm per 100 ml can be present in the reduced state; in this case the person will be hypoxic but not cyanotic. The undersurface of the tongue is a reliable area to check for central cyanosis due to heart or lung disease[1] (cyanosis due to abnormal peripheral circulation does not occur here).

Carbon Dioxide Transport

Carbon dioxide is a by-product of tissue metabolism. It is transported in the blood in three forms— *attached to hemoglobin, as dissolved carbon dioxide,* and *as bicarbonate*. It is carried in the form of carbaminohemoglobin attached to reduced hemoglobin. Carbon dioxide is much more soluble in plasma than oxygen and, as a result, larger quantities are carried in the extracellular fluid as bicarbonate (60 to 70%) and in the dissolved form (about 10%). The remainder of the carbon dioxide is transported as carbaminohemoglobin. How dissolved carbon dioxide and bicarbonate influences acid–base balance is discussed in Chapter 23.

Blood Gases

To accurately measure blood gases, arterial blood is required. Venous blood is not used because venous levels of oxygen and carbon dioxide reflect the metabolic requirements of the tissues rather than the gas exchange properties of the lungs. The PO_2 of arterial blood is normally above 80 mm Hg, and the PCO_2 in the range of 35 to 45 mm Hg.

In summary, oxygen and carbon dioxide rely on the lungs for exchange with the external environment and on the blood for transport between the lungs and the tissues. Oxygen is transported in two forms—dissolved in the plasma and attached to hemoglobin. Hemoglobin is an efficient carrier of oxygen, and about 98 to 99% of oxygen is transported in this manner. Carbon dioxide is carried in three forms—as carbaminohemoglobin, dissolved carbon dioxide, and bicarbonate. Seventy to eighty percent of carbon dioxide in the plasma is in bicarbonate or dissolved form.

:Respiratory Failure

Respiratory insufficiency is a condition in which respiratory function is inadequate to meet body needs during exertion. Respiratory failure occurs when the lungs are unable to adequately oxygenate the blood and/or prevent undue retention of carbon dioxide, even at rest. Respiratory failure can develop acutely in persons whose lungs previously had been normal, or may be superimposed on chronic disease of the lung or chest wall. It has been reported that obstructive lung disease accounts for about one-third of the cases of acute respiratory failure in intensive care units.[2]

As a general rule, respiratory failure refers to a PO_2 level of 50 mm Hg or less, and hypercarbia (hypercapnia) to a PCO_2 level greater than 50 mm Hg. These values are not altogether reliable when dealing with persons who have chronic lung disease, because many of these persons are alert and functioning with blood gas levels within the abnormal range. Table 20-1 compares the normal values for blood gases with those of respiratory failure.

Causes

Respiratory failure is not a specific disease. It is associated with a number of disorders in which the lungs fail to deliver sufficient oxygen to the arterial blood or to remove sufficient carbon dioxide. These conditions include impaired ventilation due to up-

Table 20-1   Blood Gases in Respiratory Failure as Compared With Normal Values

Arterial Blood Gas Value	Normal Value	Respiratory Failure
PO_2	above 80 mm Hg	50 mm Hg or less
PCO_2	35 to 45 mm Hg	50 mm Hg or above

per airway obstruction, weakness or paralysis of the respiratory muscles, chest wall injury, and disease of the pulmonary airways and lungs. Respiratory failure can also arise when diffusion of gases across the alveolar capillary membrane is impeded. The causes of respiratory failure are summarized in Table 20-2; many are discussed in other parts of the text.

Manifestations

Respiratory failure may be seen in previously healthy persons as the result of acute disease or trauma involving the respiratory system, or may develop in the course of a chronic respiratory disease. The presenting signs and symptoms are different in each of these situations. The common manifestations of respiratory failure are *hypoxemia* and *hypercarbia*.

Hypoxemia. In hypoxemia blood oxygen levels are insufficient to meet oxidative requirements. Signs and symptoms can be divided into two groups (see p. 267). First are the compensatory mechanisms such as those caused by activation of the sympathetic nervous system. These include tachycardia, anxiety, peripheral vasoconstriction, diaphoresis, and a mild increase in blood pressure. Those in the second group are caused by nervous system hypoxia and somewhat resemble alcohol intoxication—for example, muscular incoordination, euphoria, loss of judgment, extreme restlessness, delirium, and eventually coma. The signs and symptoms of hypoxemia are listed in the chart on page 267. Although there may be cyanosis, it is not usually a reliable sign.

Hypoxemia may be insidious in onset and its symptoms may be attributed to other causes, particularly in chronic lung disease. It has been my observation that decreased sensory function, such as impaired vision or fewer complaints of pain, is often an early sign of hypoxia. This is probably because the involved neurons have the same need for high levels of oxygen as do other parts of the nervous system. In one case, that of an elderly man with chronic lung disease who was hospitalized for a respiratory tract infection, the earliest signs of hypoxia were impaired vision and muscle incoordination. These gave rise to difficulty in reading his mail and in feeding himself. Although he had been able to read the fine print in the newspapers (when wearing his glasses) upon admission to the hospital, the restlessness and anxiety following the early visual problems were attributed to his concern over his eyesight; a tranquilizer was prescribed and it was

Table 20–2 Causes of Respiratory Failure

Category of Impairment	Examples
Impaired Ventilation	
Upper airway obstruction	Laryngospasm
	Foreign body aspiration
	Tumor of the upper airways
	Infection of the upper airways (e.g., epiglottitis)
Weakness or paralysis of the respiratory muscles	
	Drug overdose
	Injury to the spinal cord
	Poliomyelitis
	Guillain-Barré syndrome
	Muscular dystrophy
	Disease of the brain stem
Chest wall injury	Rib fracture
	Burn eschar
Disease of the lower airways and lungs	Chronic obstructive lung disease
	Restrictive lung disease
	Severe pneumonia
	Atelectasis
Impaired Diffusion	
Pulmonary edema	Left heart failure
	Inhalation of toxic materials
Respiratory distress syndrome	Respiratory distress syndrome in the newborn
	Adult respiratory distress syndrome (shock lung)

Signs and Symptoms of Hypoxemia

Arterial blood gas levels below 50 mm Hg

Tachycardia

Mild increase in blood pressure

Diaphoresis

Confusion

Delirium

Difficulty in problem solving

Loss of judgment

Euphoria

Sensory impairment

Mental fatigue

Drowsiness

Stupor and coma (late)

Hypotension (late)

Bradycardia (late)

suggested that he might need new glasses when he left the hospital. It was not until after he had lapsed into coma that the severity of the hypoxia was fully appreciated.

Hypercarbia.   Carbon dioxide has a direct vasodilatory effect on many blood vessels and a sedative effect on the nervous system. When the cerebral vessels are dilated, headache will develop. The conjunctiva are hyperemic and the skin flushed. Hypercarbia has nervous system effects similar to those of an anesthetic—hence the term "carbon dioxide narcosis." There is progressive somnolence, disorientation and, if untreated, coma. Mild to moderate increases in blood pressure are common. The signs and symptoms of hypercarbia are summarized in the chart below. The body adapts to chronic increases in

Signs and Symptoms of Hypercarbia

Headache

Conjunctival hyperemia

Flushed skin

Increased sedation

Drowsiness

Disorientation

Coma

Tachycardia

Diaphoresis

Mild to moderate increase in blood pressure

blood levels of carbon dioxide, hence persons with chronic hypercarbia may not develop symptoms until the PCO_2 is markedly elevated. Elevated levels of PCO_2 are characterized by respiratory acidosis, discussed in Chapter 23.

Treatment

Treatment of respiratory failure is directed toward correcting the cause and relieving the hypoxemia and hypercarbia, and for this purpose a number of treatment modalities are available, including establishment of an airway, use of bronchodilators, antibiotics for respiratory infections and others. Controlled oxygen therapy and mechanical ventilation are measures that are used in treating blood gas abnormalities associated with respiratory failure.

Oxygen therapy.   Oxygen may be given by nasal cannula, catheter, Venturi mask, and mask–bag combination. The oxygen must be humidified as it is being administered. The flow rate (liters per minute) is based on the arterial PO_2. The rate must be carefully monitored in persons with chronic lung disease because marked increases in PO_2 (above 60 mm Hg) are apt to depress the ventilatory drive. There is also danger of oxygen toxicity with high concentrations of oxygen. Continuous breathing of high concentrations can lead to diffuse parenchymal lung injury. Persons with normal lungs begin to experience respiratory symptoms ranging from substernal distress to paresthesias, nausea and vomiting, general malaise, and fatigue after breathing 100% oxygen (at 1 atmosphere) for 6 to 30 hours.[3]

Mechanical ventilation.   Should oxygen therapy and other conservative methods prove ineffective, in situations where the PO_2 cannot be maintained at 50 mm Hg and respiratory acidosis is out of control, use of a mechanical ventilator may be a life-saving measure. Mechanical ventilators are of two types—pressure-controlled units and volume-controlled units. The pressure-controlled ventilator delivers a tidal volume determined by the airway pressure while the flow rate is being controlled. The volume-controlled ventilator delivers a preselected tidal volume while the pressure is monitored. The tidal volume and respiratory rate are adjusted to maintain ventilation at a given minute volume. A nasotracheal, orotracheal, or tracheotomy tube is inserted into the trachea to provide the patient with the airway needed for mechanical ventilation.

In summary, respiratory failure is a condition in which the lungs fail to adequately oxygenate the blood or prevent undue retention of carbon dioxide. The causes of *respiratory failure are many: it may arise acutely in persons with previously healthy lungs or may be super-imposed in chronic lung disease. It is generally defined as a PO_2 of 50 mm Hg or less and a PCO_2 of 50 mm Hg or more. Hypoxemia incites sympathetic nervous system responses such as tachycardia and produces symptoms similar to those of alcohol intoxication. Hypercarbia causes vasodilatation of blood vessels, including those in the brain, and has an anesthetic effect (carbon dioxide narcosis).*

:Alterations in Red Blood Cells

Although the lungs provide the means for gas exchange between the external and internal environments, it is the hemoglobin in the red blood cells that transports oxygen to the tissues. The red blood cells also function as carriers of carbon dioxide and participate in acid–base balance (Chapter 23). In this section, the structure and function of the red blood cell are discussed. Anemia and polycythemia, two important disorders of red cell function, are also presented.

Structure of the Red Blood Cell

The mature red blood cell is called an *erythrocyte*. Red cells are concave, spherical disks (Fig.20-3). This shape serves to increase the surface area available for

Figure 20–3.   Scanning micrograph of normal red blood cells (X 5000). The normal concave disk appearance of these cells is apparent. (Courtesy of STEM Laboratories and Fischer Scientific Company)

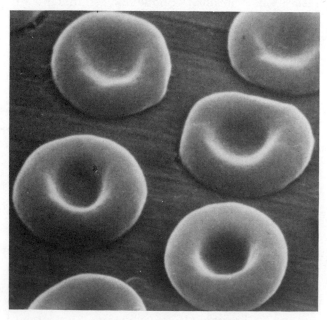

diffusion of oxygen and allows for changes in cell volume and shape without rupturing its membrane.

Red Blood Cell Production and Its Regulation

Erythropoiesis is the production of red blood cells. After birth, the red cells are produced in the red bone marrow. Until the age of five years, almost all bones produce red cells to meet growth needs. Following this period, there is a gradual decline in bone marrow activity, and after age 20, red cell production takes place mainly in the membranous bones of the vertebrae, sternum, ribs, and pelvis. With this lessened activity, the red bone marrow is replaced with fatty yellow bone marrow.

The red cells derive from the erythroblasts, which are continously being formed from the primordial stem cells in the bone marrow. In developing into a mature red cell, the primordial stem cell moves through a series of stages—*erythroblast* to *normoblast* to *reticulocyte*, and finally to *erythrocyte* (Fig. 20-4). Hemoglobin synthesis begins at the erythroblast stage and continues until the cell becomes an erythrocyte. During its transformation from normoblast to reticulocyte, the red blood cell loses its nucleus. Maturation of reticulocyte to an erythrocyte takes about 24 to 48 hours, and during this process the red cell loses its mitochondria and ribosomes along with its ability to produce hemoglobin and engage in oxidative metabolism. Most maturing red cells enter the blood as reticulocytes. Normally about 1% of the red blood cells are generated from bone marrow each day, and therefore the reticulocyte count serves as an index of the erythropoietic activity of the bone marrow.

Erythropoiesis is determined for the most part by tissue oxygen needs. *Hypoxia* is the main *stimulus* for red cell production. Hypoxia does not, however, act directly on the bone marrow. Instead, red cell production by the bone marrow is regulated by *erythropoietin*, sometimes called the erythropoietic factor. Erythropoietin, a glycoprotein with a molecular weight of 39,000 to 70,000, is released in response to hypoxia, although the precise mechanism of erythropoietin formation is unclear. It is known that erythropoietin levels are lower in persons with impaired kidney function and in those who have had a kidney removed. It is thought that the kidney, when exposed to hypoxia, releases an enzyme—renal erythropoietic factor—which converts a circulating plasma protein into erythropoietin.

It takes several days for erythropoietin to effect release of red blood cells from the bone marrow, and it is only after 5 or more days that red blood cell production reaches maximum. Since red blood cells are released into the blood as reticulocytes, the percentage of these cells in relation to the total red blood cell count is higher when there is a marked increase in red blood cell production. In some severe anemias, for example, the reticulocytes may account for as much as 30 to 50% of the total.[4] There are some situations where red cell production is so accelerated that numerous normoblasts appear in the blood.

The Lifespan of the Red Blood Cell

The red blood cells have a lifespan of about 4 months or 120 days. As the red blood cell ages, a number of changes occur. The metabolic activities within the cell decrease; enzyme activity falls off; and there is a decrease in ATP, potassium, and membrane lipids. Normally the rate of red cell destruction (1% per day) is equal to red cell production, but in some conditions, such as hemolytic anemia, the cell's lifespan may be shorter.

Laboratory Tests

The red cells can be studied by means of a sample of blood (Table 20-3). The *red blood cell count (RBC)* measures the *total number* of RBC in a cubic millimeter of blood. The *percentage of reticulocytes* (normally about 1%) provides an index of the rate of red cell production. The *hemoglobin* (grams per 100 ml of blood) measures the *hemoglobin content* of the blood. The major components of the blood are the red cell mass and plasma volume. The *hematocrit* measures the volume of red cell mass in 100 ml of plasma volume. To determine the hematocrit, a sample of blood is placed in a glass tube, which is then cen-

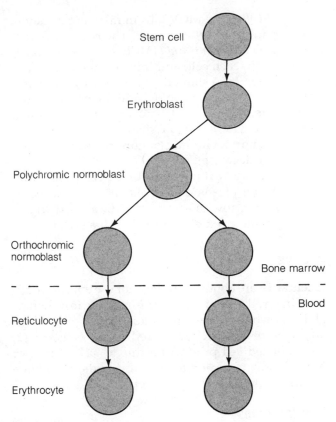

Figure 20–4. Diagram showing the red blood cell development.

trifuged to separate the cells and the plasma. The hematocrit may be deceptive, since it varies with the quantity of extracellular fluid present, rising with dehydration and falling with overexpansion of the extracellular fluid volume.

The word *corpuscle* means little body. The *mean corpuscular volume (MCV)* reflects the *volume or size*

Table 20-3 Standard Laboratory Values for Red Blood Cells

Test	Normal Values	Significance
Red blood cell count (RBC)		
Men	4.2 to 5.4 million/cu m	The number of red cells in the blood
Women	3.6 to 5 million/cu m	
Reticulocytes	0.1% to 1.5% of total RBC	Rate of red cell production
Hemoglobin (Hgb)		
Men	14 to 16.5 gm/100 ml	The hemoglobin content of the blood
Women	12 to 15 gm/100 ml	
Hematocrit (Hct)		
Men	40 to 50/100 ml	The volume of cells in 100 ml of blood
Women	37 to 47/100 ml	
Mean corpuscular volume (MCV)	85 to 100 cu U	Size of the red cell
Mean corpuscular hemoglobin concentration (MCHC)	31 to 35 gm/100 ml	Amount of hemoglobin in the red cell

of the red cells. The MCV falls in microcytic anemia and rises in macrocytic anemia. The *mean corpuscular hemoglobin concentration (MCHC)* is the *amount of hemoglobin* in each cell, and it is decreased in hypochromic anemia. A stained red cell study gives information about the size, color, and shape of the red blood cells. They may be normocytic (of normal size), microcytic (of small size), or macrocytic (of large size); normochromic (of normal color) or hypochromic (of decreased color).

Bone marrow function in blood cell production is studied by means of the *bone marrow smear*, in which the marrow is aspirated with a short, rigid, sharp-pointed needle equipped with a stylet.

Anemia

Anemia is an abnormally low total number of circulating red blood cells, abnormally low hemoglobin, or both. In anemia, there may be (1) excessive loss or destruction of red blood cells, or (2) deficient red cell production due to lack of iron or other elements related to erythropoiesis, or to bone marrow failure.

Manifestations

Anemia interferes with oxygen transport to the tissues and, unlike respiratory failure, causes hypoxia but not hypercarbia. Its effects on body function depend significantly on its severity and its rapidity of development. In anemia due to acute hemorrhage, there may be circulatory collapse with a 30% decrease in red cell mass.[5] On the other hand, the body tends to adapt to slowly developing anemia, and the loss of red cell mass may be considerable yet without signs and symptoms.

The signs and symptoms of anemia include those of any underlying disorder and those due to the anemia itself. Lack of red cells in the superficial vessels causes pallor of the skin, mucous membranes, conjunctiva, skin folds, and nail beds. In extreme cases the skin may appear yellow due to lack of reddish pigment. Decreased oxygen transport gives rise to fatigue, syncope, dyspnea, angina, and organ dysfunction. The body tries to compensate by increasing cardiac output; but this can cause palpitations, wide pulse pressure, and heart murmurs. Anemia is more serious in persons with other pathology, such as heart disease.

Excessive red cell losses

Increased red cell loss is due to one of two causes—bleeding, acute or chronic, in which iron and other components of the erythrocyte are lost; and hemo-

lysis (breakdown) of cells within the body, with retention of iron and other blood components.

Blood loss. Blood loss can be acute or chronic. In the *acute form*, there is risk of hypovolemia and shock, rather than anemia. The red cells are normal, but movement of fluid into the vascular compartment causes hemodilution and a fall in the red blood cell count and hemoglobin. The hypoxia due to blood loss stimulates red cell production by the bone marrow. If iron stores are normal, the red cells that were lost are soon replaced. *Chronic blood loss* does not affect blood volume, but rather leads to iron deficiency anemia (discussed later).

Hemolysis (abnormal destruction). By abnormal destruction is meant the destruction due to damage to the cell membrane or to the presence of abnormal hemoglobin, as in sickle cell disease. Unlike anemia due to red blood loss, in hemolytic anemia the destroyed red cell and its iron are retained in the body. The bile pigment *bilirubin* is formed as the hemoglobin molecule is broken down. The liver removes bilirubin from the blood. When the rate of red cell destruction is abnormally high, bilirubin may accumulate in the blood causing *jaundice*, a yellowish discoloration of the skin. In continued hemolytic anemia, there will be hyperplasia of bone marrow as the body attempts to retain the red cells. As a result, the number of reticulocytes in the blood rises.

Hemolysis of red cells due to *damage to the red cell membrane* can be caused by mechanical destruction of red cells such as that imposed by prosthetic cardiac ball valves, hereditary abnormalities of red cell membrane (hereditary spherocytosis or congenital hemolytic anemia), or immune mechanisms. The *Coombs' test* detects the presence of immune globulins (or complement) on the surface of the red cell. A *direct Coombs' test* detects the antibody on red blood cells. In this test red cells, which have been washed free of serum, are mixed with Coombs' antiserum. The red cells will agglutinate if the specific immune globulins or other proteins attach to the red cell membrane. The direct Coombs is positive in autoimmune hemolytic anemia, erythroblastosis fetalis (Rh disease of the newborn), transfusion reactions, and following exposure to certain drugs such as large doses of penicillin, cephalothin, and the antihypertensive drug alpha-methyldopa. The *indirect Coombs' test* detects the presence of antibody in the serum, and is positive in the presence of specific antibodies resulting from previous transfusions or pregnancy.

Sickle cell anemia is largely a disease of blacks, affecting approximately 50,000 Americans, and can present as either sickle cell trait (heterozygote) or sickle cell disease (homozygote). About one out of every ten black Americans is estimated to carry the trait.[6] In sickle cell anemia, there is a defect of the β-chain of the hemoglobin molecule, with an abnormal substitution of a single amino acid. Sickle hemoglobin (HbS) is inherited as a recessive trait. In the heterozygote only about 40% of the hemoglobin is HgS, whereas in the homozygote almost all of the hemoglobin is HbS. Sickle cell trait is not a mild form of sickle cell anemia, although in severe hypoxia, persons with sickle cell trait may experience some sickling.

In the homozygote, the HbS becomes sickled when deoxygenated. These deformed red blood cells obstruct blood flow in the microcirculation. In order for sickling to occur, one HbS molecule must interact with another HbS molecule. Thus the person with sickle cell trait who has 60% HbA has little tendency to sickle except in hypoxia. Fetal hemoglobin does not interact with HbS and therefore the child with sickle cell anemia does not usually begin to experience the effects of the sickling until sometime after 4 to 6 months of age when the fetal hemoglobin has been replaced by HbS.

Factors which precipitate sickling are exertion, infection, other illnesses, hypoxia, acidosis, dehydration, or even such trivial incidents as reduced oxygen tension induced by sleep. Hardly an organ is spared in sickle cell anemia. Affected persons develop severe anemia, painful crises, organ damage, and chronic hyperbilirubinemia. A painful crisis results from vessel occlusion and can appear suddenly in almost any part of the body. The common sites are the abdomen, the chest, and the joints. Infarctions due to sluggish blood flow may cause chronic damage to the liver, spleen, heart, kidney, and other organs. The hyperbilirubinemia often leads to production of pigment stones in the gall bladder.

At present, there is no known cure or therapeutic regimen that prevents the problems associated with sickle cell anemia, and treatment is largely supportive. There is an emphasis on avoiding situations that precipitate sickling episodes, such as infections, cold exposure, severe physical exertion, acidosis, and dehydration. Genetic counseling may be of value in family planning.

The *thalassemias* are inherited disorders of synthesis of either the α or β-chains of hemoglobin A, as an autosomal dominant trait. A person may be heterozygous for the trait and have a mild type of thalassemia or be homozygous and have the full-blown disease. The deficit of HbA may range from mild to severe, and with a microcytic, hypochromic anemia. Along with the HbA deficiency, there is abnormally high production of the HbB chain, leading to the precipitation of aggregates (Heinz bodies) within the red cell. In some way, these aggregates damage the red cell membrane, causing hemolysis.

The survival of children with homozygous β-thalassemia depends on blood transfusions. Two types of α thalassemia predominate. In one, hemoglobin Bart's syndrome (hydrops fetalis), synthesis of α chains is absent, so the hemoglobin in affected babies does not release oxygen, and the babies are either stillborn or die soon after birth. The other type, H hemoglobin disease, is less severe, and affected persons often live a relatively normal life, requiring transfusions intermittently.

Deficient red cell production
Production of red cells or hemoglobin can be abnormally low due to iron deficiency, vitamin B_{12} deficiency, folic acid deficiency, or impaired bone marrow function.

Iron deficiency anemia. In iron deficiency anemia there is a decrease in serum iron. The red cells are also decreased, and are microcytic, hypochromic, and often malformed in shape (poikilocytosis). Membrane changes may predispose to hemolysis, causing further loss of red cells.

Body iron is repeatedly reused. When red cells become senescent and are broken down, their iron is released and reused in the production of new red cells. The normal diet contains about 12 to 15 mg iron of which normally only 5% to 10% is absorbed. In iron deficiency, the absorption increases. Normally, less than 1 mg iron is lost from the body daily. About 30% of body iron is stored in the bone marrow, the spleen, muscle, and other organs; the remainder is present in the form of hemoglobin.

In the adult, a blood loss of 2 to 4 ml per day is the usual reason for an iron deficiency.[7] This blood loss may be due to gastrointestinal bleeding, such as occurs with peptic ulcer, intestinal polyps, hemorrhoids, or malignancy. Excessive aspirin intake may cause undetected gastrointestinal bleeding. In women, blood is lost during menstruation. Each milliliter of blood contains 0.5 mg iron, and the average menstrual flow is about 44 ml, with a loss of 22 mg of iron.[7] Although cessation of menstruation spares iron loss in the pregnant woman, iron requirements increase at this time; expansion of the mother's blood volume requires about 480 mg of additional iron, and the growing fetus, about 390 mg.[7]

A child's growth places extra demands on the body: blood volume increases, with a greater need for iron. Iron requirements are proportionally higher in infancy (3 to 24 months) than at any other age, though childhood and adolescence also bring higher requirements.

The signs and symptoms of iron deficiency anemia are related to the cause and impairment of oxygen transport and lack of hemoglobin. Dependent upon its severity, there may be fatigability, palpitations, dyspnea, angina, and tachycardia. Late signs are waxy pallor, brittle hair and nails, smooth tongue, and sores in the corners of the mouth. A poorly understood symptom is pica, the bizarre compulsive eating of ice or dirt, that sometimes is seen. Also there may be extreme dysphagia.

The treatment of iron deficiency anemia is directed toward controlling chronic blood loss, increasing dietary intake of iron, and administering supplemental iron. Parenteral iron may be given if oral forms are not tolerated. Special care is required when administering an iron preparation (Imferon) intramuscularly; it must be injected deeply by pulling the skin to one side before inserting the needle (Z track) to prevent leakage, with skin discoloration.

Megaloblastic anemias. Megaloblastic anemias are characterized by a mean corpuscular volume above 100, with increase in red cell size due to abnormalities of maturation in the bone marrow. There may be a vitamin B_{12} deficiency (pernicious anemia) or a folic acid deficiency. (One form of megaloblastic anemia, unresponsive to either vitamin B_{12} or folic acid therapy, is not discussed here.) Because megaloblastic anemias develop slowly, there are often few symptoms until the anemia is far advanced.

Vitamin B_{12} (*cyanocobalamin*) is an essential nutrient, required for synthesis of DNA; when it is deficient, there is failure of nuclear maturation and cell division, especially of the rapidly proliferating red cells. Moreover, when B_{12} is deficient, the red cells that are produced are abnormally large, have flimsy membranes, and are oval in shape rather than being of the normal biconcave disk shape. The resulting condition is called pernicious anemia. These odd-shaped cells have a short life span that can be measured in weeks rather than months. Pernicious anemia is also accompanied by neurologic changes in which degeneration of the dorsal and lateral columns of the spinal cord causes symmetrical paresthesias of the feet and fingers, which eventually progress to spastic ataxia.

Absorption of vitamin B_{12} in the intestine re-quires the presence of *intrinsic factor*, which is produced by the gastric mucosa. Intrinsic factor binds to vitamin B_{12} in food and protects it from the enzymatic actions of the gut. As discussed in Chapter 37, production of intrinsic factor is impaired in chronic gastritis (in which there are atrophic changes in the gastric mucosa) and following total removal of the stomach. Treatment consists of intramuscular injections of vitamin B_{12}.

Folic acid is also required for red cell maturation, and its deficiency produces the same type of red cell changes that occur in pernicious anemia. Folic acid deficiency does not, however, induce the neurologic manifestations that are seen in pernicious anemia. Folic acid is readily absorbed from the intestine. It is found in vegetables (particularly the green leafy types), fruits, cereals, and meats. However, much of the vitamin is lost in cooking. The most common cause of a folic acid deficiency is malnutrition, especially in association with alcoholism, and it is also seen with malabsorption syndromes, such as sprue. Pregnancy increases the need for folic acid by five to ten times, so that a deficiency can occur at this time. Poor dietary habits, anorexia, and nausea are other reasons for a folic acid deficiency during pregnancy. Several groups of drugs may contribute to a deficiency, also. Primidone, phenytoin, and phenobarbital—drugs used to treat seizure disorders—predispose to a deficiency by interfering with its absorption. Triamterene (a diuretic) and methotrexate (a folic acid analogue used in treatment of cancer) are other drugs that impair the action of folic acid by blocking its conversion to the active form.

Bone marrow depression

Bone marrow depression or failure usually is an outcome of stem cell dysfunction with failure to produce leukocytes and thrombocytes, as well as erythrocytes. True red cell aplasia can occur, but is rare. *Aplastic* refers to a failure to grow or develop, and it describes this type of anemia. In aplastic anemia the senescent (old) red cells that are destroyed and leave the circulation are not replaced. With aplastic anemia, there is failure to replace the senescent red cells that are destroyed and leave the circulation, although the cells that remain are of normal size and color. At the same time, because the leukocytes, particularly the neutrophils, and the thrombocytes have a short life span, a deficiency of these cells usually is apparent before the anemia becomes severe.

Aplastic anemia can occur at any age. It may be insidious in onset, or it may strike with suddenness and great severity. There is weakness, fatigability, and pallor. Thrombocytopenia (decrease in the number of platelets) develops and leads to purpura; and the decrease in neutrophils increases susceptibility to infection.

Among the causes of bone marrow depression are exposure to radiation, infections, and chemical agents that are toxic to bone marrow. The best-documented of the identified toxic agents are benzene, the antibiotic chloramphenicol, and the alkylating agents and antimetabolites used in the treatment of cancer (Chap. 7). Bone marrow depression due to exposure to a chemical agent may sometimes be an idiosyncratic reaction, that is, it affects only certain susceptible persons. Such reactions are often severe, and sometimes irreversible and fatal. Although aplastic anemia can develop in the course of many infections, it is seen most often in viral hepatitis and miliary tuberculosis. In about half the cases there is no known cause, and these are termed "idiopathic aplastic anemia."[8]

The treatment of aplastic anemia includes avoidance of the offending agent and prevention of infection and trauma. Deficient blood cells may be replaced by transfusions. Transplantation of bone marrow is a relatively recent procedure, and may be tried in selected cases. In radiation and many drug-

induced aplastic anemias, there is gradual recovery of bone marrow function once the offending agent has been discontinued.

Transfusion therapy

Transfusion therapy provides the means for (1) replacing deficient red cell mass in the blood and thereby improving oxygen transport and (2) volume replacement. It consists of the transfusion of whole blood or one of its components. In modern blood banking, only the needed components are administered rather than whole blood.[9] In this way a single unit of blood can supply components for more than one person, and there is less risk to recipients because they are not being exposed to antigens or other foreign substances contained in the unneeded portion of the blood. This discussion focuses on the administration of whole blood or the red cell component. Plasma or its components (platelets, granulocytes, albumin, clotting factors) may be administered separately. Table 20-4 describes the red cell components that are used for transfusion.

Blood transfusions must be carefully typed (ABO and Rh type) and carefully crossmatched before they are administered. Failure to do so may

Table 20–4   Red Blood Cell Components Used in Transfusion Therapy

Component	Preparation	Advantages
Whole blood	Drawn from the donor. Anticoagulants are added, usually acid-citrate-dextrose or citrate-phosphate-dextrose. Stored at 1° to 6°C until used or expiration date is reached.	Useful in blood loss. Does not require additional preparation except for typing and crossmatching. Contains both red cells and colloids that are in the plasma.
Packed red cells	Red cells are separated from the plasma of whole blood.	Can replace whole blood transfusion when red cells are needed. Minimizes exposure to potentially dangerous materials in the plasma such as potassium, various allergens, and free hemoglobin. Also reduces the danger of volume overload.
Buffy coat-poor red cells	The buffy-coat is the white layer that lies above the red cells when whole blood is centrifuged. It is removed in addition to the plasma.	Removes the leukocytes and platelet antigens and reduces the risk of nonhemolytic febrile reactions.
Washed red cells	Packed red cells are washed by special centrifuge method using normal saline.	Further lessens the antigens in sensitized persons. Cost is high and the cells must be used within 24 hours to avoid bacterial contamination.
Frozen red cells	Red cells are mixed with glycerol to prevent ice crystals from forming and rupturing the cell membrane. Cells must be washed before they have been thawed in preparation for administration.	Lessens the risk of febrile reactions and decreases the sensitization to the HLA antigens on the lymphocytes. Eliminates hepatitis risk. Used in kidney transplant recipients and other high-risk individuals. Costly and takes too long to prepare for use in emergency transfusions.

Data obtained from Reich PR: Blood Groups II: Pathology and Transfusion Therapy. In Beck WS: Hematology, 2nd ed, pp 317-334. Cambridge, MIT Press, 1977.

cause a fatal blood transfusion reaction. In crossmatching, cells and serum from donor and recipient are selectively combined and observed for agglutination following direct mixing, addition of a high-protein solution to promote agglutination, and addition of Coombs' reagent following thorough washing of the red cells (direct Coombs').

ABO types. There are four major ABO blood types as determined by the presence or absence of two types of red cell antigens (A and B). Persons who have no red cell antigens are classified as having type O blood, those with A antigens as type A blood, those with B antigens as type B blood, and those with AB antigens as type AB blood (Table 20-5). The ABO blood types are genetically determined. The type O gene is apparently functionless in production of a red cell antigen. Each of the other genes is expressed by the presence of a strong antigen on the red blood cell. Six genotypes and four blood types stem from the four gene types.

Normally, the body does not develop antibodies to its own tissues or blood cells. When an ABO antigen is not present on the red cell, antibodies develop in the plasma. Thus persons with type A antigens on their red cells develop type B antibodies in their serum; persons with type B antigens develop type A antibodies in their serum; and persons with type O blood develop both type A and type B antibodies. The ABO antibodies are usually not present at birth, but begin to develop two to eight months following birth and reach maximum at about eight to ten years of age.[10]

Blood transfusion reactions. The seriousness of blood transfusion reactions prompts the need for extreme caution when blood is administered. Care should be taken to ensure proper identification of the recipient and transfusion source. Once the transfusion has been started, careful observation for signs of a transfusion reaction is imperative.

The most critical transfusion reaction is that between the antibody of the recipient's serum and the antigen on the donor's red cells. The signs and symptoms of such a reaction include sensation of heat along the vein where the blood is being infused, flushing of the face, urticaria, headache, pain in the lumbar area, chills and fever, constricting pain in the chest, cramping pain in the abdomen, nausea and vomiting, tachycardia, hypotension, and dyspnea. The transfusion should be stopped immediately should any of these signs occur. Access to the vein should be maintained, since it may be necessary to administer intravenous medications. The blood must be saved for studies to determine the cause of the reaction. One of the complications of a blood transfusion reaction is oliguria and renal shutdown. The urine should be examined for hemoglobin, urobilinogen, and red blood cells.

Rh types. Blood to be transfused must also be typed for Rh type. The Rh type is coded by a triple-gene complex: Cc, Dd, and Ee. The Rh (positive) factors— C, D, and E—are inherited as dominant mendelian traits so that if either of the two chromosomes carrying these genes contains one or more of these dominant genes, the antigen will be present on the red cell. To be Rh-negative (to lack the red cell Rh antigens), it is necessary that none of the dominant (C, D, or E) genes be present. Unlike serum antibodies for the ABO blood types that develop spontaneously after birth, development of the Rh antibodies requires exposure to one or more of the Rh factors or their protein products. This means that transfusion of Rh-positive blood into a person with Rh-negative blood who has never been exposed to the Rh positive factor will have no immediate consequences, because it takes several weeks to build antibodies. After several weeks a reaction might occur, but it is usually mild. If, however, subsequent transfusions of Rh-positive blood are given to the person who has now become sensitized, there may be a severe immediate reaction.

Erythroblastosis fetalis, or hemolytic disease of the newborn, occurs in Rh-positive infants of Rh-negative mothers who have been sensitized by previous pregnancies in which the infants are Rh positive, or by blood transfusions of Rh-positive blood. The Rh-negative mother usually becomes sensitized during the first few days following delivery. During this time the antigens from the placental site are released into the maternal circulation. Because the development of the antibodies requires several weeks, the first Rh-positive infant of an Rh-negative mother is usually not affected. Infants with Rh-negative blood have no antigens on their red cells to react with the maternal antibodies and are also not affected.

Table 20–5   ABO System for Blood Typing

Genotype	Red Cell Antigens	Blood Type	Serum Antibodies
OO	none	O	AB
AO	A	A	B
AA	A	A	B
BO	B	B	A
BB	B	B	A
AB	AB	AB	none

Once an Rh-negative mother has been sensitized, the *Rh antibodies* from her blood are *transferred to the baby through the placental circulation.* These antibodies react with the red cell antigens of the Rh-positive infant, causing agglutination and hemolysis. This leads to severe *anemia* with compensatory hyperplasia and enlargement of the blood-forming organs, including the spleen and liver, in the fetus. Liver function may be impaired, with decreased production of albumin and development of a generalized edema called *hydrops fetalis.* *Bilirubin* levels in the blood are abnormally high due to red cell hemolysis, and with these elevated levels there is danger that the bilirubin will precipitate into neuronal tissue and cause destructive changes; this condition is called *kernicterus.*

Not all babies born to Rh-negative mothers are Rh-positive, and those that are Rh-negative are not likely to develop erythroblastosis. If, for example, the father carries a complex of both Rh-positive and Rh-negative genes, there is a chance that the baby will be Rh-negative.

Three recent advances have served to decrease the threat to babies born to Rh-negative mothers: (1) the prevention of sensitization, (2) the intrauterine transfusion to the affected fetus, and (3) the exchange transfusion. Injection of *Rh immune globulin* (gamma globulin containing Rh antibody) prevents sensitization in Rh-negative mothers who have given birth to an Rh-positive infant if administered within 72 hours of delivery. The Rh immune globulin must be given after each delivery (or abortion) of an Rh-positive infant to prevent sensitization—once sensitization has developed, the immune globulin is of no known value. In the past, about 20% of erythroblastotic fetuses died in utero. It is now possible to increase their chances of survival by studying the *amniotic fluid* to determine whether *intrauterine blood transfusions* are necessary. If the specimen of amniotic fluid indicates that the fetus is erythroblastotic, the intrauterine transfusions will be given. *Exchange transfusions* are given after birth. In this technique, 10 to 20 ml of the infant's blood is removed and replaced with an equal amount of type O, unsensitized Rh-negative blood. This procedure is repeated until twice the blood volume of the infant has been exchanged. The purpose of the exchange transfusion is to prevent hyperbilirubinemia with consequent damage to the brain.

Polycythemia

Polycythemia is an abnormally high total red blood cell mass. It is categorized as relative, primary, or secondary. In *relative polycythemia* the hematocrit

rises due to loss of blood volume without a corresponding decrease in red cells. *Polycythemia vera (primary polycythemia)* is a proliferative disease of the bone marrow characterized by an absolute increase in total red blood cell mass and volume. It is seen most commonly in men aged 40 to 60 years. *Secondary polycythemia* results from an increase in the level of erythropoietin. This elevation is related to living at high altitudes and to chronic heart and lung disease, both of which cause hypoxia. Smoking more than one and a half packs of cigarettes daily may also cause secondary polycythemia.

In polycythemia vera, signs and symptoms are those related to increased blood viscosity and hypermetabolism—increase in red cell count, hemoglobin, and hematocrit. The increased blood volume gives rise to hypertension. There may be complaints of headache, inability to concentrate, and some difficulty in hearing. There is a plethoric appearance, or dusky redness—even cyanosis—particularly of the lips, fingernails, and mucous membranes. Because of the increased blood flow, the person may experience itching and pain in the fingers or toes, and the hypermetabolism may induce night sweats and weight loss. With the elevated blood viscosity and stagnation of blood flow, thrombosis and hemorrhage are possible.

Relative polycythemia is corrected by increasing the extracellular fluid volume. Treatment of secondary polycythemia focuses on relieving the hypoxia. For example, the use of continuous low-flow oxygen therapy is a means of correcting the severe hypoxia that occurs in some persons with chronic obstructive lung disease. This form of treatment is thought to relieve the pulmonary hypertension and polycythemia, and delay the onset of cor pulmonale. The goal in primary polycythemia is a reduction in blood viscosity. This can be done by phlebotomy (withdrawal of blood) or chemotherapy or radiation to suppress bone marrow function.

In summary, the lungs provide for gas exchange between the external and internal environments, and the red blood cells transport oxygen to the tissues. Red blood cells, which have a life span of about 120 days, are produced in the bone marrow. Their production is regulated by erythropoietin, a glycoprotein that is released in response to hypoxia. The precise mechanism of erythropoietin formation is unclear; its levels are decreased in persons in renal failure. Anemia describes a condition in which there is a decrease in red cell mass. It may be caused by a loss of red cells as occurs with acute or chronic blood loss, or may result from the abnormal destruction of red cells that occurs in hemolytic anemia. The production of red blood cells may be impaired by a *deficiency of iron, vitamin B_{12}, or folic acid. Bone marrow depression also impairs red cell production. Polycythemia describes a condition in which there is an increase in red blood cell mass. It may be relative in type, with red cell mass increased due to loss of vascular fluid; primary, with proliferative changes in the bone marrow; or secondary with elevation of erythropoietin levels due to hypoxia.*

:Study Guide

After you have studied this chapter, you should be able to meet the following objectives:

: : State the factors that determine oxygen dissolubility in plasma.

: : Describe the transport of oxygen by hemoglobin.

: : Describe the structure of hemoglobin.

: : Explain the significance of *shift to the right* vs. *shift to the left* in the oxygen-hemoglobin dissociation curve.

: : Compare a condition in which cyanosis would be a significant finding with one in which cyanosis would not be of clinical significance.

: : Explain why blood gases cannot be measured accurately by means of venous blood.

: : Explain the pathology of respiratory failure by citing clinical examples.

: : Describe the clinical manifestations of hypoxemia and hypercarbia.

: : Trace the development of a red cell from erythroblast to erythrocyte.

: : Describe changes in the red blood cell as it ages.

: : Describe the excessive red cell loss that is characteristic of anemia.

: : Explain the cause of sickling in sickle cell anemia.

: : Explain the pathology of iron deficiency anemia.

: : Describe the relationship between vitamin B_{12} and megaloblastic anemia.

: : Explain the physiologic basis of bone marrow depression.

: : Explain the importance of crossmatching before transfusing blood.

: : Describe the pathophysiology involved in erythroblastosis fetalis.

: : Compare polycythemia vera and secondary polycythemia.

:References

1. Brannin PK: Physical assessment in acute respiratory failure. Crit Care Q 1:27-41, 1979
2. Rogers RM, Weiler C, Ruppenthal B: The impact of intensive care unit on survival of patients with acute respiratory failure. Heart Lung 1:475-480, 1973
3. Pierce AK: Oxygen toxicity. Basics of RD 1(2), 1972
4. Guyton A: Textbook of Medical Physiology, 6th ed, p. 59. Philadelphia, WB Saunders, 1981
5. Wallerstein RO: Blood. In Krupp MA, Chatton M: Current Medical Diagnosis and Treatment, p. 292. Los Altos, California, 1980
6. Proc First National Sickle Cell Educational Symposium, p. 6. Department of Health, Education and Welfare, 1976
7. Beck WS: Hematology, 2nd ed, p. 129. Cambridge, MIT Press, 1977
8. Robbins SL, Cotran R: Pathologic Basis of Disease, p. 739. Philadelphia, WB Saunders, 1979
9. Reich PR: Blood groups II: Pathology and transfusion therapy. In Beck WS: Hematology, 2nd ed, p. 322. Cambridge, MIT Press, 1977
10. Guyton A: Textbook of Medical Physiology, 6th ed, p. 85. Philadelphia, WB Saunders, 1981

:Suggested Readings

Respiratory failure

Berger AJ, Mitchell RA, Severinghaus JW: Medical progress: Regulation of respiration (first of three parts). N Engl J Med 297(2):92-97, 1977

Berger AJ, Mitchell RA, Severinghaus JW: Medical progress: Regulation of respiration (second of three parts). N Engl J Med 297(3):138-142, 1977

Berger AJ, Mitchell RA, Severinghaus JW: Medical progress: Regulation of respiration (third of three parts). N Engl J Med 297(4):194-201, 1977

Cherniack NS: The control of breathing in COPD. Chest 77(2):291-293, 1980

Fromm G: Using basic laboratory data to evaluate patients with acute respiratory failure. Crit Care Q 1:43-51, 1979

Koss JA, Christoph C: Oxygen therapy and other respiratory therapy in acute respiratory failure. Crit Care Q 1:53-63, 1979

Martin RJ: The treatment of acute respiratory failure without mechanical ventilation. Med Times 106(7):31-37, 1978

Radwan L, Defmats H: Variations of arterial oxygen and carbon dioxide tensions during 24 hours in chronic respiratory insufficiency. Scand J Respir Dis 55:99-104, 1974

Rhodes ML: Acute respiratory failure in chronic obstructive lung disease. Crit Care Q 1:1-14, 1979

Rogers RM: Acute respiratory failure: How to recognize it quickly—how best to handle it. Med Times 106(7):26-30, 1978

Seriff NS, Khan F, Lazo BL: Acute respiratory failure: Current concepts of pathophysiology and management. Med Clin North Am 57(6):1539-1551, 1973

Tisi GM: Strategies of care in acute respiratory failure. Med Times 107(5):43-51, 1979

Alterations in red cell structure and function

Axelson JA, LoBuglio AF: Immune hemolytic anemia. Med Clin North Am 64(4):597, 1980

Brewer GJ: Inherited erythrocyte metabolic and membrane disorders. Med Clin North Am 64(4):579, 1980

Crosby WH: Red cell mass: Its precursors and its perturbations. Hosp Pract 15, No. 2:71-81, 1980

Forget BG: Hemolytic anemias: Congenital and acquired. Hosp Pract 15, No. 4:67-78, 1980

Goldstein M: The aplastic anemias. Hosp Pract 15, No. 5:85-96, 1980

Hamilton E: Intrauterine transfusion for Rh disease: A status report. Hosp Pract 13(8):113-124, 1978

Katz AJ: Transfusion therapy: Its role in the anemias. Hosp Pract 15, No. 6:77-84, 1980

McFarlane J: Sickle cell disorders. Am J Nurs 77:1948-1954, 1977

McFee JG: Iron metabolism and iron deficiency during pregnancy. Clin Obstet Gynecol 22(4):788-808, 1979

Nimeh N, Bishop RC: Disorders of iron metabolism. Med Clin North Am 64(4):631-644, 1980

Scott RB: Reflections on the current status of the national sickle cell disease program in the United States. J Nat Med Assoc 71(7):679-681, 1979

Shohet SB, Ness PM: Hemolytic anemias: Failure of the red cell membrane. Med Clin North Am 60(5):913-932, 1976

Silver BJ, Zuckerman KS: Aplastic anemia: Recent advances in pathogenesis and treatment. Med Clin North Am 64(4):607-629, 1980

Trubowitz S: The management of sickle cell anemia. Med Clin North Am 60(5):933-944, 1976

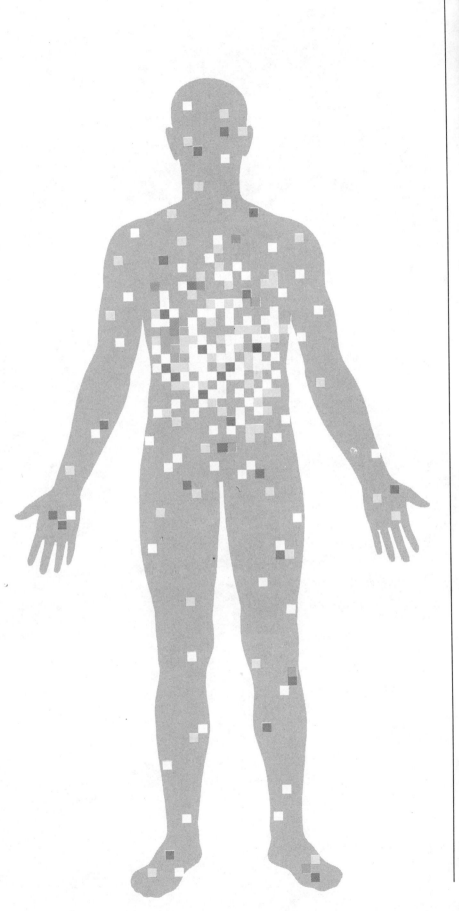

Alterations in Composition and Regulation of Body Fluids

Fluids are essential components of a biologic system. Body fluids vary in amount and composition, according to their location and purpose. Although water is the major component of body fluids, the fluids also contain dissolved gases, electrolytes, nutrients, plasma proteins, and metabolic wastes. The content of this unit is divided into four sections: (1) introductory concepts, (2) alterations in body fluids and electrolytes, (3) acid–base disorders, and (4) alterations in the distribution of body fluids.

Fluid distribution
Electrical properties
Concentration effects
Regulation of fluids and electrolytes

21

Body Fluids and Electrolytes: Introductory Concepts

The composition and distribution of body fluids are constantly changing. This chapter introduces the reader to concepts related to electrical, mechanical, and chemical forces that affect the movement, distribution, and composition of body water and electrolytes.

:Fluid Distribution

Body fluids are distributed between two body compartments. The *intracellular compartment* contains the fluid within all of the body's billions of cells (Fig. 21-1). The *extracellular compartment* contains all of the fluid located outside of the cells. Included in the extracellular compartment are the *interstitial fluids* (fluids that surround the cells), *the intravascular fluids*, cerebral spinal fluid, and fluid contained within the various body spaces such as the pleural cavity and the joint spaces. Even the water contained in the anterior chamber of the eye is considered to be extracellular fluid.

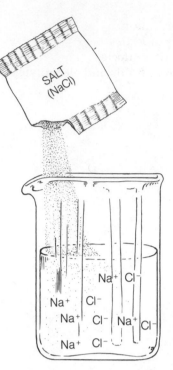

Figure 21–2. Dissociation of chemical compounds into ions.

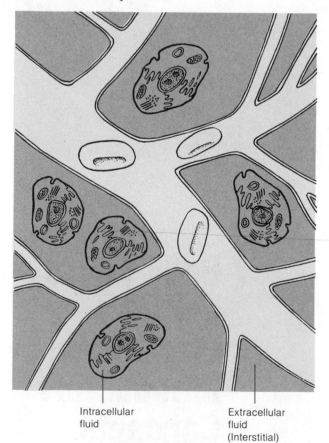

Figure 21–1. Distribution of body water—the extracellular space includes the vascular compartment and the interstitial spaces.

Intracellular fluid

Extracellular fluid (Interstitial)

:Electrical Properties

Body fluids contain both water and chemical compounds. In solution, these chemical compounds can either remain intact or separate in a process known as *dissociation*. *Electrolytes* are compounds that dissociate in solution to form *charged particles* or *ions*. For example, a sodium chloride molecule dissociates to form a positively charged sodium (Na^+) and a negatively charged chloride (Cl^-) ion (Fig. 21-2). Substances such as glucose and urea remain intact and are called *nonelectrolytes*.

Positively charged ions are called *cations* because they are attracted to the *cathode* of a wet electric cell. Similarly, negatively charged ions are called *anions* because they are attracted to the *anode* (Fig. 21-3). The ions found in body fluids carry either one charge (*a monovalent ion*) or two charges (*a divalent ion*). Table 22-6 lists the major electrolytes of the body fluids.

The location of electrolytes is influenced by their electrical charge. You will recall that *ions* with *like* charges *repel* and that *ions* with *opposite* charges *attract*. This attraction or repulsion can cause electrolytes to move from one body compartment to another. In other words, an excess of positively charged ions in a body compartment would tend to attract

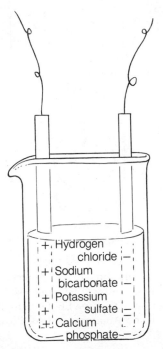

Figure 21–3.   In a wet cell, cations go to the negative pole and anions go to the positive pole. (Adapted from Metheny N, Snively WD: Nurses' Handbook of Fluid Balance, 3rd ed. Philadelphia, JB Lippincott, 1979)

negatively charged ions in an attempt to balance the electrical charge.

In general, the positive charge from one cation is no different from the positive charge of another; for example, the positive charge from a sodium ion is equivalent to the positive charge from a potassium ion. As a general rule, however, the total number of cations in the body equals the total number of anions.

The unit that expresses the charge equivalency of a given weight of an electrolyte is the milli-equivalent per liter (mEq/l). The number of milli-equivalents in a substance can be derived from the following formula:

$$mEq/l = \frac{mg/100 \ ml \times 10 \times valence}{atomic \ weight}$$

The International System of Units expresses electrolytes as millimoles per liter (mmol/l).

$$mmol/l = \frac{mEq/l}{valence}$$

This means that one mEq will equal one mmol of a monovalent electrolyte. Laboratory reports of serum electrolytes and electrolyte composition of intravenous solutions and other medications are expressed as either mEq/l or mmol/l.

:Concentration Effects

In a biologic system, the concentration of dissolved particles in a solution influences water movement and controls cell size. *Diffusion* is the movement of charged or uncharged particles along a *concentration gradient*. The addition of sugar to a container of water is an example of diffusion. Initially, the concentration of sugar will be greatest at the point where it comes in contact with the water. Moments later, however, the sugar will have diffused so that its concentration has been equalized throughout the container. *Many small molecules move from one body compartment to another along a concentration gradient.*

Most of the membranes in the body are semipermeable. This means they allow water and small uncharged particles to diffuse freely through their pores, while partially or completely preventing the passage of charged ions and large molecules. Water diffuses through a semipermeable membrane moving from the side with the least number of nondiffusible particles to the side that has the greater number (Fig. 21-4). The pressure due to water movement is called the *osmotic pressure*. The osmotic activity or work potential that dissolved particles exert in drawing water from one side of the membrane to another is measured through a unit called a *milliosmol* (mOsm/l).

Figure 21–4.   Movement of water across a semipermeable membrane. Water movement is from the side that has the lesser number of nondiffusible particles to the side that has the greater number.

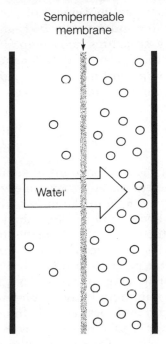

One gram mol of a nondiffusible
and nonionizable substance
is equal to 1 osmol.

A milliosmol is equal to one-thousandth of an osmol. If a substance dissociates to form two ions, then 0.5 gram mol of the substance will equal 1 osmol. Each nondiffusible particle, large or small, is equally effective in its ability to pull water through a semipermeable membrane. Thus the osmotic activity of a solution is determined by the number, rather than the size, of the dissolved particles.

Osmotic activity of a solution may be expressed as either osmolarity or osmolality. Osmolarity refers to the osmolar concentration in one liter of solution (mOsm/l); whereas osmolality refers to the osmols dissolved in one kilogram of water (mOsm/kg H$_2$O). Although the terms *osmolarity* and *osmolality* are often used interchangeably, most clinical laboratories report osmotic activity as osmolality. The normal serum osmolality of body serum is approximately 280 mOsm/l.

The movement of water across a cell membrane due to osmosis can cause the cell to either *swell* or *shrink* (Fig. 21-5). By definition, a *hypertonic* solution is one that causes a cell to *shrink* or become *crenated*. A *hypotonic* solution causes a cell to *swell*. An *isotonic* solution is one that *does not* cause cells to *either shrink or swell*.

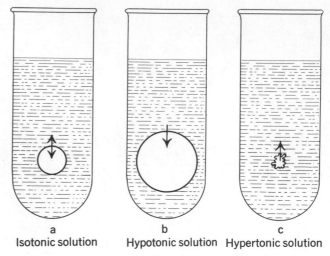

a
Isotonic solution
b
Hypotonic solution
c
Hypertonic solution

Figure 21–5. Osmosis—(*a*) red cells undergo no change in size in isotonic solutions, (*b*) they increase in size in hypotonic solutions, and (*c*) they decrease in size in hypertonic solutions. (Chaffee EE, Greisheimer EM: Basic Physiology and Anatomy, 3rd ed. Philadelphia, JB Lippincott, 1974)

these mechanisms for easier understanding of the subject.

In summary, water and electrolytes are essential components of the intracellular and extracellular compartments. The precise regulation of the fluid and electrolyte composition within the body compartments is controlled by electrical (ionic) forces, chemical (diffusion) gradients, and the osmotic movement of water.

:Regulation of Fluids and Electrolytes

There is a continual movement of water and electrolytes both into and out of the body and among the various body structures and compartments. As a general rule, the level of body water and electrolytes present at any given time is directly related to the amount taken into the body minus the amount lost from the body.

$$\begin{array}{c} \text{level of water} \\ \text{or electrolyte} \end{array} = \begin{array}{c} \text{amount} \\ \text{taken in} \end{array} - \begin{array}{c} \text{amount lost} \\ \text{from the body} \end{array}$$

For example, the total amount of sodium chloride present in the body at any given time will reflect the oral and/or parenteral intake minus what has been lost from the body through skin, kidney, and bowel.

As a method for approaching the study of fluids and electrolytes, it is recommended that the reader consider (1) the purpose or function that water or a given electrolyte serves in overall body function, (2) the basal or minimum body requirements, (3) the sources of gain and loss, and (4) the mechanisms responsible for regulating body levels of water or specific electrolytes. The causes and manifestations of fluid and electrolyte imbalances can be related to

:Study Guide

After you have studied this chapter, you should be able to meet the following objectives:

: : Differentiate between the intracellular compartment and the extracellular compartment.

: : Define *electrolyte*.

: : State the formula for deriving the number of milliequivalents in a substance.

: : Explain the term *concentration gradient*.

: : State the parameters that determine the level of body water and electrolytes.

:Suggested Readings

Chaffee EE, Lytle IM: Basic Physiology and Anatomy, 4th ed, p 500. Philadelphia, JB Lippincott, 1980

Guyton AC: Textbook of Medical Physiology, 6th ed, pp 358, 391. Philadelphia, WB Saunders, 1981

Metheny NM, Snively WD: Nurses' Handbook of Fluid Balance, 3rd ed. Philadelphia, JB Lippincott, 1979

22

Alterations in Body Fluids and Electrolytes

Body fluids consist of water and electrolytes. The precise regulation of these fluids within a very narrow physiologic range is essential to life. Normally, the volume and composition of these fluids remain relatively constant in the presence of a wide range of changes in intake and output. Environmental stresses and disease states often increase losses, impair intake, and otherwise interfere with mechanisms that regulate body fluid volume and composition. This chapter is divided into two parts: the first part is concerned with changes in fluid volume and the second part with changes in the electrolyte composition of body fluids.

:Water

The body is largely water, therefore, body water is usually expressed as a percentage of body weight. Total body water varies with age, decreasing from infancy to old age. In the full-term infant, body water constitutes as much as 75% to 80% of body weight, whereas body water accounts for only 60% to 70% of body weight in the adult. The premature infant has greater amounts of body water, the elderly person much less. Because fat is essentially water free, obesity tends to decrease the percentage of water that the body contains, sometimes reducing these levels to values as low as 45% of body weight.

In the previous chapter it was pointed out that body fluids are divided between the intracellular and extracellular compartments. The intracellular compartment contains about two-thirds of the body's water and the extracellular compartment about one-third. In the adult, intracellular water constitutes about 45% of body weight and extracellular fluid about 15% (Fig. 22-1).

Despite its greater body-water content, the infant is more likely to develop fluid imbalances than the adult. This is because the infant has both a higher metabolic rate and a larger surface area in relation to its body mass than an older child or adult. Also, the infant has more difficulty in concentrating its urine because its kidney structures are immature. This means that the infant has greater skin and urine losses and that more water is needed to transport metabolic wastes. The infant, therefore, both ingests and excretes relatively greater volumes of water than the adult. For example, an infant may exchange one-half of its extracellular fluid volume in a single day, whereas an adult exchanges only about one-sixth of this volume during the same period of time. By the third year of life, the percentages and distribution of body water in the young child approach those of the adult.

Figure 22–1. Diagram showing fluid compartments in the adult. Fluid in the intracellular compartment constitutes about 45% of body weight, whereas fluid in the extracellular compartment constitutes about 15% of body weight. Fluid from the extracellular compartment moves into the gastrointestinal tract, skin, lungs, and kidneys.

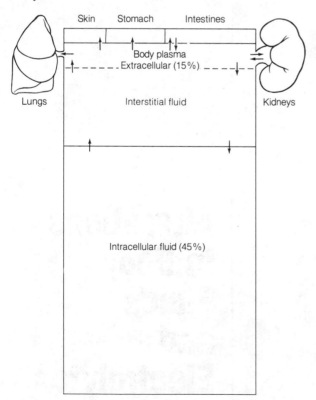

Functions in Water

Because of its ubiquitous nature, the functions of water in the human body are many (see chart p. 287). Water adds to the structure of the body; acts as a transport vehicle; lubricates and cushions; acts to hydrolyze food in the digestive system; and is necessary for chemical reactions that occur within the cell.

It is water that gives the body its *structure*. One has only to compare the dry and wrinkled skin of an elderly person with that of a child to become aware of the extent to which water contributes to the overall form and appearance of the body. Water adds a resiliency to the skin and underlying tissues that is often referred to as *skin or tissue turgor*. Tissue turgor is assessed by pinching a fold of skin between the thumb and forefinger. Normally, the skin immediately returns to its normal configuration when the fingers are released. A loss of 3% to 5% of body

Functions of Water

Provides form for body structures

Acts as a transport vehicle for
    Nutrients
    Electrolytes
    Blood gases
    Metabolic wastes
    Heat
    Electrical currents

Provides insulation

Aids in the hydrolysis of food

Acts as a medium and reactant for chemical
    reactions

Acts as a lubricant

Cushions and acts as a shock absorber

---

water causes the resiliency of the skin to be lost and the tissue will remain raised for several seconds.

The transport of body nutrients, wastes, electrical currents, and heat, depends on fluid movement both in the interstitial spaces and in the vascular compartment. In relation to *body temperature*, water not only transports heat from the inner core of the body to the periphery where it can be released into the external environment, but it also *insulates* the body against changes in the external temperature. Were it not for the insulation afforded the body by its water content, the body would be much like a rock, gaining heat during the day and losing it at night.

Water *hydrolyzes* food eaten, breaking it down into particles that can be digested and then absorbed across the gastrointestinal tract wall. Additionally, many of the *chemical reactions* that occur within the body require water as a medium or reactant.

Water also lubricates and cushions. Synovial fluid lubricates the joints, and pericardial fluid prevents the heart from rubbing against the pericardial sac. The act of swallowing would be difficult, if not impossible, were it not for the lubricating properties of the mucus that lines the gastrointestinal tract. The

cerebral spinal fluid acts to cushion the brain. During pregnancy, amniotic fluid acts as a shock absorber and protects the delicate fetus.

Water Requirements

Regardless of age, all normal individuals require approximately 100 ml of water per 100 calories metabolized. This means that a person expending 1800 calories requires approximtely 1800 ml of water for metabolic purposes. Metabolic rate increases with fever and there is a 13% increase in metabolic rate for every 1°C (7%/1°F) increase in body temperature.

Water Gains

The main source of water gain is that which is absorbed from the gastrointestinal tract; this includes water obtained from fluids, ingested foods, tube feedings, and sometimes from water used in rectal irrigation. Water gain also includes water derived from cellular oxidation of foodstuffs. This quantity varies from 150 ml to 250 ml depending on the rate of metabolism. Sources of water gain are summarized in Table 22-1.

Water Losses

Water losses occur through the *kidney, skin, lungs,* and *gastrointestinal tract* (Table 22-1). Even when oral and parenteral intake has been withheld, the kidneys continue to produce urine as a means of ridding the body of metabolic wastes. The urine output that is required to eliminate these wastes is called the *obligatory urine output.* The obligatory urine loss is about 300 ml to 500 ml per day.

Water losses that occur from the skin and respiratory tract are termed *insensible water losses* because the individual is not aware that they are occurring. Under normal conditions, water vapor lost from the skin and lungs approximates 500 ml per square meter of surface area per day. Skin losses include the water that continually diffuses through the pores in

---

Table 22-1 Sources of Body Water Gains and Losses in the Adult

Gains		Losses	
		Urine	1500 ml
Oral intake		Insensible losses	
As water	1000 ml	Lungs	300 ml
In food	1300 ml	Skin	500 ml
Water of oxidation	200 ml	Feces	200 ml
Total	2500 ml	Total	2500 ml

the skin as well as the water lost in the process of sweating. Respiratory losses consist of water vapor that is withdrawn from the mucous membranes to humidify the inspired air and then is lost to the environment during expiration. For readers who have lived in a cold climate, the frosty breath that they see on a cold day is evidence of water losses that occur with respiration.

Regulation of Body Water

Two physiologic mechanisms assist in regulating body water levels; one of these is *thirst* and the other is the *kidney's ability to concentrate urine*. Thirst is primarily a regulator of intake, and renal concentrating mechanisms a regulator of output. Both mechanisms respond to changes in extracellular volume and osmolality.

Thirst

The thirst center is located in the lateral preoptic area of the hypothalamus (Fig. 22-2). Nerve cells, called osmoreceptors, which are located in or near the thirst center, respond to changes in extracellular osmolality by either swelling or shrinking. Thirst occurs when an increase in extracellular osmolality causes these cells to shrink. Thirst is one of the

earliest symptoms of water loss, occurring when water loss is equal to 2% of body weight.

The most common cause of thirst is an increase in the osmotic concentration of the extracellular fluids. A second cause of thirst is severe hypokalemia which causes significant defects in the kidneys' ability to concentrate urine. This then results in polyuria followed by polydipsia. Hypokalemia is known to stimulate prostaglandin E synthesis. Inasmuch as prostaglandin E is known to stimulate thirst, it is also possible that polydipsia secondary to hypokalemia is mediated by prostaglandins. A third cause of thirst is a decrease in blood volume which may or may not be associated with a decrease in serum osmolality. Thirst is one of the earliest symptoms of hemorrhage, often being present long before other signs of blood loss begin to appear. Lastly, dryness of the mouth produces a sensation of thirst that is not necessarily associated with the body's state of hydration, for example, the thirst that a lecturer experiences as the mouth dries during speaking. It is interesting to note that in animal experiments in which salivary secretion was blocked, excessive drinking did not occur unless the animals were eating food.[1] This same effect has been reported in humans with salivary glands that did not secrete saliva, suggesting that the lubricating properties of water are needed for swallowing food.

Pathology of thirst.   Excessive thirst is called polydipsia. Polydipsia is normal when it accompanies conditions of water deficit. Although infrequent, a water excess can occur as the result of excess intake that is unrelated to need. An example of excessive water intake occurs in psychogenic polydipsia. Persons afflicted with this disorder drink water in excess of what the kidneys can excrete. A 1977 news story related the fatal outcome of a 29-year-old woman with a diagnosis of chronic schizophrenia who was drinking four gallons of water a day to "cleanse her body of cancer."[2]

Renal concentrating mechanisms

The kidney controls the concentration of most of the constituents in body fluids, including water and electrolytes. Each kidney has about one million functional units called nephrons (Fig. 22-3). Water and electrolytes are filtered from the blood in the *glomerulus* and are then selectively reabsorbed in the *tubules*. The rate at which water and electrolytes can be removed from the body is determined by renal blood flow and the glomerular filtration rate; urine output declines during shock as renal blood flow falls. As the urine filtrate moves through the tubule,

Figure 22–2.   Diagram of the center of the hypothalamus and pituitary gland which are involved in water balance.

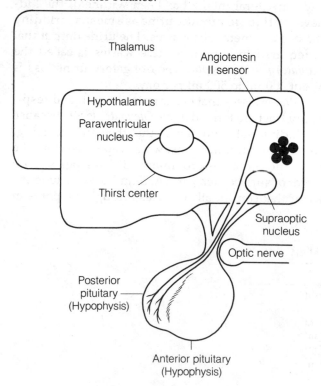

Thalamus

Angiotensin II sensor

Hypothalamus

Paraventricular nucleus

Thirst center

Supraoptic nucleus

Optic nerve

Posterior pituitary (Hypophysis)

Anterior pituitary (Hypophysis)

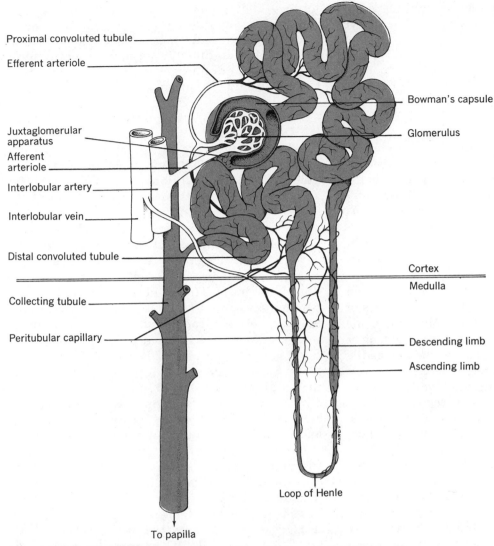

Proximal convoluted tubule

Efferent arteriole

Juxtaglomerular apparatus

Afferent arteriole

Interlobular artery

Interlobular vein

Distal convoluted tubule

Collecting tubule

Peritubular capillary

Bowman's capsule

Glomerulus

Cortex

Medulla

Descending limb

Ascending limb

Loop of Henle

To papilla

Figure 22–3. Diagram of the kidney nephron. Water and electrolytes are
filtered in the glomerulus and are reabsorbed in the tubular structures.
(Chaffee EE, Lytle IM: Basic Physiology and Anatomy, 4th ed.
Philadelphia, JB Lippincott, 1980)

water and electrolytes that are needed for maintaining the volume and composition of body fluids are reabsorbed into the extracellular fluid and those that are not needed are excreted in the urine.

The reabsorption of water by the kidney is regulated by the *antidiuretic hormone* (ADH). The antidiuretic hormone is synthesized by cells in the supraoptic and paraventricular nuclei of the hypothalamus (Fig. 22-2). The hormone is transported along a neural pathway (the hypophyseal tract) to the neurohypophysis (posterior pituitary) and is then stored for future release. A rise in ADH levels causes increased reabsorption of water from the distal tubules and collecting ducts of the kidney. As

with thirst, ADH levels are controlled by *volume* and *osmolar* changes in the extracellular fluids. *Osmoreceptors* in the hypothalamus sense changes in extracellular osmolality and stimulate production and release of ADH. A small increase in serum osmolality of 1 to 2% is sufficient to cause ADH release. Likewise, stretch receptors in the *great veins*, *atria*, and *carotid sinus area* sense changes in blood volume or blood pressure and input from these receptors aids in regulation of ADH release.

Stress situations tend to cause an increase in ADH release. Severe pain, trauma, surgery, certain anesthetic agents, and some analgesic drugs increase ADH levels. Nicotine stimulates ADH release. Alcohol, on the other hand, inhibits ADH release. Table 22-2 lists drugs that are known to affect ADH release.

Pathology of ADH levels.

There are two important conditions that serve to alter ADH levels: diabetes insipidus and inappropriate secretion of ADH. Because of their effect on water balance, both of these conditions are discussed in this chapter.

Diabetes insipidus means "tasteless diabetes" as opposed to diabetes mellitus or "sweet diabetes." Diabetes insipidus occurs because of a defect in the synthesis or release of ADH (*central diabetes insipidus*) or because the kidney does not respond to ADH (*nephrogenic diabetes insipidus*). About 60% of diabetes insipidus seen clinically results from tumors or lesions in the hypophyseal tract.[3] Temporary diabetes insipidus can result following surgery in the area of the hypophyseal tract, or head injury. A person with diabetes insipidus excretes large quantities of urine, usually 3 to 15 liters per day. This large urine output is accompanied by excessive thirst; as long as the thirst mechanism is normal and fluid is readily available there is little or no alteration in fluid levels in persons with diabetes insipidus. *The danger arises when the condition develops in an unconscious person*, since an inadequate fluid intake rapidly leads to hypertonic dehydration and increased serum osmolality.

The treatment of central diabetes insipidus consists of treating any underlying disorder and supplying the body with pharmacologic preparations that contain the missing hormone. These preparations must be administered parenterally or nasally; they are not given by mouth because they are destroyed in the gastrointestinal tract. New nonhormonal forms of therapy have been recently introduced. Thiazide diuretics and the oral hypoglycemic agent chlorpropamide cause marked reduction in urine volume. Thiazide diuretics are now the specific form of therapy for nephrogenic diabetes insipidus. Chlorpropamide has no effect on this form of diabetes insipidus.

The syndrome of inappropriate secretion of ADH (SIADH) is characterized by a continued secretion of ADH in the presence of a decreased serum osmolality; this leads to a marked retention of water in excess of sodium (dilutional hyponatremia). The *urine osmolality is high* and *serum osmolality low*. *Serum sodium, hematocrit,* and *blood urea nitrogen* are all *decreased* due to expansion of the extracellular fluid volume. The increased plasma volume leads to an increase in the glomerular filtration rate which causes further increases in sodium loss. Serum sodium levels may fall from a normal value of 142 mEq per liter to values of 120 to 110 mEq per liter. Delirium, convulsions, coma, and death may occur as serum sodium levels fall to these low levels.

The first report of SIADH was made in the late 1950s in association with lung cancer; since that time the condition has been linked to various chest and central nervous system lesions. *Tumors*, particularly *bronchogenic carcinoma*, are known to produce and release ADH independent of hypothalamic control. *Disease and injury to the central nervous system* can trigger an inappropriate release of ADH. *Drugs* induce SIADH in different ways; some drugs are thought to *increase hypothalamic production and release*, while others are believed to act directly on the *renal tubules to potentiate the action of ADH*.

Treatment for SIADH is primarily directed toward reduction in water intake. Mannitol and furo-

Table 22-2 Drugs That Affect ADH Levels

Drugs That Decrease ADH Levels/Action	Drugs That Increase ADH Levels/Action
Demeclocycline	Acetaminophen
Ethanol	Analgesics (morphine and meperidine)
Glucocorticoids	Anesthetics (most)
Lithium carbonate	Antipsychotic tranquilizers
Morphine antagonists	Cancer drugs (vincristine and cyclophosphamide)
Norepinephrine	Carbamazepine
Phenytoin	Chlorpropamide
Reserpine, chlorpromazine	Clofibrate
	Isoproterenol
	Nicotine
	Phenobarbital
	Thiazide diuretics (chorothiazide)
	Tricyclic antidepressants

semide may be given to promote diuresis. Lithium and the antibiotic demeclocycline inhibit ADH action and have recently been used with some success in the treatment of SIADH.

Alterations in Fluid Volume

Body-fluid levels are dependent upon both sodium and water balance. Water provides about 90% to 93% of the volume of body fluids and sodium salts comprise 90% to 95% of the solute in the extracellular fluids. This means that the total volume of fluid in the extracellular compartment is controlled by the osmotic effect of sodium. The concentration of sodium, on the other hand, is determined by the water volume. There are two major types of alterations in extracellular fluid: one is an alteration in both sodium and water (isotonic contraction or expansion of the extracellular fluid volume), and the other is a disproportionate alteration in extracellular fluid as it relates to sodium concentration (dilutional hypo- and hypernatremia).

Extracellular fluid volume deficit

An extracellular fluid volume deficit occurs when there is a reduction in body water. It can consist of an isotonic depletion of body fluids or as a situation in which water losses are in excess of sodium losses. There are two main causes of an extracellular fluid deficit: (1) decrease in intake of fluids and electrolytes, and (2) an increased loss. The extracellular fluid compartment is the source of all body secretions, including sweat, urine, and gastrointestinal secretions. This means that excessive losses of any of these fluids affords the potential for extracellular fluid deficit (Table 22-3).

Table 22-3   Extracellular Fluid Deficit

Causes	Signs and Symptoms
Decreased fluid intake	**Acute weight loss (% of total weight)**
Unconsciousness or inability to express thirst	Mild extracellular deficit: 2% loss
Oral trauma or inability to swallow	Moderate extracellular deficit: 2-5% loss
Impaired thirst mechanism	Severe extracellular deficit: 6% or more loss
Withholding fluids for therapeutic purposes	
	Thirst
Increased fluid losses	
	Decreased urine output
Gastrointestinal losses	In water deficit
Vomiting	Increased urine osmolality
Diarrhea	Increased specific gravity
Gastrointestinal suction	In sodium and water deficit
Fistula drainage	Normal specific gravity and osmolality
Urine losses	Low sodium chloride content
Diuretic therapy	
Osmotic diuresis (hyperglycemia)	**Decreased plasma volume**
Adrenal insufficiency	Increased serum osmolality
Salt-wasting renal disease	Increased hematocrit
Skin losses (salt and water)	Increased BUN
Fever	
Exposure to hot environment	**Decreased vascular volume**
Burns and wounds that remove skin	Tachycardia
Third space losses (sodium and water)	Weak and thready pulse
Intestinal obstruction	Postural hypotension
Edema	Decreased vein filling and vein refill time
Ascites	Hypotension and shock
Burns (first several days)	
	Decreased volume in extracellular spaces
	Depressed fontanel in an infant
	Sunken eyes and soft eyeballs
	Loss of intracellular fluid
	Dry skin and mucous membrane
	Cracked and fissured tongue
	Decreased salivation and lacrimation
	Neuromuscular
	Weakness
	Fatigue

Increased surface losses. The skin acts as an exchange surface for body heat and as a vapor barrier to prevent water from leaving the body. Body surface losses of sodium and water increase when there is excessive sweating or when large areas of the skin have been damaged. Fever and hot weather increase sweating. During heavy exercise in a hot environment, sweat losses may exceed 3.5 liters per hour.[4] Both respiratory rate and sweating are usually increased as body temperature rises. As much as 3 liters of water may be lost in a single day as a result of fever. Burns are another cause of excess fluid loss. Evaporative losses range from 0.8 to 2.6 ml per kg percent burn area. This loss can approach a level of 6 to 8 liters per day.[5]

Gastrointestinal losses. There is a continual exchange of fluid between the extracellular compartment and the lumen of the gastrointestinal tract. In a single day, 8 to 10 liters of extracellular fluid is secreted into the gastrointestinal tract; most of this fluid is reabsorbed as the bowel contents move toward the anus. Vomiting and diarrhea interrupt the reabsorption process and in some situations lead to increased secretion of fluid (in excess of 8 to 10 liters) into the gastrointestinal tract; the presence of irritating or hypertonic contents increases the movement of fluid into the bowel, exaggerating fluid losses. In many forms of diarrhea, the rate of fluid secretion into the gastrointestinal tract is increased due to the osmotic or irritating effects of the causative agent. In Asiatic cholera, death can occur within a matter of hours as irritating substances formed by the cholera organism cause excessive amounts of fluid to be secreted into the bowel; these fluids are then lost as vomitus or diarrheal fluid.

Third space losses. Third space losses refer to the sequestering of extracellular fluids in an area that is physiologically unavailable to the body—in the serous cavities or the lumen of the gut. For example, fluid deficits can develop in intestinal obstruction as water and electrolytes become pooled in the distended bowel. The capillaries that supply the third space often have an increased permeability and there is a concomitant movement of plasma proteins into the sequestered area. The osmotic gradient associated with the presence of these colloids causes additional water to move into the third space area.

Increased urinary losses. The kidney normally regulates the volume and solute concentration of the extracellular fluid—promoting diuresis in situations of fluid excess and conserving fluids when extracellular fluid volume is decreased. Extracellular fluid deficit can result from osmotic diuresis or the injudicious use of diuretic therapy. In hyperglycemia, serum sodium is diluted as the osmotic effects of the elevated glucose cause water to be pulled out of body cells. The presence of glucose in the urine filtrate prevents reabsorption of water by the renal tubules; this causes increased losses of both sodium and water. The degree of hyponatremia, or serum sodium decrease, resulting from hyperglycemia can be estimated by assuming a 1.6 mEq per liter decrease in serum sodium for every 100 mg per 100 ml rise in blood sugar above normal values.[6]

Signs and symptoms of fluid volume deficit

The signs and symptoms of fluid deficit are closely associated with the functions of water that were discussed in the first part of the chapter. A discussion of signs and symptoms associated with extracellular fluid deficit is complicated by the fact that fluid deficit may present as an isotonic depletion of fluid volume or as a situation in which water losses exceed sodium loss. The signs and symptoms presented in this section of the chapter consider both situations.

Body weight. A decrease in body weight is one of the best indicators of fluid loss. One liter of water weighs 1 kilogram or 2.2 pounds. A mild extracellular fluid deficit exists when weight loss equals 2% of body weight; in a person weighing 68 kilograms or 150 pounds this percent of weight loss equals 1.4 liters of water. Severe fluid deficit exists when weight loss is in excess of 6% of body weight. To be accurate, weight must be measured at the same time each day, with equal amounts of clothing being worn. Because extracellular fluid is trapped within the body in persons with third space losses, body weight may not decrease when extracellular fluid loss occurs for this reason.

Intake and output imbalance. Intake and output affords a second method for assessing fluid balance. Although these measurements provide insight into the causes of fluid imbalance, they are often inadequate in measuring actual losses and gains. This is because accurate measurements of intake and output are often difficult to obtain and because insensible losses are difficult to estimate. Pflaum reported a mean error in intake and output calculations of 800 ml per day when compared to daily weight measurements.[7]

Thirst. Thirst is an early symptom of water deficit, occurring when water losses are equal to 1% to 2% of body weight. Unfortunately, infants and persons who are unconscious or who cannot communicate are unable to express this need. Also, thirst is not always present in isotonic fluid deficit which is caused by sodium depletion.

Urine output.   Urine output usually decreases and urine osmolality and specific gravity increase during periods of water deficit. An exception to this rule occurs in situations in which the fluid deficit occurs as a result of renal mechanisms in situations where the kidneys' ability to concentrate urine has been impaired or when diuresis occurs for other reasons. Normally, the ratio of urine osmolality to serum osmolality in a 24-hour urine sample exceeds 1, and after an overnight fast should be greater than 3 to 1. A dehydrated patient (one who has a loss of water) may have a urine osmolality that exceeds 1000 mOsm per kg. In persons who have difficulty concentrating their urine, i.e., those with diabetes insipidus or chronic renal failure, the urine to serum ratio is often less or equal to one. Urine specific gravity compares the weight of urine to that of water, providing an index for solute concentration. A change in specific gravity of 1.010 to 1.020 (water is considered to be 1.000) is an increase of 400 mOsm per kg. In the sodium-depleted state, the kidney will usually try to conserve sodium; urine specific gravity will be normal and urine sodium and chloride concentrations will be low.

Serum osmolality and concentrations of extracellular constituents

The normal serum osmolality is 275 to 295 mOsm per liter. Because the serum in the extracellular compartment is roughly 90% to 93% water, the concentration of blood cells and other solutes will increase as extracellular water decreases. This is true of hematocrit and blood urea nitrogen (BUN). Serum sodium will also increase when fluid deficit is due primarily to a water loss.

Vascular volume.   Arterial and venous volumes decline during periods of fluid deficit. There is a change in both the pulse and blood pressure that occurs as the volume in the arterial system declines. Heart rate is increased and the pulse becomes weak and thready. Postural hypotension is an early sign of fluid deficit, characterized by a blood pressure that is at least 10 mm Hg lower in the sitting and standing position than it is when lying down. When volume depletion becomes severe, signs of shock and vascular collapse appear. On the venous side of the circulation, the veins become less prominent and venous

refill time increases. A simple test to determine venous refill time consists of compressing the distal end of a vein on the dorsal aspect of the hand (when the hand is not in the dependent position). The vein is then emptied by "milking" the blood toward the heart. Normally, the vein will refill almost immediately when the occluding finger is removed. When venous volume is decreased, as is true in fluid deficit, venous refill time will increase.

Extracellular fluid spaces.   Fluid in all of the body spaces is decreased in fluid deficit. Although most body spaces are not visible, a decrease in cerebral spinal fluid in the infant causes depression of the anterior fontanel. Likewise, the eyes assume a sunken appearance and feel softer than normal when the fluid content in the anterior chamber of the eye is decreased.

Cellular fluids.   As fluid is lost from the extracellular compartment in excess of solute, the osmolarity of the extracellular fluid becomes hypertonic in relation to the fluid in the intracellular compartment. When this happens, water is pulled out of body cells. The skin and mucous membranes become dry and there is a decrease in the activity of the cells in the salivary and lacrimal glands. The tongue becomes dry and fissured. Swallowing is difficult. A reliable method for testing for dryness of the mouth is to place your finger on the mucous membranes where the gums and the cheek meet. When a fluid deficit is present, you will find that your finger does not glide easily because of the dryness. This method works well in infants and in persons who are unresponsive.

One of the most serious aspects of a fluid deficit is the *dehydration of brain and nerve cells*. Generalized muscle weakness, muscle rigidity, and muscle tremors often occur in severe fluid deficit as water is removed from cells in the nervous system. Delirium, hallucinations, and maniacal behavior may also develop in situations of severe fluid deficit.

Body temperature.   Dehydration is known to produce a rise in body temperature. Part of this elevation in temperature probably results from a lack of available fluid for sweating. It also appears that dehydration has a direct effect on the hypothalamus, since dehydration can cause fever even in a cold environment. Body temperature may reach 105°F when dehydration is severe.[8]

In summary, an isotonic fluid deficit is characterized by a reduction in the extracellular fluid volume that is caused by a loss of both sodium and water. Extracellular fluid volume deficit causes thirst; decreased urine output and specific gravity, decreased vascular volume, and signs related to loss of fluid from the cellular compartment. The causes and manifestations of extracellular fluid volume deficit are summarized in Table 22-3.

Extracellular fluid excess (isotonic)

In extracellular fluid excess, sodium and water are retained and there is an isotonic expansion of fluid in the extracellular compartment.

Causes of extracellular fluid excess.

Extracellular fluid excess is generally caused by conditions that favor the retention of sodium and water, such as heart failure, cirrhosis of the liver, and kidney disease (Table 22-4). Circulatory overload can occur during administration of intravenous fluids or blood; this is particularly true when blood is given to a patient with a normal blood volume. The elderly and patients with heart disease require careful observation because even small amounts of blood may overload the circulatory system. Although extracellular fluid excess often accompanies disease, this is not always the case. For example, there is a compensatory increase in extracellular fluid that occurs during hot weather, and premenstrual fluid retention that is caused by hormonal changes.

Manifestations of extracellular fluid excess.

Development of edema is characteristic of extracellular fluid excess.* Just as weight is a good indicator of extracellular fluid deficit, so also is weight gain a good indicator of fluid excess. In situations where

---

*The causes and mechanisms associated with edema are discussed in Chapter 24.

fluid excess occurs gradually, edema fluid may mask weight loss that is due to actual loss of tissue mass; this often happens in debilitating disease states and in starvation. The edema associated with excess extracellular fluid may be generalized or it may be confined to dependent areas of the body such as the legs and feet. Often the eyelids are puffy when the person awakens. When excess fluid accumulates in the lungs, there is shortness of breath, complaints of dyspnea, rales, and a productive cough. An increase in vascular volume causes the pulse to have a full and bounding quality.

In summary, an extracellular fluid volume excess describes an isotonic expansion of the extracellular compartment. It is seen in conditions that favor reabsorption of sodium and water by the kidney. Although extracellular fluid excess is frequently seen in disease states, it can occur as a compensatory mechanism during hot weather or as an indication of cyclic changes in hormonal balance, such as premenstrual fluid retention. The causes and manifestations of extracellular fluid excess are summarized in Table 22-4.

:Electrolytes

Although water provides volume for body fluids, it is the electrolytes that contribute to the function of these fluids. Electrolytes serve many functions. They (1) assist in regulating water balance, (2) participate in acid–base regulation, (3) contribute to enzyme reactions, and (4) play an essential role in neuromuscular activity. This section focuses on the alterations in body function that are associated with disturbances in sodium, potassium, calcium, phosphate, and magnesium balance. Alterations in bicar-

---

Table 22-4   Extracellular Fluid Excess

Causes	Signs and Symptoms
Excess sodium and water intake	**Acute weight gain (in excess of 5%)**
Excess dietary intake	**Increased extracellular fluid**
Medications or home remedies containing sodium	Pitting edema of the extremities
Administration of parenteral solutions which	Puffy eyelids
contain sodium	Pulmonary edema
Decreased renal losses	Shortness of breath
Renal disease	Rales
Increased mineralocorticoid levels	Dyspnea
Aldosterone	Cough
Glucocorticoids	Full and bounding pulse
Congestive heart failure	Venous distention
Cirrhosis	

Table 22-5   Concentration of Intracellular and Extracellular Electrolytes

Electrolyte	Intracellular Concentration (mEq/liter)	Extracellular Concentration (mEq/liter)
Sodium	10	137–147
Potassium	141	3.5–5.0
Chloride	4	100–106
Bicarbonate	10	24–31
Phosphate	75	1.7–3.6
Calcium	1	4.5–5.3
Magnesium	58	1.5–2.5

bonate and chloride concentrations are discussed in Chapter 23.

There are marked differences in the composition of intracellular and extracellular electrolytes (Table 22-5). The reader will note that the sodium concentration is greatest in the extracellular compartment, whereas potassium is concentrated within the cells. Blood tests measure electrolytes and therefore represent the concentration of electrolytes in the extracellular compartment rather than the intracellular compartment. This means that blood tests do not always provide an accurate index of intracellular electrolytes such as potassium.

Alterations in Sodium Balance

Sodium affects many body functions. Regulation of serum sodium is essential for maintaining (1) the osmolality of the extracellular fluids, (2) normal neuromuscular function, (3) acid–base balance, and (4) numerous vital chemical reactions. As the major cation in the extracellular compartment, sodium and its attendant anions (chloride and bicarbonate) account for about 93% of the osmotic activity that is present in the extracellular fluids. Sodium is a component of sodium bicarbonate and, as such, is highly important in regulating acid–base balance.

Sodium gains

Sodium intake is normally derived from dietary sources. Body needs can usually be met by as little as 500 mg per day.* In the United States, average salt intake is about 6 to 15 grams per day or 12 to 30 times the daily requirement. Other sources of sodium are intravenous saline infusions and medications that contain sodium. An often-forgotten source of sodium is the sodium bicarbonate or other sodium-containing home remedies that are used to treat upset stomach or other ailments. Sodium ingestion in

_____
*In the absence of sweating

excess of what the kidneys can excrete is an unlikely occurrence in healthy individuals, probably because taste prohibits this from occurring and because of the kidneys' remarkable ability to regulate sodium. Sodium excess has occurred, however, in persons receiving intravenous saline infusions and in persons unable to monitor their oral intake. The accidental substitution of salt for sugar in infant formulas has been known to produce severe hypernatremia, causing brain damage and death.

Sodium losses

The body loses sodium through the kidneys, skin, and gastrointestinal tract. The kidneys are extremely efficient in regulating sodium output, and when sodium intake is limited or conservation of sodium is needed, the kidneys are able to reabsorb almost all of the sodium that has been filtered by the glomerulus. This results in an essentially sodium-free urine. Conversely, urinary losses of sodium will increase as intake is increased. For practical purposes, the 24-hour urinary excretion of sodium is assumed to be equal to sodium intake.

Renal losses. Alterations in kidney function can cause either an increase or a decrease in sodium losses. Sodium deficit with an accompanying loss of extracellular fluid occurs in salt-wasting kidney disease. On the other hand, many forms of kidney disease cause sodium retention. A decrease in renal blood flow causes increased sodium retention via the renin–angiotensin–aldosterone mechanism. Sodium retention is therefore increased in nonrenal diseases that lead to a decrease in renal blood flow. In congestive heart failure, renal blood flow is decreased because the heart does not pump properly.

Skin losses. Although skin losses of sodium are usually negligible, sweat losses can be extensive during exercise and periods of exposure to a hot environment. A person who sweats profusely can lose as much as 15 to 20 grams of sodium per day; this amount decreases to as little as 3 to 5 grams with acclimatization.[9] Loss of skin surface, such as occurs in extensive burns, also leads to excessive skin losses of sodium.

Gastrointestinal losses. Sodium moves freely between the extracellular fluid and the contents of the gastrointestinal tract. In the upper part of the gastrointestinal tract, the concentration of sodium is very similar to that of plasma. Sodium is reabsorbed as the contents of the gut move through the lower part of the bowel, so that the concentration of sodium in the stool is normally only about 32 mEq per liter. Sodium losses increase with vomiting, diarrhea, fistula drainage, and gastrointestinal suction. Irrigation of gastrointestinal tubes with distilled water removes sodium from the gastrointestinal tract as do repeated tap water enemas.

Regulation of serum sodium levels

The normal serum concentration of sodium ranges from 135 to 147 mEq per liter. It is important for the reader to recognize that serum sodium values reflect the *concentration* of sodium in the extracellular fluids, *expressed as mEq per liter*, rather than an *absolute amount*. This means that dehydration will cause the concentration of sodium to increase even though the total amount of sodium that the body contains has not been changed. Likewise, fluid excess will cause sodium levels to decrease even though sodium has not been lost from the body.

Aldosterone. Renal reabsorption of sodium by the kidney is largely regulated by aldosterone levels. Aldosterone is a mineralocorticoid (remember that sodium and potassium are minerals) hormone which is produced by the adrenal cortex. The hormone promotes the reabsorption of sodium and the secretion of potassium by cells in the distal tubule of the kidney while allowing potassium to be lost in the urine. Several mechanisms, including the following, are known to control aldosterone levels: (1) extracellular sodium concentrations, (2) extracellular potassium levels, (3) angiotensin II, and (4) the adrenocorticotropic hormone (ACTH). A reduction in renal blood flow increases aldosterone via the renin–angiotensin mechanism. Although aldosterone increases sodium reabsorption by the kidney and thereby contributes to what might be termed the "short-term" regulation of sodium balance, it seems to play only a minor role in the long-term regulation of sodium levels. This is because an

increase in sodium reabsorption via the aldosterone mechanism ultimately leads to an increase in vascular volume which causes an increase in renal blood flow and glomerular filtration rate, with a subsequent decrease in renin release.

Addison's disease is a condition of chronic adrenal insufficiency in which there is unregulated loss of sodium in the urine with increased retention of potassium. The *glucocorticoids* from the adrenal cortex also have mineralocorticoid activity. *Cushing's syndrome* characterizes a condition in which there are increased levels of glucocorticoids. The fact that these hormones increase salt and water retention helps to explain why persons who are being treated with drugs that contain exogenous forms of these hormones often develop hypertension and edema.*

Sodium deficit (hyponatremia)

Sodium deficit (hyponatremia) occurs when the sodium concentration falls below 130 mEq per liter. Sodium deficit may constitute an actual loss of sodium from the body or it may occur because of dilution of sodium in the extracellular fluid. Usually sodium is lost from the body in excess of water. Although the discussion in this chapter focuses on dilutional hyponatremia the reader is reminded that sodium deficit may present with a decrease in extracellular or vascular volume.

Causes of sodium deficit. Normally, homeostatic mechanisms make it almost impossible to produce an increase in body water when renal function is adequate and ADH and aldosterone levels are normal. Excess water is retained, however, when a person has an *elevation in ADH levels*. Although infrequent, water excess can occur as the result of *excessive water intake*. As was mentioned earlier in the chapter, the drinking of water in excess of that which the kidneys can excrete occurs in patients with *psychogenic polydipsia*. Water intoxication in the psychiatric patient may be aggravated by treatment with antipsychotic drugs that increase ADH levels.

Excessive sodium losses occur with excessive sweating, gastrointestinal losses, and diuresis. Excessive sweating in hot weather leads to loss of sodium and water. Hyponatremia develops when fluids lost in sweating are replaced by the drinking

*The reader is referred to Chapter 33 for a more complete discussion of the adrenal cortical hormones.

Table 22-6 Dilutional Hyponatremia

Causes	Signs and Symptoms
Excess water intake or gain	**Laboratory values**
Administration of excess sodium-free parenteral solutions	Serum sodium below 137 mEq/liter
Psychogenic polydipsia	Decreased serum osmolality
Ingestion of tap water during periods of sodium deficit	Dilution of other blood components, including chloride, hematocrit and BUN
Repeated administration of tap water enemas	
Decreased water losses	**Increased water content of brain and nerve cells**
Kidney disease which impairs urine concentration	Headache
Increased ADH levels	Depression
Trauma, stress, pain	Personality changes
SIADH	Confusion
Use of medications which increase ADH release	Apprehension and feeling of impending doom
	Lethargy
	Stupor
	Coma
	Convulsions
	Gastrointestinal disturbances
	Anorexia
	Abdominal cramps
	Diarrhea
	Increased intracellular fluid
	Fingerprinting over sternum

of tap water.* Repeated administration of tap water enemas or frequent irrigation of gastrointestinal tubes with distilled water leads to removal of sodium chloride from the gastrointestinal tract. Salt depletion also occurs with adrenal insufficiency and diuresis due to vigorous use of diuretics (see Table 22-6).

Manifestations of sodium deficit. In dilutional hyponatremia, the osmotic pressure of the extracellular fluids becomes less than that in the cells and water moves out of the extracellular compartment into the cells. The signs and symptoms of hyponatremia depend on the rapidity of onset and severity of the sodium dilution. If the condition develops slowly, signs and symptoms are usually not apparent until serum sodium levels approach 125 mEq per liter. The brain and nervous system are the most seriously affected by increases in intracellular water, and neurologic signs and symptoms progress rapidly once serum sodium levels fall below 120 mEq per liter. Swelling of the brain can cause headache, mental

depression, apprehension, personality changes, gross motor weakness, and even hemiplegia. Convulsions and coma occur when serum sodium levels reach extremely low levels. An acute increase in intracellular water is often of sudden onset and should be suspected in any postoperative or post-trauma patient who suddenly behaves in a bizarre fashion.

An increase in intracellular water produces another interesting finding. The increased intracellular water content causes tissues to have a plastic consistency that is similar to that of modeling clay. This permits fingerprinting of the skin. If you roll your finger over the sternum, your fingerprint will become visible on the patient's skin. This is different from the tissue indentation that occurs with pitting edema.

In summary, dilutional hyponatremia describes a condition in which the sodium concentration of the extracellular fluids is decreased. It can occur as the result of excess water retention or because sodium is lost from the body in excess of water losses. The decrease in serum osmolality that accompanies sodium deficit causes water to move into body cells. Many of the detrimental effects of dilutional hyponatremia are due to swelling of body cells, particularly those in the central nervous system. The causes and manifestations of hyponatremia are summarized in Table 22-6.

---

*Salt tablets (0.5 g per 500 ml water) may be used to replace excessive sweat losses. Oral electrolyte solutions, such as Gatorade (Stokely Van Camp), Sportade punch concentrate (Becton, Dickinson) and Bike Half-time Punch Mix (Kendall) can also be used to replace water and electrolytes lost through excessive perspiration.

Sodium excess (hypernatremia)

Sodium excess (hypernatremia) occurs when sodium levels rise above 150 mEq per liter. Serum sodium excess almost always follows a loss in body fluids that contain more water than sodium.* This can occur (1) in diabetes insipidus where urinary losses of water are increased, (2) when respiratory losses are increased as during tracheobronchitis, (3) in situations of watery diarrhea, or (4) when osmotically active tube feedings are given with inadequate amounts of water. Generally hypernatremia, with an accompanying water deficit, will stimulate thirst and increase water intake. Hypernatremia is therefore more apt to occur in infants and persons who are unable to express their thirst or obtain water to drink. The unconscious person is particularly at risk for developing hypernatremia (see Table 22-7).

The *clinical manifestations* of hypernatremia are largely related to an increase in serum osmolality; this causes water to be pulled out of body cells. With hypernatremia urine output is decreased due to renal conserving mechanisms. Thirst is excessive. Body temperature is frequently elevated and the skin becomes warm and flushed. The mucous membranes are dry and sticky and the tongue is rough and dry. The subcutaneous tissues assume a firm and rubbery texture. Vascular volume decreases, the pulse becomes rapid, and the blood pressure drops. Most significantly, water is pulled out of cells in the central nervous system; this causes decreased reflexes, agitation, and restlessness. Coma and convulsions may develop as hypernatremia progresses. Permanent brain damage has occurred in infants recovering from severe hypernatremia.

In summary, hypernatremia occurs when the concentration of sodium levels in the extracellular fluid rises above 150 mEq per liter. The increase in sodium concentration causes the extracellular fluid to be hypertonic in relation to the intracellular fluid. Water is pulled out of all body cells including the skin and mucous membranes. In the central nervous system, neural function is impaired due to cellular dehydration. The causes and manifestations of hypernatremia are summarized in Table 22-7.

Alterations in Potassium Balance

Potassium is the major cation in the intracellular compartment. Potassium affects many body functions and (1) contributes to maintenance of intra-

---

*The reader will note that the causes and manifestations of hypernatremia are similar to those of water deficit.

Table 22-7 Dilutional Hypernatremia

Causes	Signs and Symptoms
Excess sodium intake	**Laboratory findings**
Rapid or excess administration of sodium chloride parenteral solutions	Serum sodium above 147 mEq/liter
Excess oral intake	Increased serum osmolality
Decreased extracellular water	**Thirst**
Increased water losses	**Urine output**
Diuretic therapy	Oliguria or anuria
Adrenal cortical hormone excess	High specific gravity
Diabetes insipidus	
Tracheobronchitis	**Intracellular dehydration**
Watery diarrhea	Skin and mucous membranes
Hypertonic tube feedings	Skin dry and flushed
Decreased water intake	Mucous membranes dry and sticky
Unconsciousness or inability to relate thirst	Tongue rough and dry
Oral trauma or inability to swallow	Subcutaneous tissue
Impaired thirst mechanism	Firm and rubbery
Withholding of water for therapeutic reasons	Central nervous system
	Agitation and restlessness
	Decreased reflexes
	Maniacal behavior
	Convulsions and coma
	Increased body temperature
	Decreased vascular volume
	Tachycardia
	Decreased blood pressure
	Weak and thready pulse

cellular osmolality, (2) is necessary for neuromuscular control and the precise regulation of skeletal, cardiac, and smooth muscle activity, (3) influences acid–base balance, and (4) participates in many intracellular enzyme reactions. For example, potassium contributes to the intricate chemical reactions that transform carbohydrates into energy, change glucose into glycogen, and convert amino acids to proteins.

Gains and losses

Potassium intake is normally derived from dietary sources. In healthy individuals, potassium balance can usually be maintained by a daily dietary intake of 50 to 100 mEq. Additional amounts of potassium are needed during periods of trauma and stress. The kidney is the main source of potassium loss. Normally about 80% to 90% of potassium losses occur in the urine with the remaining losses occurring in the stool and sweat.

Regulation of body potassium levels

Potassium is essentially an intracellular cation. This means that serum levels of potassium which normally range from 3.5 to 5.0 mEq per liter will not always reflect the intracellular potassium content; however, they do accurately reflect the concentration in the extracellular fluid. Potassium moves freely between the interstitial and vascular compartments. When body cells are injured or when cellular activity becomes catabolic, potassium is released into the extracellular compartment and is then lost in the urine. Subsequently, following chronic potassium deficiency, the kidneys' ability to conserve potassium improves and the loss is reduced to as little as 5 mEq per liter. When this happens, plasma levels of potassium are likely to remain within normal levels even though total body potassium has decreased. On the other hand, plasma potassium levels tend to fall when tissue breakdown ceases and cellular activity becomes anabolic causing potassium to move back into the cellular compartment. This is because potassium is needed for glycogen storage and protein synthesis.

Potassium–hydrogen ion exchange. The hydrogen ion concentration (pH) of the extracellular fluid contributes to the compartmental shift of potassium. In acidosis, the movement of hydrogen ions into body cells is used as a means of buffering pH changes in the extracellular fluids. Generally, the plasma potassium concentration rises 0.6 mEq per liter for each 0.1 unit fall in blood pH. When a hydrogen ion moves into the cell another positively charged ion

(potassium) must leave.* This means that potassium tends to move out of the intracellular compartment in acidosis and into the intracellular compartment in alkalosis.

Plasma potassium levels also affect pH at the kidney level where potassium and hydrogen compete for excretion in exchange for reabsorbed sodium. When the extracellular concentration of potassium is high, tubular secretion of potassium into the urine is increased and hydrogen excretion is decreased. Conversely, when extracellular concentrations of potassium are low, tubular secretion of potassium into the urine is decreased and hydrogen ion secretion is increased; this tends to lead to metabolic alkalosis.

Aldosterone regulation of potassium levels. Aldosterone plays an important role in regulating extracellular potassium concentrations. Urinary losses of potassium increase under the influence of aldosterone, whereas sodium retention is increased. The feedback regulation of aldosterone levels, in turn, is strongly regulated by plasma potassium levels; for example, an increase in potassium ion concentration of less than 1 mEq per liter will cause aldosterone levels to triple. Furthermore, this increased secretion will continue for as long as the elevated potassium levels are present.

Pathology of aldosterone secretion or production. Primary aldosteronism is caused by a tumor in the cells of the adrenal cortex (in the zona glomerulosa) that secrete aldosterone. Excess secretion of aldosterone by the tumor cells causes severe potassium losses and a decrease in serum potassium levels. Patients with this disorder may develop muscle paralysis as a result of the low serum levels of potassium. Adrenal insufficiency (Addison's disease) causes the opposite effect; these patients have elevated serum potassium levels due to an aldosterone deficiency.

Potassium deficit (hypokalemia)

Hypokalemia refers to a decrease in serum potassium levels below 3.5 mEq per liter. Because potassium moves freely between the intracellular and extracellular compartments, hypokalemia can occur as the result of a loss of total body potassium or because extracellular potassium has moved into the intracellular compartment. Usually both intracellular and extracellular potassium concentrations are decreased simultaneously.

---

*The reader is reminded that cations must equal anions.

Causes of potassium deficit. Potassium deficit can occur for three reasons: (1) inadequate intake, (2) excessive losses, or (3) extracellular potassium has moved into body cells (Table 22-8).

The kidneys are unable to conserve potassium and even in time of great need the kidneys continue to excrete potassium. This means that a potassium deficit can develop rather quickly if intake is inadequate. Unfortunately, intake is frequently impaired at the time that potassium losses are increased, as following surgery or during prolonged diarrhea. The elderly are particularly likely to develop a potassium deficit. This is because they often have poor eating habits as a consequence of living alone; they have limited income which makes buying of foods high in potassium difficult; they have difficulty in chewing many of the foods which have a high potassium content because of poorly fitting dentures; or they may have problems with swallowing. Furthermore, medical problems in the elderly often require treatment with drugs, such as the diuretics, that tend to increase potassium losses.

The kidney is the main source of potassium loss and normally about 80% to 90% of potassium losses occur in the urine with the remaining losses occurring in the stool and sweat. Unfortunately, the kidneys do not have the homeostatic mechanisms needed to conserve potassium during decreased intake. An adult on a potassium-free diet will continue to lose approximately 5 to 15 mEq of potassium daily. Following trauma, and in stress situations, urinary losses of potassium are greatly increased, sometimes approaching levels of 150 to 200 mEq per day. Diuretic therapy (with the exception of spironolactone

Table 22-8 Potassium Deficit

Causes	Signs and Symptoms
Inadequate intake	**Laboratory values**
Inability to eat	Serum potassium below 3.5 mEq/liter
Diet deficient in potassium	**Skeletal muscles**
Administration of potassium-free parenteral solutions	Fatigue
	Muscle tenderness or paresthesias
Excessive gastrointestinal losses	Weakness
Vomiting	Muscle flabbiness
Diarrhea	Paralysis
Suction	
Fistula	**Cardiovascular system**
	Postural hypotension
Excessive renal losses	Increased sensitivity to digitalis
Diuretic phase of renal failure	Arrhythmias
Diuretic therapy (except triamterene and spironolactone)	**Gastrointestinal tract**
Increased mineralocorticoid levels	Anorexia
Cushing's syndrome	Vomiting
Primary aldosteronism	Abdominal distention
Treatment with glucocorticoid hormones	Paralytic ileus
Intracellular shift	**Respiratory muscles**
During treatment for diabetic acidosis	Shortness of breath
Alkalosis, either metabolic or respiratory	Shallow breathing
	Kidneys
	Polyuria
	Low osmolality and specific gravity of urine
	Nocturia
	Thirst
	Central nervous system function
	Confusion
	Depression
	Acid–base balance
	Metabolic alkalosis

and triamterene) results in additional urinary losses of potassium.

Although potassium loses through the skin and gastrointestinal tract are usually minimal, these losses can become excessive under certain conditions. For example, burns increase surface losses of potassium and sweat losses can become markedly increased in persons who are acclimated to a hot climate. In other situations, gastrointestinal losses become excessive; this occurs with vomiting and diarrhea and in situations where gastrointestinal suction is being used.

Manifestations of potassium deficit.   Potassium deficit results in impaired function of skeletal, cardiac, and smooth muscle. Often the signs and symptoms of potassium deficit are gradual in onset and for that reason go undetected for a considerable period of time.

Renal function.   Important abnormalities of renal function occur in hypokalemia. The kidneys are unable to concentrate urine normally. Urine output is increased and serum osmolality and specific gravity are increased. The patient complains of polyuria, nocturia, and thirst.

Gastrointestinal function.   Hypokalemia causes numerous signs and symptoms associated with gastrointestinal function. These include anorexia, nausea, vomiting, abdominal distention, absent bowel sounds, and paralytic ileus. When gastrointestinal symptoms occur gradually and are not severe, they often serve to impair potassium intake.

Neuromuscular function.   Neuromuscular signs and symptoms appear when serum potassium levels fall to approximately 2.5 mEq per liter. Muscle weakness appears first, followed by paralysis. Leg muscles, particularly the quadriceps, are most prominently affected. Some patients complain of muscle tenderness and paresthesias rather than weakness. In chronic potassium deficiency, actual muscle atrophy may occur and contribute to muscle weakness. Familial periodic paralysis is a disorder in which episodes of hypokalemia cause attacks of flaccid paralysis that last from a few minutes to several hours. The paralysis may be precipitated by situations that reduce serum potassium levels, such as a high carbohydrate meal or administration of insulin, epinephrine, or glucocorticoid drugs. The paralysis is often reversed by potassium therapy. Severe hypokalemia may affect the respiratory muscles. When

this happens, the diaphragm is usually affected earlier than the intercostal muscles.

Cardiovascular function.   Potassium deficiency also affects cardiovascular function. Postural hypotension is common. *Of particular importance is the fact that hypokalemia increases the risk of digitalis toxicity.* The dangers associated with digitalis toxicity are compounded in patients who are receiving both digitalis and diuretics. Serious cardiac arrhythmias that result from hypokalemia are described in Figure 22-4.

Treatment of potassium deficit.   Potassium deficits are treated by increasing the intake of foods high in potassium content—meats, dried fruits, fruit juices (particularly orange juice), and bananas. The reader is referred to a nutrition text for a description of foods that are high in potassium. Potassium supplements are prescribed for persons whose intake of potassium is insufficient in relation to losses. This is particularly true of persons who are on diuretic therapy and who are taking digitalis.

Potassium is given intravenously when the oral route is not tolerated or when rapid replacement is needed. The rapid infusion of a concentrated potassium solution has been known to cause death due to cardiac arrest. It is suggested that all health personnel who assume responsibility for administering intravenous solutions containing potassium be fully aware of all the precautions pertaining to its dilution and flow rate. Pharmacology texts, drug company package inserts, fluid and electrolyte texts, and pharmacists serve as useful resources for this information.

In summary, potassium is the major cation in the intracellular compartment. Potassium is ingested in the diet and excreted in the urine. The kidneys are relatively inefficient in potassium conservation, and urinary losses continue even when intake has been curtailed; these losses are accentuated in persons on diuretic therapy. Potassium is essential for normal function of skeletal, cardiac, and smooth muscle. Hypokalemia occurs when potassium levels fall below 3.5 mEq per liter. The causes and manifestations of potassium deficit are summarized in Table 22-8.

Potassium excess (hyperkalemia)

Hyperkalemia refers to blood levels of potassium that are in excess of 5.5 mEq per liter. In general it can be said that serum potassium excess occurs whenever potassium gains exceed losses.

Causes of potassium excess. The major causes of potassium excess are (1) renal failure, (2) adrenal insufficiency, and (3) excess potassium gains due to tissue trauma or intravenous administration of potassium at a rate that exceeds the kidneys' ability to control serum potassium levels (Table 22-9). It is seldom possible to increase intake of potassium to the point of causing hyperkalemia when sufficient aldosterone is present and renal function is adequate. An exception to this rule exists when potassium solutions are being infused intravenously—*severe and fatal incidents of hyperkalemia have resulted from intravenous infusion of potassium. Intravenous solutions containing potassium should never be started until urine output has been assessed and renal function deemed to be adequate*; this is because the kidneys control potassium losses. Movement of potassium out of body cells into the extracellular fluids also affords the potential for elevation of blood potassium. For example, burns and crushing injuries cause potassium to be liberated into the extracellular fluid. Often these same injuries cause a decrease in renal function which contributes to the development of hyperkalemia.

Manifestations of potassium excess. The signs and symptoms of potassium excess are closely related to the alterations in neuromuscular function that accompany potassium imbalance. Many of these manifestations are similar to those which were described for hypokalemia. While the mechanisms responsible for the altered neuromuscular function observed in hypo- and hyperkalemia are different, the end results are similar. The first symptom associated with hyperkalemia is often a paresthesia; this may appear when potassium levels reach 6 mEq per liter. The most serious effect of hyperkalemia is cardiac arrest. The electrocardiographic changes that occur with alterations in serum potassium levels are described in Figure 22-4.

Treatment of potassium excess. The treatment of potassium excess focusses on (1) decreasing or curtailing intake, (2) increasing renal excretion, and (3) increasing cellular uptake. Decreased intake can be accomplished by restricting dietary sources of potassium. It should be mentioned here that most of the salt substitutes contain potassium chloride as their major ingredient and should not be given to patients

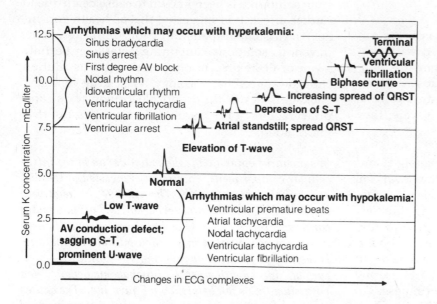

Figure 22–4. ECG changes at various levels of serum potassium concentration. (Krupp MA, Chatton MJ (eds): Current Medical Diagnosis and Treatment. Copyright 1974, Lange Medical Publications, Los Altos, CA)

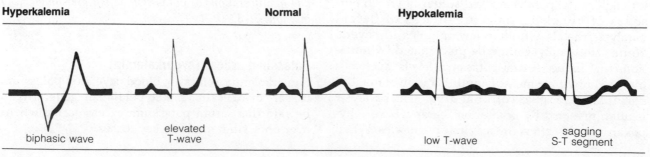

Table 22-9   Potassium Excess

Causes	Signs and Symptoms
Excess intake or gain	**Laboratory values**
Excessive oral intake	Serum potassium above 5.5 mEq/liter
Excessive or rapid parenteral infusion	**Neural and skeletal muscle activity**
Tissue trauma, early burns, and massive crushing injuries	Paresthesias
Decreased renal losses	Weakness and dizziness
Renal failure	Muscle cramps
Adrenal insufficiency	**Smooth muscle activity of the gastrointestinal tract**
Addison's disease	Nausea, diarrhea
Potassium-sparing diuretics (spironolactone and triamterene)	Intestinal colic and gastrointestinal distress
	Cardiac electrophysiology
	Peaked T waves, depressed ST segment
	Depressed P wave and widening of QRS
	Cardiac arrest

with renal problems. Increasing potassium output is often more difficult. Persons with renal failure may require hemodialysis or peritoneal dialysis to reduce serum potassium levels. A sodium polystyrene sulfonate resin may also be used to remove potassium ions from the colon. The sodium ions in the resin are replaced by potassium ions and then the potassium-containing resin is excreted in the stool.

Emergency methods usually focus on measures that cause serum potassium to move into the cell. Intravenous infusion of insulin and glucose is sometimes used for this purpose.

In summary, serum potassium excess is of concern in patients with renal failure and adrenal insufficiency. Hyperkalemia can also occur during rapid infusion of intravenous fluids that contain potassium. Cardiac arrest is a dreaded complication of potassium excess. The causes and manifestations of potassium excess are described in Table 22-9.

Calcium and Phosphate

There is a close link between regulation of calcium and of phosphate ions in the body. A change in the concentration of one ion leads to a change in the concentration of the other. Therefore, calcium and phosphate are discussed together in this chapter.

Calcium and phosphate salts are deposited in the organic matrix of bone—bone is essentially 30% matrix and 70% salts. In the extracellular fluid the concentration of calcium and phosphate is reciprocally regulated—when calcium levels are high, phosphate levels are low and *vice versa*. Normal serum levels of calcium (9.0 to 10.6 mg per dl) and

phosphate (3.0 to 4.5 mg per dl) have a product of approximately 35. This reciprocal relationship is important because the concentrations of calcium and phosphate are considerably greater than those required to cause precipitation. Precipitation of calcium and phosphate salts is normally prevented by inhibitors that are present in most tissues.

Gains and losses

Calcium and phosphate enter the body through the gastrointestinal tract, are stored in bone, and are excreted through the kidney. The major source of calcium is milk and milk products. Phosphate is derived from many sources, including milk and meats. Only about 30% to 50% of dietary calcium is absorbed in the duodenum and upper jejunum; the remainder is excreted in the stool. Phosphate, on the other hand, is absorbed exceedingly well.

Normally, the kidney controls calcium and phosphate losses. The two ions are filtered in the glomerulus and are selectively reabsorbed in the renal tubules. The amount of phosphate that is lost in the urine is directly related to phosphate concentrations in the blood. When serum phosphate levels rise above a critical level, the rate of phosphate loss in the urine reflects blood phosphate levels. Calcium excretion is reciprocally related to phosphate excretion. In renal failure, phosphate excretion is impaired and as a result serum calcium levels decline as blood phosphate levels rise.

Regulation of calcium and phosphate

Serum calcium and phosphate are regulated by vitamin D, parathyroid hormone, and calcitonin. The body contains a supply of exchangeable calcium that is in equilibrium with calcium in the extracellular fluids. Most of this exchangeable calcium is found in bone. It is this exchangeable pool that serves as a storage site for calcium. Movement of calcium between the blood and the exchangeable pool is rapid—it usually occurs within minutes to 1 hour. The regulation of phosphate levels is closely linked to calcium metabolism. The phosphate ion is freely absorbed from the intestine, and changing the serum phosphate levels to as high as three to four times the normal value does not seem to have an immediate effect on body function.

Vitamin D.   Vitamin D has a potent effect on calcium absorption from the intestine and aids in both deposition and mobilization of calcium and phosphate from bone. Vitamin D exists in several forms. Cholecalciferol results from ultraviolet radiation of 7-dehydrocholesterol in the skin. A synthetic vitamin D, ergocalciferol, is formed by irradiation of ergosterol. Both forms of vitamin D must be converted to the active form of vitamin D (1,25-dihydroxycholecalciferol) before it can accomplish these functions. Vitamin D is activated by processes that occur in the liver and kidney. This means that severe diseases of the liver and kidney may impair the activation of vitamin D and lead to defects in calcium metabolism.

Parathyroid hormone (PTH).   Parathyroid hormone is produced by the four parathyroid glands which are located on the surface of the thyroid gland. The actions of the hormone are directed toward maintaining serum calcium levels; the stimulus for PTH release is a decrease in serum calcium. The physiologic actions of the hormone include (1) stimulation of calcium and phosphate reabsorption from bone, (2) increased activation of vitamin D, (3) stimulation of renal tubular reabsorption of calcium, and (4) increased loss of phosphate due to decreased tubular reabsorption. The increase in renal excretion of phosphate is necessary to rid the body of the phosphate that has been released from the bone as calcium was reabsorbed.

Calcitonin.   The hormone calcitonin (sometimes called thyrocalcitonin) is secreted by the parafollicular (C) cells in the thyroid gland. Calcitonin inhibits calcium mobilization from bone and thus tends to lower serum calcium in a manner that is opposite that of PTH. Its release is stimulated by hypercalcemia. *Paget's disease* is characterized by continuous destruction of bone. The rapid turnover rate of bone in persons with this disease is often suppressed by administration of calcitonin.

Alterations in Calcium Balance

Calcium can be found in several forms in the body. Ninety-nine percent of body calcium is found in bone where it provides the strength and stability for the collagen and ground substance that form the structural matrix of the skeletal system. The other 1% is located in the tissues and extracellular fluids. The calcium salts in bone serve as a reservoir of tissue and serum calcium.

Extracellular calcium exists in three forms. About 50% of serum calcium is bound to plasma proteins and cannot pass through the capillary wall to leave the vascular compartment. Five percent of serum calcium is combined with substances such as citrate, phosphate, and sulfate. This form is not ionized. The remaining 45% of serum calcium is ionized. It is the ionized calcium that is able to leave the capillary and enter the intercellular spaces, and it is this form of calcium that is physiologically important.

Serum calcium serves a number of functions. First, ionized calcium helps to maintain the permeability of cell membranes. Nerve cell membranes are less permeable and less excitable when sufficient ionized calcium is present. Second, calcium participates in a number of enzyme reactions. Third, calcium aids in blood clotting. The calcium ion is required for all but the first two steps of the intrinsic pathway for blood coagulation. Removal of ionized calcium is often used as a method to prevent clotting in blood that has been removed from the body. For example, citrate is often used to prevent clotting in blood that is to be used in tranfusion. Fortunately, calcium ion concentrations in the body never fall to levels that affect blood clotting.

The normal level of serum calcium (4.5 to 5.5 mEq per liter or 2.25 to 2.75 mmol per liter) can be misleading because it usually measures all three forms of calcium. First, the proportion of ionized to unionized calcium is affected by pH. The ionization of calcium is increased in acidosis and decreased in alkalosis. Second, plasma protein levels determine how much calcium can be carried in the blood. It has been estimated that there is a 0.8 mg per 100 ml decrease in serum calcium for every 100 g per 100 ml decrease in serum albumin below the normal values.[10]

Calcium deficit (hypocalcemia)

Serum calcium levels are protected by bone stores and do not usually require a continual daily intake. The causes of hypocalcemia, or deficit in ionized calcium are (1) impaired ability to mobilize calcium from bone stores, (2) abnormal binding of calcium so that greater proportions of calcium are in the unionized form, (3) abnormal losses of calcium by the kidney, and (4) decreased absorption of calcium from the intestine (Table 22-10).

Causes of calcium deficit. The ability to mobilize calcium from bone stores is impaired in hypoparathyroidism. A PTH deficiency occurs in primary hypoparathyroidism and in accidental surgical removal of the parathyroid glands during thyroid surgery. All patients who have had a thyroidectomy should be observed for signs of calcium deficit during the early postoperative period. A pseudohypoparathyroidism occurs when there is end-organ refractoriness to parathyroid hormone.

The electrolyte or ionized form of calcium is decreased as serum calcium binds to plasma proteins or other substances. For example, serum pH affects the ionization of calcium; ionization is increased in acidosis and decreased in alkalosis. As mentioned previously, citrate combines with calcium and is often used as an anticoagulant for blood transfusions. Theoretically, excess citrate in donor blood could combine with the calcium in the recipient's blood, causing hypocalcemia and tetany. Normally, however, the liver removes the citrate from the blood within a matter of minutes and this does not occur. Therefore, when blood transfusions are given at a slow rate (less than 1 liter per hour in the adult) there is little danger of hypocalcemia due to citrate binding.[11] Hypocalcemia is a common finding in acute pancreatitis. A fall in serum calcium below 7 mg per 100 ml portends a poor prognosis in acute pancreatitis. It is not known whether the calcium is precipitated in the pancreas as a result of fat necrosis or whether calcium is sequestered elsewhere.

There is an inverse relationship between calcium and phosphate excretion by the kidney. Phosphate is retained in renal failure, causing serum calcium levels to decrease and PTH levels to increase. Hypocalcemia and hyperphosphatemia occur when the glomerular filtration rate falls below 25 to 30 ml per minute, the normal being 100 to 120 ml per minute.

Intestinal absorption of calcium is decreased when there is a deficiency of vitamin D. Vitamin D deficiency due to lack of intake is seldom seen today because many foods are fortified with vitamin D. Vitamin D deficiency is more apt to occur in malabsorption states, such as biliary obstruction, pancreatic insufficiency, and celiac disease in which there is impaired ability to absorb fat and fat-soluble vitamins. Vitamin D (inactivated form) is stored in the liver. In subsequent steps the liver and the kidneys convert inactive vitamin D to the activated form (1,25-dihydroxycholecalciferol). Vitamin D remains in the body only a short time once it has been activated. This means that patients with renal failure will have problems with absorption of calcium because of impaired activation of vitamin D. Fortunately, the activated form of the hormone has been synthesized and is now available (calcitriol) for use in treatment of calcium deficit in patients with renal failure.

Table 22-10 Calcium Deficit

Causes	Signs and Symptoms
Decreased serum gains	**Laboratory values**
Intestinal malabsorption	Serum calcium below 4.5 mEq/liter
Rapid dilution of plasma by parenteral administration of calcium-free solutions	
Hypoparathyroidism	**Increased nerve excitability**
Vitamin D deficiency (or impaired activation of vitamin D)	Paresthesias, especially numbness or tingling
	Skeletal muscle cramps
Increased serum losses	Abdominal spasms and cramps
Sequestering of calcium in tissue, e.g., massive infections of subcutaneous tissue	Hyperactive reflexes
	Carpopedal spasm
Decreased ionization (alkalosis or rapid correction of acidosis)	Tetany
	Laryngeal spasm
Citrate binding due to excessive administration of citrated blood	Positive Chvostek's test
	Positive Trousseau's test
Acute pancreatitis	
Hyperphosphatemia (in renal insufficiency)	
Decrease in plasma protein levels	

Manifestations of calcium deficit. Acute hypocalcemia ordinarily causes no significant signs and symptoms aside from those associated with neural excitability. This is because tetany will lead to death before other effects can develop. Ionized calcium stabilizes neuromuscular excitability. In severe hypocalcemia, increased neuromuscular excitability can cause tetany, laryngeal spasm, convulsions, and death. Both the Chvostek and the Trousseau signs are utilized to observe for an increase in neuromuscular excitability and tetany. The Chvostek's sign is elicited by tapping the face just below the temple at the point where the facial nerve emerges. Tapping the face over the facial nerve causes spasm of the lip, nose, or face when the test is positive. An inflated blood pressure cuff is used to test for Trousseau's sign. The cuff is inflated to a point which temporarily occludes the circulation of the hand, usually for a period of one to five minutes. Contraction of the fingers and hands (carpopedal spasm) indicates the presence of tetany.

Treatment of calcium deficit. The treatment of calcium deficit is directed toward increasing intake or absorption from the intestine. One glass of milk contains about 300 mg of calcium. An intravenous infusion containing calcium gluconate is used when tetany is present or anticipated. The active form of vitamin D is administered when liver or kidney mechanisms needed for hormone activation are impaired.

In summary, hypocalcemia describes a decrease in serum levels of ionized calcium. Although the body has large stores of calcium that are located in bone, it is the ionized calcium in the blood that is active as electrolytes. It is the electrolyte form of calcium that is essential to the control of neuromuscular function. In hypocalcemia, there is danger of increased neuromuscular activity and development of tetany. The causes and manifestations of calcium deficit are summarized in Table 22-10.

Calcium excess (hypercalcemia)

A serum calcium excess (hypercalcemia) results from excessive bone reabsorption and from intestinal absorption that exceeds the ability of the kidney to excrete the excess calcium ions (Table 22-11).

The most common causes of increased bone reabsorption (or destruction) are neoplasms, hyperparathyroidism, and prolonged immobility. There

Table 22-11   Calcium Excess

Causes	Signs and Symptoms
Increased serum gains	**Serum calcium above 5.5 mEq/liter**
Increased intestinal absorption	**Altered neural and muscular activity**
Excessive vitamin D	Muscle weakness and atrophy
Excessive calcium in diet	Ataxia, loss of muscle tone
Milk–alkali syndrome	Lethargy
Increased bone absorption	Stupor and coma
Immobility	Personality or behavioral changes
Increased levels of parathyroid hormone	**Associated with increased bone absorption**
Malignant neoplasms including leukemia and lymphomas	Deep bone pain
Decreased losses	Pathologic fractures
Excessive parathyroid hormone	**Renal**
	Polyuria
	Flank pain
	Signs of kidney stones
	Increased losses of sodium and potassium
	Cardiovascular
	Hypertension
	Shortening of the QT interval, AV block on electrocardiogram
	Gastrointestinal
	Anorexia
	Nausea
	Vomiting
	Constipation

are a number of malignant tumors, including carcinoma of the lung, kidney, bone, and ovaries that have been associated with hypercalcemia. Some tumors actually destroy the bone, while others produce a parathyroid-like hormone. Intestinal absorption of calcium increases with excessive doses of vitamin D. Fortunately, the liver can store vitamin D and it is reported that 1000 times the normal quantities can be ingested with only a threefold increase in serum levels of the active vitamin.[12] Another cause of excessive calcium absorption is the milk–alkali syndrome. The milk–alkali syndrome occurs in patients with peptic ulcers who are being treated with excessive amounts of milk and alkaline antacids, particularly calcium carbonate preparations. Excess calcium carbonate taken without milk has also been known to produce an increase in calcium levels.

Manifestations of calcium excess. The signs and symptoms associated with calcium excess originate from three sources: (1) a decrease in neuromuscular activity, (2) reabsorption of calcium from bone, and (3) exposure of the kidney to high concentrations of calcium. Neural excitability is decreased in hypercalcemia. There may be a dulling of consciousness, stupor, weakness, and muscle flaccidity. Acute psychoses are common when calcium levels rise above 16 mg per 100 ml. The heart responds to elevated levels of calcium with increased contractility and ventricular arrhythmias. Digitalis causes these responses to be accentuated. High calcium concentrations in the urine impair the ability of the kidney to concentrate urine by interfering with the action of ADH. This causes salt and water diuresis and an increased sensation of thirst. Hypercalciuria also predisposes to the development of renal calculi.

Hypercalcemic crisis describes an acute increase in serum calcium levels above 8 to 9 mEq per liter or (4 to 4.5 mmol per liter). In hypercalcemic crisis, polyuria, excessive thirst, volume depletion, fever, altered levels of consciousness, azotemia (nitrogenous wastes in the blood), and a disturbed mental state accompany other signs of calcium excess. Symptomatic hypercalcemia is associated with a high mortality rate; death is often due to cardiac arrest.

Treatment of calcium excess. Treatment of calcium excess is usually directed toward correcting or controlling the condition that is causing the disorder. Diuretics and sodium chloride can be administered in emergency treatment of hypercalcemia. Corticosteroids and mithramycin are used to treat hypercalcemia due to malignancy.

In summary, elevation of serum calcium levels predisposes to extraskeletal calcification, including the development of nephrolithiasis or kidney stones. A more serious effect of calcium excess is depression of neuromuscular activity and increased myocardial irritability. Hypercalcemic crisis describes an acute increase in serum calcium levels. Serum calcium levels are increased in neoplastic disease conditions that destroy bone, in immobility, and in situations of increased PTH levels. The causes and manifestations of calcium excess are summarized in Table 22-11.

Phosphate

Phosphate is an integral part of all body tissues. About 85% of phosphorus is located in bone; most of the remaining 15% is located intracellularly. In the adult, the normal serum phosphate level is 3.0 to 4.5 mg per 100 ml of plasma. These values are slightly higher in children (4.0 to 7.0 mg per 100 ml).

The functions of phosphate can be grouped into four categories: (1) phosphate plays a major role in bone formation; (2) phosphate is essential to metabolic processes, i.e., it is incorporated into adenosine triphosphate (ATP) as well as into enzymes needed for glucose, fat, and protein metabolism; (3) phosphate is an essential component of several vital parts of the cell, being incorporated into the nucleic acids and into the cell membrane; and (4) phosphate acts as an acid–base buffer in the extracellular fluid and in renal excretion of hydrogen ions. Delivery of oxygen by the red cell depends on organic phosphates in ATP and 2,3-diphosphoglycerate (2,3-DPG). Phosphate is also needed for normal function of other blood cells, including the white cells and platelets.

Phosphate deficit (hypophosphatemia)

Only recently has the importance of phosphate depletion been recognized. Phosphate depletion is associated with antacid use, malnutrition, alcoholism, ketoacidosis, alkalosis, and hyperthyroidism. Antacids that contain aluminum hydroxide, aluminum carbonate, and calcium carbonate bind with phosphate, causing increased phosphate losses in the stool. Aluminum hydroxide is sometimes used therapeutically to decrease phosphate levels in chronic renal failure. Alcoholism is commonly recognized as a cause of hypophosphatemia. One study reports that 42% of alcoholic patients who were admitted to hospital had low serum phosphate levels.[13] The mechanisms underlying hypophosphatemia in the alcoholic are not clearly understood; it may be related to malnutrition or to hypomagnesemia. Malnutrition and diabetic ketoacidosis increase phosphate excretion and phosphate loss from the body. Refeeding of malnourished patients increases phosphate incorporation into nucleic acids and phosphorylated compounds in the cell. The same thing happens when diabetic ketoacidosis is reversed with insulin therapy. The intracellular shift of phosphate causes serum phosphate levels to drop. Parathyroid hormone decreases serum phosphate levels through a different mechanism: it causes increased renal excretion of phosphate. Alkalosis has an indirect effect on serum phosphate levels. The increase in pH causes increased binding of calcium, which in turn leads to a decrease in ionized calcium and an increase in release of PTH.

Manifestations of phosphate deficit. Hypophosphatemia causes signs and symptoms related to altered neural function, disturbed musculoskeletal function, and hematologic disorders. Neural manifestations include intentional tremors, paresthesias, hyporeflexia, stupor, coma, and seizures (Table 22-12). Anorexia and dysphagia can occur. There may be muscle weakness, stiffness of the joints, bone pain, and osteomalacia. Red cell metabolism is impaired in phosphate deficiency; the cells become rigid and have increased hemolysis and diminished ATP and 2,3-DPG levels. There is impairment of chemotaxis and phagocytosis by white blood cells. Platelet function is also disturbed.

Treatment of phosphate deficit. Treatment of hypophosphatemia includes replacement therapy. This may be accomplished with dietary sources high in phosphate (one glassful of milk contains about 250 mg phosphate) or with oral or intravenous replacement solutions. Phosphate supplements are usually contraindicated in hypercalcemia and renal failure. Treatment with phosphate supplements can lead to disseminated calcification.

Phosphate excess (hyperphosphatemia)

Hyperphosphatemia usually results from renal failure or a decrease in PTH. Hyperphosphatemia has been reported in children following use of a single sodium phosphate/biphosphate enema.[14]

Hyperphosphatemia is associated with a decrease in serum calcium; thus many of the signs and symptoms of a phosphate excess may be related to a calcium deficit (see Table 22-10).

In summary, phosphorus is an important constituent of all body tissues. Phosphates are linked to metabolic processes, to formation of nucleic acids, and to red cell function. Phosphate deficiency occurs in chronic malnutrition, alcoholism, and diabetic acidosis. The causes and manifestations of phosphate deficit are summarized in Table 22-12.

Table 22–12 Phosphate Deficit

Causes	Signs and Symptoms
Increased loss from the gastrointestinal tract	**Altered neural function**
Antacids (aluminum and calcium)	Intention tremor
Severe diarrhea	Ataxia
Lack of vitamin D	Paresthesias
	Hyporeflexia
Increased renal excretion	Confusion
Alkalosis	Stupor
Hyperparathyroidism	Coma
Diabetic ketoacidosis	Seizures
Renal tubular defects	
	Altered musculoskeletal function
Decreased intake	Muscle weakness
Malnutrition	Joint stiffness
	Bone pain
Alcoholism	Osteomalacia
Increased movement into the cell	**Gastrointestinal symptoms**
Intravenous hyperalimentation	Anorexia
Recovery from malnutrition	Dysphagia
Administration of insulin for ketoacidosis	
	Hematological disorders
	Hemolytic anemia
	Platelet dysfunction with bleeding disorders
	Impaired function of white blood cells

Alterations in Magnesium Balance

Magnesium is the fourth most abundant cation in the body. Fifty percent of the total magnesium content of the body is stored in bone, while 49% is contained in body cells and the remaining 1% is dispersed in the extracellular fluids. The normal serum concentration of magnesium is 1.5 to 2.5 mEq per liter.

Gains and losses

The average American diet contains about 180 mg to 300 mg of magnesium. All green vegetables contain abundant amounts of magnesium. Although controversial, it is generally agreed that the minimum daily requirement for magnesium in the adult is 250 mg (150 mg in the infant and 400 mg in pregnant or lactating women).[15] Magnesium is absorbed from the intestine and excreted by the kidney. Calcium and magnesium compete for absorption in both the intestine and renal tubules, i.e., factors that increase calcium absorption will cause a decrease in magnesium absorption. Although the mechanisms are unclear, there appears to be a relationship between the actions of PTH and magnesium levels. Hyperparathyroidism increases renal excretion of magnesium. It has also been suggested that the action of PTH in regulating calcium metabolism is impaired in hypomagnesemia, i.e., hypomagnesemia is associated with hypocalcemia.[16]

Functions of magnesium

Only recently has the importance of magnesium to the overall function of the body been fully recognized. The functions of magnesium can be grouped in three categories. First, magnesium acts as a cofactor in many enzyme reactions, particularly those that involve transfer of a phosphate group. Second, magnesium exerts an effect similar to that of calcium on neuromuscular function, in that neuromuscular activity is increased when magnesium levels are decreased. Third, magnesium deficiency is associated with both a potassium and a calcium deficiency state. Renal excretion of potassium is increased in magnesium deficiency. The actions of PTH in maintaining normal serum calcium levels appear to be impaired in hypomagnesemia.

Magnesium deficit (hypomagnesemia)

One of the most common causes of hypomagnesemia is alcoholism. Alcohol ingestion seems to promote a magnesium deficiency that is unrelated to dietary intake. Magnesium levels are also decreased in conditions that cause malabsorption, in malnutrition, and in patients receiving parenteral hyperalimentation in which there is inadequate magnesium. Excessive intake of calcium will also impair magnesium absorption by competing for the same transport site. Magnesium losses are increased in diabetic ketoacidosis, diuretic therapy, and hyperaldosteronism (Table 22-13).

The signs and symptoms of magnesium deficit are characterized by an increase in neuromuscular irritability. Tremors, athetoid or choreiform movements, positive Babinski, Chvostek or Trousseau signs, tachycardia, hypertension, and ventricular arrhythmias are signs and symptoms associated with the increase in neuromuscular irritability.

Table 22-13   Magnesium Deficit

Causes	Signs and Symptoms
Impaired intake or absorption	**Laboratory findings**
Alcoholism	Serum magnesium less than 1.4 mEq/liter
Malabsorption	**Neuromuscular hyperirritability**
Small-bowel bypass	Athetoid or choreiform movements
Malnutrition or starvation	Positive Babinski sign
Parenteral hyperalimentation with inadequate mg^{++}	Nystagmus
High dietary intake of calcium without concomitant increase in mg^{++}	Tetany
	Positive Chvostek or Trousseau signs
Increased losses	**Cardiovascular manifestations**
Diabetic ketoacidosis	Tachycardia
Diuretic therapy	Hypertension
Hyperparathyroidism	Ventricular arrhythmias
Hyperaldosteronism	
Magnesium-wasting renal disease	

Magnesium excess (hypermagnesemia)

Magnesium excess is rare. When it does occur it is usually related to renal insufficiency or to injudicious use of magnesium sulfate as a laxative. Hypermagnesemia causes sedation of the nervous system with muscle weakness, confusion, and respiratory paralysis. There is a decrease in blood pressure and the electrocardiogram shows an increase in the PR interval, a broadening of the QRS complex, and elevation of the T wave.

In summary, although magnesium is the fourth most abundant cation in the body, only recently has its importance been recognized. Hypomagnesemia occurs in alcoholism and malnutrition. The causes and manifestations of magnesium deficit are described in Table 22-13.

:Study Guide

After you have studied this chapter, you should be able to meet the following objectives:

: : Explain why water is essential to life, by summarizing its functions in the body.

: : State the source(s) of water gain and of water loss.

: : Describe the means by which thirst is manifested.

: : Explain how ADH regulates renal reabsorption of water.

: : Compare the pathophysiological defect in diabetes insipidus with that in SIADH.

: : Describe the pathology of extracellular fluid volume deficit with reference to its manifestations in the skin, gastrointestinal tract, the third space, and the urinary tract.

: : Relate the signs and symptoms of fluid volume deficit to the functions of water.

: : Describe the effect of fluid deficit on arterial and venous volumes and on brain and nerve cells.

: : Relate the causes of extracellular fluid excess to its clinical manifestations.

: : Describe the role of the kidneys in regulation of serum sodium.

: : State the effect of renal disease on serum sodium.

: : Compare Cushing's syndrome with Addison's disease with reference to serum aldosterone level.

: : State the criterion for hyponatremia.

: : Relate the causes of hyponatremia to its clinical manifestations.

: : Describe the clinical manifestations of hypernatremia.

: : State the functions of potassium.

: : Describe the relationship of pH to potassium balance.

: : Describe the feedback regulation of serum aldosterone.

: : List the causes of potassium deficit.

: : State the sources of potassium loss.

: : Relate hypokalemia to its clinical manifestations in four major body systems.

: : State the role of the kidneys in regulation of serum potassium.

: : Compare hypokalemia and hyperkalemia.

: : Explain the interaction between serum calcium and serum phosphate.

: : Describe the role of vitamin D in regulation of serum calcium and phosphate.

: : Compare the physiologic actions of PTH and calcitonin.

: : List the functions of serum calcium.

: : Describe the clinical manifestations of decreased serum calcium gains compared with those of increased serum calcium losses.

: : Describe the clinical manifestations of hypercalcemic crisis.

: : List the functions of phosphate.

: : Relate the causes of hypophosphatemia to its clinical manifestations.

: : State the relationship between hyperphosphatemia and serum calcium.

: : Describe the neuromuscular manifestations of hypomagnesemia.

:References

1. Guyton A: Textbook of Medical Physiology, p 441. Philadelphia, WB Saunders, 1981
2. Lawrence SV: Woman's death by water intoxication ruled suicide. Clin Psych News 5:3, 1977
3. Baker AB, Baker LH: Clinical Neurology, Vol 2. In Haymaker W, Anderson E (eds): Disorders of the Hypothalamus and Pituitary Gland, pp 18, 24, 25. Hagerstown, Harper & Row, 1976
4. Guyton A: Textbook of Medical Physiology, p 392. Philadelphia, WB Saunders, 1981

5. Pruit BA: Other complications of burn injury. In Artz CP et al: Burns, p 518. Philadelphia, WB Saunders, 1979

6. Katz MA: Hyperglycemia-induced hypernatremia—Calculations of expected serum sodium depression. N Engl J Med 293:843, 1975

7. Pflaum SS: Investigation of intake–output as a means of assessing body fluid balance. Heart Lung 8, No. 3:498, 1979

8. Goldberger E: A Primer on Water, Electrolytes, and Acid–Base Syndromes, 6th ed, p 34. Philadelphia, Lea & Febiger, 1980

9. Guyton A: Textbook of Medical Physiology, p 890. Philadelphia, WB Saunders, 1981

10. Goldberger E: A Primer on Water, Electrolytes, and Acid–Base Syndromes, 6th ed, p 326. Philadelphia, Lea & Febiger, 1980

11. Guyton A: Textbook of Medical Physiology, p 89. Philadelphia, WB Saunders, 1981

12. Guyton A: Textbook of Medical Physiology, p 974. Philadelphia, WB Saunders, 1981

13. Stein JH, Smith WO, Ginn HE: Hypophosphatemia in acute alcoholism. Am J Med Sci 252:78, 1966

14. Davis RF, Eichner J, Archie W et al: Hypocalcemia, hyperphosphatemia and dehydration following a single hypertonic phosphate enema. J Pediatr 90, No. 3:484, 1977

15. Metheny NM, Snively WD: Nurses' Handbook of Fluid Balance, p 79. Philadelphia, JB Lippincott, 1979

16. Sodeman WA, Sodeman TM: Pathologic Physiology, p 993. Philadelphia, WB Saunders, 1980

:Suggested Readings

Fluid balance

Anderson BJ: Antidiuretic hormone: Balance and imbalance. J Neurosurg Nurs 11, No. 2:71, 1979

Coleman P: Antidiuretic hormone: Physiology and pathophysiology—A review. J Neurosurg Nurs 11, No. 4:199, 1979

Grant M, Kubo WM: Assessing a patient's hydration status. Am J Nurs 75, No. 8:199, 1975

Hays RM: Principles of ion and water transport in the kidney. Hosp Pract 13, No. 9:79, 1978

Humes DH, Narins RG, Brenner BM: Disorders of water balance. Hosp Pract 14, No. 3:133, 1979

Kee JL: Clinical implications of laboratory studies in critical care. Crit Care Quart 2:1, 1979

Kubo WM, Grant MM: The syndrome of inappropriate secretion of antidiuretic hormone. Heart Lung 7, No. 3:469, 1978

Kubo WR: Fluid and electrolyte problems. Crit Care Update 19, 1979

Newsome HH Jr: Vasopressin: Deficiency, excess and the syndrome of inappropriate antidiuretic hormone secretion. Nephron 23:125, 1979

Ricci MM: Water and electrolyte metabolism in patients with intracranial lesions. J Neurosurg Nurs 9, No. 4:165, 1979

Rosenbaum JF, Rothman JS, Murray GB: Psychosis and water intoxication. Clin J Psych 40:287, 1979

Twombly M: The shift into third space. Nursing 78:38, 1978

Wilson RF: Tips on managing fluid and electrolyte problems. Consultant:31, 1977

Sodium balance

Adlard JM, George JM: Hyponatremia. Heart Lung 7, No. 4:587, 1978

Arieff AI, Francisco L, Massry S: Neurological manifestations and morbidity of hyponatremia: Correlation with brain and electrolytes. Medicine 55, No. 2:121, 1976

Burke MD: Electrolyte studies. 1. Sodium and water. Postgrad Med 64, No. 4:147, 1978

Levy M: The pathophysiology of sodium balance. Hosp Pract 13, No. 11:95, 1978

Moses AM, Miller M: Drug-induced hyponatremia. N Engl J Med 291, No. 23:1234, 1974

Potassium balance

Cohen J: Disorders of potassium balance. Hosp Pract 15, No. 1:119, 1979

Nardone DA, McDonald WJ, Girard DE: Mechanisms of hypokalemia: Clinical correlation. Medicine 57, No. 5:435, 1978

Zeluff GW, Suki WN, Jackson D: Hypokalemia—Cause and treatment. Heart Lung 7, No. 5:854, 1978

Calcium, magnesium, and phosphate balance

Chan JCM: Clinical disorders of calcium, phosphate, magnesium and hydrogen ion metabolism. Urology 13, No. 2:122, 1979

Fitzgerald F: Clinical hypophosphatemia. Ann Rev Med 29:177, 1978

Hipkin LJ: Hyperparathyroidism. Nurs Times 1430, 1977

Iseri LT, Freed J, Bures AR: Magnesium deficiency and cardiac disorders. Am J Med 58:837, 1975

Juan D: Differential diagnosis of hypercalcemia. Postgrad Med 66, No. 4:72, 1979

Juan D: Hypocalcemia. Arch Inter Med 139:1166, 1979

Kreisber RA: Phosphorus deficiency and hypophosphatemia. Hosp Pract 12, No.3:121, 1977

Recker RR, Saville PD: Hypercalcemia and hypocalcemia in clinical practice. Hosp Med 15, No. 9:74, 1979

Roberts A: Systems of life. Calcium homeostasis: Regulation. Nurs Times 75:center pages, 1977

Roberts A: Systems of life. Calcium homeostasis: Clinical disorders. Nurs Times 75:center pages, 1979

Zeluff GW, Suki WN, Jackson D: Hypercalcemia—Etiology, manifestations and management. Heart Lung 9, No. 1:146, 1980

Zeluff GW, Suki WN, Jackson D: Depletion of body phosphate—Ubiquitous, subtle, dangerous. Heart Lung 6, No. 3:519, 1977

23

Acid–Base Balance

Normal body function is dependent upon precise regulation of acid–base balance. The metabolic activities that take place in the body require regulation of pH so that enzyme systems and chemical reactions can proceed at an optimal rate. Both hydrogen and carbon dioxide are formed in the metabolic processes that transform carbohydrates, fats, and proteins into cellular energy. Carbonic acid, resulting from dissolved carbon dioxide, is called a respiratory acid because it is eliminated through the lungs. All of the other acids formed in the body or that enter the body through the gastrointestinal tract or parenteral route are referred to as metabolic acids.

Many conditions, pathologic and otherwise, afford the potential for altering body pH. This chapter focuses on metabolic and respiratory-induced changes in acid–base balance.

:Regulation of pH

The symbol pH refers to the concentration of hydrogen ions, or more specifically to the negative logarithm (p) of the hydrogen (H^+) in milliequivalents per liter. The hydrogen ion and carbon dioxide content of the body are normally regulated so that the pH of the extracellular fluids is maintained within the narrow range of 7.35 to 7.45.

Carbon Dioxide

Carbon dioxide content of the blood is transported in three forms: (1) attached to hemoglobin, (2) dissolved carbon dioxide (PCO_2), and (3) bicarbonate (HCO_3^-) (see Fig. 23-1). Normally, about 23% of the

Figure 23–1.   Mechanisms of carbon dioxide transport. (From Guyton AC: Textbook of Medical Physiology, 5th ed. Philadelphia, WB Saunders, 1976)

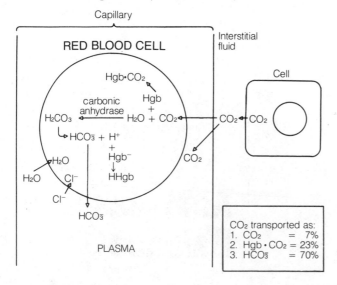

carbon dioxide is transported in the red blood cell where it is attached to the hemoglobin molecule. A small percentage of carbon dioxide dissolves in the plasma to form the volatile acid, carbonic acid (H_2CO_3), and the rest of the carbon dioxide is carried as the bicarbonate ion. Collectively, dissolved carbon dioxide and bicarbonate constitute about 77% of the carbon dioxide that is transported in the extracellular fluid.

Carbon dioxide content in blood can be calculated using the *solubility coefficient* for carbon dioxide. Under normal physiologic conditions, this coefficient has been shown to have a value of 0.03. This means that the H_2CO_3 content of the venous blood, which has a PCO_2 value of 45 mm Hg, will be 1.35 mEq per liter ($45 \times .03 = 1.35$).

Carbon dioxide also combines with water to form *bicarbonate* ($CO_2 + H_2O = H^+ + HCO_3^-$). This reaction is catalyzed by the enzyme carbonic anhydrase, which is present in large quantities in the red blood cell and in other tissues of the body. The rate of the reaction between carbon dioxide and water is increased about 5000 times by the presence of carbonic anhydrase. Were it not for this enzyme, the reaction would occur too slowly to be of any significance. Base bicarbonate is formed when the cations sodium, potassium, calcium, and magnesium combine with the bicarbonate ion.

Hydrogen Ions

Metabolic acids are the main source of hydrogen ions in the body. There are several metabolic acids that we are concerned with in this chapter. Lactic acid is formed when there is insufficient oxygen available to convert metabolic end-products to water and carbon dioxide. The ketoacids are metabolic acids that are produced when carbohydrates are not available for use in cell metabolism or when cells are unable to use carbohydrates, e.g., in diabetes mellitus.

Control of pH

The body has two major mechanisms for controlling pH. One is the regulation of pH by renal and respiratory mechanisms which act to selectively release hydrogen and carbon dioxide into the external environment. The other is a system for buffering excess acid and alkali to protect the body against extreme changes in pH.

Respiratory mechanisms
The respiratory system plays a major role in regulation of dissolved carbon dioxide. This is accomplished through changes in ventilation, that is,

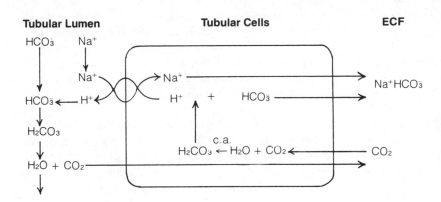

Figure 23–2.   Diagram of hydrogen ion (H^+) secretion and bicarbonate ion (HCO_3^-) retrieval in a renal tubular cell. Carbon dioxide (CO_2) diffuses into the tubular cell from the blood where it combines with water in a carbonic anhydrase (c.a.) catalyzed reaction which yields carbonic acid (H_2CO_3). The H_2CO_3 dissociates to form H^+ and HCO_3^-. The H^+ is secreted into the tubular fluid in exchange for Na^+. The Na^+ and HCO_3^- enter the extracellular fluid. (From Chaffee EE, Lytle IM: Basic Physiology and Anatomy, 4th ed. Philadelphia, JB Lippincott, 1980)

larger amounts of carbon dioxide are released into the air at high ventilation rates.

Renal mechanisms

The kidneys can produce an acid or an alkaline urine as a means for controlling pH. This is accomplished through secretion of hydrogen ions into the tubular fluid and reabsorption of bicarbonate ions into the extracellular fluid (Fig. 23-2). The process of hydrogen ion secretion begins when carbon dioxide moves into the tubular cell. The carbon dioxide combines with water in a carbonic anhydrase-catalyzed reaction that yields a bicarbonate ion and a hydrogen ion. The bicarbonate ion is then absorbed into the extracellular fluid and the hydrogen ion is secreted into the tubular fluid in a coupled reaction that involves the reabsorption of a sodium ion. The hydrogen ion, once it enters the tubular fluid, combines with a bicarbonate ion to form carbon dioxide and water. The water then passes into the urine and the carbon dioxide diffuses back into the tubular cells.

Normally, only a few hydrogen ions remain in the tubular fluid for passage into the urine. This is because the tubular secretion of hydrogen ions is

roughly equal to the number of bicarbonate ions that are filtered in the glomerulus. When excess carbon dioxide is present, as occurs during periods of decreased ventilation, hydrogen ion secretion will exceed bicarbonate filtration and the urine will become acidic. On the other hand, filtration of bicarbonate in excess of hydrogen ion secretion produces an alkaline urine. An extremely acid urine is damaging to the structures in the urinary tract. Therefore, the maximum decrease in pH that the kidneys can excrete is 4.5; this limits the number of hydrogen ions that the kidneys can excrete.

The kidney uses two other buffer systems for excreting hydrogen ions when the need to eliminate acids exceeds the pH limits of the urine. One of these buffer systems is the phosphate buffer system and the other is the ammonia buffer system.

The *phosphate buffer system* consists of monohydrogen phosphate (HPO_4^{--}) and dihydrogen phosphate ($H_2PO_4^-$). The combination of H^+ with HPO_4^{--} to form $H_2PO_4^-$ allows the kidney to increase its excretion of hydrogen ions (Fig. 23-3).

The *ammonia buffer system* allows the hydrogen ion to combine with ammonia (NH_3) to form an ammonium ion (NH_4^+). The ammonium ion is ex-

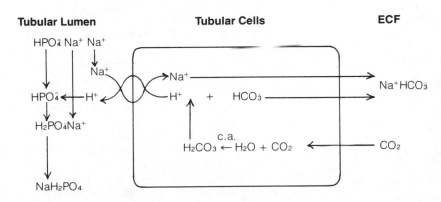

Figure 23–3.   Diagram of the renal phosphate buffer system. The monohydrogen phosphate ion (HPO_4^{--}) enters the renal tubular fluid in the glomerulus. A H^+ combines with the HPO_4^{--} to form $H_2PO_4^-$ and is then excreted into the urine in combination with a Na^+. The HCO_3^- moves into the extracellular fluid along with the Na^+ that was exchanged during secretion of the H^+. (From Chaffee EE, Lytle IM: Basic Physiology and Anatomy, 4th ed. Philadelphia, JB Lippincott, 1980)

creted in the urine as ammonium chloride (Fig. 23-4). Ammonia is synthesized by the renal tubules from amino acids. In contrast to the rapidly occurring changes in respiration that compensate for pH changes, the renal ammonia buffer system requires two to three days to become optimally effective.

The phosphate and ammonia systems have a twofold effect in returning pH toward a more normal value in acidosis. You will note in Figures 23-3 and 23-4 that these two buffer systems not only remove a hydrogen ion from the extracellular fluid, but they also have the added effect of adding a bicarbonate ion to the blood buffer pool by converting carbon dioxide to bicarbonate.

The blood buffer systems

The ability of the body to maintain the pH of the extracellular fluids within the physiologic range is dependent upon blood buffer systems. These buffers are immediately available for combination with excess acids and alkalis and thus prevent large changes in pH from occurring. The body has several blood buffer systems—the phosphate, hemoglobin, and bicarbonate systems. Of these systems, the bicarbonate buffer system assumes the major role in regulation of extracellular pH.

A buffering system consists of a weak acid and the alkali salt of that acid or a weak base and its acid salt. In the bicarbonate buffer system, carbon dioxide combines with water to form the weak acid, carbonic acid ($CO_2 + H_2O = H_2CO_3$). The carbonic acid dissociates into a bicarbonate (HCO_3^-) ion and a hydrogen (H^+) ion. The alkali salt of carbonic acid is sodium bicarbonate (Na HCO_3). The bicarbonate buffer system is unique in that its acid is volatile and can be released into the air through the respiratory system.

Determination of pH

The pH of the extracellular fluid is determined by the bicarbonate to carbonic acid ratio and the degree to which carbonic acid dissociates to form a hydrogen

and a bicarbonate ion. The dissociation constant (K) is used to describe the degree to which an acid dissociates. The symbol pK refers to the negative logarithm of the dissociation constant. At normal body temperature the pK for the bicarbonate buffer system is 6.1. The use of a negative logarithm for the dissociation constant allows pH to be expressed as a positive value.

The Henderson–Hasselbalch equation computes the serum pH by using the logarithm of the dissociation constant and the logarithm of the bicarbonate and dissolved carbon dioxide ratio. In its simplest form this equation states that

$$pH = pK + \log \frac{HCO_3}{H_2CO_3}$$

As a point of emphasis, it is the ratio rather than the absolute values for bicarbonate and carbonic acid that determines pH. Let us consider two examples to emphasize this point. The first situation uses normal serum values and the second uses increased concentrations of both bicarbonate and carbonic acid.

Situation 1

pH 7.4 = 6.1 + log

$$\frac{27 \text{ mEq/liter } HCO_3}{1.35 \text{ mEq/liter } H_2CO_3}$$

ratio 27:1.35 = 20:1*

Situation 2

pH 7.4 = 6.1 + log

$$\frac{48 \text{ mEq/liter } HCO_3}{2.40 \text{ mEq/liter } H_2CO_3}$$

ratio 48:2.5 = 20:1*

These examples demonstrate that pH will remain relatively stable over a wide range of changes in bicarbonate and carbonic acid concentrations as long as the ratio values for the two concentrations

---

*The log of 20 is 1.3.

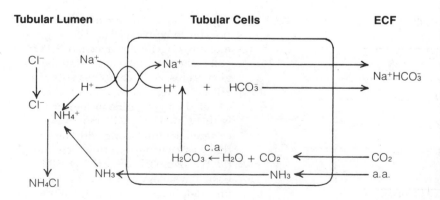

Tubular Lumen   **Tubular Cells**   **ECF**

Figure 23–4. Diagram of the ammonia buffer system in a renal tubular cell. The tubular cell synthesizes ammonia (NH_3) from amino acids (a.a.). The NH_3 is secreted into the tubular fluid where it combines with a H^+ to form an ammonium ion (NH_4^+). The ammonium ion combines with chloride for excretion in the urine. The HCO_3^- moves into the extracellular fluid along with the Na^+ that was exchanged during secretion of the H^+. (From Chaffee EE, Lytle IM: Basic Physiology and Anatomy, 4th ed. Philadelphia, JB Lippincott, 1980)

approach a ratio value of 20 to 1. Plasma pH will decrease when the ratio is less than 20 to 1 (for example, the log of 10 is 1; when the ratio of HCO_3 to H_2CO_3 is equal to 10, the pH of the blood will be 7.1) and it will increase when the ratio is greater than 20 to 1.

Correction Versus Compensation

There are two mechanisms for regulating pH changes. One mechanism corrects the underlying cause and the other compensates for the disorder.

Correction of acid–base disorders requires that the primary causative factor be controlled or corrected. Improved ventilation is a corrective measure in respiratory acidosis. In diabetic ketoacidosis, administration of insulin is corrective in that it prevents further breakdown of fats with formation of organic acids.

Compensation for acid–base disorders can be either respiratory or renal. The respiratory system can compensate for changes in pH by either increasing or decreasing ventilation. Respiratory compensation is rapid but it is seldom complete. The kidney, as mentioned earlier, compensates for pH changes by producing either an acid or an alkaline urine. It normally takes longer to recruit renal compensatory mechanisms than it does respiratory mechanisms. Renal mechanisms are more efficient, however, since they continue to operate until the pH has returned to normal or near normal levels.

Compensatory mechanisms usually provide a means to control pH in situations where correction is impossible or when it cannot be immediately achieved. Often compensatory mechanisms are interim measures which permit survival while the body attempts to correct the primary disorder. It is important for the reader to recognize that compensation requires the use of mechanisms that are different from those that caused the primary disorder. In other words, the lungs cannot compensate for respiratory acidosis that is caused by lung disease, nor can the kidneys compensate for metabolic acidosis that occurs because of kidney failure. The body can, however, use renal mechanisms to compensate for respiratory-induced changes in pH and it can use respiratory mechanisms to compensate for metabolically induced changes in acid–base balance.

Effects of potassium on pH regulation

Potassium and hydrogen are interchangeable cations that move freely between the intracellular and extracellular compartments. This means that excess hydrogen ions can move into the intracellular compartment for buffering. When this happens potassium moves out of the cell into the extracellular fluids. Conversely, in hypokalemia potassium moves out of the cell into the extracellular fluid and hydrogen moves into the cell; this causes alkalosis.

Hydrogen and potassium also compete for excretion into the urine. In the distal tubules of the kidney, potassium or hydrogen is secreted into the tubular fluid as sodium is reabsorbed into the extracellular fluid. For example, in hypokalemia, there are fewer potassium ions available for secretion into the urine, which means that there will be a predominance of hydrogen-ion secretion into the urine. This tends to cause alkalosis since the secreted hydrogen ions are removed from the extracellular fluid. On the other hand, hyperkalemia tends to cause pH to decrease as the kidney secretes potassium ions in excess of hydrogen ions.

Effects of chloride on pH regulation

Chloride and bicarbonate can substitute for each other when there is need for anion exchange. For example, serum bicarbonate levels normally increase as chloride is secreted into the stomach following a heavy meal, causing what is termed the postprandial alkaline tide. Later as the chloride is reabsorbed from the intestine, the pH returns to normal. Hypochloremic alkalosis refers to an increase in pH which is induced by a decrease in serum chloride levels. Hyperchloremic acidosis occurs when excess levels of chloride are present.

:Methods for Assessing pH Changes

The terms acidemia and alkalemia refer only to the pH of the blood as measured on a pH meter and give little information about the cause of the acid–base disorder. It was pointed out earlier that pH can be relatively normal within a wide range of changes in dissolved carbon dioxide and base bicarbonate levels. A number of laboratory tests can be used to provide a better description of acid–base disorders.

Carbonic acid levels.   As mentioned previously, carbonic acid levels can be determined from blood gas measurements using the PCO_2 and the solubility coefficient for carbon dioxide (normal arterial PCO_2 is 38 to 42 mm Hg).

Bicarbonate.   More than 95% of the carbon dioxide content is in the form of bicarbonate. The serum bicarbonate level can be determined from the carbon dioxide content in the blood. The normal range of values for venous bicarbonate is 24 to 33 mEq per liter.

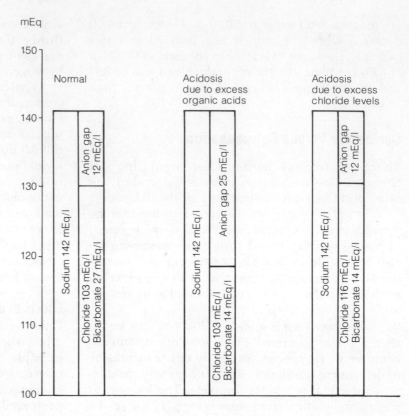

Figure 23–5.   Diagram of anion gap in acidosis due to excess metabolic acids and excess serum chloride levels. Anions such as phosphates, sulfates, and organic acids increase the anion gap because they replace bicarbonate (this assumes there is no change in sodium content).

Base excess or deficit.   Base excess or deficit measures the level of all the buffer systems in the blood—hemoglobin, protein, phosphate, and bicarbonate. The normal base excess is assigned a value of 0. Base excess or deficit describes the amount of a fixed acid or base that must be added to a blood sample to achieve a pH of 7.4 (normal −2.5 to +2.5 mEq per liter). For practical purposes, base excess is a measurement of bicarbonate excess or deficit. A positive result (bicarbonate excess) indicates metabolic alkalosis and a negative result (bicarbonate deficit) indicates metabolic acidosis.

The anion gap.   The anion gap describes the difference between the sodium ion concentration and the sum of the measured anions (Cl^- and HCO_3^-). This difference represents the concentration of anions such as phosphates, sulfates, organic acids, and proteins that are present in the extracellular fluid (Fig. 23-5). Normally, the anion gap is about 12 mEq per liter. (A value of 16 mEq is normal if the potassium concentration is used to calculate the anion gap.)

:Alterations in Acid–Base Balance

The terms acidosis and alkalosis describe the clinical conditions that arise as the result of changes in pH, dissolved carbon dioxide, and bicarbonate concentrations. Acidosis and alkalosis occur as both primary defects and as compensatory conditions. A *primary defect* refers to the initiating event that caused the acid–base disorder. The *compensatory state* is the result of homeostatic mechanisms that attempt to prevent large changes in pH. A primary defect in acid–base balance can be either *respiratory* or *metabolic* in origin. Cell metabolism regulates carbon dioxide (and bicarbonate). Therefore, primary alterations in the bicarbonate portion of the bicarbonate–carbonic acid ratio are referred to as metabolic acid–base disorders (Fig. 23-6). Carbonic acid is a volatile acid that is eliminated from the body through the respiratory tract. It follows that primary disorders of the carbonic acid portion of the bicarbonate–carbonic acid ratio are classified as respiratory pH disorders.

Both primary and compensatory mechanisms often are operational in acid–base disorders. For example, a patient may have a primary metabolic acidosis due to an accumulation of ketoacids and a compensatory respiratory alkalosis due to increased ventilation. Figure 23-7 illustrates the PCO_2, bicarbonate, and pH changes that occur in acute and chronic disorders of acid–base balance.

Most of the *manifestations* of acid–base disorders fall into three main categories: (1) those associated with the primary disorder that caused the pH disturbance, (2) those related to the altered pH, and

↓ HCO₃⁻ Metabolic acidosis represents a decrease in bicarbonate
    (HCO₃ deficit)
↑ H₂CO₃ Respiratory acidosis represents an increase in carbonic acid
    (H₂CO₃ excess)
↑ HCO₃⁻ Metabolic alkalosis represents an increase in bicarbonate
    (HCO₃ excess)
↓ H₂CO₃ Respiratory alkalosis represents a decrease in carbonic acid
    (H₂CO₃ deficit)

Figure 23–6. Primary defects in acid–base balance.

(3) those that occur because of the body's attempt to compensate for the altered pH. Many of the alterations in body function which are associated with acid–base disturbances are directly related to the pH change and its effect on the excitability of the nervous system. The hydrogen ion tends to stabilize the nerve membrane rendering it less excitable. The ionization of serum calcium is also affected by changes in pH and this too contributes to the excitability of the nervous system. For example, ionization of serum calcium is increased in acidosis, and this tends to decrease nerve excitability. Conversely, alkalosis causes a decrease in ionized calcium levels with a resultant increase in neural excitability.

Figure 23–7. Diagram of acute and chronic acid–base disorders as determined by PCO₂, bicarbonate, and pH values. (Adapted from Masoro EJ, Siegel PD: Acid–Base Regulation: Its Physiology, Pathophysiology and Interpretation of Blood Gas Analysis. Philadelphia, WB Saunders, 1977)

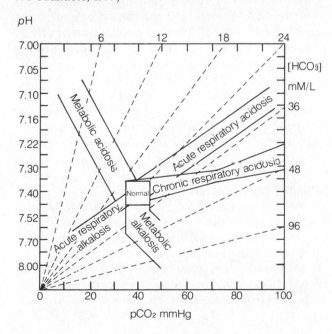

Metabolic Acidosis

Metabolic acidosis refers to a primary deficit in base bicarbonate. In metabolic acidosis, the pH falls below 7.35, and the plasma bicarbonate decreases to less than 24 mEq per liter. The causes of metabolic acidosis can be divided into two groups. The first group is characterized by disorders that cause an increase in metabolic acids (lactic acid and ketoacids). Patients in this group have an increased anion gap due to an accumulation of unmeasured metabolic acids. The second group has a decreased serum bicarbonate; persons in this group have an increased chloride level and a normal anion gap. The causes of metabolic acidosis are described in Table 23–1.

Metabolic acids tend to accumulate and increase when (1) metabolic demands are in excess of carbohydrate stores or when body cells are not able to use carbohydrates normally, (2) body cells are forced to metabolize carbohydrates without a sufficient supply of oxygen, or (3) the kidneys are unable to excrete metabolic acids.

Formation of ketoacids

The production of the metabolic ketoacids is increased when carbohydrate stores are low or when the body cannot use available carbohydrates as a fuel. When this happens, the body is forced to mobilize fatty acids as a means of producing ketones which are then used in the metabolic process. Ketone production is high during periods of *fasting*, *starvation*, and *uncontrolled diabetes mellitus*.* Ketoacidosis also develops in persons who are following a ketogenic diet for weight control or for other purposes. The ketogenic diet is high in fat content and low in carbohydrates.

---

*The reader is referred to Chapter 34 (Control of Metabolism) and Chapter 35 (Diabetes Mellitus) for additional information on the metabolic events that surround ketone production.

Table 23-1 Metabolic Acidosis

Laboratory Findings

Primary Defect (Uncompensated)		Compensation
pH	Bicarbonate	PCO$_2$
Decreased	Decreased	Decreased

Causes	Manifestations
Increase in metabolic acids (increased anion gap) Excess production of metabolic acids Fasting and starvation Ketogenic diet Diabetic ketoacidosis Lactic acidosis Alcoholic ketoacidosis Salicylate poisoning Decreased loss of metabolic acids Renal failure **Increase in bicarbonate loss (normal anion gap)** Loss of intestinal secretions Diarrhea Intestinal suction Intestinal or biliary fistula Decreased renal losses Renal tubular acidosis Treatment with acetazolamide Increased chloride levels Abnormal chloride reabsorption by the kidney Sodium chloride infusions Treatment with ammonium chloride Parenteral hyperalimentation	**Altered gastrointestinal function** Anorexia Nausea Vomiting Abdominal pain **Depression of neural function** Weakness Lethargy General malaise Confusion Stupor Coma Depression of vital functions **Skin** Warm and flushed **Signs of compensation** Kussmaul breathing Acid urine Increased ammonia in urine Increased serum potassium

Salicylate toxicity

Salicylates cause two types of acid–base disorders. Initially, the salicylates cause stimulation of the respiratory center with marked hyperventilation and development of respiratory alkalosis. Renal mechanisms compensate for the increased pH by causing increased excretion of the bicarbonate ion and other basic salts. Salicylates also interfere with carbohydrate metabolism which leads to an increased production of metabolic acids; this usually occurs several hours after acute intoxication.

Formation of lactic acid

The accumulation of lactic acid in the body occurs for two reasons: (1) because of excess lactic acid production, and (2) because of decreased removal of lactic acid from the blood by the liver. Lactic acid is produced during periods of anaerobic metabolism when cells do not receive sufficient oxygen for converting body fuel sources to carbon dioxide and

water. Blood flow to skeletal muscles, liver, and other tissues is decreased during shock and heart failure. Lactic acid also accumulates during periods of excess oxygen need, such as, during strenuous exercise when blood flow and oxygen delivery cannot keep pace with the increased needs of the exercising muscle. Since the liver removes lactic acid from the blood and converts it to glucose, lactic acidosis can occur in liver disease or in situations that impair the liver's ability to convert lactic acid to glucose.

Impaired renal function

The excretion of metabolic acids occurs through the kidney. In renal failure there is loss of both glomerular and tubular function with retention of nitrogenous wastes and metabolic acids. Bicarbonate losses are increased when renal tubular cells are unable to secrete hydrogen ions or when bicarbonate reabsorption is decreased. In a condition called renal tubular acidosis, there is normal glomerular function but the tubular secretion of hydrogen or reabsorption of bicarbonate is abnormal. Treatment with the drug acetazolamide (Diamox) also leads to increased renal losses of bicarbonate. This drug, which is an inhibitor of carbonic anhydrase, interferes with the formation of carbonic acid in the renal tubular cells; this leads to increased losses of bicarbonate, sodium, and chloride.

Gastrointestinal losses of bicarbonate

Intestinal secretions have a high bicarbonate concentration. Consequently, excess losses of bicarbonate occur with increased losses of intestinal secretions, as in severe diarrhea, small bowel or biliary fistula drainage, ileostomy drainage, and intestinal suction. In diarrhea of microbial origin, bicarbonate is secreted into the bowel to neutralize the metabolic acids that are produced by the organisms causing the diarrhea.

Hyperchloremic acidosis

When the anion gap is within normal limits, there is a reciprocal relationship between serum chloride concentrations and serum bicarbonate levels; when chloride levels are elevated, the bicarbonate concentration will be decreased. Hyperchloremic acidosis can occur as the result of abnormal reabsorption of chloride by the kidney or as the result of treatment with chloride-containing medications (sodium chloride, amino acid–chloride hyperalimentation solutions, and ammonium chloride). Ammonium chloride is broken down into an ammonium (NH_4) and a chloride ion. The ammonium ion is converted to urea in the liver. This leaves the chloride ion free to react with hydrogen to form hydrochloric acid. The administration of intravenous sodium chloride or parenteral hyperalimentation solutions that contain an amino acid–chloride combination can cause acidosis in a similar manner.

The signs and symptoms of metabolic acidosis

The signs and symptoms of metabolic acidosis usually begin to appear when plasma bicarbonate is 20 mEq per liter (mmol per liter) or less. These signs and symptoms fall into the three categories which were mentioned earlier in the chapter.

The *first category* of signs and symptoms is related to the *primary disorder*. With diabetic ketoacidosis there is an increase in blood and urine sugars and the breath has the characteristic smell of acetone. In patients in renal failure, blood urea nitrogen and tests of renal function are abnormal.

The *second category* of symptoms relates to alterations in body function that result from a *decrease*

in pH. These signs and symptoms occur regardless of the cause of the pH disorder. A patient with metabolic acidosis will often complain of weakness, fatigue, general malaise, and a dull headache. There may also be anorexia, nausea, vomiting, and abdominal pain. The anorexia associated with mild metabolic acidosis may be viewed as advantageous for persons who are trying to lose weight through use of a ketogenic diet. On the other hand, the gastrointestinal symptoms may be misleading in a patient with undiagnosed diabetes mellitus. For example, such a patient may be thought to have gastrointestinal "flu" or some other form of abdominal pathology, such as appendicitis.

Neural activity becomes depressed as pH declines. As acidosis progresses there is a decreased level of consciousness and stupor and coma develop. The skin is often warm and flushed because the skin vessels become less responsive to the vasoconstrictor input from the sympathetic nervous system. Tissue turgor is impaired and the skin is dry in situations where fluid deficit accompanies acidosis. When the pH falls to 7.0 the heart also becomes unresponsive to the catecholamines (norepinephrine and epinephrine). At this point both heart rate and cardiac output decrease. Acidosis develops rapidly following cardiac arrest—both lactic acid and carbonic acid accumulate. Therefore, it is necessary to infuse sodium bicarbonate during cardiopulmonary resuscitation procedures.

A *third group* of signs and symptoms seen in metabolic acidosis are those related to recruitment of renal and respiratory compensatory mechanisms. When renal mechanisms are operative, the urine pH will decrease and urine ammonia levels will rise. The respiratory system compensates by increasing ventilation; this is accomplished through deep and often rapid respirations called *Kussmaul breathing*. Kussmaul breathing removes carbon dioxide from the blood as evidenced by a low PCO_2. For descriptive purposes, it can be said that Kussmaul breathing resembles the hyperpnea of exercise—the person appears to have been running.

Treatment of metabolic acidosis

The treatment of metabolic acidosis focuses on correction of the condition that caused the disorder and on restoration of fluid and electrolytes that have been lost from the body.

Lactic Acidosis

Lactic acidosis is a rare but serious form of metabolic acidosis. Because of its clinical importance and because it is not discussed elsewhere in the book, lactic acidosis is discussed separately in this chapter. Lactic acid is the end-product of anaerobic metabolism of glucose. Although the normal person produces lactate ions, they are removed by the liver and converted to pyruvate so that they can be converted to glucose or oxidized in the citric-acid cycle. This means that they do not accumulate in the extracellular fluid. There is the potential for development of lactic acidosis during periods of excess production or when lactate is not removed from the blood.

Lactic acidosis is seen most frequently in situations in which there is acute cellular hypoxia, such as shock or severe heart failure. The condition is also seen in severe liver failure, pulmonary insufficiency, and pulmonary edema. Although lactate levels rise during severe exercise, the blood is usually promptly cleared of the excess lactic acid when the activity is stopped. The oral hypoglycemic drug, phenformin (DBI), is known to cause lactic acidosis by interfering with the liver's ability to convert lactate to glucose. Phenformin has been withdrawn from general use, although it is still available for investigational purposes. Lactic acidosis can also occur following ingestion of a number of toxic agents, including the salicylates, ethylene glycol, paraldehyde, and methanol. Ethanol also interferes with the liver's ability to remove lactate from the blood, and when consumed in large amounts affords the potential for causing lactic acidosis.

Arterial lactate concentrations are elevated (about 2 mEq per liter) in lactic acidosis, the serum pH is decreased, and the anion gap is increased. Furthermore, urine tests of acetone are usually negative or only slightly positive. The intravenous infusion of methylene blue, which facilitates the conversion of lactic acid to pyruvic acid, is sometimes used in the treatment of lactic acidosis. Sodium bicarbonate may also be given to correct the acidosis; this drug is the treatment of choice in cardiac arrest.

In summary, metabolic acidosis describes a condition characterized by a decrease in extracellular pH and base bicarbonate. The causes and manifestations of metabolic acidosis are summarized in Table 23-1. Metabolic acidosis can be caused by an accumulation of metabolic acids or an excessive loss of base bicarbonate. The anion gap is increased when acidosis is due to increased levels of metabolic or organic acids and it is usually within normal limits when acidosis is due to excess loss of bicarbonate ions. The body compensates for metabolic acidosis by increasing the respiratory losses of carbon dioxide, and when possible, by increasing urinary excretion of hydro-

gen ions. In general, the signs and symptoms of metabolic acidosis reflect the cause of the disorder, a decrease in neural function resulting from the fall in pH, and changes in respiration and urine composition that are associated with the body's attempt to correct and maintain the pH within a normal physiologic range.

Metabolic Alkalosis

Metabolic alkalosis refers to a primary increase in base bicarbonate. In metabolic alkalosis, serum pH is above 7.45, plasma bicarbonate is above 29 mEq per liter, and base excess is above +2.5 mEq per liter.

Bicarbonate increase

An increase in bicarbonate-ion concentration can occur as the result of (1) excessive ingestion of alkaline drugs, (2) rapid decrease in extracellular fluid volume, or (3) rapid correction of compensated respiratory acidosis. The medicinal use of sodium bicarbonate or other alkaline salts increases bicarbonate intake. The milk–alkali syndrome occurs in patients with peptic ulcer who are being treated with excessive amounts of milk and alkaline antacids. Renal reabsorption of sodium and bicarbonate is increased when there is a sudden decrease in extracellular fluid volume; this is called *contraction alkalosis* and can occur in the course of diuretic therapy. Respiratory acidosis causes a compensatory loss of hydrogen and chloride ions in the urine along with retention of base bicarbonate. If the cause of the respiratory acidosis is corrected abruptly, metabolic alkalosis may develop.

Loss of hydrogen and chloride

Hydrogen and chloride losses are increased (1) during vomiting or gastric suctioning, (2) in hypokalemia, and (3) with excess levels of aldosterone. Vomiting and gastric suctioning remove both hydrogen and chloride from the body, causing an increased retention of sodium bicarbonate. In hypokalemia, renal excretion of hydrogen is increased as the kidney focuses on conserving potassium. Chloride and potassium losses are also increased with excessive use of organic mercurial, thiazide, and loop diuretics (furosemide and ethacrynic acid). Increased aldosterone levels cause increased reabsorption of sodium and bicarbonate while causing increased urinary losses of potassium and chloride to occur.

Signs and symptoms of metabolic alkalosis

The signs and symptoms of metabolic alkalosis are related to the primary cause of the disorder, to the associated changes in pH, and to accompanying decreases in potassium. Anorexia, nausea, and vomiting often occur as the result of metabolic alkalosis. Alkalosis causes increased excitability of the nervous system. Consequently, the patient may be confused and mentally unreliable. Hypertonic reflexes, tetany, and carpopedal spasm may occur. Metabolic alkalosis may also lead to a compensatory hypoventilation with development of respiratory acidosis. The pH of the urine is usually increased as the kidney attempts to decrease pH levels.

The treatment of metabolic alkalosis

The treatment of metabolic alkalosis is usually directed toward correcting the condition that has caused the disorder. Potassium chloride is often administered when there is a potassium deficit.

In summary, metabolic alkalosis reflects an increase in base bicarbonate and is characterized by an increase in pH, serum bicarbonate, and base excess. The causes and manifestations of metabolic alkalosis are summarized in Table 23-2. Metabolic alkalosis can be caused by an increase in bicarbonate gain or a decrease in hydrogen and chloride levels. In contrast to metabolic acidosis which causes depression of the nervous system, metabolic alkalosis causes an increase in neural excitability; this is evidenced by hypertonic reflexes, tetany, and carpopedal spasm. Neural manifestations are dependent upon the pH changes that have occurred.

Respiratory Acidosis

Respiratory acidosis is due to an accumulation of carbonic acid or dissolved carbon dioxide. In respiratory acidosis plasma pH is below 7.35 and PCO_2 is above 50 mm Hg.

Respiratory acidosis can occur as an acute or a chronic disorder in acid–base balance. The causes of respiratory acidosis include any respiratory problem that impairs ventilation. Acute respiratory infections, narcotic or bicarbonate overdose, chest injuries, and pulmonary edema are examples of conditions that lead to acute respiratory acidosis. Acute respiratory acidosis can also result from breathing air that has a high carbon dioxide content. Chronic obstructive lung disease causes chronic respiratory acidosis.

An *acute episode* of severe respiratory acidosis in a person suffering from chronic lung disease often results in what is called *"carbon dioxide narcosis."* Carbon dioxide narcosis occurs in patients in whom the respiratory center in the brain has become adapted to increased levels of carbon dioxide. In these patients, the decreased oxygen content of the blood serves as the major stimulus for respiration. If oxygen is administered at a flow rate which is sufficient to suppress the stimulus, the rate and depth of respiration will decrease and the carbon dioxide content of the blood will increase. The signs and symptoms of carbon dioxide narcosis are varied.

Table 23-2   Metabolic Alkalosis

Laboratory Findings

Primary Defect (Uncompensated)		Compensation
pH	Bicarbonate	PCO_2
Increased	Increased	Increased

Causes	Manifestations
Increase in gain of bicarbonate	**Altered gastrointestinal function**
Ingestion of sodium bicarbonate or alkaline salts	Anorexia
Milk–alkali syndrome	Nausea
Contraction alkalosis (loss of body fluids)	Painless vomiting
Increase in hydrogen ion loss	**Increased excitability of the nervous system**
Loss of chloride (hydrogen) with bicarbonate retention	Confusion
Vomiting	Hyperactive reflexes
Gastric suctioning	Muscle hypertonicity
Increased potassium loss with hydrogen retention	Tetany
Diuretic therapy	Convulsions
Excessive levels of adrenal cortical hormones	
Decreased potassium intake	**Signs of compensation**
Increased potassium losses	Decreased rate and depth of respiration
	Increased urine pH

There may be psychological disturbances, including irritability, depression, euphoria, paranoia, and hallucinations. Muscle twitching may occur and reflexes may be decreased or absent. As the PCO_2 rises, there is an impairment of consciousness that can range from lethargy to coma. Paralysis of the extremities may occur and there may be respiratory depression. Less severe forms of acidosis are often accompanied by such signs as a warm and flushed skin, headache, weakness, and tachycardia.

Chronic respiratory acidosis is often seen in patients with chronic respiratory problems; it is often accompanied by varying degrees of hypoxia. Weakness and a dull headache are common manifestations of chronic respiratory acidosis.

The treatment of acute and chronic respiratory acidosis is directed toward improving ventilation.

In summary, respiratory acidosis occurs when there is impaired ventilation and retention of carbon dioxide. In respiratory acidosis the pH of the blood is below 7.35 and the PCO_2 is above 50 mm Hg. The causes and manifestations of respiratory acidosis are summarized in Table 23-3. An acute episode of respiratory acidosis is referred to as carbon dioxide narcosis. It can occur in patients with chronic lung disease in whom the respiratory center has adapted to the increased levels of carbon dioxide; administration of high concentrations of oxygen to these patients can result in a decreased ventilation rate that causes a sudden increase in carbon dioxide.

Respiratory Alkalosis

Respiratory alkalosis is caused by a decrease in dissolved carbon dioxide or a carbonic acid deficit. In respiratory alkalosis, the pH is above 7.45, arterial PCO_2 is below 35 mm Hg, and serum bicarbonate levels are usually below 24 mEq per liter. Since respiratory alkalosis can be of sudden origin, changes in bicarbonate level may not occur before correction has been accomplished.

The causes of respiratory alkalosis focus on situations that produce hyperventilation. Hyperventilation means that the respiratory rate is in excess of that needed to maintain normal PCO_2 levels and should not be confused with the hyperpnea that occurs with exercise. The most common cause of hyperventilation is anxiety. Other causes of hyperventilation are fever, oxygen lack, early salicylate toxicity, and encephalitis. Salicylate toxicity and encephalitis produce hyperventilation by directly

Table 23-3 Respiratory Acidosis

Laboratory Findings

Primary Defect (Uncompensated)		Compensation
pH	PCO_2	Bicarbonate
Decreased	Increased	Increased

Causes	Manifestations
Increased carbon dioxide inhalation	**Depression of neural function**
Breathing air that is high in carbon dioxide content	Headache
	Weakness
Decreased ventilation	Confusion and disorientation
Depression of the central nervous system	Behavioral changes
Drug overdose	Depression
Head injury	Paranoia
Diseases of the airways or lungs	Hallucinations
Bronchial asthma	Tremors
Emphysema	Paralysis
Chronic bronchitis	Stupor and coma
Respiratory distress in the newborn	
Pneumonia	**Skin**
Pulmonary edema	Warm and flushed
Disorders of chest wall or respiratory muscles	**Compensatory mechanisms**
Paralysis of respiratory muscles	Increased loss of hydrogen in the urine
Chest injuries	(metabolic alkalosis)
Treatment with curare	

Table 23-4   Respiratory Alkalosis

Laboratory Findings

Primary Defect (Uncompensated)		Compensation
pH	PCO$_2$	Bicarbonate
Increased	Decreased	Decreased

Causes	Manifestations

Increased ventilation (hyperventilation)
   Stimulation of respiratory center
      Elevated blood ammonia
      Salicylate toxicity
      Encephalitis
      Anxiety
   Reflex stimulation
      Hypoxemia
   Lung disease that reflexly stimulate ventilation
      Local lung lesions
   Mechanical ventilation
	Increased excitability of the nervous system
	   Numbness and tingling of fingers and toes
	   Dizziness, panic, and lightheadedness
	   Tetany
	   Positive Chvostek's and Trousseau's signs
	   Convulsions

stimulating the respiratory center. Hyperventilation can also occur during anesthesia or with use of mechanical ventilatory devices.

The *signs and symptoms* of respiratory alkalosis are associated with hyperexcitability of the nervous system. There is often a feeling of lightheadedness, dizziness, tingling, and numbness of the fingers and toes. There may also be sweating, palpitations, panic, air hunger, and dyspnea. Chvostek's and Trousseau's signs may be positive and tetany and convulsions may occur. Since carbon dioxide provides the stimulus for short-term regulation of respiration, short periods of apnea may occur in persons with acute episodes of hyperventilation.

The treatment of respiratory alkalosis focuses on measures to increase the PCO$_2$. Attention is directed toward correcting the disorder that caused the overbreathing. Rebreathing of small amounts of expired air (breathing into a paper bag) may prove useful in restoring PCO$_2$ levels in persons with anxiety-produced respiratory alkalosis.

In summary, respiratory alkalosis occurs from overbreathing. There is an increase in pH above 7.45 and a decrease in PCO$_2$ levels to a value below 35 mm Hg. The causes and manifestations of respiratory alkalosis are summarized in Table 23.4. There is hyperexcitability of the nervous system in respiratory alkalosis. The most common cause of respiratory alkalosis is anxiety, although it can be caused by other conditions that increase the respiratory rate.

:Study Guide

After you have studied this chapter, you should be able to meet the following objectives:

: : Describe carbon dioxide transport.

: : Describe the role of the respiratory system in control of pH.

: : Describe hydrogen ion secretion by renal mechanisms.

: : Describe the renal phosphate buffer system and the ammonia buffer system.

: : Describe the blood buffer systems.

: : State the Henderson-Hasselbalch equation and explain its use.

: : Compare corrective vs. compensatory mechanisms for regulation of changes in pH.

: : Describe the role of potassium in pH regulation.

: : Explain the postprandial alkaline tide.

: : Define the *anion gap*.

: : Describe a clinical situation involving an acid–base disorder in which both primary and compensatory mechanisms might be active.

: : Describe the effect of metabolic acidosis on the renal and gastrointestinal systems.

: : Categorize the following signs and symptoms of metabolic acidosis: Kussmaul breathing, odor of acetone on the breath, decrease in heart rate and output.

: : State the cause of lactic acidosis.

: : List the causes of metabolic alkalosis.

: : Describe the clinical manifestations of metabolic alkalosis.

: : Explain the relationship between respiratory disorders and respiratory acidosis.

: : Explain the relationship between hyperventilation and respiratory alkalosis.

:Suggested Readings

Arruda JAL, Kurtzman NA: Metabolic acidosis and alkalosis. Clin Nephrol 7, No. 5:201, 1977

Broughton JD: Understanding blood gases. In Hudak C et al: Critical Care Nursing, 2nd ed. Philadelphia, JB Lippincott, 1977

Chan JCM: Acid–base, calcium, potassium and aldosterone metabolism in renal tubular acidosis. Nephron, 23:152, 1979

Cohen S, Miller M, Sherman RL: Metabolic acid–base disorders: Part 1—Chemistry and physiology. Am J Nurs 77, No. 10:1619, 1977

Cohen S, Miller M, Sherman RL: Metabolic acid–base disorders. Am J Nurs 78, No. 1:87, 1978

Frohlich ED: Pathophysiology, 2nd ed., p 287. Philadelphia, JB Lippincott, 1976

Goldberger E: A Primer of Water, Electrolyte and Acid–Base Syndromes, 6th ed. Philadelphia, Lea & Febiger, 1980

Guyton AC: Textbook of Medical Physiology, 6th ed., p 448. Philadelphia, WB Saunders, 1981

Hassan H: Hypercapnia and hyperkalemia. Anaesthesia 34:897, 1979

Lum LC: Respiratory alkalosis and hypocarbia. Chest Heart Stroke J, 3:31, 1978/1979

Martinez–Maldonado M, Sanchez–Montserrat R: Respiratory acidosis and alkalosis. Clin Nephrol 7, No. 5:191, 1977

Metheny NM: Nurses' Handbook of Fluid Balance, 3rd ed. Philadelphia, JB Lippincott, 1979

Sabatini S, Arruda JA, Kurtzman NA: Disorders of acid–base balance. Med Clin North Am 62, No. 6:1223, 1978

24

Alterations in Distribution of Body Fluids: Edema

Normally, about 5% of the total body water is contained in the interstitial, or tissue, spaces. This water acts as a transport vehicle for gases, nutrients, wastes, and other materials that need to be transported between body cells and the vascular compartment. Interstitial fluid also provides a reservoir from which vascular volume can be maintained during periods of hemorrhage or loss of vascular volume. A tissue gel, or sponge-like material composed of large quantities of mucopolysaccharides, fills the tissue spaces and aids in the even distribution of interstitial fluid. This tissue gel decreases with age and is thought to account in part for the wrinkled appearance that occurs with aging.

Several factors contribute to alterations in the distribution of extracellular water. Because of the nonspecific nature of these alterations and the frequency with which they occur, this chapter focuses on *increases* in interstitial fluid or *edema*.

:Regulation of Interstitial Fluid Volume

The interchange of cellular and vascular fluid occurs at the capillary level, with fluid leaving the capillary bed, traversing the interstitial spaces, and entering the cell and *vice versa*. Normally, there is a continuous movement of fluid between the capillary bed and the interstitial spaces. A state of equilibrium exists as long as equal amounts of fluid both enter and leave the interstitial spaces. White blood cells, plasma proteins, and other molecules which are too large to reenter the capillary rely on the loosely structured wall of the lymphatic vessels for return to the vascular compartment. About 10% of the filtered fluid is returned to the circulation through the lymphatics.

$$\frac{\text{fluid leaving}}{\text{the capillary}} = \frac{\text{fluid reentering}}{\text{the capillary}} + \text{lymphatic flow}$$

Capillaries are microscopic vessels one layer thick that connect the arterioles of the arterial system with venules of the venous system. Small cuffs of smooth muscle, the precapillary sphincters, are positioned at the arterial end of the capillary. The smooth muscle tone of the arterioles, venules, and precapillary sphincters serves to control blood flow through the capillary bed (see Figure 24-1).

There are two types of mechanisms that control movement of capillary fluid—outward and inward forces (Fig. 24-1). The outward forces, those that cause fluid to move out of the capillary into the tissue spaces, include (1) the capillary filtration (or capillary) pressure, (2) the negative tissue fluid pressure, and (3) the colloid osmotic pressure exerted by plasma proteins that are in the tissue spaces. The inward movement of fluid is controlled largely by the colloid osmotic pressure within the capillary.

Figure 24–1. Diagram of the forces that control movement of fluid between the capillary bed and tissue spaces. (From Chaffee EE, Lytle IM: Basic Physiology and Anatomy, 4th ed. Philadelphia, JB Lippincott, 1980)

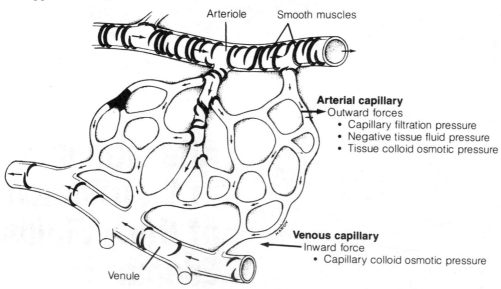

Capillary Filtration Pressure

The capillary filtration pressure is the pushing force that forces water through the capillary pores into the interstitial spaces. Capillary filtration pressure reflects the arterial pressure, the venous pressure, and the hydrostatic effects of gravity (Fig. 24-2).

The *arterial pressure* decreases as blood moves away from the heart. Nevertheless, the pressure at the arterial end of the capillary is normally higher than the pressure at the venous end of the capillary. This pressure difference, or gradient, contributes to the exchange of fluid at the capillary level. *Venous pressure* is freely transmitted back to the capillary because there are no sphincters at this end of the capillary. This means that increases in venous pressure, such as those that occur with heart failure, will eventually lead to an increase in intracapillary pressure. Capillary pressure also reflects changes in *capillary volume*. Capillary volume is controlled by the precapillary flow (tone of the precapillary sphincters and the arterioles that supply the capillary) and the postcapillary (venule and small vein) resistances. Selective constriction of the venules will cause capillary pressures to rise, whereas constriction of the arterioles and precapillary sphincters leads to a decrease in pressure. The pressure due to gravity is called the *hydrostatic pressure*. In a person in the standing position, the weight of the blood in the vascular column causes an increase of 1 mm Hg in pressure for every 13.6 mm of distance from the heart.* Gravity has no effect on blood pressure in a person in the recumbent position because the blood vessels are then at the level of the heart. Often the terms capillary pressure and hydrostatic pressure are used interchangeably; this is because of the passive nature of pressure in the capillary bed. In this chapter, for purposes of discussion, hydrostatic pressure is considered to be the result of gravity and is presented separately from other factors that affect capillary pressure.

Colloid Osmotic Pressure

Colloids are particles that become evenly dispersed when placed in solution, much as cream particles become dispersed when milk is homogenized. The term *colloid osmotic pressure* is used to distinguish the osmotic effects of the colloids from those of the

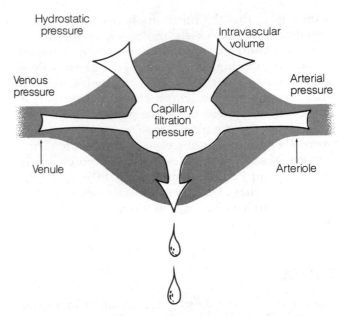

Figure 24-2.   Diagram of forces that influence capillary filtration pressure.

dissolved crystalloids such as sodium. The plasma proteins are large colloid molecules that disperse in the blood and occasionally escape into the tissue spaces. Because the capillary membrane is almost impermeable to the plasma proteins, these particles exert a force that draws fluid into the capillary and offsets the pushing force of the capillary filtration pressure. The plasma contains a mixture of plasma proteins, including albumin, the globulins, and fibrinogen. Albumin, which is the smallest and most abundant of the plasma proteins, accounts for about 70% of the total osmotic pressure. The reader is reminded that it is the number, and not the size of the particles in solution, that controls the osmotic pressure. One gram of albumin (molecular weight 69,000) contains almost six times as many molecules as one gram of fibrinogen (molecular weight 400,000).†

Lymph Flow

Normally, slightly more fluid leaves the capillary than can be reabsorbed at the venous end. This excess fluid is returned to the circulation by way of the lymph channels; almost all body tissues have lymph channels. The structure of the lymph capillary

---

*The hydrostatic pressure in the veins of an adult male can reach a level of 90 mm Hg. This pressure is then transmitted to the capillary bed.

---

†The normal values for the plasma proteins are (1) albumin 4.5 g per 100 ml, (2) globulins 2.5 g per 100 ml, and (3) fibrinogen 0.3 g per 100 ml.

is unique in that the junctions between the endothelial cells of the vessels are loosely connected to form valves and are attached by anchoring filaments to the surrounding tissue (Fig. 24-3). These valves allow fluid to enter the lymph channel. Once the fluid has entered the lymph channel, however, it cannot leave because the valve prevents backward flow. The anchoring filaments serve to pull the valve open when there is an increase in tissue fluid. Contraction of smooth muscles in the lymph channels (lymph pump) causes lymph fluid to empty into veins in the chest. Compression of tissues and muscle movements contributes to movement of fluid in the lymph channels.

:Edema

Edema refers to excess interstitial fluid in the tissues. Edema is not a disease. Rather, it is the manifestation of altered physiologic function.

Causes of Edema

Alterations in physiologic function that lead to edema are (1) increases in capillary filtration pressure, (2) decreases in capillary colloid osmotic pressure, (3) increases in capillary permeability, and (4) obstruction to lymph flow. Edema can occur in healthy as well as sick individuals, for example, the swelling of the hands and feet that occurs in hot weather. The causes of edema are summarized in Table 24-1.

Figure 24–3. Special structure of the lymphatic capillaries that permits passage of substances of high molecular weight back into the circulation. (From Guyton AC: Textbook of Medical Physiology, 5th ed. Philadelphia, WB Saunders, 1976)

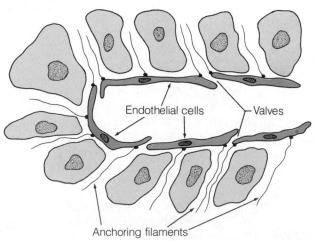

Table 24-1   Causes of Edema

Increased capillary pressure

Arteriolar dilatation
  Allergic responses (hives and angioneurotic edema)
  Inflammation
Venous obstruction
  Hepatic obstruction
  Heart failure
  Thrombophlebitis
Increased vascular volume
  Heart failure
  Increased levels of adrenal cortical hormones
  Increased premenstrual sodium retention
  Pregnancy
  Environmental heat stress
Effects of gravity
  Prolonged standing

Decreased colloid osmotic pressure

Decreased production of plasma proteins
  Liver disease
  Starvation or severe protein deficiency
Increased loss of plasma proteins
  Protein-losing kidney diseases
  Extensive burns

Increased capillary permeability

Inflammation
Immune responses
Neoplastic disease
Tissue injury and burns

Lymphatic obstruction

Infection or disease of the lymphatic structures
Surgical removal of lymph nodes

Increased capillary pressure

Edema develops when there is an increase in capillary pressure that causes excess movement of fluid from the capillary bed into the interstitial spaces. Among the factors that cause an increase in capillary pressures are (1) decreased resistance to flow through the arterioles and capillary sphincters that supply the capillary bed, (2) increased resistance to outflow at the venous end of the capillary bed, (3) increased extracellular fluid volume associated with an increase in intravascular volume, and (4) increased gravitational forces. In hives and other allergic or inflammatory conditions, localized edema develops because of a histamine-induced dilatation of the precapillary sphincters and arterioles that supply the swollen area. Impaired venous outflow from the capillary causes a retrograde increase in capillary pressure. Thrombophlebitis, or the presence of venous blood clots, leads to edema of the affected part. In right-sided heart failure, blood dams up throughout the entire systemic venous system, causing organ congestion and edema of the dependent extremities. Increased reabsorption of sodium and water by the kidney leads to an increase in extracellular volume with an increase in capillary pressure and subsequent movement of fluid into the tissue spaces. In hot weather there is dilatation of the superficial blood vessels and an increase in sodium and water retention which causes swelling of the hands and feet. Edema of the ankles and feet becomes more pronounced during periods of prolonged standing when the forces of gravity are superimposed on the heat-induced vasodilatation and the increase in extracellular fluid volume.

Decreased colloid osmotic pressure

The plasma proteins exert the osmotic force that is needed to move fluid back into the capillary from the tissue spaces. Edema develops when plasma protein levels become inadequate due to abnormal losses or inadequate production. The glomerulus of the kidney nephron is a network of capillaries. In certain conditions, these capillaries may become permeable to the plasma proteins. When this happens, large amounts of plasma proteins are filtered out of the blood and then lost in the urine. An excess loss of plasma proteins also occurs when large areas of skin are injured or destroyed. Edema is a frequent problem during early stages of a burn, resulting from both capillary injury and loss of plasma proteins.

Plasma proteins are synthesized from amino acids. In starvation and malnutrition, edema develops because of a lack of amino acids for use in plasma proteins production. In starvation, edema may actually mask loss of tissue mass. Finally, since plasma proteins are synthesized in the liver, severe liver dysfunction causes decreased plasma protein synthesis with development of edema and ascites. Liver disease also contributes to edema formation by causing obstruction to venous flow through the portal circulation and through impaired metabolism of hormones, such as aldosterone, which increase sodium retention.

It is now possible to measure the colloid osmotic pressure of the plasma (normal 25.4).[1] Infusion of albumin can be used to raise colloidal osmotic pressure as a means of restoring intravascular volume or reversing interstitial fluid losses.

Increased capillary permeability

In situations of increased capillary permeability, the capillary pores become enlarged or the integrity of the capillary wall is destroyed. Injury due to burns, mechanical distention, inflammation, and immune responses are known to increase capillary permeability. Once an increase in capillary permeability has been established, plasma proteins and other osmotically active materials leak out into the interstitial spaces and perpetuate the accumulation of tissue fluid.

Obstruction of lymphatic flow

The osmotically active plasma proteins and other large particles rely on the lymphatics for movement back into the circulatory system from the interstitial spaces. Lymphedema occurs when there is obstruction to lymph flow. Malignant involvement of lymph structures or removal of lymph nodes at the time of cancer surgery are common causes of lymphedema. Another cause of lymphedema is infection. Elephantiasis (filariasis) is a tropical infection in which nematodes of the super-family Filarioidea invade the lymph nodes, causing massive swelling of a body part. This infection has been reported to cause a single leg to swell to such proportions that it weighs almost as much as the rest of the body.

Effects of Edema

The effects of edema are determined largely by its location. Edema of the brain, larynx, and lung is an acute, life-threatening situation. On the other hand, swelling of the ankles and feet is often insidious in onset and may or may not be associated with disease. Edema may interfere with movement, limiting motion or making opening of the eyes difficult. Edema can also be disfiguring. In terms of psychological effects and self-concept, edema often causes a distortion of body features, creating problems in obtaining proper-fitting clothing and shoes.

At the tissue level, edema increases the distance for diffusion of oxygen, nutrients, and wastes. Edematous tissues are usually more susceptible to injury and to development of ischemic tissue damage, including pressure sores. The skin of a severely swollen finger can act as a tourniquet, shutting off blood flow to the finger.

In chronic edema, the tissue spaces become stretched "like an old balloon" so that less filtration pressure is needed to push fluids into the interstitial spaces. The stretching of the tissue spaces makes correction or permanent reversal of edema difficult.

Pitting Edema

Pitting edema occurs when the accumulation of interstitial fluid exceeds the absorptive capacity of the tissue gel. In pitting edema, the tissue water is mobile and can be translocated with pressure exerted by a finger. Imagine, if you will, a sponge that is supersaturated with water. To test for pitting edema, the observer applies firm finger pressure to the edematous areas. Pitting edema is present if an indentation remains after the finger has been removed.

Nonpitting Edema

Nonpitting edema usually represents a situation in which serum proteins that have accumulated in the tissue spaces coagulate. Often the area is firm and discolored. Brawny edema describes a type of nonpitting edema in which the skin becomes thick and hardened. Nonpitting edema is seen most frequently following local infection or trauma.

Assessment Measures

Methods for assessing edema include visual inspection, including the use of digital pressure to determine the degree of pitting that is present. Pitting edema is evaluated on a scale of $+1$ to $+4$. Daily weight is also a useful index of interstitial fluid gain. A third assessment measure involves measuring the circumference of an extremity (or the abdomen).

Treatment of Edema

The treatment of edema is usually directed toward (1) maintaining life in situations in which the swelling involves vital structures, (2) correcting or controlling the cause, and (3) preventing tissue injury. Diuretic therapy is often used to treat edema. The reader is again reminded that edema is not always associated with disease and that normal compensatory increases in tissue fluid may respond to such simple measures as elevating the feet.

Elastic support stockings and sleeves are applied to increase the resistance to the outward flow of fluid from the capillary. These support devices are often prescribed in situations such as lymphatic or venous obstruction and are most efficient if applied before the tissue spaces have filled with fluid, as in the morning before the effects of gravity have caused fluid to move into the ankles.

:Accumulation of Fluid in the Serous Cavities

The serous cavities are potential spaces which are located in strategic body areas where there is continual movement of body structures—the joints, the pericardial sac, and the pleural cavity. The exchange of extracellular fluid between the capillaries, the interstitial spaces, and the potential space of the serous cavity is similar to capillary exchange mechanisms that exist elsewhere in the body. The potential spaces are closely linked with lymphatic drainage systems. The milking action of the moving structures continually forces fluid and plasma proteins back into the circulation, keeping these cavities empty. One of the factors that contribute to fluid accumulation in a potential space is obstruction to lymph flow.

The prefix *hydro-* may be used to indicate the presence of excessive fluid, as, for example, in hydrothorax, which means excessive fluid in the pleural cavity. Or the term *effusion* may be used, as, for example, in pleural effusion, referring to an accumulation of fluid in the pleural cavity.

The fluid accumulated in a serous cavity may be either serous or exudative. A frequent cause of fluid accumulation in serous cavities is infection. In infection, white cells and cellular debris collect and obstruct lymph flow causing osmotically active proteins to accumulate. A second cause of fluid accumulation is a malignant tumor; malignant tumors may invade the lymph channels that drain the serous cavity, and thus contribute to fluid accumulation.

Ascites is an accumulation of fluid in the peritoneal cavity. Because of its location in reference to the portal circulation, the peritoneal cavity is more susceptible to excess fluid accumulation than are other body cavities. This is because anytime there is a significant increase in pressure in the liver sinusoids, serum exudes through the capillaries on the surface of the liver and passes into the peritoneal cavity. Congestive heart failure, cirrhosis, and carcinoma of the liver are examples of conditions that obstruct hepatic blood flow and cause fluid to move into the peritoneal cavity. Since the portal vein receives blood from the peritoneal surface, portal hypertension creates an increase in the filtration pressure of the capillaries that line the peritoneal cavity.

Excess fluid may be aspirated or removed from a serous cavity. The term paracentesis refers to removal of fluid through a puncture site. Usually a needle or similar instrument is inserted into the cavity and the fluid is withdrawn. Analysis of the fluid for the presence of infectious organisms and malignant cells often aids in diagnosis of the disease responsible for the fluid accumulation.

In summary, edema refers to an excess accumulation of interstitial fluids that results from a disruption in fluid movement between the capillary and tissue spaces.

Edema occurs in healthy as well as sick individuals. The physiologic mechanisms that predispose to edema formation are (1) increased capillary pressure, (2) decreased capillary colloidal osmotic pressure, (3) increased capillary permeability, and (4) obstruction of lymphatic flow. The effect that edema exerts on body function is determined by its location—cerebral edema can be a life-threatening situation, whereas swollen feet can be a normal discomfort that accompanies hot weather.

:Study Guide

After you have studied this chapter, you should be able to meet the following objectives:

: : Describe the role of the capillaries in regulating interstitial fluid volume.

: : Explain the use of the term *colloid osmotic pressure*.

: : Describe lymph flow.

: : Describe the pathologic basis of increased capillary pressure.

: : Explain the relationship betwen plasma protein levels and edema formation.

: : List causes of increased capillary permeability.

: : State the clinical manifestations of lymphedema.

: : Compare pitting edema and nonpitting edema.

: : State the goal in treatment of edema.

: : Explain why the serous cavities are referred to as *potential spaces*.

:Reference

1. Morissette MP: Colloid osmotic pressure: Its measurement and clinical value. Can Med Assoc J 116:897, 1977

:Suggested Readings

Burch E: Cardiac edema. Consultant April, 227, 1980
Guyton AC: Textbook of Medical Physiology, ed 6, pp 358, 370. Philadelphia, WB Saunders, 1981

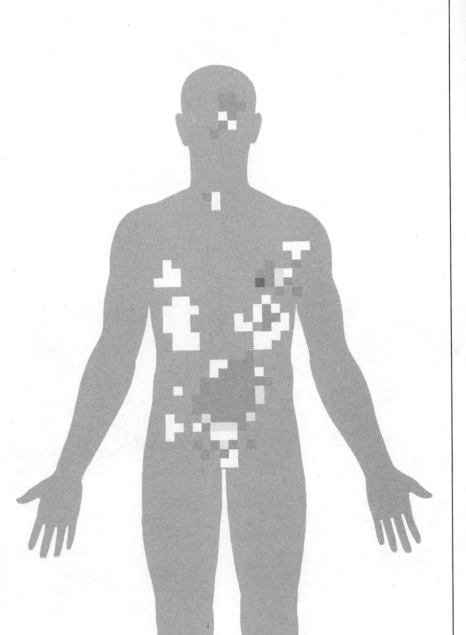

IV

Alterations in Genitourinary Function

The genitalia, reproductive structures, and the urinary system are collectively called the genitourinary system. The urinary system provides the means for elimination of metabolic wastes and regulation of the composition of body fluids. The reproductive structures and associated secondary sex characteristics are important during all phases of the life cycle. During childhood and adolescence they contribute to psychological development and help to shape the self-concept. While the primary function of the reproductive system is procreation, the sex act itself is a pleasurable experience and ranks among the basic needs.

The genitourinary system is subject to the same pathological processes that affect other organs in the body. Anatomically, the reproductive structures are located in close proximity to the structures of the urinary system and therefore pathology of one system often affects the other. This unit focuses on normal and altered function of the (1) urinary system, (2) male reproductive system, and (3) the female genitourinary system.

25

Control of Renal Function

It is no exaggeration to say that the composition of the blood is determined not so much by what the mouth takes in, but by what the kidneys keep (Homer W. Smith, *From Fish to Philosopher*). The kidneys are two remarkable organs. Each is smaller than a man's hand, yet in one day they filter about 1700 liters of blood and combine its waste products into about 1 liter of urine. As a part of their function, the kidneys filter dissolved particles from the blood and selectively reabsorb those that are needed to maintain the normal composition of the internal body fluids. Substances not needed for this purpose pass into the urine. In regulating the volume and composition of body fluids, the kidney performs both excretory and endocrine functions. This chapter discusses the structure and function of the kidneys, the action of diuretics, and tests of renal function.

:Kidney Structure and Function

The kidneys are two bean-shaped structures that are located in the back of the abdominal cavity (Fig. 25-1). The longitudinal fissure, in the central concave portion of the kidney, is called the *hilus*. It is here that blood vessels and nerves enter and leave the kidney. The *ureters*, which connect the kidney with the bladder, also enter the kidney in the hilus.

On longitudinal section, the outer third of the kidney can be seen to have a brownish-red hue. This is the *cortex* (Fig. 25-2). The *medulla* consists of light-colored, cone-shaped masses, the renal pyramids. The free ends of the pyramids form a papilla, which opens into the *renal pelvis*. The renal pelvis is made up of calyces, which drain the upper and lower halves of the kidney. The calyces, in turn, unite with the renal pelvis at the upper end of the ureter.

Each kidney is composed of over a million functional units called *nephrons*, and each nephron consists of a *glomerulus* and a *tubule* (Fig. 25-3). The glomerulus consists of a network of capillaries encased in a thin-walled sac, *Bowman's capsule*. Fluid and particles from the blood are filtered through the membrane of the glomerulus into Bowman's capsule. Bowman's capsule extends to form the tubules of the nephron. Water, nutrients, electrolytes, and other substances are reabsorbed from the glomerular filtrate as it passes through the tubules. Finally, fluid from the tubules flows into the *collecting duct*, which collects fluid from several nephrons. The collecting duct, in turn, empties into the renal pelvis.

The nephron is supplied by *two capillary beds*, a

Figure 25–1. Diagram of the kidneys, ureter, and bladder. (From Chaffee EE, Greisheimer EM: Basic Physiology and Anatomy, 3rd ed. Philadelphia, JB Lippincott, 1974)

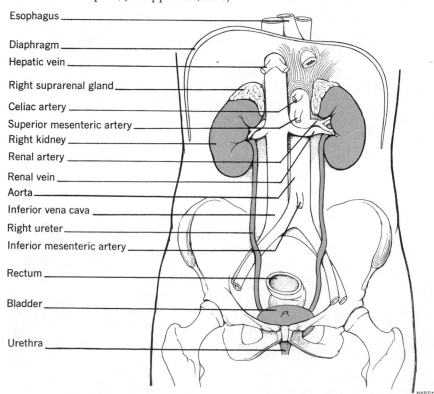

Esophagus

Diaphragm

Hepatic vein

Right suprarenal gland

Celiac artery

Superior mesenteric artery

Right kidney

Renal artery

Renal vein

Aorta

Inferior vena cava

Right ureter

Inferior mesenteric artery

Rectum

Bladder

Urethra

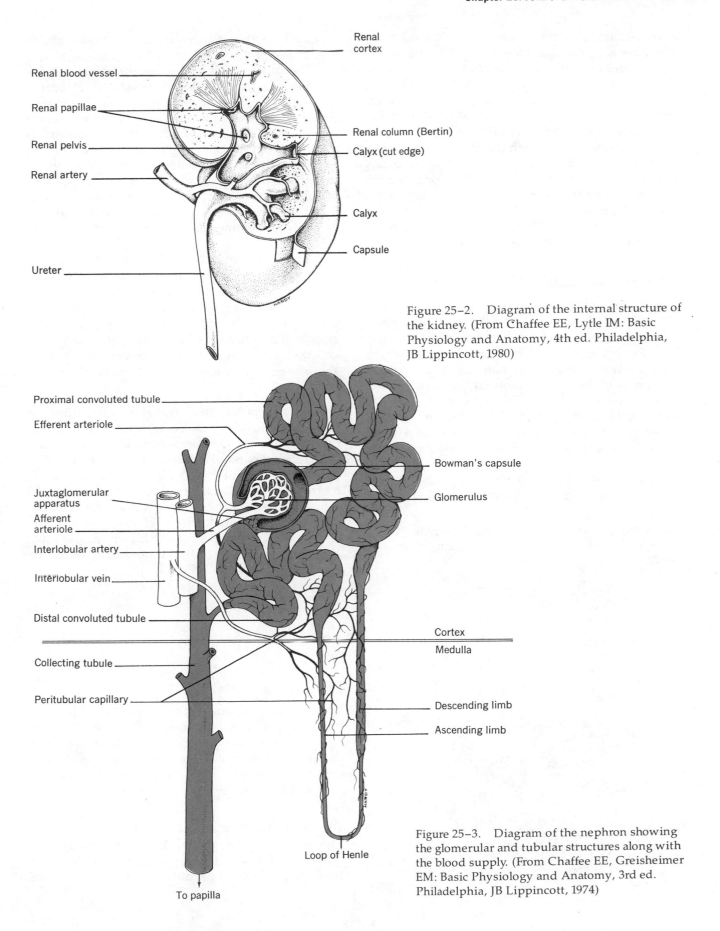

Renal cortex

Renal blood vessel

Renal papillae

Renal column (Bertin)

Renal pelvis

Calyx (cut edge)

Renal artery

Calyx

Capsule

Ureter

Figure 25–2.   Diagram of the internal structure of the kidney. (From Chaffee EE, Lytle IM: Basic Physiology and Anatomy, 4th ed. Philadelphia, JB Lippincott, 1980)

Proximal convoluted tubule

Efferent arteriole

Bowman's capsule

Juxtaglomerular apparatus

Glomerulus

Afferent arteriole

Interlobular artery

Interlobular vein

Distal convoluted tubule

Cortex

Medulla

Collecting tubule

Peritubular capillary

Descending limb

Ascending limb

To papilla

Loop of Henle

Figure 25–3.   Diagram of the nephron showing the glomerular and tubular structures along with the blood supply. (From Chaffee EE, Greisheimer EM: Basic Physiology and Anatomy, 3rd ed. Philadelphia, JB Lippincott, 1974)

glomerulus, and a *peritubular network*. The glomerulus is a unique high-pressure capillary filtration system that is located between two arterioles, the *afferent* and *efferent* arterioles. The reader will note in Figure 25-3 that the low-pressure reabsorptive system of the peritubular capillary network arises from the efferent arteriole. Blood entering the nephron must pass through the glomerular capillary network before it enters the peritubular capillary system. This arrangement has implications with reference to kidney failure, since blood flow to the tubular capillary network is impaired when there is a decrease in or obstruction to flow through the glomerular capillary network.

Excretory Functions

Filtration

Filtration is the process whereby fluids and small particles are removed from the blood. The location of the glomerulus, between two arterioles, allows for maintenance of a high-pressure filtration system. The *capillary filtration pressure* in the glomerulus is about two to three times as high as that of other capillary beds in the body. The filtration pressure and the glomerular filtration rate are regulated by the constriction or relaxation of the afferent and efferent arterioles. During strong sympathetic stimulation, which causes marked constriction of the afferent arteriole, the filtration pressure is reduced to the

Figure 25–4. Diagram of the glomerular capillary membrane, showing the endothelial, basement membrane, and epithelial layers.

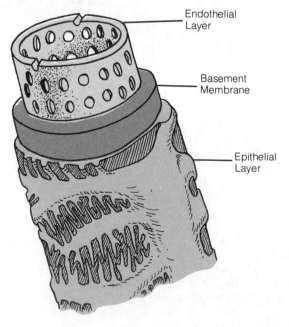

Endothelial Layer

Basement Membrane

Epithelial Layer

point where the glomerular filtration rate falls to almost zero.

The capillary membrane of the glomerulus is composed of three layers: (1) the endothelial layer of the capillary, (2) the basement membrane, and (3) a layer of epithelial cells that line Bowman's capsule (Fig. 25-4). Glomerular capillary permeability is about 100 to 1000 times as great as that of capillaries elsewhere in the body. All three layers allow water and dissolved particles, such as electrolytes, to leave the blood and pass rapidly into Bowman's capsule. Blood cells and plasma proteins are too large to pass through the glomerular membrane of a healthy kidney.

Normally about 125 ml of fluid is filtered each minute (glomerular filtration rate). This amount can vary from a few milliliters to as high as 200 ml per minute. Under normal conditions only about *1 ml of the 125 ml that was filtered by the glomerulus is excreted as urine*. The other 124 ml is reabsorbed in the tubular structures. This means that the average output is about 60 ml per hour or 1440 ml per day.

Glomerular filtration rate. The glomerular filtration rate (GFR) provides a measure to assess renal function, and can be measured clinically by collecting timed samples of blood and urine. Creatinine, a product of creatine metabolism by the muscle, is filtered by the kidney but not reabsorbed in the renal tubule. Therefore, one of the substances that are measured in calculating the GFR is creatinine. The clearance rate for such a substance is the amount that is completely cleared by the kidney in 1 minute. The formula is expressed as follows:

$$C = \frac{UV}{P}$$

where C = clearance rate
 U = urine concentration
 V = urine volume
 P = plasma concentration

The normal creatinine clearance is 115 to 125 ml per min and is corrected for body surface area. The test may be done on a 24-hour basis with blood drawn at the time the urine collection is completed. In another method two 1-hour urine samples can be collected with a blood sample drawn between.

Tubular reabsorption and secretion

The filtrate from the glomerulus passes through the (1) proximal tubule, (2) loop of Henle, (3) distal tubule, and (4) collecting duct before it reaches the pelvis of the kidney (see Fig. 25-3). In the process of reabsorption, water, sodium, and other substances leave the lumen of the tubule and enter the blood. Secretion, on the other hand, is the process by which substances pass from the blood into the lumen of the tubule. Some solutes, such as glucose and amino acids, are completely reabsorbed. About 99% of the filtered water is reabsorbed, while some substances are poorly reabsorbed or not reabsorbed at all. Only 50% of urea is reabsorbed, and the kidney does not reabsorb any creatinine. Electrolyte reabsorption is generally determined by need.

The urine-concentrating ability of the kidney. The kidney is able to produce either a dilute or a concentrated urine as a means of controlling the composition and volume of the extracellular fluids. Two mechanisms come into play: an increased solute concentration in the medullary area surrounding the collecting tubules, and the selective permeability of the collecting tubules, which is controlled by the antidiuretic hormone (ADH). In about one-fifth of the tubules, the loop of Henle and the peritubular capillary (the vasa recta) descend into the renal medulla. Here a countercurrent mechanism controls water and solute flow, as a result of which water is kept out of the peritubular area surrounding the tubules, and sodium and urea are retained. As a consequence of these processes, a high concentration of these osmotically active particles collects in the interstitium of this portion of the kidney (Fig. 25-5). This portion of the kidney surrounds the collecting tubules, and it is here that the presence of these osmotically active particles facilitates the ADH-mediated reabsorption of water.

The permeability of the collecting tubules is *controlled by ADH.* During periods of dehydration, the kidney plays a major role in maintaining water balance. *Osmoreceptors* in the hypothalamus sense the increase in extracellular osmolality and stimulate release of *ADH from the posterior pituitary.* The collecting tubules, under the influence of ADH, become *permeable to water.* Once the permeability of the collecting tubules has been established, water moves out of the tubular lumen and into the interstitium of the medullary area, where it enters the peritubular capillaries for return to the vascular system. This serves to increase vascular volume, leading to production of a concentrated urine. In the absence of ADH, the renal tubules remain impermeable to water and a dilute urine is formed.

The *specific gravity* (or osmolality) of urine varies with its concentration of solutes. Urine specific gravity provides a valuable index of the hydration

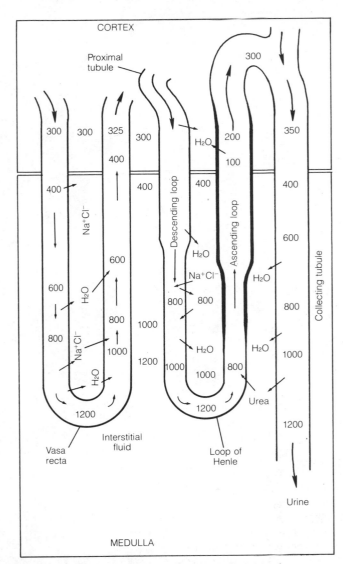

Figure 25–5.   The counter-current mechanism for concentrating urine. Antidiuretic hormone controls the permeability of the collecting tubule.

status and functional ability of the kidneys. Although there are more sophisticated methods for measuring specific gravity, it can be easily measured using an inexpensive piece of equipment called an urinometer (Fig. 25-6 *A&B*). Healthy kidneys can produce a concentrated urine with a specific gravity of 1.030 to 1.040. During periods of marked hydration, the specific gravity can approach 1.000. With diminished renal function, there is a loss of renal concentrating ability, and the urine specific gravity may fall to levels of 1.006 to 1.010. These low levels are particularly significant if they occur during periods that follow a decrease in water intake (e.g., during the first urine specimen on arising in the morning).

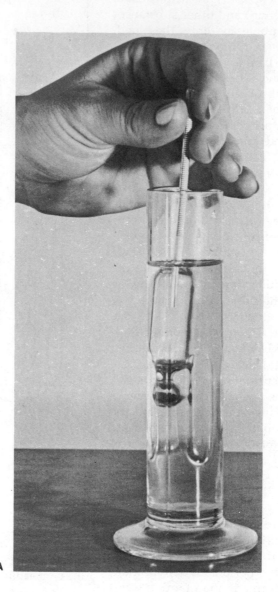
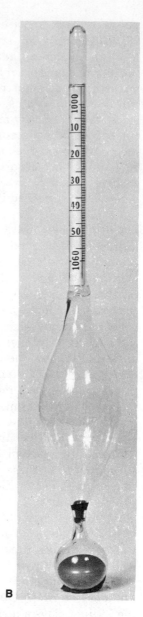

Figure 25–6. (*A*) Urinometer that is used for measuring the specific gravity of urine; (*B*) Urinometer scale. (From Metheny NM, Snively WD Jr: Nurses' Handbook of Fluid Balance, 3rd ed. Philadelphia, JB Lippincott, 1979)   **A**   **B**

Sodium and potassium regulation. About 65% of the glomerular filtrate is reabsorbed in the proximal tubule. Sodium and potassium chloride traverse the cells in the proximal tubule and are pumped, in an energy-requiring process, into the intercellular spaces, where they are absorbed into the peritubular capillaries. Water movement accompanies the movement of these osmotically active particles. Another 25% of sodium and potassium chloride is absorbed as the filtrate passes through the tubular structures in the loop of Henle.

Sodium reabsorption in the distal tubule is highly variable and is dependent upon the presence of *aldosterone*. In the presence of aldosterone, almost all of the sodium from the distal tubular fluid is reabsorbed, and the urine becomes essentially sodium-free. Virtually no sodium is reabsorbed from the distal tubule in the absence of aldosterone. The remarkable ability of the distal tubular cells to alter sodium reabsorption in relation to changes in aldosterone allows the kidney to excrete urine with sodium levels that range from a few tenths of a gram to 30 to 40 grams.

Regulation of extracellular potassium is accomplished through an aldosterone-mediated secretion of potassium into the tubular fluid. Normally only about 70 mEq of potassium is delivered to the distal tubule each day, yet the average person consumes this much and more potassium in the diet. The secretory transport of potassium into the tubular fluid is, therefore, extremely important in regulating extracellular potassium levels. Potassium can also be reabsorbed in the distal tubule and collecting tubules. Usually, however, potassium secretion exceeds reabsorption. In the absence of aldosterone, potassium secretion becomes minimal and, in this situation, potassium reabsorption exceeds secretion, causing blood levels of potassium to increase.

Endocrine Function

At present it is known that the kidney is concerned with either producing or activating renin, erythropoietin, and vitamin D.

Renin is released by special cells located near the glomerulus (juxtaglomerular cells) in response to a reduction in the glomerular filtration rate or as a result of sympathetic stimulation (Fig. 25-7). Renin combines with *angiotensinogen*, a plasma protein that circulates in the blood, to form *angiotensin I*, which is subsequently converted to *angiotensin II*. *Angiotensin II* is a potent *vasoconstrictor* and *stimulator* of *aldosterone release*. The role of the renin–angiotensin–aldosterone mechanism in control of blood pressure is discussed in Chapter 12.

Erythropoietin is released in response to hypoxia. It acts on bone marrow to stimulate production and release of red blood cells (Chap. 20). Although the role of the kidney in erythropoietin production is not fully understood, it is believed that the kidney responds to hypoxia by producing a substance or enzyme that converts a circulating plasma protein to an active form of *erythropoietin*. As a result, persons with chronic hypoxia often have in-

Figure 25–7. Drawing of the renal capsule showing the close contact of the distal tubule with the afferent arteriole and the macula densa and juxtaglomerular apparatus. (From Ham AW, Cormack DH: Histology, 8th ed. Philadelphia, JB Lippincott, 1979)

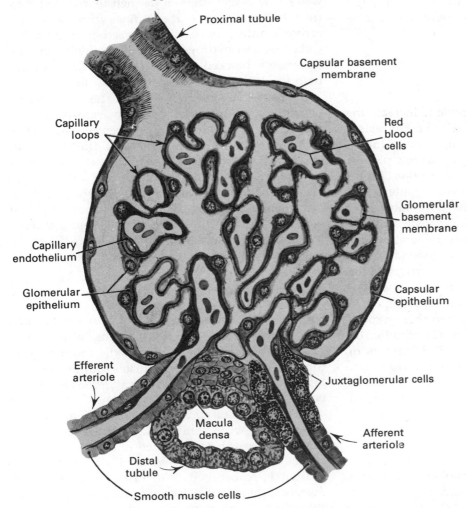

creased red blood cell levels (polycythemia) due to increased erythropoietin levels. This occurs in persons with congestive heart failure, chronic lung disease, or in those living at a high altitude.

Vitamin D is activated in the kidney. Cholecalciferol (vitamin D_3) is transformed to 25-hydroxycholecalciferol in the liver and then converted to active 1,25-dihydroxycholicalciferol in the kidney. The role of vitamin D in calcium metabolism is discussed in Chapter 22.

In summary, the kidneys perform both excretory and endocrine functions. In the process of excreting wastes, the kidneys filter the blood and then selectively reabsorb those materials that are needed to maintain a stable internal environment. The kidneys (1) rid the body of metabolic wastes, (2) regulate fluid volume, (3) regulate the composition of electrolytes, (4) assist in maintaining acid–base balance, (5) aid in regulation of blood pressure through the renin–angiotensin–aldosterone mechanism and control of extracellular fluid volume, (6) regulate red blood cell production through erythropoietin, and (7) aid in calcium metabolism by activating vitamin D.

:Action of Diuretics

In some disease states, it is desirable to increase the urine output through the use of diuretics. Diuresis is the rapid passage of urine through the kidneys. Water reabsorption in the kidneys is largely passive and is dependent upon sodium reabsorption. Therefore, most diuretics exert their action by interfering with sodium reabsorption. Only those substances that have a direct impact on the kidney are regarded as diuretics. For example, digitalis preparations increase urine output in persons with heart failure by increasing cardiac output, renal blood flow, and the glomerular filtration rate, but are not diuretics. Because of their mechanism of action, it is logical to include a discussion of diuretics in this chapter. There are four types of diuretics: (1) osmotic, (2) inhibitors of urine acidification, (3) inhibitors of sodium transport, and (4) aldosterone antagonists. Table 25-1 describes the sites and mechanisms of action and untoward effects of these classes of diuretics. See Figure 25-8.

Osmotic Diuretics

Osmotic diuretics such as mannitol are substances that are filtered in the glomerulus, but not reabsorbed in the tubules. Because they are not reab-

sorbed, they serve to increase the osmolality of the tubular filtrate and cause a decrease in water reabsorption. The osmotic diuretics maintain a high urine volume following a hemolytic reaction, or ingestion of toxic substances, such as salicylates or barbiturates, that are excreted in the urine. Osmotic diuretics have a dehydrating effect on body tissues and may be useful in reducing intracranial or intraocular pressure. In diabetes mellitus, the renal tubular cells are unable to reabsorb all of the glucose that is filtered in the glomerulus, and this glucose acts as an osmotic diuretic.

Inhibitors of Urine Acidification

Acetazolamide (Diamox), a *carbonic anhydrase inhibitor,* impairs the reaction that converts carbon dioxide and water to bicarbonate and hydrogen ions. Bicarbonate is poorly absorbed in the renal tubules; rather, it combines with hydrogen that is secreted into the tubule to form carbon dioxide and water. The carbon dioxide is then reabsorbed into the tubular cells where it combines with water, in a carbonic anhydrase-catalyzed reaction, to form bicarbonate and hydrogen ions. When hydrogen ion secretion is blocked by the action of acetazolamide, both the bicarbonate ion and the sodium ion that accompany it are lost in the urine. The loss of bicarbonate results in a mild systemic acidosis, and as this occurs the kidney resumes secreting hydrogen ions, overcoming the effect of the carbonic anhydrase inhibition. Therefore, the action of acetazolamide is of short duration, and this drug has been replaced by more effective diuretics, such as the thiazides. Acetazolamide also decreases the formation of aqueous humor and the formation of cerebral spinal fluid, and it continues to be used for that purpose.

Inhibitors of Sodium Transport

Sodium reabsorption occurs in the proximal tubule, the ascending loop of Henle, in the tubular area between the ascending loop of Henle and the distal tubule where aldosterone regulates sodium and potassium exchange. Diuretics that alter sodium transport can act at any of these levels.

Mercurial diuretics (e.g., mercaptomerin and meralluride) act to inhibit enzymes needed for sodium transport that are located in the *proximal convoluted tubules,* where 70% to 80% of the filtered sodium is reabsorbed. With use of the mercurial diuretics, there is also decreased reabsorption of the chloride ion, causing excess chloride losses in the

Table 25-1   Diuretic Actions*

Diuretic	Site of Action	Untoward Actions
Osmotic diuretics	Cause water diuresis by creating an osmotic gradient which serves to hold water in the tubular fluid; osmotic diuretics are filtered in the glomerulus but not reabsorbed in the tubule	Dehydration and electrolyte imbalance
Inhibitors of urine acidification (carbonic anhydrase inhibitors)	Impair hydrogen ion secretion in the tubular exchange system where sodium reabsorption is linked to hydrogen secretion	Increase potassium and bicarbonate losses; cause systemic acidosis
Mercurial diuretics	Prevent sodium reabsorption in the proximal tubule	Sodium depletion due to site of action; excess chloride loss can lead to hypochloremic alkalosis
Aldosterone antagonists	Blocks sodium reabsorption in the potassium–sodium exchange site of the distal tubule	Can increase potassium levels
Thiazide diuretics	Prevent sodium reabsorption at the site between ascending loop of Henle and aldosterone-governed site	Cause increased potassium loss; may increase uric acid levels and impair glucose metabolism
Furosemide and ethacrynic acid	Prevent sodium reabsorption in the active transport site of the ascending loop of Henle	Increase potassium losses and uric acid retention; ethacrynic acid has been associated with eighth nerve damage and deafness

*The reader is referred to a pharmacology text for specific examples of each of these diuretics.

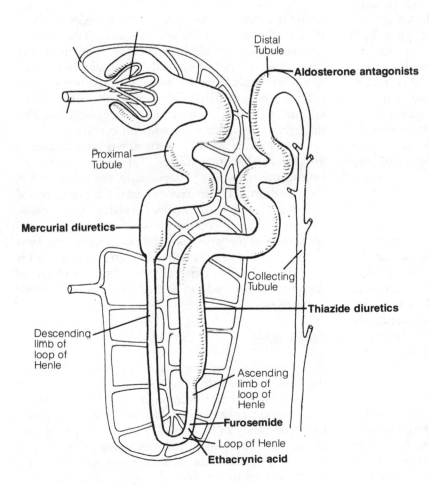

Figure 25–8.   Sites where diuretics exert their action. (From Rodman MJ, Smith DW: Pharmacology and Drug Therapy in Nursing, 2nd ed. Philadelphia, JB Lippincott, 1979)

urine with a resultant development of hypochloremic alkalosis. The mercurial diuretics are poorly absorbed from the gastrointestinal tract and they almost always cause gastrointestinal irritation. Therefore, they are given by injection.

Thiazide diuretics (e.g., chlorothiazide [Diuril] and hydrochlorothiazide [Hydro-Diuril]) exert their action by preventing the reabsorption of sodium in the area of the tubular structures located *between the ascending loop of Henle and the distal tubular site*, where aldosterone exerts its action. The thiazides cause increased loss of potassium in the urine, uric acid retention, and some impairment of glucose tolerance. They are given orally and are very suitable for long-term therapy.

Furosemide (Lasix) and *ethacrynic acid* (Edecrin) are sometimes called *loop diuretics* because they exert their major effect on sodium reabsorption occurring in the *ascending loop of Henle*. About three-fourths of the sodium remaining after passage through the proximal tubule is absorbed in the ascending loop of Henle. This means that diuretics that act at these sites can cause potent diuresis. Impairment of sodium reabsorption in the loop of Henle causes a decrease in the osmolarity of the interstitial fluid surrounding the collecting ducts and further impedes the kidney's ability to concentrate urine. Both of these drugs cause potassium loss, increase uric acid retention, and tend to impair glucose tolerance. Both drugs also afford the potential for development of hypovolemia. Ethacrynic acid is associated with eighth nerve damage and deafness. Because of its ability to produce arteriolar vasodilatation and diuresis when given intravenously, furosemide is often administered in emergency treatment of pulmonary edema.

Aldosterone Antagonists

Spironolactone (Aldactone) and *triamterene (Dyrenium)* are *aldosterone antagonists* which act by blocking the action of aldosterone on the distal tubular exchange site. In this way they increase the loss of sodium in the urine while enhancing potassium retention. Because of this action, these diuretics are sometimes called *potassium sparing diuretics*. Spironolactone, in particular, has the potential for causing hyperkalemia.

In summary, diuretics are drugs that increase urine output. Diuretics, with the exception of osmotic diuretics, exert their action by altering sodium transport. Osmotic diuretics are filtered in the glomerulus and reabsorbed in the tubules. They act by increasing the osmolarity of tubular fluid. Inhibitors of urine acidification, such as

acetazolamide, prevent bicarbonate reabsorption and with it accompanying sodium reabsorption. The mercurial and thiazide diuretics, as well as furosemide and ethacrynic acid, inhibit sodium transport at different tubular sites. The aldosterone antagonists, spironolactone and triamterene, block the action of aldosterone in the distal tubule. These diuretics decrease sodium reabsorption while causing potassium retention. They are sometimes called potassium sparing diuretics.

:Tests of Renal Function

The function of the kidneys is to filter the blood, selectively reabsorb those substances that are needed to maintain the constancy of body fluid, and excrete metabolic wastes. Therefore, the composition of the urine and blood provides valuable information about the adequacy of renal function. Radiological tests, endoscopy, and renal biopsy are procedures that afford a means of viewing the gross and microscopic structures of the kidneys and urinary system.

Urinalysis

Urine is a clear, amber-colored fluid which is about 95% water and 5% dissolved solids. The kidneys normally produce about 1.5 liters of urine a day. Normal urine contains metabolic wastes and few, if any, plasma proteins, blood cells, and glucose molecules. Urine tests can be performed on a single urine specimen or on a 24-hour urine sample. Table 25-2 describes urinalysis values for normal urine.

Casts are molds of the distal nephron lumen. A gel-like substance called Tamm and Horsfall mucoprotein, which is formed in the tubular epithelium, forms the matrix of casts. Casts composed of this gel but devoid of cells are called *hyaline casts*. These casts tend to develop when the protein concentration of the urine is high (as in nephrotic syndrome) and urine osmolality is high and urine pH is low. The inclusion of granules or cells in the matrix of the protein gel leads to formation of various other types of casts.

Blood Tests

Blood tests can provide valuable information about the kidney's ability to remove metabolic wastes from the blood and to maintain normal electrolyte and pH composition of the blood. Normal blood values are listed in Table 25-3. Serum potassium, phosphate blood urea nitrogen (BUN), and creatinine tend to increase in renal failure. Serum calcium, pH, and bicarbonate tend to decrease in renal failure. The

Table 25-2 Normal Values for Routine Urinalysis

General Characteristics and Measurements	Chemical Determinations	Microscopic Examination of Sediment
Color: yellow–amber; indicates a high specific gravity and small output of urine.	Glucose—negative	Casts negative— occasional hyaline casts
Turbidity: clear	Ketones—negative	Red blood cells negative
Specific gravity: 1.015–1.025 with a normal fluid intake	Blood—negative	Crystals negative
pH: 4.6–8; average person has a pH of about 6 (acid)	Protein—negative	White blood cells negative
	Bile-bilirubin— negative	

From Fishbach F: A Manual of Laboratory Diagnostic Tests, p 112. Philadelphia, JB Lippincott, 1980.

Table 25-3 Normal Blood Chemistry Levels

Substance	Normal Value
BUN	8.0 mg/100 ml to 25.0 mg/100 dl
Creatinine	0.5 mg/dl to 1.5 mg/dl
Sodium	137 mEq/l to 147 mEq/l
Chloride	100 mEq/l to 106 mEq/l
Potassium	3.5 mEq/l to 5 mEq/l
Carbon dioxide (CO_2 content)	24 mEq/l to 30 mEq
Calcium	4.5 mEq/l to 5.3 mEq
Phosphate	1.7 mEq/l to 3.6 mEq
Uric acid	3.0 mg/100 ml to 8.5 mg/100 ml
pH	7.35 to 7.45

effect of renal failure on the concentration of serum electrolyte and metabolic end-products is discussed further in Chapter 27.

Cystoscopy

Cystoscopy provides a means for direct visualization of the urethra, bladder, and urethral orifices. It relies on the use of a cystoscope, an instrument with a lighted lens. The cystoscope is inserted through the urethra into the bladder. Biopsy specimens, small stones, lesions and small tumors, and foreign bodies can be removed from the urethra, bladder, and ureters by this means.

Radiological Examination

X-ray films often provide information about urinary tract structures. *Computerized axial tomography* (scanner) refers to x-ray films taken by rotating tubes which sharply delineate tissue at any level they radiate. Tomography may be used to outline the kidney and detect tumors therein. A radiopaque iodine contrast medium allows for visualization of urinary structures. The dye can be introduced into the urinary system or through a vein. An *intravenous pyelogram* (IVP) allows for x-ray visualization of the renal calyces, renal pelvis, and ureters as the dye is excreted by the kidneys. During *retrograde pyelography*, a cystoscope is used to introduce dye into the ureters.

In summary, urinalysis and blood tests which measure levels of byproducts of metabolism and electrolytes provide information about renal function. A cystoscope is used for direct visualization of the urethra, bladder, and ureters. Radiological methods are a means by which the structure of the renal calyces, pelvis, ureters, and bladder can be outlined.

:Study Guide

After you have studied this chapter, you should be able to meet the following objectives:

: : Describe the anatomy of the normal kidney.

: : State the purpose of renal filtration.

: : Explain the formula $C = \dfrac{UV}{P}$

: : Explain the renal mechanisms for concentrating the urine.

: : Describe the function of ADH.

: : Describe the role of aldosterone in regulation of sodium and potassium.

: : Explain the endocrine function of the kidneys.

: : State the basis for the action of osmotic diuretics.

: : Describe the actions of acetazolamide.

: : Explain why mercaptomerin and meralluride alter sodium transport.

: : Describe the effects of furosemide and ethacrynic acid.

: : State another term for aldosterone antagonists and give one example of an aldosterone antagonist.

: : Name and describe three tests of renal function.

:Suggested Readings

Bauman J, Chinard F: Renal Function: Physiological and Medical Aspects. St. Louis, CV Mosby, 1975

Chaffee EE, Lytle IM: Basic Physiology and Anatomy, ed. 4, p 480. Philadelphia, JB Lippincott, 1980

Crowe LR, Hatch FE: Evaluating Renal Function. Postgrad Med 62(1):58, 1977

Guyton AC: Textbook of Medical Physiology, ed. 6, pp 403, 420. Philadelphia, WB Saunders, 1981

Hausler MR, McCair TA: Basic and clinical concepts related to vitamin D metabolism and action. N Engl J Med 297:974, 1041, 1977

Stein JR: Hormones and the kidney. Hosp Pract 14(7):91, 1977

26

Alterations in Renal Function

In 1975, an estimated 80,000 to 110,000 deaths were due to renal diseases. During that same period another 1.2 million Americans were afflicted with nonfatal but disabling urological disorders such as urinary tract infections, kidney stones, and obstructive disorders. The number of persons with chronic and disabling renal disease has increased, in part because of recent advances in dialysis and renal transplant methods which are now keeping persons alive who would formerly have died of renal failure. In 1972, Congress enacted PL 92–603, section 2991, which extended Medicare coverage to 95% of all persons with terminal renal failure as a means of covering at least part of the dialysis and renal transplant costs for these persons. In 1977, 32,656 persons were receiving dialysis, and 4450 renal transplants were done.[1]

The urinary tract is subject to much the same types of disorders as other parts of the body, including developmental defects, infections, altered immune responses, and neoplasms. The kidney filters blood from all parts of the body, and while many forms of renal disorders originate within the kidney, there are some that arise as a consequence of disease or functional states, such as hypertension and diabetes, of other systems of the body. This chapter discusses each of these categories of urinary tract disease, and Chapter 27 discusses acute and chronic renal failure. The effects of other disease conditions, such as hypertension, shock, and diabetes mellitus, are discussed in other sections of the text.

:Congenital Disorders of the Kidney

About 10% of persons are born with potentially significant malformations of the urinary system.[2] Unlike other organs, which develop in a direct and continuous process, the kidneys evolve through the differentiation of three sets of excretory organs, with the third set remaining as the permanent kidneys. In the process of development, the secretory or nephronic components of the kidney develop independently of the collecting system, and the two then are joined. It is during these complex stages of development that structural abnormalities may occur. The permanent kidneys develop early in the fifth week of gestation and begin to function about 3 weeks later. The urine produced by the fetal kidneys mixes with the amniotic fluid, and the fetus drinks it and reabsorbs it through the gastrointestinal tract. In renal agenesis, in which the kidneys fail to develop, the amount of amniotic fluid is very small. In other defects, which impair swallowing by the fetus, there are excessive amounts of amniotic fluid.

Congenital defects of the kidneys include developmental defects and metabolic and enzyme defects which involve tubular transport, such as cystinuria. The discussion in this section is restricted to developmental defects, including agenesis, hypoplasia, dysplasia, and polycystic kidney disease.

Unilateral agenesis of the kidneys is relatively common and persons with this defect are often unaware of its presence as long as the single kidney functions normally. *Agenesis of both kidneys* is rare. It is incompatible with life, and infants with this defect are either stillborn or die shortly after birth. In renal *hypoplasia*, the kidneys do not develop to normal size. As with agenesis, hypoplasia more commonly affects only one kidney. When both kidneys are affected, there is progressive development of renal failure and children with this condition often die of renal failure unless sustained on dialysis.

Fusion of the kidneys at the midline results in what is called a *horseshoe kidney*. This abnormality occurs in about 1 out of 600 persons. It usually does not cause problems unless there is an associated defect in the renal pelvis or kidney that favors obstruction to renal flow.

The most common of the renal developmental disorders is due to *dysplasia*, which results from abnormal differentiation of the renal structures during the embryonic period along with cyst formation. Dysplastic defects account for about 20% of urinary tract malformations and commonly occur along with other types of congenital defects of the lower urinary tract.[3] One example of renal dysplasia is multicystic kidney, which is associated with atresia or obstruction of the ureter. It is tempting to believe that this kidney defect results from obstructed urine flow.

Polycystic disease of the kidneys is characterized by the presence of *bilaterally* enlarged and cyst-filled kidneys. Polycystic kidney disease is categorized into infantile or adult types. *Infantile polycystic kidney disease* is inherited as an autosomal recessive trait. The kidneys are nonfunctional at birth, and fetuses with this defect are stillborn, or if born alive usually die shortly thereafter. The *adult form of polycystic kidney disease* is fairly common, affecting about 1 in 500 persons. It is manifested as an autosomal dominant trait. The disease is characterized by enlarged, palpable, cyst-filled kidneys which can reach the size of a football. The disease usually gives rise to signs of renal failure, during the third or fourth decade of life, although some persons may begin to have symptoms in their teens and others not until they reach 70 or 80 years of age. In the members of an affected family, polycystic kidney disease tends to cause kidney failure at the same age, so families in whom it becomes manifest early in life are more aware of the family history than those in whom the disease becomes manifest later in life. A very common early symptom is a dull, aching pain of the abdomen or back, which is thought to be caused by pressure from the large cysts. Persons with polycystic kidney disease often have cysts in the liver, and intracranial aneurysms. Although the liver cysts seldom cause problems, the intracranial aneurysms may have serious consequences, especially if coupled with hypertension. Fifteen percent of deaths in persons with polycystic kidney disease are caused by these aneurysms.[4]

In summary, approximately 10% of persons are born with potentially significant malformations of the urinary system. These abnormalities can range from bilateral renal agenesis, which is incompatible with life, to hypogenesis of one kidney, which usually causes no problems unless the function of the single kidney is impaired. Polycystic kidney occurs as the result of an inherited trait. Infantile polycystic kidney is inherited as a recessive trait and results in nonfunctional kidneys which are present at birth. The adult form of polycystic kidney disease is inherited as an autosomal dominant trait and is not manifested until later in life.

:Urinary Tract Infections

Urinary tract infections are the second most common type of bacterial infections seen by the physician (respiratory tract infections being first). More women than men have urinary tract infections; about 20% of all women will develop at least one urinary tract infection during their lifetime.[1] These infections range from simple bacteriuria (bacteria in the urine) to severe kidney involvement with irreversible loss of kidney function. *Cystitis* is an infection of the bladder and *pyelonephritis*, an infection of the kidney pelvis and interstitium. Of all patients who must go on dialysis to sustain life, 13% to 22% have infections as the cause of their situation.[1]

Bacteriuria

Normal urine is clear amber in color, and has a distinctive aroma. Bacteria convert urea to ammonia, increasing the pH of the urine and causing it to have a strong and pungent smell. Although nor-

mally these changes occur in urine that has been allowed to stand for a period of time, they are also present in the freshly voided urine of persons with a urinary tract infection. Depending upon the type and extent of infection, the urine may contain mucus shreds and may be discolored, thick, and cloudy.

The presence of 100,000 or more organisms per milliliter of urine is consistent with bacteriuria. There are three types of methods commonly used to detect the presence of bacteria in the urine: microscopic examination of the sediment from a centrifuged sample of urine, urine culture, and chemical tests.

Four chemical tests are available to detect the presence of bacteria in the urine: (1) the nitrate (Griess) test, based on the reduction of nitrate to nitrite by the bacteria, (2) the glucose oxidase test, which relies on the removal of residual glucose in the urine by bacterial action, (3) the catalase test, which detects the presence of enzymes produced by the bacteria, and (4) the reduction of tetrazolium salts by the bacteria after standardized incubation of voided urine. Of these, the nitrate test (or nitrate test combined with tetrazolium salts) is done most widely in this country. Individual test strips (Microstix–Nitrite or Bac–U–Dip) are available for home use or in screening programs. The test is most reliable if done on the first morning specimen, since incubation time in the bladder is needed for bacterial reduction of nitrate to nitrite, and should be carried out on three consecutive mornings.[5] Positive findings are usually confirmed by microscopic or culture methods.

Care is needed in collecting urine specimens so that the samples are representative of bladder urine, i.e., the sample must be examined and cultured promptly. Specimens kept for longer than 1 hour must be refrigerated to prevent the contaminating organisms from multiplying. Catheterized specimens, once common, have been largely replaced by *clean voided specimens*. To obtain a clean voided specimen, the area around the urethral meatus is carefully cleansed and a midstream specimen is obtained by having the person void directly into a sterile container. This method is usually adequate, and eliminates the risk of introducing organisms into the bladder during insertion of a catheter. In infants, a suprapubic needle aspiration may be done when there is indication of bacteriuria.

Pyuria, the presence of pus cells (polymorphonuclear leukocytes) in the urine, has long been believed to represent infection of the urinary tract; however, about 50% of persons with bacteriuria do not have significant pyuria.

Host resistance and contributing factors

Most urinary tract infections ascend the urinary tract through the urethra; occasionally, the entrance may be through the blood stream or lymphatics. Obstruction and reflux of urinary flow are important contributing factors in the development of urinary tract infections.

The urine formed in the kidney and found in the bladder is normally sterile, whereas the distal portion of the urethra often contains pathogens. The bacteria responsible for most urinary tract infections are *Escherichia coli* (*E. coli*), Enterobacter, Klebsiella, Pseudomonas, and Proteus. It has been estimated that 80% to 90% of all initial urinary tract infections are caused by *E. coli*, while persons who have been treated with antimicrobial drugs or have been subjected to catheterization or other urological procedures are more apt to have other organisms, such as Proteus or enterocoli, as the causative pathogens.

In women, the urethra is short and in close proximity to the vagina and rectum, offering little protection against entry of microorganisms into the bladder. There is a peak incidence of these infections in the 15-to-24-year age group, suggesting that hormonal and anatomic changes associated with puberty as well as sexual activity contribute to urinary tract infections. The role of sexual activity in the development of urethritis and cystitis is controversial. The well-documented "honeymoon cystitis" suggests that sexual activity may contribute to such infections in susceptible women. Various preventive measures have been recommended for sexually active women who are bothered with frequent urinary tract infections. These measures include drinking a glassful or two of water and emptying the bladder soon after intercourse on the assumption that this will wash the bacteria out of the urethra and bladder. Women are also more likely to develop urinary tract infections during pregnancy, possibly due to related anatomic and physiological changes. For example, the ureters and renal pelvis dilate during most normal pregnancies.

In men, the length of the urethra and the antibacterial properties of the prostatic fluid provide some protection from ascending urinary tract infections until about age 50. After this age, prostatic hypertrophy becomes more common, and with it there may be obstruction and urinary tract infection.

One common cause of urinary tract infections is reflux or obstruction of urine flow. Under normal conditions, bacteria are removed from the bladder with each voiding. The bladder mucosa has antibacterial properties which further protect against urinary tract infections, and host factors including phagocytosis aid in the removal of bacteria from the urinary tract. Thus, inability to empty the bladder completely with each voiding impedes removal of bacteria from the bladder.

In women, a *urethrovesical reflux* can occur during coughing and sneezing, causing the urine to be squeezed into the urethra with increased abdominal pressure, then to flow back into the bladder as the pressure decreases. This also happens when the act of voiding is abruptly interrupted for any reason. Since the urethral orifice is frequently contaminated with bacteria, the reflux mechanism may cause bacteria to be drawn back into the bladder.

A second reflux mechanism can occur at the level of the bladder and the ureter. This is called the *vesicoureteral reflux*. It is commonly seen in children with urinary tract infections, and is believed to arise from congenital defects of length, diameter, muscle, or innervation of the submucosal segment of the ureter.[6] It is also seen in adults with obstruction to bladder outflow. There is a question whether the renal scarring that is often observed in association with vesicoureteral reflux is due primarily to infection or to the pressure and presence of urine constituents that reflux into the kidney.

Urinary catheters are tubes made of rubber or plastic. They are inserted through the urethra into the bladder for the purpose of urinary drainage. They are a source of urethral irritation, and provide a means for entry of microorganisms into the urinary tract. Indwelling catheters are used in about 10% of patients admitted to general hospitals.[5] A *closed drainage system* (closed to the entrance of air and other sources of contamination) and careful attention to perineal care (cleansing of the area around the urethral meatus) will help to prevent infection in persons who require an indwelling urinary catheter. Careful handwashing and early detection and treatment of urinary tract infections are also essential. When an indwelling catheter is employed, the risk of infection is increased with use of broad-spectrum antibiotics and catheter irrigations—in fact hospital patients themselves are cited as the most frequent reservoir of infection.[7] The Center for Disease Control[7] recommends that patients with urinary catheters not share a room unless special requirements for intensive care make this necessary. This recommendation follows the observation that an increased incidence of urinary tract infections has been reported in catheterized patients sharing a room.

Cystitis

An acute episode of cystitis is characterized by frequency of urination (sometimes as often as every 20 minutes), lower abdominal discomfort, with burning and pain on urination (dysuria). There may also be systemic signs of infection, with fever and generalized malaise. If there are no complications, the symptoms disappear within 48 hours. This type of cystitis is mainly a disorder of young women.

Pyelonephritis

Acute pyelonephritis is a bacterial infection of the kidney and renal pelvis. In its earliest stages it is characterized by inflammatory foci which are interspersed throughout the renal interstitium. Small abscesses may form on the surface of the kidney. In time the lesions are replaced by scar tissue. Among the factors contributing to the development of acute pyelonephritis are catheterization and urinary tract instrumentation, vesicoureteral reflux, pregnancy, preexisting renal disease, and diabetes mellitus.

The onset of acute pyelonephritis is usually abrupt, with chills and fever, headache, back pain, tenderness over the costovertebral angle, and general malaise. It is now possible to localize the site of both upper and lower urinary tract infections by detecting the presence of *antibody coating* on the bacteria.[8] Antibody coating is an immune response of the kidney and is easily detected by the immunofluorescence test. The finding of leukocyte casts in the urine indicates that the infection is in the kidney rather than the lower urinary tract.

Chronic pyelonephritis is both chronic and progressive. There is scarring and deformation of the renal calyces and pelvis. Essentially the disorder appears to involve a bacterial infection superimposed on obstructive abnormalities or the vesicoureteral reflux. The condition may cause many of the same symptoms as acute pyelonephritis, or its onset may be insidious. Loss of tubular function and the ability to concentrate urine gives rise to polyuria and nocturia, and mild proteinuria is common. Severe hypertension is often a contributing factor in the progress of the disease. Chronic pyelonephritis is a significant cause of renal failure.

Treatment of Urinary Tract Infections

The usual treatment of *acute* urinary tract infections consists of administration of anti-infectives such as the sulfonamides, and increased fluids. Although symptoms often regress within 48 hours, treatment is usually continued for a week to 10 days. Phenazopyridine is a local urinary analgesic that relieves many of the discomforts of cystitis. It is available both as a component of many urinary anti-infectives and as a specific drug. It imparts a red-

dish-orange cast to the urine. The patient should be so informed, to avoid any needless worry.

Chronic infections are more difficult to treat. Since they are often associated with obstructive uropathy or reflux flow of urine, diagnostic tests are usually performed to detect such abnormalities. When possible, the condition causing the reflux flow or obstruction is corrected.

Early diagnosis and treatment are essential to preventing permanent kidney damage. Screening of high-risk groups and attention to care of patients with indwelling catheters are important measures. Pregnant women and persons with diabetes or renal problems who are at risk for developing urinary tract infections can be followed in the physician's office. The availability of reliable diagnostic tests makes screening of large populations possible. Although not a common practice, it would be feasible to screen school age girls since it has been estimated that 5 to 6% of girls will have at least one episode of bacteriuria between the time of entering first grade and graduation from high school.[5]

In summary, urinary tract infections are the second most frequent cause of bacterial infection seen by the practicing physician. These infections range from bacteriuria to severe kidney infections that ultimately cause irreversible kidney damage. Most urinary tract infections ascend from the urethra and bladder, and urinary obstruction and reflux are factors predisposing to their development.

:Obstructive Disorders

Urinary obstruction can occur in persons of any age and can involve any of the urinary tract structures from the renal tubules to the urinary meatus. Ninety percent of obstructions are located below the level of the glomeruli, and most cause impairment of urine flow. Obstruction to urine flow can result from developmental defects, calculi, normal pregnancy, benign prostatic hypertrophy, infection and inflammation with development of scar tissue, and neurologic disorders such as spinal cord injury and diabetic neuropathy.

The effects of urinary obstruction are threefold: (1) a heightened susceptibility to infection, (2) a greater likelihood that calculi will develop, and (3) permanent kidney damage. The extent of these effects is determined by its severity and its duration.

Hydronephrosis is a dilatation of the renal pelvis with progressive renal atrophy caused by obstruction to urine flow through the ureter or lower parts of the urinary tract (Fig. 26-1). At autopsy, hydronephrosis is found in 3% to 4% of adults and 2% of

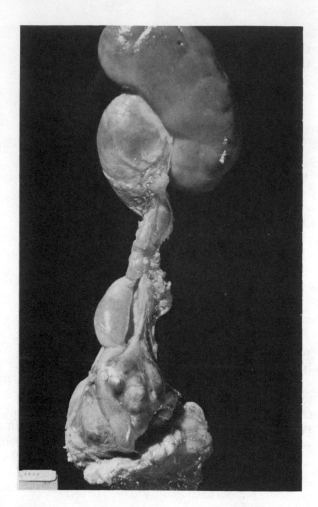

Figure 26–1. Hydroureter caused by ureteral obstruction in a woman with cancer of the uterus.

children.[3] It causes increased pressure in the renal pelvis, which is transmitted back to the collecting ducts and other renal structures, interfering with blood flow and glomerular filtration. If obstruction is complete, serious and irreversible kidney damage occurs after about 3 weeks; if incomplete, about 3 months.[9]

Diagnosis is made on the basis of intravenous pyelography, cystography, or cystoscopy. Other than measures to assess renal failure, there are no screening tests of blood or urine by which the extent of obstruction can be determined.

Urolithiasis

At least 1% of persons in the United States develop urolithiasis, at an annual cost for treatment of $47.3 million.[3] Moreover, about one-third of persons who have recurrent upper urinary tract calculi will even-

tually lose a kidney. Although stones can form in any part of the urinary tract, most develop in the kidney (Fig. 26-2). A small stone may become trapped in a minor calyx and cause no symptoms. However, occasionally a stone will fill the entire renal pelvis; its shape gives it the name—*staghorn* stone. Stones passing into the ureter obstruct urine flow, causing colicky pain. Bladder stones are seen more frequently in elderly men, and often are associated with prostatic hypertrophy.

The usual cause of stones is an increased concentration of the constituents that make up the stones. In persons who form stones there is supersaturation of these constituents; this causes precipitation and crystallization. It is believed that there are inhibitory factors present in the kidneys, and when these inhibitors are deficient stone formation is more likely.

Calcium stones (oxalate or phosphate), magnesium ammonium phosphate stones, uric acid stones, and cystine stones comprise the four types of renal stones. The causes and treatment measures for

Figure 26–2. Locations where renal calculi may form.

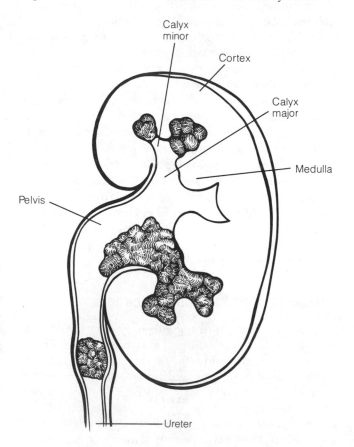

Calyx minor

Cortex

Calyx major

Medulla

Pelvis

Ureter

Table 26-1   Composition, Contributing Factors, and Treatment of Kidney Stones

Type of Stone	Contributing Factors	Treatment
Calcium (oxalate and phosphate)	Hypercalcemia and hypercalciuria Immobilization Hyperparathyroidism Vitamin D intoxication Diffuse bone disease Milk–alkaline syndrome Renal tubular acidosis	Treatment of underlying conditions Thiazide diuretics Increased fluid intake
	Hyperoxaluria Intestinal bypass surgery	
Magnesium Ammonium phosphate (struvite)	Urea-splitting urinary tract infections	Treatment of urinary tract infection Acidification of the urine Increased fluid intake
Uric acid (urate)	Formed in acid urine with pH of approximately 5.5 Gout High-purine diet	Increased fluid intake Allopurinol for hyperuricosuria Alkalinization of urine
Cystine	Cystinuria (inherited disorder of amino acid metabolism)	Increased fluid intake Alkalinization of urine

each of these types of stones are described in Table 26-1. By far the largest number of kidney stones (80 to 90%) are calcium—calcium oxalate, calcium phosphate, or a combination of the two. Calcium stones are usually associated with increased blood and urinary concentrations of calcium. Excessive bone reabsorption caused by immobility, bone disease, hyperparathyroidism, and renal tubular acidosis are all predisposing contributory conditions. Very high oxalate concentrations in the blood and urine may promote formation of oxalate stones. *Magnesium ammonium phosphate* (struvite) stones are caused by the urea-splitting action of bacteria. Staghorn stones are almost always associated with urinary tract infections and a persistently alkaline urine. The presence of gout, along with a high concentration of uric acid, increases development of uric acid stones. Unlike radiopaque calcium stones, uric acid stones are not visible on x-ray film. *Cystine stones* are rare. They are seen in cystinuria in which there is a genetic defect of renal transport of cystine.

Renal Colic

Symptoms
The presence of renal stones may give rise to renal colic. The symptoms of renal colic are due to stones that are 1 to 5 cm in diameter, which are able to move into the ureter and cause obstruction of urine flow. Classic ureteral colic is manifested by acute, excruciating pain in the flank and upper outer quadrant of the abdomen on the affected side. It may radiate to the lower abdominal quadrant, the bladder area, the perineum, and to the scrotum in the male. The skin may be cool and clammy, and there is often nausea and vomiting. The colicky nature of the pain, which comes and then subsides, is due to the ball-valve action of the stone. An intravenous pyelogram is usually used as a means of confirming the diagnosis and determining the location of the stone.

Treatment
Treatment of acute renal colic is supportive for the most part. It includes measures to relieve the pain and promote passage of the stone, and prevent urinary tract infection and renal damage. An occasional stone will necessitate surgery for removal. All urine should be strained during an attack of renal colic in the hope of retrieving the stone for chemical analysis. Long-term treatment measures are directed toward preventing further stone formation; the type of stone and the factors that contributed to its formation need to be identified. This information, along with a careful history and laboratory tests, affords the basis of long-term measures.

In summary, obstruction of urine flow can occur at any level of the urinary tract. Developmental defects, normal pregnancy, infection and inflammation, urolithiasis, and neurologic defects are all predisposing factors. Obstructive disorders tend to increase urinary tract infection and calculi, and can cause permanent damage to renal structures.

:Inflammation and Immune Responses

The kidney is subject to inflammation caused by altered immune responses, drugs and other chemicals, toxins, and radiation. Inflammation can cause primary changes in the glomerulus, tubules, or interstitium. This section discusses drug-induced nephritis and glomerular disease.

Drug-Induced Nephritis

Drug-induced nephritis is an idiosyncratic reaction, marked by an acute tubulointerstitial nephritis, with damage to the tubules and to the interstitium. It was initially observed in patients who were sensitive to the sulfonamide drugs, but currently it is more frequently observed to result from use of methicillin and other synthetic antibiotics, as well as furosemide and the thiazides, in persons who are sensitive to these drugs. The condition begins about 15 days after exposure to the drug (the period may vary from 2 to 40 days).[9] At the onset there is fever, eosinophilia, hematuria, mild proteinuria, and in about one-fourth of cases a rash. In about 50% of the cases oliguria and signs of acute renal failure develop. Withdrawal of the drug is usually followed by complete recovery, but there may be permanent damage in some cases, usually those of older persons. Drug nephritis may not be recognized in its very early stage because it is a rare occurrence.

Chronic analgesic nephritis, which is seen in relation to analgesic abuse, causes interstitial nephritis with renal papillary necrosis.[9] When first observed, it was attributed to phenacetin, a then-common ingredient of over-the-counter pain medications containing aspirin, phenacetin, and caffeine. Although phenacetin is no longer contained in these preparations, it has been suggested that other ingredients such as aspirin and acetaminophen may also contribute to the disorder. How much analgesic it takes to produce papillary necrosis is not known; ingestion of 2 to 30 kg of these analgesic compounds over a period of years has been known to result in papillary necrosis.[10] Headache, anemia, gastrointestinal symptoms, and hypertension are associated with the condition.

Diseases of the Glomerulus

Within the glomeruli, the capillary network of the kidneys, blood is filtered and the urine filtrate formed. The glomerular membrane is composed of three layers: (1) the endothelial layer lining the capillary, (2) the basement membrane, and (3) a layer of epithelial cells forming the outer surface of the capillary and lying adjacent to Bowman's capsule. The membrane is selectively permeable, allowing water, electrolytes, and dissolved particles such as glucose and amino acids to enter, and preventing larger particles, such as the plasma proteins and blood cells, from entering the urine filtrate.

Diseases of the glomeruli disrupt glomerular filtration and alter the capillary membrane so that it is permeable to plasma proteins and blood cells. Because the glomerulus lies in a strategic position between the afferent and efferent arterioles that connect with the peritubular capillaries, glomerular disease affords the potential for impairing blood flow to structures supplied by these vessels.

Glomerulonephritis refers to inflammation of the glomerulus. It is now accepted that immune mechanisms are probably responsible for most forms of glomerulonephritis. Acute proliferative glomerulonephritis, rapidly progressive glomerulonephritis, and the nephrotic syndrome are the most frequently seen manifestations of glomerulonephritis.

Acute proliferative glomerulonephritis

The most commonly recognized form of acute proliferative glomerulonephritis is that which follows infections by strains of group A, beta-hemolytic streptococci. In this situation, there is an abnormal immune reaction, causing immune complexes to become entrapped in the glomerular membrane, inciting an inflammatory response. There follows proliferation of the endothelial cells lining the glomerulus and the mesangial cells lying between the endothelium and epithelium of the capillary membrane. The capillary membrane swells and is then permeable to plasma proteins and blood cells. While the disease is seen primarily in children, adults of any age can be affected, too.

This type of glomerulonephritis follows a streptococcal infection by about 10 days to 2 weeks—the time needed for formation of antibodies. As the glomerular membrane swells, oliguria is one of the early symptoms. Salt and water retention gives rise to edema, particularly of the face and hands, and frequently, hypertension. Proteinuria and hematuria (protein and red cells in the urine) follow from the increased capillary permeability. The hematuria imparts a smoky hue to the urine. In fact, in a child, the "cola"-colored urine may be the first sign of the disorder.

Treatment of acute poststreptococcal glomerulonephritis is largely symptomatic. The acute symptoms usually begin to subside in about 10 days to 2 weeks, although in some children the proteinuria may persist for several months. The immediate prognosis is favorable, and approximately 95% recover spontaneously. The outlook is less favorable for adults. About 60% recover completely. In the remainder of cases, the lesions resolve eventually but there may be permanent kidney damage.

Rapidly progressive glomerulonephritis

This type of glomerulonephritis is relatively rare, accounting for less than 2% of cases of glomerulonephritis. Often the disease is preceded by an upper respiratory tract or flu-like syndrome. *Antiglomerular basement membrane antibodies* develop early in the course. There is extensive inflammation and proliferation of the epithelial layer of the glomerular membrane that lines Bowman's capsule. Clinically, there is an insidious onset of signs related to fluid retention and uremia. Ultimately, dialysis or renal transplant is required, because the outlook for recovery is poor.

Goodpasture's syndrome is a form of rapidly progressive glomerulonephritis in which antiglomerular membrane antibodies bind to both lung and kidney tissue, giving rise to pulmonary hemorrhage and glomerulonephritis.

The nephrotic syndrome

The nephrotic syndrome is not a single disease but rather a complex of symptoms. It is manifested by excessive permeability of the glomerular membrane to the plasma proteins (particularly albumin), and in some cases with progressive loss of nephrons.

There is massive proteinuria, with a daily loss of 3.5 gm or more of protein. There is an associated *hypoalbuminemia* (less than 3 gm per 100 ml), *generalized edema*, and *hyperlipidemia*. The edema is due to a decrease in capillary colloidal osmotic pressure which accompanies the loss of plasma proteins. Both cholesterol and triglyceride levels are usually increased, as part of the hyperlipidemia. It is believed that the hyperlipidemia results from compensatory increases in the production of albumin by the liver which serves as a stimulus for increased synthesis of low-density lipoproteins. Because of the elevated levels of cholesterol and triglycerides, persons with the nephrotic syndrome run an increased risk of developing atherosclerosis. The loss of immunoglobulins in the urine is believed to increase susceptibility to infection, especially infection due to the staphylococcus and the pneumococcus.

Nephrosis can occur as a result of primary glomerular disease or secondary to glomerular

A. **Normal**

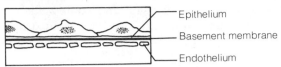

B. **Acute proliferative glomerulonephritis**

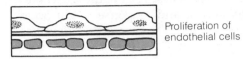

C. **Rapidly proliferating glomerulonephritis**

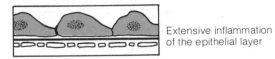

D. **Minimal change disease**

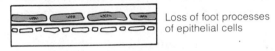

E. **Membranous glomerulonephritis**

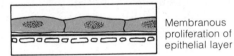

Figure 26–3. Changes in the glomerular membrane that occur with acute proliferative glomerulonephritis, rapidly progressive glomerulonephritis, minimal change nephrosis, and membranous glomerulonephritis.

changes that result from systemic diseases such as diabetes mellitus or lupus erythematosus. Among the primary glomerular diseases that give rise to the nephrotic syndrome are minimal change disease, focal sclerosis, membranous glomerulonephritis, and proliferative membranous glomerulonephritis.

Minimal change disease, or *lipoid nephrosis*, is characterized by diffuse loss of the foot processes in the epithelial layer of the glomerular membrane. Although an immune mechanism has not been identified in this type of glomerulonephritis, there is increasing evidence that one does exist. It is the main form of nephrotic syndrome in children, with a peak incidence in those 2 to 3 years of age. Approximately 75% of children with the nephrotic syndrome have this form. It is highly responsive to glucocorticosteroids, and in 90% of cases is completely reversed by a fairly short course of oral glucocorticosteroid therapy. Nevertheless, some children have further relapses, and some will become "steroid-dependent." The long-term prognosis is, however, generally good, with complete remission in many cases.

Focal sclerosis takes its name from the fact that it affects only portions of the glomerulus. It accounts for about 10% to 15% of cases of nephrosis. There is persistent proteinuria, and response to glucocorticoids is poor. Renal failure ensues within 10 years of diagnosis, in more than 50% of the cases.

Membranous glomerulonephritis is characterized by a progressive thickening of the glomerular wall on the epithelial side. Although it can develop at any age, it is more common after age 40. It is thought that this form of the disease results from an immune complex phenomenon. Approximately 10% of persons with lupus erythematosus also have membranous glomerulonephritis. Various infections such as syphilis, malaria, or hepatitis-B virus, exposure to heavy metals, and certain tumors are associated with the condition. However, in most cases the underlying cause is unknown.

The first indications of the presence of disease are hypoalbuminemia and hyperlipidemia, and the course of the disease varies from case to case. In 70 to 90% of cases the changes are irreversible, progressing finally to renal failure, within 2 to 20 years.

Membranoproliferative glomerulonephritis involves membranous changes of the epithelial layer of the glomerulus and proliferative changes in the mesangium. It accounts for 10% to 15% of cases of idiopathic nephrotic syndrome. The course is relentlessly progressive, with chronic renal failure developing within 10 years, in some 50% of cases.

Diabetic glomerulosclerosis

Diabetic glomerulosclerosis is the most important manifestation of diabetic nephropathy. In the *diffuse* form of diabetic glomeruloscerosis, there is diffuse thickening of the entire basement membrane. In the *nodular* form, also known as Kimmelstiel-Wilson's sydnrome, there is a nodular deposition of hyaline in the mesangial portion of the glomerulus. The clinical picture includes recurrent proteinuria, with slow but steady progression to renal failure.

In summary, in addition to infection, the kidney is subject to a number of inflammatory responses due to chemicals and drugs. These inflammatory responses can involve the glomerulus, tubular structures, and interstitium of the kidney. The various types of glomerulonephritis are believed to result from immune responses.

Neoplasms

Cancer of the kidney accounts for 1% to 2% of all cancers. The average age at diagnosis is 55 to 65 years. The most frequent manifestations are costovertebral pain, a palpable mass, and hematuria. Unfortunately, renal cancer tends to metastasize before giving rise to local signs and symptoms. Treatment usually consists of nephrectomy and, if the cancer is not too far advanced, postoperative irradiation.

Wilms' tumor (nephroblastoma)

Wilms' tumor is one of the most common malignant tumors of children; 70% of cases occur in children under 5 years of age.[10] Epithelial, muscle, and bone tissue are components of the tumor. The common presenting signs are a large abdominal mass and hypertension. Treatment involves surgery, chemotherapy, and radiotherapy (the tumor is radiosensitive). Two-year survival rates have increased to about 90% with this aggressive plan of treatment.

In summary, cancer of the kidney is relatively rare in the adult. However, one type of renal cancer—Wilms' tumor, an undifferentiated type of cancer—accounts for 70% of all cancers of early childhood.

:Study Guide

After you have studied this chapter, you should be able to meet the following objectives:

: : Explain the basis of congenital malformations of the urinary system.

: : Explain what is meant by the term *clean voided specimen*.

: : Explain why urinary tract infections are more common in women than in men.

: : Describe three measures aimed at reducing urinary infections due to the use of urinary catheters.

: : State the symptoms of cystitis.

: : Compare acute pyelonephritis and chronic pyelonephritis.

: : Define *hydronephrosis*.

: : Describe the relationship between the concentration of mineral salts in the body and the development of urinary calculi.

: : List appropriate treatment measures for acute renal colic.

: : Explain the occurrence of drug nephritis.

: : Compare acute proliferative glomerulonephritis and rapidly progressive glomerulonephritis.

: : Describe the general clinical manifestations of the nephrotic syndrome and name three diseases that are representative of the syndrome.

: : Describe the form of diabetic nephropathy known as diabetic glomerulosclerosis.

: : Describe a renal cancer found most frequently in young children.

:References

1. Report of the Coordinating Committee: Research Needs in Nephrology and Urology, Vol 1. National Institute of Health, National Institute of Arthritis, Metabolism, and Digestive Disorders, Public Health Service, 1978. DHEW Publication No. (NIH) 78–1481

2. Holiday MA: Developmental abnormalities of the kidney in children. Hosp Pract 13(6):101, 1978

3. Report of the Coordinating Committee: Research Needs in Nephrology and Urology, Vol 5, p 3. National Institute of Health, National Institute of Arthritis, Metabolism, and Digestive Disorders, Public Health Service. DHEW Publication No. (NIH) 78–1485

4. Chester AC, Harris JP, Schreiner GE: Polycystic kidney disease. American Family Practitioner 16(6):95, 1977

5. Kunin C: Detection, Prevention and Management of Urinary Tract Infections, ed 3, pp 41, 99, 157. Philadelphia, Lea & Febiger, 1979

6. Hodson J, Kincaid–Smith P: Reflux Nephrology, p 3. New York, Masson Publishing, 1979

7. Center for Disease Control: Epidemics of nosocomial urinary tract infections caused by multiple resistant gram-negative bacilli: Epidemiology and control. J Infect Dis 133(3):363–366, 1976

8. Jones SR, Smith JW, Sanford JP: Localization of urinary tract infections by detection of antibody-coated bacteria in urine sediment. N Engl J Med 290(11):591, 1974

9. Robbins SL, Cotran RS: Pathologic Basis of Disease, pp 1160, 1161. Philadelphia, WB Saunders, 1979

10. Frank I: Urological and male genital cancers. In Rubin P (ed): Clinical Oncology, ed 5, p 142. American Cancer Society, 1978

:Suggested Readings

Buckley RM, McGucking M, MacGregor RR: Urine bacterial counts after sexual intercourse. New Engl J Med 298(6):321–324, 1978

Charlton CA: The urethral syndrome. Practitioner 223:333–337, 1979

Coe F: Nephrolithiasis: Causes, classification and management. Hosp Prac 16(4):33–45, 1981

Coe FL: Treatment and prevention of renal stones. Consultant 18(10):47–50, 1978

Coltman K: Urinary tract infections: New thoughts on an old subject. Practitioner 223:351, 1979

Cornfeld D: Nephrosis in childhood. Hospital Medicine 14(3):98–111, 1978

Derrick FC, Carter WC: Kidney stone disease. Postgrad Med 66(4):115–125, 1979

Donadio JV: Glomerulonephritis: Approach to diagnosis and treatment. Hospital Medicine 14(4):36–33, 1978

Fairly KF, Whitworth JA: Problems in the treatment of urinary tract infections. Drugs 19:190–194, 1980

Galloway E, Glassman AB, Haley WE: Acute glomerulonephritis. Am J Med Technol 45(8):694–700, 1979

Gleckman RA: Recurrent urinary tract infections. Postgrad Med 65(2):156–159, 1979

Glossock RJ: The nephrotic syndrome. Hosp Pract 14(11):105–129, 1979

Grob PR: Urinary tract infections in general practice. Practitioner 221(8):237–244, 1978

Harding GKM, Marrie TJ, Ronald AR et al: Urinary tract infection localizing in women. JAMA 240(11):1147–1150, 1976

Hirszel P: A new approach to primary glomerulonephritis. Med Times 107(10):77–85, 1979

Juliani L: Acute glomerulonephritis. Nursing '79 9(9):40–45, 1979

Kaplan RA: Renal calculi. Hospital Medicine 14(8):52–67, 1978

Kleeman CR et al: Kidney stones. West J Med 132(4):313–332, 1980

Kunin C, Polyak F, Postel E: Periurethral bacterial flora in women. JAMA 243(2):134–139, 1980

Kurtz S: UTI in the elderly: Seeking solutions for special problems. Geriatrics 10:97–102, 1980

Lach PA, Elster AB, Roghmann KJ: Sexual behavior and urinary tract infection. Nurse Pract 5:27–32, 1980

Loening SA, Smiley JW, Smith CL: Kidney stones—suspicion to therapy. Patient Care 14:26+, 1980

Mayer T: UTI in the elderly: How to select the treatment. Geriatrics 3:67–77, 1980

Mowad JL: Pyuria: Guide to management. Hospital Medicine 15(12):34–37, 1979

Nagar D, Wathen RL: Nephrotic syndrome. Primary Care 6(3):541–560, 1979

Nemoy NJ: Axioms on renal calculi. Hospital Medicine 15(2):8–19, 1979

Pagana KD: The intrigue and challenge of Goodpasture's syndrome. Heart Lung 9(4):699–706, 1980

Rector FC, Cogan MJ: The renal acidosis. Hosp Pract 15(4):99–111, 1980

Robinson RL: Laboratory findings in the differential diagnosis of acute renal failure. Critical Care Quarterly 32(4):87–98, 1979

Sabbath LD: Urinary tract infections in the female. Obstet Gynecol 55(5):162s–165s, 1980

Shapiro SR, Santamarina A, Harrison JH: Catheter-associated urinary tract infections: Incidence and a new approach to prevention. J Urol 112(11):659–663, 1974

Turek M: Urinary tract infections. Hosp Pract 15(1):49–58, 1980

Vogel CH: Postobstructive diuresis. Nursing '79 9(3):50–56, 1979

Walther PC, Lamm D, Kaplan GW: Pediatric urolithiases: A ten-year review. Pediatrics 65(6):1068–1072, 1980

Wilson DR: Renal function during and following obstruction. Annu Rev Med 28:329–339, 1977

27

Renal Failure

Renal failure describes the situation in which the kidneys fail to remove the metabolic end-products from the blood and to regulate the electrolyte and pH balance of the extracellular fluids. The underlying cause may be renal pathology, systemic disease, or urological defects of nonrenal origin. Chronic renal failure is the end result of irreparable damage to the kidney. It is slowly developing, usually over a number of years. By contrast, acute renal failure is abrupt in onset and is often reversible if recognized early and treated appropriately.

Azotemia

The term azotemia means an abnormally high level of nitrogenous wastes (blood urea nitrogen, uric acid, and serum creatinine) in the blood. Its presence reflects renal inability to filter these waste products from the blood, and it is found in both acute and chronic renal failure. It may be symptomless.

Urea

Urea is an end-product of protein metabolism. The normal adult produces 25 gm to 30 gm per day,[1] but the quantity rises when a high-protein diet is consumed, when there is excessive tissue breakdown, or in the presence of gastrointestinal bleeding. In the presence of gastrointestinal bleeding, the blood protein is broken down in the intestine and the urea is absorbed into the blood. The kidneys, in their role of regulators of blood urea nitrogen (BUN) levels, filter the urea in the glomeruli and then reabsorb it in the tubules. This allows for maintenance of a normal BUN, which is in the range of 8 mg to 25 mg per 100 ml of blood. Blood urea nitrogen becomes concentrated during periods of dehydration and its excretion is markedly decreased when the glomerular filtration rate drops. The renal tubules are permeable to urea, which means that the longer the tubular fluid remains in the kidney, the greater the reabsorption of urea into the blood. Hence, only small amounts of urea are reabsorbed into the blood when the glomerular filtration rate is high; whereas, relatively large amounts of urea are returned to the blood when the glomerular filtration rate is reduced.

Creatinine

Creatinine is a product of *creatine* metabolism in muscles and, therefore, its formation and release is relatively constant and is proportional to the amount of muscle mass that is present. Since creatinine is filtered in the glomeruli but not reabsorbed in the tubules, its blood values depend closely on the glomerular filtration rate. In addition to its use in calculating the glomerular filtration rate (Chap. 25), the creatinine level is useful in estimating the functional capacity of the kidney (Fig. 27-1). The creatinine value for a woman with a small frame is approximately 0.5 mg per 100 ml of blood; for a normal adult man, about 1.0 mg per 100 ml of blood, and for a muscular man about 1.4 mg per 100 ml of blood. A normal serum creatinine usually is indicative of normal renal function. If the value doubles, the glomerular filtration rate—and renal function—probably have fallen to half their normal state. A rise in blood creatinine level to three times the normal value suggests that there is a 75% loss of renal function, and with creatinine values of 10 mg per 100 ml or more, it can be assumed that about 90% of renal function has been lost.

Figure 27-1. Relationship between percentage of renal function and serum creatinine levels. (Drawn from data in Mitch WE, Walser M: A simple method of estimating progression of chronic renal failure. Lancet 1326: December 18, 1976)

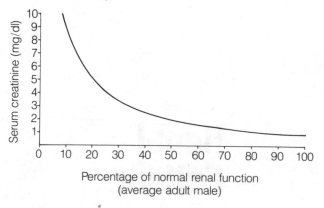

:Acute Renal Failure

Acute renal failure refers to an acute suppression of renal function. The true incidence of acute renal failure is unknown, but it is thought to affect at least 10,000 persons annually in the United States.[2] The mortality is, unfortunately, about 60%. This is probably because older persons and those with severe illness and trauma are being kept alive by respirators and other extraordinary means until renal failure supervenes.

Causes of acute renal failure

Conditions responsible for acute renal failure are usually described as being prerenal, intrarenal, and postrenal (Table 27-1). This classification aids in identifying and treating the cause of the disorder.

Table 27-1   Causes of Acute Renal Failure

Prerenal

Hypovolemia
  Loss of gastrointestinal tract fluid
  Hemorrhage
  Fluid sequestration (e.g., burns)

Septicemia
  Septic shock

Heart failure

Interruption of renal blood flow due to surgery,
  and other causes

Intrarenal

Prolonged renal ischemia

Exposure to nephrotoxic agents
  Aminoglycosides (e.g., gentamicin, kanamycin, colistin)
  Heavy metals (e.g., lead, mercury)
  Organic solvents (e.g., carbon tetrachloride,
    ethylene glycol)
  Radiopaque contrast media
  Sulfonamides

Acute glomerulonephritis

Intratubular obstruction
  Uric acid crystals
  Hemolytic reactions (e.g., blood transfusion reactions)
  Precipitated proteins resulting from multiple myelomas
  Rhabdomyolysis

Acute inflammatory conditions
  Acute pyelonephritis
  Necrotizing papillitis

Postrenal

Ureteral obstruction (e.g., calculi, tumors)

Bladder outlet obstruction (e.g., prostatic hypertrophy,
  urethral structures)

Prerenal conditions. Prerenal causes of acute renal failure consist of those conditions that impair renal blood flow. This is the most common form of acute renal failure and is considered to be reversible if the basis of renal hypofunction can be identified and corrected within 24 hours.

The kidneys normally filter about 20% to 25% of the cardiac output. With a loss of blood volume or cardiac failure, this large blood flow to the kidneys may be sharply reduced. When the afferent arterial pressure falls much below 60 to 70 mm Hg, glomerular filtration ceases and little or no urine is formed. Thus, one of the early manifestations of prerenal failure is a sharp decrease in urine output. Normally, the ratio of serum BUN to creatinine is about 20 to 1, but in acute renal failure, there is a disproportionate elevation in BUN compared with serum creatinine. This is because the low glomerular filtration rate allows more time for smaller particles, such as urea, to filter back into the blood. Creatinine, being larger

and nondiffusible, remains in the tubular fluid and the total amount of creatinine that is filtered, even though small, is excreted in the urine.

Intrarenal conditions. Intrarenal causes of acute renal failure can be grouped into five categories: ischemia, injury to the glomerular membrane (acute glomerulonephritis), acute tubular necrosis, intratubular obstruction, and acute pyelonephritis and necrotizing papillitis. Acute glomerulonephritis is discussed in Chapter 26 as is pyelonephritis.

Intratubular obstructions are due to the accumulation of casts and cellular debris, secondary to severe *hemolytic reactions* or *myoglobinuria*. Skeletal and cardiac muscle contains myoglobin, which accounts for their rubiginous color. Myoglobin corresponds to hemoglobin in function, serving as an oxygen reservoir within the muscle fibers. Myoglobin is not normally found in the serum or urine. It has a low molecular weight of 17,000; should it escape into the circulation, it is rapidly filtered in the glomerulus. Myoglobinuria is most commonly due to muscle trauma, but may result from extreme exertion, hyperthermia, sepsis, prolonged seizures, potassium or phosphate depletion, and alcoholism or drug abuse. Hemoglobin may also escape into the glomerular filtrate when serum levels are markedly increased due to a severe hemolytic reaction. Both myoglobin and hemoglobin cause discoloration of the urine, ranging from the color of tea to red, brown, or black.

Acute tubular necrosis is characterized by destructive changes in the tubular epithelium, due to *ischemia* or *exposure to nephrotoxic agents*. Shock and heart failure, to name two such events, cause prerenal failure, tend to cause renal ischemia, and if allowed to progress, can produce tubular necrosis. As a rule, the blood supply to a normal kidney can be interrupted for about 30 minutes without inflicting damage to the kidney,[3] but in acute trauma, sepsis, and heart failure, for example, the interruption in blood flow is often both more severe and of longer duration.

Several drugs and other chemicals, including organic solvents and heavy metals such as lead and mercury, can injure the renal tubular structures. The aminoglycosides, a group of antibiotics of which gentamicin, kanamycin, and colistin are examples, are all capable of impairing renal function. Several factors contribute to aminoglycoside toxicity, including a decrease in the glomerular filtration rate, which often occurs in the elderly, a preexisting renal disease, hypovolemia, and concurrent administration of other drugs which have a nephrotoxic effect.

Contrast media used during cardiac catheterization and intravenous cholangiography, for example, may also be nephrotoxic. The risk of renal damage due to radiopaque contrast media is greatest in elderly persons, in persons with diabetes mellitus, and in persons who for one reason or another are susceptible to kidney disease.

Postrenal conditions.   Obstruction of the urinary system at any point from the renal calyces to the urinary meatus is the cause of postrenal failure. Prostatic hypertrophy is the most frequent underlying problem. It can also be caused by ureteral obstruction in persons who have only one functioning kidney. Obstructive uropathy is responsible for about 10% of cases of acute renal failure.[4]

Clinical manifestations

The manifestations of acute renal failure are frequently superimposed on the signs and symptoms exhibited by the condition that caused the kidney failure—heart failure, shock, prostatic hypertrophy, and others. Since acute renal failure is potentially reversible, it is important that early signs be recognized so that appropriate treatment measures can be instituted promptly.

Acute renal failure causes marked impairment in elimination of nitrogenous wastes, water, and electrolytes. Its course is frequently divided into two phases: the oliguric and the diuretic phase.

Oliguric phase.   During the oliguric phase, urine output is greatly reduced. The magnitude of the azotemia that develops depends largely on urine output and on the degree of protein breakdown that is taking place. Although oliguria is usually associated with acute renal failure, there are situations in which urine output will be nearly normal, as when intrarenal dysfunction impairs the ability of the renal tubular structures to concentrate the urine. In severe oliguria, in which there is increased tissue breakdown, the BUN, creatinine, potassium, and phosphate levels in the serum increase rapidly, and metabolic acidosis develops. Fluid retention gives rise to edema, water intoxication, and pulmonary congestion. If the period of oliguria is prolonged, hypertension frequently develops and with it, signs of uremia. When untreated, the neurological manifestations of uremia progress from neuromuscular irritability to convulsions, somnolence, and finally, coma and death. Hyperkalemia is usually asymptomatic until serum levels of potassium rise above 6.0 to 6.5 mEq per liter, at which point characteristic electrocardiographic changes and signs of muscle weakness are seen. Gastrointestinal bleeding and infection are serious complications of acute renal failure.

Diuretic phase.   The diuretic phase of acute renal failure usually begins within a few days to 6 weeks of the oliguria, indicating that the nephrons have recovered to the point where urine excretion is possible. Diuresis usually occurs before renal function has returned to normal. Consequently, BUN, serum creatinine, potassium, and phosphate may remain elevated or continue to rise even though urine output is increased. In some cases, the diuresis may be due to impaired nephron function and may cause excessive loss of water and electrolytes.

Treatment

A major concern in treatment of acute renal failure is identifying and correcting the cause, by improving renal perfusion or discontinuing nephrotoxic drugs. Fluids are carefully regulated in an effort to maintain normal fluid volume and electrolyte concentrations. Adequate caloric intake is needed to prevent breakdown of body proteins which increase nitrogenous wastes. Parenteral hyperalimentation may be used for this purpose. Since infection is a major cause of death in persons with acute renal failure, constant vigilance is needed to prevent infection. Dialysis may be indicated when nitrogenous wastes and water and electrolyte balance cannot be kept under control by other means.

In summary, acute renal failure describes an acute reversible suppression of kidney function. It is generally classified as being prerenal, intrarenal, or postrenal in origin. Typically, it progresses through an oliguric phase during which urine output is markedly diminished and fluid and end-products of metabolism accumulate. During the second phase, that of diuresis, urine output increases as renal function begins to return. Usually, correction of the azotemia follows diuresis.

:Chronic Renal Failure

Chronic renal failure differs from acute renal failure in that it represents progressive and irreversible destruction of kidney structures. In end-stage renal disease, the kidneys are often shrunken and evidence of the underlying disease process has been obscured by the scar tissue and destructive changes that have occurred. Chronic renal failure can result from various conditions, including all of the renal diseases discussed in Chapter 26. Regardless of the cause, the consequences of nephron destruction culminate in progressive deterioration of the filtration, reabsorptive, and endocrine functions of the kidney. The rate of destruction differs from case to case, and may range from several months to many years. In its final stages, chronic renal failure involves virtually every body organ and structure.

Uremia, which literally means urine in the blood, is the term used to describe the clinical manifestations of end-stage renal failure. It is different from azotemia, which refers to the accumulation of nitrogenous wastes in the blood but which can occur without symptoms.

The person with uremia looks sick. The body is emaciated and there is extreme muscle wasting. A smell of urine clings to the body. The skin is a sallow-brown color. It is dry and, because of the uncontrolled itching, there are bruises and scratch marks everywhere. In the end, crystals of urea and other metabolic wastes, which are present even in the perspiration—the uremic frost—begin to precipitate on the skin. The respirations are deep and sighing and there is evidence of mild dyspnea. Anorexia, nausea, and vomiting are present and there is no desire for food. The tongue and mucous membranes are dry and cracked. Belching and hiccoughs are common. Often there is the fetid smell of digested blood on the breath—the result of gastrointestinal tract ulceration and bleeding. While initially there was a burning sensation on the feet, this has been replaced by numbness, paresthesias, muscle cramps, and twitching. Muscle weakness is often overwhelming and there is lethargy and difficulty in concentrating. Soon coma will develop and then death will ensue.

As recently as 20 years ago, most patients in chronic renal failure progressed to the uremic stage, then died. But today, through dialysis and renal transplantation, patients in end-stage renal failure not only survive, but may lead productive lives. In many such cases, the patients die not of uremia, but of complications, such as cardiovascular disease.

Signs of renal failure do not begin to appear until there has been extensive loss of function in both kidneys. This must be true, since many persons survive an entire lifetime with only one kidney, many of them unaware of this fact. Or a person in end-stage renal disease may receive a healthy kidney from a close relative, such as a parent or sibling, leaving the donor with only one kidney.

The kidney has tremendous adaptive capabilities. As nephrons are destroyed, the remaining nephrons undergo adaptive changes by which they compensate for the lost nephrons. In the pro-

cess, each of the remaining nephrons filters more solute from the blood. Since these solute particles are osmotically active, they cause additional water to be lost in the urine. Along with this, the kidneys lose their ability to concentrate the urine. One of the earliest signs of renal failure is *isosthenuria*—polyuria with excretion of urine that is almost isotonic with plasma. Since the few remaining nephrons constitute the functional reserve of the kidney, when the function of these remaining nephrons is disrupted, renal failure progresses rapidly.

All forms of renal failure are characterized by a marked reduction in the glomerular filtration rate. There are four stages in the progression of renal failure: renal impairment, renal insufficiency, renal failure, and uremia.[5] *Renal impairment* occurs when the glomerular filtration rate falls to 40% to 50% of normal. *Renal insufficiency* represents a reduction in the glomerular filtrate to a level of 20% to 40% of normal. During this stage, there is azotemia and mild anemia. *Renal failure* develops when the glomerular filtration rate drops to about 10% of normal. *Uremia* is the final stage and is characterized by symptomatology of renal failure.

Manifestations of chronic renal failure

The signs and symptoms of renal failure can be divided as follows: (1) derangements in the chemical, electrolyte, and fluid balance that result directly from impaired nephron function and (2) the associated alterations in function in other parts of the body. These changes are summarized in Table 27-2.

Alterations in body fluids. One of the earliest signs of impaired renal function is the inability of the kidneys to regulate the concentration of the urine. In renal failure, the specific gravity of the urine becomes fixed (1.008 to 1.012) and varies little from specimen to specimen. Polyuria and nocturia are common. The first morning specimen is usually best for assessing the kidneys' ability to concentrate the urine, since this usually represents a period of time when fluid intake is minimal.

Renal ability to *regulate sodium excretion* is lost as renal function declines. Normally, the kidneys tolerate large variations in sodium intake (from 1 mEq to 900 mEq) while maintaining normal serum levels of sodium.[6] As renal function begins to fail, the kidneys lose the ability to excrete large amounts of sodium and to conserve small amounts. Consequently, ingestion of excess sodium tends to cause hypertension and edema. Likewise, volume depletion and further decreases in the glomerular filtration rate occur when sodium intake is restricted or excess

Table 27-2 Alterations in Body Function That Occur with Chronic Renal Failure

Body System	Altered Function	Manifestation
Body Fluids	Compensatory changes in tubular function	Fixed specific gravity of urine; polyuria and nocturia
	Decreased ability to synthesize ammonia and conserve bicarbonate	Metabolic acidosis
	Inability to excrete potassium	Hyperkalemia
	Inability to regulate sodium excretion	Salt wasting or sodium retention
	Impaired ability of the kidney to excrete phosphate	Hyperphosphatemia
	Hyperphosphatemia and inability of the kidney to activate vitamin D	Hypocalcemia and increased levels of parathyroid hormone
Hematopoietic	Impaired synthesis of erythropoietin and effects of uremia	Anemia
	Impaired platelet function	Bleeding tendencies
Cardiovascular	Activation of renin–angiotensin mechanism, increased vascular volume, and failure to produce vasodepressor substances	Hypertension
	Fluid retention and hypoalbuminemia	Edema
	Excess extracellular fluid volume, anemia	Congestive heart failure; pulmonary edema
	Elevated BUN	Uremic pericarditis
Gastrointestinal	Liberation of ammonia	Anorexia, nausea, vomiting
	Decreased platelet function and increased gastric acid secretion due to hyperparathyroidism	Gastrointestinal bleeding
Neurological	Fluid and electrolyte imbalance	Headache
	Increase in metabolic acids and other small, diffusible particles, such as urea	Signs of uremic encephalopathy: lethargy, decreased alertness, loss of recent memory, delirium, coma, seizures, asterixis, muscle twitching, and tremulousness
		Signs of neuropathy: restless-leg syndrome, paresthesias, muscle weakness, and paralysis
Osteodystrophy	Hyperphosphatemia	Osteomalacia
	Hypocalcemia	Osteoporosis
	Hyperparathyroidism	Bone pain and tenderness
		Spontaneous fractures
	Calcium × phosphate product greater than 60	Metastatic calcifications
Skin	Salt wasting	Dry skin and mucous membranes
	Anemia	Pale, sallow complexion
	Hyperthyroidism	Pruritus
	Decreased platelet function and bleeding tendencies	Ecchymosis and subcutaneous bruises
	High concentration of metabolic end-products in body fluids	Uremic frost
		Odor of urine on skin and breath
Genitourinary	Impaired general health	
	Decreased testosterone	Impotence and loss of libido
	Decreased estrogen	Amenorrhea and loss of libido

sodium is lost from the body due to diarrhea or vomiting.

Regulation of serum *phosphate levels* requires a daily urinary excretion of an amount equal to that ingested in the diet. With deteriorating renal function excretion of phosphate falls, and the phosphate level rises. Because of this, the serum calcium level must fall in order for the body to maintain the normal calcium × phosphate product (discussed in Chapter 22). This fall in serum calcium due to the hyperphosphatemia in turn acts as a stimulus for parathyroid release; there is then reabsorption of calcium from the bones. The unrelieved hypocalcemia results in hyperplasia of the parathyroids.

The kidneys control *vitamin D activity* by converting the inactive form of vitamin D (25-hydroxycholecalciferol) to its active form (1,25-dihydroxycholecalciferol). In renal failure, however, the hypocalcemia is aggravated by the lack of vitamin D.

Phosphate-binding antacids are frequently administered to treat the hypocalcemia and hyperphosphatemia. They act by increasing fecal losses of phosphate and thereby reducing its absorption from the gastrointestinal tract. At the same time, milk and foods high in phosphate content are eliminated from the diet. In renal failure there is a rise in the plasma magnesium level. Since many antacids contain magnesium, these should not be given to treat the hyperphosphatemia. Once the phosphate level has been reduced, the active form of vitamin D (calcitriol) may be given for the hypocalcemia—there is a danger that tissue precipitation will occur if vitamin D is given before the phosphate level has been brought down.

About 90% of *potassium excretion* is through the kidneys. In renal failure, there is an increase in potassium excretion by each nephron as the kidney adapts to a decrease in the glomerular filtration rate. As a result, hyperkalemia usually does not develop until kidney function is severely compromised. Because of this adaptive mechanism, it is not usually necessary to restrict potassium intake in chronic renal failure until urinary output is less than 1000 ml per day and the glomerular filtration rate has dropped below 10 ml per minute.[6]

The kidney is largely responsible for eliminating metabolic acids, which it does by secreting hydrogen ions, conserving bicarbonate, and producing ammonia, which acts as a buffer for hydrogen ions that are excreted in the urine. With a decline in renal function, these mechanisms become impaired, with *metabolic acidosis* as an almost inevitable complication. In long-term renal failure, the acidosis seems to stabilize as the disease progresses, probably as the result of the tremendous buffering capacity of bone. This buffering action is thought to increase bone reabsorption and to contribute to the skeletal defects that are present in chronic renal failure. If hypertension and edema are not a problem, the accompanying metabolic acidosis may be treated by administering appropriate doses of sodium bicarbonate.

Azotemia is an early sign of renal failure, usually seen before other symptoms become evident. Although urea is one of the first of the nitrogenous wastes to become elevated, it is unclear how urea alone causes symptoms. Gout is uncommon in renal failure, even though uric acid levels are increased. Much of the excess urate is excreted in the stool. Creatinine is not known to be toxic; its presence in the blood serves mainly as a useful indirect method for assessing the glomerular filtration rate and the extent of renal damage that has occurred.

Anemia. The kidney is the primary site of erythropoietin production. In renal failure, erythropoietin production is often insufficient to stimulate adequate red cell production by the bone marrow. Moreover, the accumulation of toxins further suppresses bone marrow red cell production, and the cells that are produced have a shortened life span. Both of these situations contribute to the anemia of chronic renal failure. This anemia, being based on lack of erythropoietin, is not relieved by dialysis. Androgenic steroids and iron supplements may be prescribed to treat this type of anemia.

Bleeding tendencies. It has been estimated that 17% to 20% of persons in chronic renal failure have a bleeding tendency.[3] Although platelet production is normal in number, their function is impaired, and this is the basis of the bleeding problem. Epistaxis, gastrointestinal bleeding, and bruising of the skin and subcutaneous tissues are seen.

Cardiovascular problems. As was stated earlier, renal failure gives rise to cardiovascular disorders, including hypertension, edema, congestive heart failure, and pericarditis.

Hypertension is a very frequent early manifestation of renal failure. This type of hypertension is believed to result from increased renin production (the renin–angiotensin mechanism) by the kidneys coupled with excess extracellular fluid volume. It is generally believed that the kidneys produce vasodepressor substances and that these may be reduced in renal disease. Even in advanced renal failure, enough functioning renal tissue remains to produce renin in quantity.[7] This hypertension is treated like other types of hypertension; generally, a diuretic along with one or more other medications is administered. In the later stages of renal failure, dialysis may be needed to maintain the extracellular fluid volume.

In chronic renal failure, the increased extracellular fluid volume consequent to sodium and water retention gives rise to edema; the associated proteinuria and hypoalbuminemia also contribute to the development of edema. The increase in extracellular fluid also contributes to congestive heart failure and pulmonary edema that occur in the late stages of uremia.

Pericarditis is seen in as many as 50% of persons with chronic renal failure,[8] due to exposure of the pericardium to metabolic end-products. A different form of pericarditis occurs in patients on dialysis, and this form, though not clearly defined as yet, is believed to be due to the effects of stress, heparinization, or infection.

Gastrointestinal disturbances.
Anorexia, nausea, and vomiting are common in uremia, and there is often a salty or metallic taste in the mouth that further depresses the patient's appetite. Ulceration and bleeding of the gastrointestinal mucosa may develop, and hiccoughs are common. The cause of the nausea and vomiting is unclear. It has been suggested that decomposition of urea by the intestinal flora may liberate ammonia, which irritates the lining of the gastrointestinal tract. Parathyroid hormone increases gastric acid secretion, and it has been proposed that this increase along with the bleeding tendency due to platelet dysfunction is a contributory factor.

Neurological disorders.
Neurological disorders, which are common in uremia, may be categorized as uremic encephalopathy and peripheral neuropathies.

The central nervous system disturbances in uremia are similar to those caused by other metabolic and toxic disorders, such as portal-systemic encephalopathy, hypoxia, and water intoxication. These manifestations are more closely related to the progress of the uremic disorder than to the level of the metabolic end-products.[9] For example, profound encephalopathy is frequent in *acute* renal failure and less frequent in *chronic* renal failure despite the more marked blood chemistry abnormalities seen in the latter. A reduction in alertness and awareness is probably the earliest and most significant indication of uremic encephalopathy. This is often followed by an inability to fix the attention, loss of recent memory, and perceptual errors in identifying persons and objects. Delirium and coma come late in the

course, and finally convulsions are the preterminal event.

Disorders of motor function are frequent accompaniments of the neurological manifestations of uremic encephalopathy. During the early stages, there is often *difficulty in performing fine movements of the extremities*; the gait becomes unsteady and clumsy. *Asterixis*—flapping movements of the hands and feet—often occurs as the disease progresses. It can be elicited by having the patient hold his arms hyperextended at the elbow and wrist, with the fingers spread apart. If asterixis is present, this position causes side-to-side flapping movements of the fingers. *Tremulousness* on movement of the extremities precedes asterixis.

Uremic encephalopathy is believed to result, at least in part, from an excess of toxic organic acids which overwhelm the normal mechanisms that prevent their entrance into the brain. The rapid reversal of the effects of uremic encephalopathy with dialysis suggests that this is the case.[9]

Neuropathy, or involvement of the peripheral nerves, is common. It affects the lower limbs more frequently than the upper, is usually symmetrical, and affects both sensory and motor function. The *restless-legs syndrome* is one of the manifestations of peripheral nerve involvement; it consists of deep creeping, crawling, prickling, and itching sensations. These sensations are usually more intense at night, and moving the legs brings relief. A burning sensation of the feet, which may be followed by muscle weakness and atrophy, is a manifestation of uremia. The uremic neuropathies usually improve with dialysis or renal transplantation.

Osteodystrophy.
Renal osteodystrophy is a condition resulting from chronic renal failure. It is characterized by derangements of serum calcium and serum phosphorus. The condition has sometimes been called *renal rickets*, because in children its manifestations resemble those of a vitamin D deficiency. The primary changes in renal osteodystrophy are *osteomalacia* and *osteoporosis*, in which there is a decrease in the calcium and phosphate content of the bone and loss of the supporting structural matrix. Increased parathyroid function causes excessive reabsorption of bone along the long bones, distal ends of the clavicle, and small bones which can be seen on x-ray films. In advanced osteodystrophy, cysts may develop in the bone, a condition called *osteitis fibrosa cystica*. The symptoms of renal osteodystrophy include pain, tenderness, and sometimes spontaneous fractures.

Soft-tissue calcification, or *metastatic calcifica-*

tion, of the cornea, arteries, subcutaneous tissues, and muscle can occur when the phosphate × calcium product rises higher than 60. This is seen after dialysis has been instituted, and is usually associated with a rapid rise in the serum calcium level which precedes a fall in the phosphate level. Calcium deposits in the eye may cause conjunctivitis and are often evidenced by what is called "band" keratopathy. Calcium deposits in the skin cause intense itching.

Skin disorders.   The skin is pale, because of the anemia, and may have a sallow, yellow-brown hue. Subcutaneous bruising is common. The skin and mucous membranes are dry because of the salt wasting. An odor of urine exudes from the body. Pruritus is common, apparently due to the hyperparathyroidism, since it is usually relieved following parathyroidectomy. In the advanced stages of uremia, urea crystals may precipitate on the skin— the result of the high urea concentration that is present in the body fluids. There are changes in the fingernails, evidenced by a dark band just behind the leading edge of the nail, followed by a white band. This is known as Terry's nails.

Genitourinary changes.   There is a reduction in testosterone and estrogen. A decrease in testicular size, male impotence, and amenorrhea are frequent findings. Relatedly, loss of libido may be a very early indication of renal failure.

Effect of renal failure on elimination of drugs

Persons with renal failure are known to have increased incidences of adverse drug reactions. Decreased elimination by the kidney allows drugs or their metabolites to accumulate in the body and requires that drug dosages be adjusted accordingly. This also means that patients with renal failure should be cautioned against the use of over-the-counter remedies.

In considering the effect of various drugs and medications on persons with renal disease, several factors about the drugs need to be taken into account: their absorption, distribution, metabolism, and excretion. The administration of large quantities of phosphate-binding antacids to control hyperphosphatemia and hypocalcemia in persons with advanced renal failure tends to interfere with the absorption of some drugs. Many drugs are bound to plasma proteins, such as albumin, for transport in the body, and the unbound portion of the drug is available to act at the various receptor sites and is free to be metabolized. Many persons have a de-

crease in plasma proteins which are used for binding and transport of drugs. In the process of metabolism, some drugs form intermediate metabolites that are toxic if not eliminated. This is true of meperidine, which is metabolized to the toxic intermediate normeperidine, which causes excessive sedation, nausea, and vomiting. Some drugs contain unwanted nitrogen, sodium, potassium, and magnesium and must be avoided in persons with renal failure. Penicillin, for example, contains potassium. Nitrofurantoin and ammonium chloride add to the body's nitrogen pool. Many antacids contain magnesium.

Treatment

The treatment of chronic renal failure can be divided into two stages: conservative management of renal insufficiency, and dialysis or renal transplantation. The conservative treatment consists of measures to prevent or retard the deterioration in renal function and to assist the body in compensating for the existing impairment. When conservative measures are no longer effective, dialysis or renal transplantation becomes necessary. The discussion in this chapter is limited to an overview of dietary management of renal failure and dialysis treatment methods. The reader is referred to specialty texts for a more complete discussion of renal failure and its management.

Dietary management.   Regulating the intake of protein, calories, sodium, potassium, and fluids is of primary importance in controlling the adverse effects of renal insufficiency. In fact, it is often possible to delay the need for dialysis or transplantation through wise manipulation of food and fluid intake. The goal of dietary treatment is to provide optimum nutrition, while maintaining tolerable levels of metabolic wastes. The specific diet that is prescribed depends on the type and severity of kidney disease that is present. Because of the severe restrictions that are placed on food and fluid intake, these diets may be complicated to prepare, and unappetizing.

Proteins.   Since proteins are broken down to form nitrogenous wastes, dietary restriction of protein is common. At present there is considerable controversy over the degree of restriction needed and the type of protein to be allowed. Usually, protein need not be restricted until renal insufficiency is relatively far advanced (glomerular filtration rate of 20 ml per minute or less). At this point, some clinicians recommend a protein intake of about 0.5 gm per kg of body weight or about 40 gm per day.[6] Other pioneers in the field of therapeutic diets for renal failure recommend a more stringent protein restriction. Giordano suggests that protein intake should be restricted to 25 gm per day or less.[10] With this more stringent limitation in protein intake, only those proteins that have a high biological value are included. Proteins with a high biological value are believed to promote the reutilization of endogenous nitrogen, decreasing the amount of nitrogenous wastes that are produced and thus ameliorating the symptoms of uremia. In reutilizing nitrogen, the proteins ingested in the diet are broken down into their constituent amino acids, to be utilized in synthesis of protein required by the body. A man weighing about 150 pounds or 70 kg synthesizes at least 150 gm of protein daily, while ingesting only about 60 gm.[10] For this to be accomplished, amino acids must be recycled, and ingestion of proteins that have a high biological value makes it possible. Almost all of the amino acids in a whole egg are utilized in synthesis of essential body proteins, so eggs are said to have a high biological value; in contrast, less than half of the amino acids in cereal proteins are reutilized. Amino acids not reutilized to build body proteins are broken down and form the end-products of protein metabolism, such as urea.

Calories.   A second consideration in the dietary management of renal failure is the provision of adequate calories in the form of carbohydrates and fats to meet energy needs. This is particularly important when the protein content of the diet is severely restricted. If sufficient calories are not available, either the limited protein in the diet goes into energy production, or body tissue itself will be used for energy purposes.

Potassium.   When the glomerular filtration rate falls to extremely low levels, regulation of potassium is seriously compromised and dietary restriction of potassium becomes mandatory. Many patients in renal failure retain the ability to excrete potassium adequately, provided their intake is not excessive. Using salt substitutes that contain potassium or ingesting fruits, fruit juice, chocolate, potatoes, or other high-potassium foods carries the risk of hyperkalemia.

Sodium.   The amount of sodium that is indicated in the diet depends on the kidneys' ability to excrete sodium and water and must be individually determined. For this assessment, the 24-hour urinary excretion of sodium is measured. Some patients will require 1 to 2 gm of sodium to prevent sodium depletion; some will require restriction to 250 mg to prevent edema and extracellular fluid excess. Generally,

renal disease of glomerular origin is more likely to contribute to sodium retention, whereas tubular dysfunction causes salt wasting.

Fluids.   As with sodium, fluid restriction varies with renal ability to excrete water. Fluid intake in excess of that which the kidneys can excrete causes circulatory overload, edema, and water intoxication. Inadequate intake, on the other hand, causes volume depletion and hypotension as well as further decreases in the already compromised glomerular filtration rate. When fluid restriction is a requirement, daily weight check and daily intake and output record will be made to determine the allowable quantity of water. It is common practice to allow a daily intake of 500 to 800 ml, which is equal to insensible (unperceived) water loss, plus a quantity equal to the previous 24-hour urine output.

Dialysis and renal transplantation.   Dialysis and renal transplantation have become accepted methods for treatment of end-stage renal disease, and because they are closely linked advances in both techniques are closely parallel. Theoretically, universal access to both types of treatment has become possible through public funding. In the United States, 32,656 persons were maintained on dialysis in 1977, and another 4450 received kidney transplants at a cost of $902 million dollars. It has been estimated that by 1984 this cost will have risen to three billion dollars.[2]

The choice between dialysis and transplantation is dictated by age, related health problems, donor availability, and personal preference. Regardless of advances in transplantation technology, dialysis will probably continue to play a major role as a treatment method for end-stage renal disease. It is life-sustaining to the patient who is awaiting a suitable kidney transplant; it is needed during the postoperative transplant period, and as a back-up form of treatment if the transplantation is unsuccessful.

Hemodialysis.   A hemodialysis system, or artificial kidney, consists of three parts—a blood compartment, a dialysis fluid compartment, and a cellophane membrane that separates the two compartments. There are several types of dialyzers, all of which incorporate these parts, and all of which function in similar fashion. The cellophane membrane is semipermeable, permitting all molecules, except blood cells and plasma proteins, to move freely in both directions—from the blood into the dialyzing solution and from the dialyzing solution into the blood. The direction of flow is determined by the concentration of the substances contained in the two solutions. Normally, the waste products and the excess electrolytes in the blood diffuse into the dialyzing solution. If there is a need to replace or add substances, such as bicarbonate, to the blood, these can be added to the dialyzing solution. (See Fig. 27-2.)

During dialysis, blood moves from an artery, through the tubing and blood chamber in the dialysis unit, thence back into the body through a vein. An arteriovenous (AV) fistula or an AV cannula provides access to both the arterial and venous systems. Heparin is used to prevent clotting within the dialysis system; it can be administered continuously, intermittently, or regionally. Most patients are dialyzed two to three times a week for 4 to 5 hours. Many persons can be managed on hemodialysis in their homes.

Peritoneal dialysis. Peritoneal dialysis operates on the same principle as hemodialysis, but in this type of dialysis, the thin serous membrane of the peritoneal cavity serves as the dialyzing membrane. A sterile dialyzing solution (usually about 2 liters) is instilled into the peritoneal cavity through a special cannula or catheter over a period of 10 to 20 minutes. The solution is then allowed to remain or "dwell" in the peritoneal cavity for variable lengths of time, at least 30 to 45 minutes, during which the metabolic end-products and extracellular fluid diffuse into the dialysate. At the end of the dwell time, the dialysate is drained by gravity out of the peritoneal cavity into a sterile bag. The procedure is repeated as necessary.

Peritoneal dialysis is effective in both acute and chronic renal failure. Less equipment is needed (unless the equipment is automated) and blood transfusion or anticoagulants are not routinely required. Persons living alone can monitor their dialysis, whereas hemodialysis usually requires that a second person assist. However, peritoneal dialysis does require more time than hemodialysis. It takes about six times as long to exchange the toxins and there is greater danger of infection (peritonitis).

In summary, chronic renal failure represents the end-stage destructive effects of many different forms of kidney disease. Regardless of the cause, the consequences of nephron destruction present in end-stage renal disease cause progressive deterioration in the filtration, reabsorptive, and endocrine functions of the kidney. In its advanced stages, renal failure affects almost every system in the body. It causes azotemia and

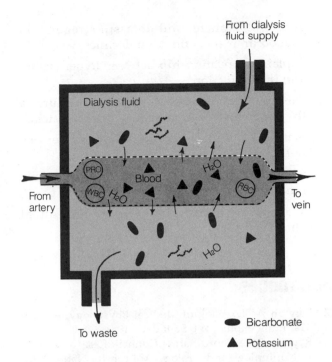

Figure 27–2. Schematic diagram of a hemodialysis system. The blood compartment and dialysis solution compartment are separated by a cellophane membrane. This membrane is porous enough to allow all of the constituents, except the plasma proteins and blood cells, to diffuse between the two compartments.

alterations in sodium and water excretion and in body levels of potassium, phosphate, calcium, and magnesium. It also causes anemia, alterations in cardiovascular function, neurological disturbances, gastrointestinal dysfunction, and discomforting skin changes. Within the past 20 years, dialysis and renal transplantation have allowed persons with what was once a fatal disorder to survive and lead a relatively normal and productive life.

:Study Guide

After you have studied this chapter, you should be able to meet the following objectives:

: : Describe the clinical manifestations of azotemia with reference to urea and creatinine.

: : Classify the following conditions according to whether they are prerenal, intrarenal, or postrenal: acute glomerulonephritis, prostatic hypertrophy, hemorrhage, septicemia, hemolytic reaction.

: : Describe the two phases that are characteristic of the course of acute renal failure.

: : Describe the alterations in serum sodium,

serum phosphate, and potassium regulation that occur as renal function declines.

: : Explain the relationship between hypertension and renal function.

: : Describe the manifestations of renal failure as they apply to four or more major body systems.

: : State the basis of drug sensitivity in persons with renal failure.

: : State the goal in dietary management of chronic renal failure.

: : Compare hemodialysis with peritoneal dialysis.

:References

1. Guyton A: Textbook of Medical Physiology, ed 6, p 424. Philadelphia, WB Saunders, 1981
2. Report of the Coordinating Council: Research Needs in Nephrology and Urology, Vol I, p 16. National Institute of Health, National Institute of Arthritis, Metabolism, and Digestive Diseases, Public Health Service, 1978. DHEW Publication No. (NIH) 78–1481
3. Leaf A, Cotran R: Renal Pathophysiology, pp 167, 204. New York, Oxford University Press, 1980
4. Schrier RW: Acute renal failure: Pathogenesis, diagnosis and management. Hosp Pract 16(3):101, 1981
5. Mitchell JC: Axioms on uremia. Hospital Medicine 14(7):6, 1978
6. Orme BM: Chronic renal failure: Guide to management. Hospital Medicine 14(1):99, 105, 1978
7. Merrill JP, Hampters CL: Uremia. N Engl J Med 282(18):1014, 1970
8. Zeluff GW, Eknoyan G, Jackson D: Pericarditis in renal failure. Heart Lung 8(6):1139, 1979
9. Raskin NH, Fishman RA: Neurological disorders in renal failure. N Engl J Med 294(3):143, 147, 1976
10. Giordano C: The role of diet in renal disease. Hosp Pract 12(11):115–119, 1977

:Suggested Readings

Bergstein JM: Acute renal failure in children. Critical Care Quarterly 1:41–51, 1978
Campbell JD, Campbell AR: The social and economic cost of end-stage renal disease. New Engl J Med 299(8): 386–392, 1978
Chambers JK: Assessing the dialysis patient at home. Am J Nurs 81(4):750–754, 1981
Eknoyan G: Axioms on acute oliguria. Hospital Medicine 13:32–33+, 1977
Finch M: Management of acute renal failure. Nursing Times 74:631–635, 1978

Fisher JW: Mechanism of anemia of chronic renal failure. Nephron 25:106–111, 1980
Lazarus JM: Uremia: A clinical guide. Hospital Medicine 15(1):52–73, 1979
Leste GW: Nondialytic treatment of established acute renal failure. Critical Care Quarterly 1:11–24, 1978
Mitchell JC: Axioms on uremia. Hospital Medicine 14(7): 6–23, 1978
Orr ML: Drugs and renal disease. Am J Nurs 81(5):969–970, 1981
Platzer H: A patient suffering from chronic renal failure. Nursing Times 76:191–195, 1980
Roberts SL: Renal assessment: A nursing point of view. Heart Lung 8(1):105–113, 1979
Robinson RL: Laboratory findings in the differential diagnosis of renal failure. Critical Care Quarterly 1:87–99, 1979
Schrier R: Acute renal failure. Kidney Int 15:205–216, 1979
Schrier RW: Acute renal failure: Pathogenesis, diagnosis and management. Hosp Prac 16(3):93–112, 1981
Shipley SL: Myoglobinuria. Heart Lung 5(6):950–953, 1976
Sorkin MI: Acute renal failure. Med Times 107(10):33–39, 1979
Stark JL: BUN/creatinine: Your keys to kidney function. Nursing '80 10(5):33–38, 1980
Szwed JJ: Pathophysiology of acute renal failure: Rationale for signs and symptoms. Critical Care Quarterly 1:1–9, 1978
Teitelbaum SL et al: Calcifediol in chronic renal failure. JAMA 235(2):164–167, 1976

28

Stephanie MacLaughlin

Structure and Function of the Male Genitourinary System

The male genitourinary system has two basic functions—urine elimination and reproduction. This chapter is concerned primarily with the structure and function of the male reproductive system. This system consists of a pair of gonads, the testes, a system of excretory ducts, and the accessory organs. The accessory organs include the penis, the bulbo-urethral glands, the prostate gland, and the seminal vesicles (Fig. 28-1).

:The Testes and Scrotum

The testes, or male gonads, are two egg-shaped structures that are located outside the abdominal cavity in the scrotum, where they are suspended by the spermatic cord. The spermatic cord is composed of the arteries, veins, lymphatics, and excretory ducts that supply the testes. The cremaster muscle that suspends the testes and forms the muscle of the scrotum is also contained in the spermatic cord. The testes are responsible for both testosterone and sperm production.

The scrotum, which houses the testes, is made up of an outer skin layer which forms rugae or folds and which is continuous with the perineum and outer skin of the thighs. Under the outer skin lies a thin layer of muscle and fascia, the *tunica dartos*. This layer contains a septum that separates the two testes.

A function of the scrotum is to *regulate the temperature of the testes*. The optimum temperature for sperm production is about two to three degrees below body temperature. If the testicular temperature is too low, the muscles within the scrotum contract,

Figure 28–1. Diagram of the structures of the male reproductive system, including the testes, the scrotum and the excretory ducts. (From Chaffee EE, Greisheimer EM: Basic Physiology and Anatomy, 3rd ed. Philadelphia, JB Lippincott, 1974)

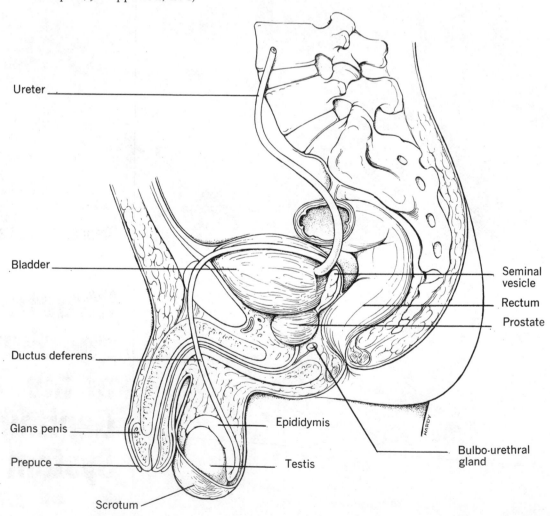

Ureter

Bladder

Ductus deferens

Glans penis

Prepuce

Scrotum

Epididymis

Testis

Seminal vesicle

Rectum

Prostate

Bulbo-urethral gland

causing the testes to be brought up tight against the body. On the other hand, when the testicular temperature rises, the muscles relax, which allows the scrotal sac to fall away from the body. Some tight-fitting undergarments hold the testes against the body and are thought to contribute to infertility by interfering with the thermoregulatory function of the scrotum. Cryptorchidism, the failure of the testes to descend into the scrotum, also exposes the testes to the higher temperature of the body.

The testes and epididymis are enclosed in a double-layered membrane, the *tunica vaginalis,* which is derived embryonically from the abdominal peritoneum. An outer covering, the *tunica albuginea,* is a tough white fibrous sheath that resembles the sclera of the eye. The tunica albuginea protects the testes and gives them their ovoid shape.

Embryologically, the testes do not develop within the scrotal sac; they develop in the abdominal cavity and then descend through the inguinal canal into a long pouch of peritoneum (which becomes the tunica vaginalis) in the scrotum during the seventh to the ninth month of fetal life. The descent of the testes is thought to be due to the male hormone, testosterone, which is very active during this stage of development. Just prior to birth, the inguinal canal closes almost completely. Failure of this canal to close predisposes to the development of an inguinal hernia later in life.

Duct System

Internally, the testes are composed of several hundred compartments or lobules (Fig. 28-2). Each lobule contains one or more coiled *seminiferous* tubules. These tubules are the site of sperm production. As the tubules lead into the *efferent ducts,* the seminiferous tubules become the *rete testes.* Ten to twenty thousand efferent ducts emerge from the rete testes to join the epididymis, which is the final site for sperm maturation. Interspersed in the connective tissue that fills the spaces between the seminiferous tubules are the epithelial cells—the *cells of Leydig*—which produce *testosterone.*

Accessory Organs

Sperm are transported through the reproductive structures by movement of the seminal fluid which is combined with secretions of the accessory sex glands, the epididymis, seminal vesicles, the prostate, and Cowper's glands. When sperm is combined with the seminal plasma it is called *semen.*

The sperm enters the epididymis from the efferent ductules in the testes. Since the sperm are

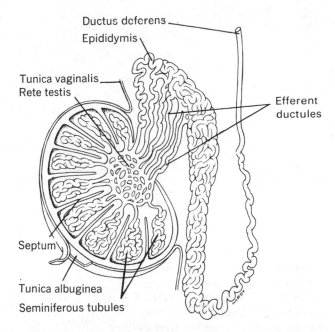

Figure 28–2. Diagram showing the parts of the testes and epididymis. (From Chaffee EE, Lytle IM: Basic Physiology and Anatomy, 4th ed. Philadelphia, JB Lippincott, 1980)

not mobile at this stage of development, peristaltic movements of the ductal walls of the epididymis aid in sperm movement. The sperm continue their migration through the *ductus deferens,* or vas deferens, and enter the *ampullae* where they are stored until they are released through ejaculation (Fig. 28-3). Sperm can be stored in the genital ducts for as long as 42 days and still maintain their fertility. The ampullae join with the *seminal vesicles* which secrete a fluid containing fructose and other substances required to nourish the sperm. The seminal vesicles lead into the *ejaculatory ducts* which enter the posterior part of the prostate, and continue through this gland until they end in the prostatic portion of the urethra. The *prostate* adds a thin, milky, alkaline fluid to the semen. The optimum pH for sperm mobilization is 6.0 to 6.5. The alkaline nature of the prostatic fluid is necessary for successful fertilization of the ovum, since both the fluid from the vas deferens and the vaginal secretions of the female are strongly acid.

The *bulbourethral,* or *Cowper's glands,* lie on either side of the membranous urethra. These glands secrete an alkaline mucus which probably aids in neutralizing acids from urine that remains in the urethra.

A man usually ejaculates about 2 ml to 5 ml of semen. The ejaculate may vary with frequency of intercourse. It is less with frequent ejaculation and

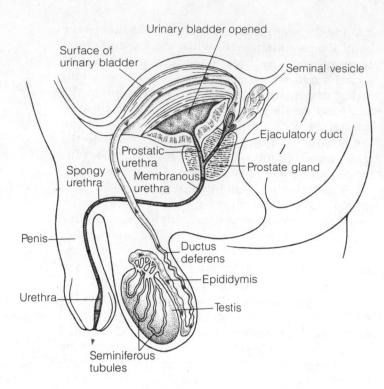

Figure 28–3.   Figure of the excretory ducts of the male reproductive system and the path that the sperm follows as it leaves the testis and travels to the urethra. (From Chaffee EE, Greisheimer EM: Basic Physiology and Anatomy, 3rd ed. Philadelphia, JB Lippincott, 1974)

may increase two to four times its normal amount following periods of abstinence. The semen that is ejaculated is largely fluid—98% fluid and only about 2% sperm.

:The Penis

The penis is the external genital organ through which the urethra passes. Anatomically, the external penis consists of a shaft which ends in a tip called the *glans* (Fig. 28-4). The loose skin of the penis shaft folds to cover the glans, forming the *prepuce* or *foreskin*. It is this cuff of skin that is removed during *circumcision*. In some situations, an adult who has not been circumcised as an infant may need to have the foreskin removed. For instance, the foreskin may become too tight and reduce blood flow or it may not be retractable for cleaning purposes. Usually circumcision is a religious (Moslem and Jewish) or social custom (United States). Most male infants in the United States are circumcised shortly after birth. The value of the procedure is controversial. It has been proposed that uncircumcised males and their sexual partners may have a higher incidence of genital cancer than those that were circumcised. This may, however, have resulted from sexual habits or

Figure 28–4.   Sagittal section of the penis, showing the prepuce, the glans, corpus cavernosum, and corpus spongiosum.

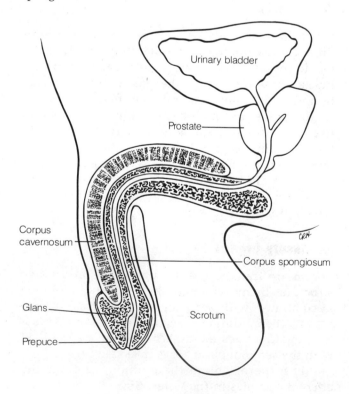

lack of hygiene, rather than lack of circumcision. One practical argument for circumcision is cleanliness. The uncircumcised male must retract his foreskin and remove any accumulation (smegma) produced by the oil glands in the foreskin. If this is not done, the resulting irritation may cause inflammation and infection. Should the inflammation become chronic, it may predispose to cancer of the penis.

The glans of the penis contains many sensory nerves, causing this to be the most sensitive portion of the penile shaft. The cylindrical body or shaft of the penis is composed of three masses of erectile tissue held together by fibrous strands and covered with skin. The two lateral masses of tissue are called the *corpora cavernosa*. The third ventral mass is called the *corpus spongiosum*. The cavernous masses are erectile tissue that distends with blood during penile erection.

In its normal flaccid state, the penis hangs down loosely. The flaccid penis is three to four inches long; the erectile penis, five to seven inches long. The penis may undergo a temporary decrease in size in situations such as cold weather, failed intercourse, or extreme exhaustion. Aging may also cause it to decrease in size. Contrary to popular belief, the size of the penis has no relationship to race, body build, sexual prowess, ability to please a woman, or frequency of intercourse.

:Spermatogenesis

The *mature sperm cell*, or *spermatozoon*, is made up of an oval head, a neck, a midpiece, and a tail (Fig. 28-5). The *head* consists mainly of nuclear material with only a small amount of cytoplasm. The cytoplasm in the head is called the *acrosome* and is believed to contain the enzymes necessary for penetration and fertilization of the ovum. The *neck* connects the head to the midpiece which is composed of a cylindrical fascicle called the axial filament. The *midpiece* is concerned with the metabolic activity, and the tail with propulsion, of the sperm.

Spermatogenesis, as mentioned earlier, occurs in the seminiferous tubules of the testes. These tubules, if placed end-to-end, would measure about 750 feet. The tubules are lined with sperm cells in various stages of development and it is these cells that eventually become the mobile spermatozoa (Fig. 28-6).

The layer of cells that lie adjacent to the tubule wall are the small unspecialized germinal cells called the *spermatogonia*. These cells undergo rapid mitotic

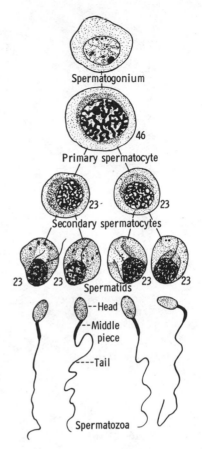

Figure 28–5. Diagram of the various stages of spermatogenesis. (From Chaffee EE, Lytle IM: Basic Physiology and Anatomy, 4th ed. Philadelphia, JB Lippincott, 1980)

division, providing a continuous source of new germinal cells. As the cells multiply the more mature spermatogonia divide into two "daughter cells" which grow in size and become the *primary spermatocytes*. These large primary spermatocytes divide by meiosis to form two smaller *secondary spermatocytes*. Each of the secondary spermatocytes, in turn, divides to form two *spermatids* or infant sperm. These spermatids burrow into the Sertoli cells, which are dispersed throughout the seminiferous tubules, until they reach maturity. As the spermatids grow to full size and increase in maturity, they move into the epididymis for final maturation and storage. Each tubule contains germ cells in various stages of development so that a continuous supply is readily available.

The entire process of spermatogenesis takes about 60 to 70 days. The sperm count in a normal ejaculate is about 100 to 400 million. *Infertility* may occur when there is an insuffient number of motile, healthy sperm.

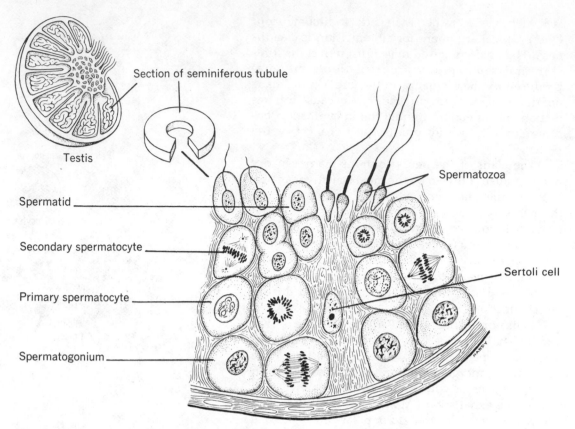

Spermatid

Secondary spermatocyte

Primary spermatocyte

Spermatogonium

Section of seminiferous tubule

Testis

Spermatozoa

Sertoli cell

Figure 28–6. A section of a seminiferous tubule, showing the various stages of spermatogenesis. (From Chaffee EE, Lytle IM: Basic Physiology and Anatomy, 4th ed. Philadelphia, JB Lippincott, 1980)

:Male Sex Hormones

The production of male sex hormones is controlled by the *gonadotropic hormones* which are produced in the anterior pituitary gland. There are two gonadotropic hormones: follicle stimulating hormone (FSH) and the interstitial cell stimulating hormone (ICSH). The ICSH is also known as luteinizing hormone (LH). The FSH acts at the level of the seminiferous tubules and is necessary for sperm production. Testosterone is produced by the interstitial cells of Leydig and is controlled by ICSH.

Androgens are male sex hormones. Testosterone is the main androgen produced in the testes. The functions of the androgens are summarized in Table 28-1. Although FSH stimulates sperm production, testosterone plays a permissive role in spermatogenesis and is needed for sperm maturation. Testosterone and other androgens function as anabolic agents in both males and females to promote protein metabolism and musculoskeletal growth. In the male, testosterone also stimulates the embryonic develop-

ment of the genital structures, the growth and development of the primary and secondary sex characteristics during puberty, and the maintenance of these characteristics during adult life.

The circulating testosterone has the effect of a negative feedback mechanism on ICSH secretion;

Table 28–1 Main Actions of Testosterone

Differentiation of the male genital tract during fetal development

Development of primary and secondary sex characteristics
 Growth and maintenance of gonadal function
 External genitalia and accessory organs
 Male voice timbre
 Male skin characteristics
 Male hair distribution

Anabolic effects
 Protein metabolism
 Musculoskeletal growth
 Subcutaneous fat distribution

Spermatogenesis (in FSH-primed tubules)
 and maturation of sperm

when testosterone levels are high, ICSH secretion is inhibited, and *vice versa*. Although the mechanism is not fully understood, it appears that spermatogenesis inhibits FSH release. It is known that failure of spermatogenesis causes an increase in FSH, whereas active spermatogenesis causes a decrease in FSH levels. If an agent could be found that would inhibit FSH and not ICSH it could be used as a male contraceptive agent. Unlike the cyclic hormonal pattern in the female, in the male FSH, ICSH, and testosterone secretion and spermatogenesis occur at relatively unchanging rates throughout adulthood.

Puberty

At the time of puberty, the male gonads and testes begin to mature and begin to carry out spermatogenesis and hormone production. Sometime around the age of 10 or 11, the adenohypophysis, or anterior pituitary, begins to secrete the gonadotropins that stimulate testicular function and cause the interstitial cells to begin producing testosterone. About the same time, hormonal stimulation induces mitotic activity of the spermatogonia and primary spermatocytes. Once cell maturation has begun, the testes begin to enlarge rapidly as the individual tubules grow. Full maturity and spermatogenesis are usually attained by age 15 or 16.

:Neural Control of the Male Sex Act

Erection and ejaculation are under the control of the autonomic nervous system. Erection can occur at all ages, even in infant boys a few hours after birth and quite elderly men. The capacity for voluntary erection usually develops with the onset of puberty.

Erection is initiated by parasympathetic fibers that originate in the second and fourth segments of the sacral cord and are transmitted by the nervi erigentes. The impulses cause dilatation of the penile arteries and compression of the penile veins. The increased blood supply to the penis and subsequent engorgement of the corpora cavernosa and the corpus spongiosum result in erection.

The process of *ejaculation* is initiated by peristaltic movements along the ductile pathways from the testes, the epididymis, the seminal vesicles, and the prostate gland. Increased pressure causes expulsion of semen. The bulbourethral glands secrete additional fluid. *Emission* of semen is brought about by sympathetic impulses that leave the spinal cord at

lumbar segments 1 and 2 and pass through the hypogastric plexus to the genitalia. Ejaculation is then caused by contraction of the muscles at the base of the penis, which are innervated by fibers of the pudendal nerve.

After ejaculation, sympathetic outflow causes vasoconstriction of the arteries of the penis, and as a result, the inflow of blood is decreased and *detumescence* or decreased penile turgor occurs. The man then passes through a refractory period during which he is unable to have an erection or ejaculation in response to sexual stimuli.

In summary, the male genitourinary system functions in both urine elimination and reproduction. The reproductive structures consist of the testes or gonads, the excretory ducts, and the accessory organs. The testes are the site of male hormone (testosterone) and sperm production. The function of the testes is regulated by the anterior pituitary gonadotropic hormones—FSH which initiates sperm production and ICSH which regulates testosterone production.

:Study Guide

After you have studied this chapter, you should be able to meet the following objectives:

: : Describe the anatomy of the testes and the scrotum.

: : Describe the anatomy of the duct system and the accessory organs.

: : Explain why circumcision may be considered a desirable practice.

: : Describe the process of spermatogenesis.

: : State the function of the androgens.

: : Describe the control of erection and ejaculation by the autonomic nervous system.

:Suggested Readings

Dunbar RE, Bush I: A Man's Sexual Health. Chicago, Budlong Press, 1976

Odell WD, Moyer DL: Physiology of Reproduction. St. Louis, CV Mosby, 1971

Schottelius BA, Schottelius DD: Textbook of Physiology. St. Louis, CV Mosby, 1978

29

Stephanie MacLaughlin

Alterations in Structure and Function of the Male Genitourinary System

The male genitourinary system is subject to structural defects, inflammation, and neoplasms, with effects on urine elimination, sexual function, and fertility. This chapter discusses disorders of the penis, the scrotum and testes, and the prostate.

:Disorders of the Penis

The penis houses the urethra and the erectile tissue, which becomes engorged with blood during sexual stimulation. Disorders of the penis include congenital and acquired defects, inflammatory conditions, and neoplasms.

Structural Defects

Hypospadias and epispadias

Hypospadias is a congenital defect present in about 1 out of every 400 to 500 male infants. In this disorder, the termination of the urethra is on the *ventral* surface of the penis. A less common defect is epispadias, in which the opening of the urethra is on the *dorsal* surface of the penis (Fig. 29-1). Both of these abnormalities are often accompanied by other congenital defects, such as undescended testicles and chordee or ventral bowing of the penis.

Surgery is required for the correction of both hypospadias and epispadias. Infants born with

Figure 29–1.   Diagram showing hypospadias and epispadias.

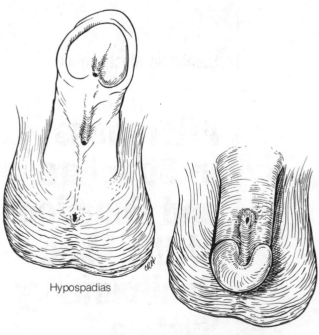

Hypospadias

Epispadias

these disorders are not circumcised since the foreskin is required in the plastic surgery done to correct the defect. When additional deformities such as chordee are present, the surgical repair procedure may be done in stages. Usually, it is suggested that surgical correction be done prior to the time that the child enters school. The adult male who has not undergone surgery will not have problems with erection or sexual function, but his semen may run out of the vagina during intercourse and thus interfere with impregnation.

Phimosis

Phimosis is a tightening of the penile foreskin, which prevents retraction of the foreskin over the glans. Although phimosis is usually congenital, it may result from inflammation, with formation of scar tissue. When the foreskin is too tight to be retracted, excess oil gland secretions and smegma accumulate under the prepuce and may cause inflammation and infection. In the adult, phimosis can prevent erection. In both children and adults, circumcision is usually the treatment of choice.

In a related condition called *paraphimosis*, the foreskin is so tight and constricted it cannot cover the glans. As with phimosis, accumulated secretions and microorganisms can cause inflammation and infection. A very tight foreskin can constrict the blood supply to the glans and lead to ischemia and necrosis.

Priapism

Priapism is a nonsexual, prolonged, painful erection which can persist for hours or days. The condition is caused by a malfunction of the posterior venous valves with a resultant trapping of blood in the corpora cavernosa; this causes the cavernosa to remain hard while the rest of the penis becomes flaccid or relaxes. If the erection persists, there is danger of thrombosis with ischemia and necrosis.

The cause of priapism is uncertain. It is most frequent in the age group of 30 to 40 years, and is seldom seen in children or in the elderly. Priapism is associated with tumors that encroach on the penile veins, injury to the penis, prolonged sexual stimulation, and diseases that impair venous drainage from the penis following erection. For instance, sickle cell disease is associated with increased incidence of priapism. Antihypertensive drugs, antianxiety medications, and testosterone have also been known to precipitate the condition.

Treatment includes application of ice packs to the penis, and sedation. Hospitalization is usually required. When this less aggressive treatment does

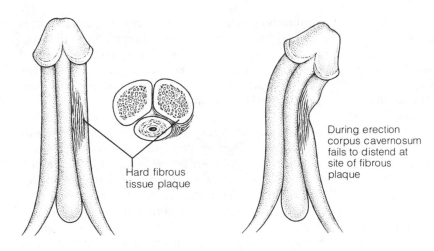

Hard fibrous
tissue plaque

During erection
corpus cavernosum
fails to distend at
site of fibrous
plaque

Figure 29–2.   Diagram showing the hard, fibrous plaque that occurs with Peyronie's disease. (Adapted from Blandy J: Lecture Notes on Urology, 2nd ed. Oxford, Blackwell Scientific Publications, 1977)

not correct the problem, shunt surgery to reroute the blood from the corpora cavernosa into veins in the corpus spongiosum may be done. It often happens that prolonged priapism gives rise to partial or complete loss of the ability to achieve an erection.

Peyronie's disease

Peyronie's disease involves a fibrous growth at the top of the penile shaft (Fig. 29-2), and is usually seen in middle-aged or elderly men. The fibrous tissue prevents lengthening of the involved area during erection, so the penis bends toward the affected area making intercourse difficult. Treatment may consist of injecting hydrocortisone into the fibrous area, administration of vitamin E, ultrasound wave therapy, or administration of fibrolytic agents, such as potassium para-aminobenzoate. The fibrous tissue can be removed surgically, although this may impair the ability to have an erection. Surgery is done when other treatment modalities fail.

Inflammatory Conditions of the Penis

Most inflammations of the penis involve the glans and prepuce and may be due to any one of several pathogenic organisms. Venereal infections—one cause of penile infections—are not discussed in this text.

Balanoposthitis

Balanoposthitis is an inflammation of the glans and prepuce due to the streptococcus, staphylococcus, coliform bacillus, or, less often, the gonococcus. It is often seen in males whose foreskin is intact, because desquamating epithelial cells, glandular secretions, and bacteria accumulate there. The surface of the glans becomes reddened, swollen, and itchy. As the

condition progresses, a yellow exudate forms, with development of superficial ulcerations on the surface of the glans.

Tumors of the Penis

Except for condyloma acuminatum and papilloma, benign tumors of the penis are relatively uncommon. Cancer of the penis is rare.

Condyloma acuminatum

Condyloma acuminatum is by far the most common form of benign penile growth. It is caused by a virus that can be transmitted to other parts of the body or to other persons, and is characterized by the presence of tumors around the foreskin. These tumors range in size from minute sessile or pedunculated growths to large masses several centimeters in diameter, not unlike raspberries in overall appearance. The lesions are easily macerated and have a foul odor. If left untreated, they tend to become ulcerated and infected. In the absence of histological examination, it is often difficult to distinguish these growths from carcinoma. They are usually treated by electrocautery or cryosurgery.

Leukoplakia of the penis

Leukoplakia is a common complication of chronic irritation and inflammation of the penis. The skin on the affected area becomes indurated and assumes a bluish-white appearance, and the foreskin is rigid and inelastic. It is considered a precancerous lesion and is significant because it can progress to squamous cell carcinoma. When histological examination reveals bizarre cell types with marked cellular disarrangement, the leukoplakia is then termed Bowen's disease or carcinoma in situ.

Cancer of the penis

Squamous cell cancer of the penis accounts for approximately 1% of male genital tumors in the United States, and it is most frequent in the age group of 45 years to 60 years. It is rare in the circumcised male; a predisposition to penile cancer appears to be linked to the irritation due to accumulated smegma under the foreskin. Many of these patients have a history of venereal disease.

The tumor is usually found on the prepuce, the glans, or the coronal sulcus. In most cases, it is a slow-growing squamous cell carcinoma, well differentiated and of low malignancy. In approximately 50% of cases, metastatic spread occurs via the lymphatics. The superficial inguinal nodes, the deep inguinal, obturator, or iliac nodes may be involved. Blood-borne metastases are rare and usually occur late in the disease.

The tumor begins as a small lump or ulcer on the penis. If phimosis is present, there may be painful swelling, purulent drainage, or difficulty in urinating. Palpable lymph nodes in the inguinal region and positive biopsy of the lesion will confirm the diagnosis. Lymphangiography may be done to assess the extent of lymphatic involvement.

Treatment methods include surgery and radiation therapy. If the lesion is confined to the prepuce, circumcision is the treatment of choice. More commonly, partial or complete penile amputation is required. Where there is no regional lymph involvement, radiation therapy is a less mutilating form of treatment. This is of particular importance to the man in whom normal sexual function and body image are psychologically important.

In summary, disorders of the penis can be either congenital or acquired. Hypospadias and epispadias are congenital defects in which there is a malposition of the urethral opening; it is located on the dorsal surface in hypospadias and on the ventral surface in epispadias. Phimosis is the condition in which the opening of the foreskin is too tight to permit retraction over the glans. Prolonged, painful, and nonsexual erection which can lead to thrombosis with ischemia and necrosis is called priapism. Peyronie's disease is characterized by growth of a band of fibrous tissue on top of the penile shaft. Cancer of the penis is relatively rare, accounting for only 1% of male genital cancers. Leukoplakia is a precancerous lesion caused by chronic irritation and inflammation of the penis.

:Disorders of the Scrotum and Testes

The tunica vaginalis is a serosa-lined sac containing the testicles and epididymis, both of which descend from the peritoneal cavity during fetal development. Defects of the scrotum and testes include cryptorchidism, disorders of the scrotal sac, vascular disorders, inflammation of the scrotum and testes, and neoplasms.

Cryptorchidism

In the fetus, the testes develop intra-abdominally, descending into the scrotum during the eighth and ninth months of gestation via the inguinal canal. Should the testes remain in the abdominal cavity or in the inguinal canal, the condition is known as *cryptorchidism* (Fig. 29-3). It is found in about 4% of prepubertal boys. Cryptorchidism may be either unilateral or bilateral, but is more common on the right side. The underlying cause is one of the following: insufficiency of hormones to stimulate descent, an inguinal canal that is too small or is occluded, or testicular abnormalities.

Uncorrected bilateral cryptorchidism leads to sterility and carries the potential for development of testicular cancer. The testicles atrophy and sterility occurs when the testes are allowed to remain in the abdominal cavity. The atrophic changes that re-

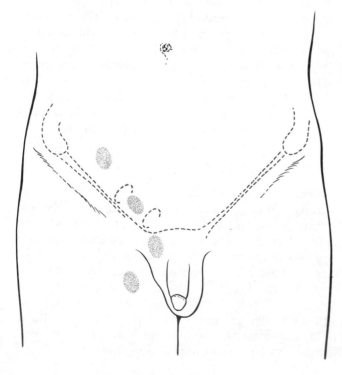

Figure 29–3. Possible locations of undescended testicles.

sult in sterility are probably due to the higher temperature to which the nonscrotal testes are exposed. If the testes are allowed to remain in the abdomen past the age of 5 or 6, there is greater risk of developing testicular cancer. The hormone chorionic gonadotropin may be administered in efforts to induce testicular descent, and should this therapy fail, surgical correction is carried out. Early surgical treatment is preferred since the testes begin to mature at about 5 years of age.

Disorders of the Scrotal Sac

A *hydrocele* is a collection of fluid in the scrotal sac. It may be congenital, due to a defect in which there is a direct communication between the tunica vaginalis and the peritoneal cavity, and if congenital, it often corrects itself spontaneously during the first year of life. In the adult, acute hydrocele may be a complication of an infectious process, such as gonorrhea, a neoplasm, or trauma to the scrotum. The tunica vaginalis may also fill with fluid in conditions such as heart failure, in which edema is widespread. The fluid is usually serous, but may become a reddish-brown with slight hemorrhage. Transillumination may be used to reveal the translucent character of the excess fluid and outline the opaque testes within the scrotal sac. Surgical drainage of the fluid may be done to prevent scrotal overheating and consequent sterility.

A *hematocele* is an accumulation of blood in the tunica vaginalis, which causes the scrotal skin to become dark red or purple in color. It may develop as the result of an abdominal surgical procedure, scrotal trauma, or a bleeding disorder.

A *spermatocele* is a painless, sperm-containing cyst which forms at the end of the epididymis. The usual cause is partial obstruction of the ducts that transport sperm from the testes to the urethra. If the cyst is bothersome, it can be evacuated with a hollow needle.

Testicular torsion

Testicular torsion is a twisting of the spermatic cord which suspends the testes. In the child, it commonly occurs after unusually rough play or violent activity; in the adult, it is associated with a large scrotum. Other related factors are incomplete descent of the testes, absence of the scrotal ligaments, or atrophy of the testes leaving them abnormally mobile within the tunica vaginalis.

The major symptom of torsion is severe pain in the scrotum and testes. The degree of twisting may vary—the cord may be only slightly twisted or may

be rotated several times. Because the blood vessels supplying the testis are encased in the spermatic cord, the twisting often interrupts the blood supply, leading to testicular atrophy or gangrene of the testis and epididymis. The degree of damage is proportional to the length of time that the blood flow has been interrupted. Immediate surgical correction provides the only means for preserving the testis when complete occlusion of the vessels has occurred. In as short a time as 4 hours, the damage may be permanent. If gangrene develops, the testis must be removed surgically. In correcting torsion, a stitch is placed to anchor the testis and prevent a recurrence, and the contralateral testis is also stitched. This is done because torsion tends to affect both testes.

Varicocele

Varicocele is characterized by varicosities of the spermatic cord veins, causing a reversal of blood flow in the internal spermatic vein. There is scrotal pain which persists when the person is supine. When the cord is palpated, tortuous scrotal veins are noted, which feel much like a "bag of worms." Palpation causes a dull ache in the cord area. Varicocele is found more often on the left side, because of the difference in the venous conformation between the right and left sides of the spermatic cord.

Varicocele is found with greatest frequency in the under-thirty age group. As it advances, it can give rise to severe testicular degeneration. This happens because the blood in the dilated venous structures has a warming effect on the testes; this interferes with spermatogenesis and leads to a reduction in sperm mobility and number of sperm produced.

The usual treatment is to have the patient bathe in cold water to cool the testes and constrict the vessels, and to have him lose weight if he is obese, since obesity tends to aggravate the problem and to make surgical intervention more difficult. Surgical treatment entails ligation of the veins in the spermatic cord. Following ligation, venous flow is maintained by the remaining scrotal vessels.

Inflammation of the Scrotum and Testes

Inflammation of the scrotum and testes can involve either the external scrotal sac or the intrascrotal contents, including the epididymis and testes.

Inflammation of the scrotum
There are certain normal characteristics of the scrotum that can be predisposing factors to inflammation of the sac. First, the scrotal rugae prevent air

circulation and evaporation of moisture from the skin surface; together with the close proximity of the anus and the urethra, this provides a favorable environment for bacterial growth. Second, the loose scrotal skin reacts to inflammation by becoming highly edematous, which in turn decreases circulation and delays healing. Third, contact of the scrotum with the thighs can cause maceration of the skin surface and prolong healing.

A common infection of the scrotum and thighs is a type of *dermatosis* called tinea cruris or "jock itch." It is characterized by reddened patches with raised scaling edges. Pruritus is common, and repeated scratching often encourages secondary infections. Obesity, excessive perspiration, poor hygiene, and tight-fitting synthetic underwear that prevents air circulation are other predisposing factors in dermatosis. Treatment consists of improved hygiene, air-drying of underclothing, and use of an antifungal agent.

Inflammation of the epididymis and testes

Inflammations of the epididymis are the most common of the intrascrotal infections, and testicular infections secondary to epididymitis are frequent. Although primary acute infections of the testes without epididymitis are relatively rare, infectious organisms can enter the testes from the vas deferens, the blood stream, or the lymphatics.

Acute epididymitis can result from a urinary tract infection or from urethritis, with the organisms traveling from the lumen of the vas deferens to the epididymis. Prostatitis can also precipitate epididymitis, in which case the organisms migrate through the seminal vesicles to the vas deferens. A nonspecific form of epididymitis results from invasion of the epididymis by common pyogenic bacteria. This occurs as a frequent complication of catheterization or surgery of the prostate gland. Symptoms of acute epididymitis include reddening, swelling, and tenderness, possibly hydrocele with edema. Since testicular tumors or torsion of the testes often mimics acute epididymitis, it is usually necessary to rule these out. Treatment includes rest, elevation of the scrotum, antibiotics, and elimination of other underlying causes.

Chronic epididymitis may occur secondary to chronic inflammation of the prostate gland. Often it is difficult to pinpoint the cause, since no distinct organisms can be isolated. Occasionally, chronic epididymitis is caused by genital tuberculosis.

Orchitis, an infection of the testes, can be precipitated by a primary infection in the genitourinary tract, such as urethritis, cystitis, or seminal vesic-ulitis. Many infections from other parts of the body spread to the testes via the blood stream or the lymphatics. Orchitis can develop as a complication of a systemic infection, such as mumps, scarlet fever, or pneumonia. Probably the best known of these is orchitis, due to the mumps virus. About 25% to 30% of males 10 years of age or older with parotitis (mumps) develop this form of orchitis.[1] The symptoms usually run their course in 7 to 10 days. Mumps orchitis causes painful enlargement of the testes, with small hemorrhages into the tunica albuginea. Microscopically, an acute inflammatory response is seen in the seminiferous tubules with proliferation of neutrophils, lymphocytes, and histiocytes, causing distention of the tubules. In severe cases in which the edema has been intense, atrophy of the germinal epithelium may occur and give rise to sterility.

Neoplasms

Tumors can arise from either the scrotum or the testes. Benign scrotal tumors are quite common and often do not require treatment. Carcinoma of the scrotum is rare and is usually linked to exposure to carcinogenic agents. On the other hand, almost all solid tumors of the testes (96%) are malignant.[2] Although testicular tumors are rare, their virulence and the fact that they develop in relatively young men make them a significant health problem.

Carcinoma of the scrotum

Cancer of the scrotum is primarily an occupational disease, linked to contact with petroleum products, such as tar, pitch, and soot. The malignancy often occurs after 20 to 30 years of exposure. In the early stages, it may appear as a small tumor or wartlike growth that eventually ulcerates. The thin scrotal wall lacks the tissue reactivity needed to block the malignant process; over half of the cases seen involve metastasis to the lymph nodes. Treatment includes wide local excision of the tumor with inguinal and femoral node dissection, since this tumor does not respond well to x-ray treatment.

Testicular cancer

Cancer of the testes accounts for about 1% of the cancers in males and for about 3% of cancers of the male urogenital system. The highest incidence of testicular cancer is found in the 20-to-40-year age group, lending it greater significance than its frequency would otherwise warrant. It is the most common cancer in men between the ages of 29 and 35. The risk of testicular cancer is greatly increased in males with cryptorchidism. It has been estimated that 1 in 20 abdominal testes and 1 in 80 inguinal testes will develop a tumor.[1] Chronic irritation of the testes, from either infection or other inflammatory processes, is also thought to increase the risk of cancer formation.

Often the first sign of testicular cancer is a slight painless enlargement of the testicle, occasionally an ache in the abdomen or groin or a sensation of dragging or heaviness in the scrotum. Frank pain may be experienced in the later stages when the tumor is growing rapidly and hemorrhaging occurs. Testicular tumors often metastasize while the primary tumor is still small and only barely palpable, in which case, the first indication of the disease is symptoms related to the organ or region to which the cancer has spread. Unfortunately, 80% to 90% of men with testicular cancer have metastatic disease by the time diagnosis is made. This is because there are only a few early symptoms and, therefore, many men delay seeing their physician until the tumor has spread.

The American Cancer Society strongly advocates that every young adult male examine his testes at least once a month as a means of early detection of this cancer, preferably after a warm bath or shower when the scrotal skin is relaxed. To do this self-examination, each testicle is examined with the fingers of both hands by rolling the testicle between the thumb and fingers to check for the presence of any lumps. If a lump, nodule, or enlargement is noted, it should be brought immediately to the attention of a physician.[3]

Testicular tumors are generally classified into four groups: (1) seminoma, (2) embryonal carcinoma, (3) teratoma and teratocarcinoma, and (4) choriocarcinoma. *Seminomas* account for 40% of testicular tumors and are the most frequent tumor associated with undescended testicles. Seminomas metastasize primarily through the lymph nodes, but also slowly through the blood stream. These tumors respond well to radiation therapy and a 92% to 96%, five-year survival rate has been reported following surgery (orchidectomy) and radiation.[3] The incidence of *embryonal carcinoma* among cancers of the testicles is 15% to 20%. These tumors are composed of variable embryonic forms of epithelial tissue. Embryonal carcinoma has a relatively grave prognosis, with a 10-year survival rate of about 35%.[2] Although radiation is the best treatment modality, eradication of the tumor usually requires a larger dose of radiation than the body can tolerate. The *teratomas* and *teratocarcinomas* account for about 20% to 25% of testicular tumors. These tumors are composed of a multitude of cell types, including tissue that resembles muscle, bone, cartilage, squamous epithelium, and brain tissue. Teratomas may occur at any age and may be either benign or malignant. In the child, a differentiated mature form of teratoma is usually benign. In the adult, the tumor may harbor foci of malignant cells. Such a teratoma is classified as a teratocarcinoma. These carcinomas are usually treated with surgery and radiation. The 10-year survival rate following treatment is about 47%.[2] *Choriocarcinoma* accounts for about 1% of all testicular cancers. These cancers metastasize while the primary tumor is still quite small. Morphologically, the tumor resembles placental tissue, and it is interesting to note that high levels of chorionic gonadotropins (the hormones responsible for a positive pregnancy test) appear in the urine of the male with choriocarcinoma. Choriocarcinoma does not respond well to treatment, and carries a 10-year survival rate of only about 11%.[2]

In summary, disorders of the scrotum and testes include cryptorchidism or undescended testicles, hydrocele, testicular torsion, and varicocele. Inflammatory conditions can involve the scrotal sac, epididymis, or testes. Tumors can arise in either the scrotum or the testes. Scrotal cancers are usually associated with exposure to petroleum products such as tar, pitch, and soot. Testicular cancer accounts for about 3% of cancers of the male genitourinary system. Testicular self-examination is recommended as a means of early detection for this form of cancer.

:Disorders of the Prostate

The prostate is a firm glandular structure that surrounds the urethra. It produces a thin, milky, alkaline secretion that aids sperm motility by helping to maintain an optimum pH. The contraction of the smooth muscle in the gland promotes semen expulsion during ejaculation.

Prostatitis

Inflammation of the prostate gland is a common condition which can be traced to a number of organisms. It may occur spontaneously or as the result of catheterization or instrumentation, or may occur secondary to other diseases of the male genitourinary system. Prostatitis may be classified as acute or chronic. About 80% of acute forms of prostatitis can be traced to strains of *E. coli* and the rest to klebsiella.[4] It is characterized by diffuse inflammation of the prostatic ducts and acini, and may progress to abscess formation. Symptoms include fever, general malaise, frequency of urination, dysuria, and pain in the groin or perineal area. There may be hematuria and rectal pain, and pain on defecation. In younger men, erections are frequently painful. Rectal examination reveals a swollen and exquisitely tender prostate.

Chronic prostatitis is probably the most common cause of relapsing urinary tract infections in the male[5] and usually occurs in middle-age or older men. It may give rise to vague perineal pain, dysuria, frequency, low-back discomfort, and prostatic tenderness, as well as a slight early morning discharge or hematuria. The chronic form often is asymptomatic. Many times, cultures of midstream urine and prostatic fluid are sterile or contain only normal bacterial flora. It is thought that in some cases the prostatitis may be due to a viral infection such as herpes simplex II, a common sexually transmitted virus.[6] If no organisms are cultured, the treatment is usually symptomatic. Prostatic massage, warm baths, and avoidance of intercourse and alcohol may be suggested.

Benign Prostatic Hypertrophy

Benign prostatic hypertrophy (BPH), or hyperplasia, is a common disorder in men over 50 years of age. Postmortem examinations have shown that 50% to 60% of men ages 40 to 59 and 95% of men over age 70 have some degree of nodular hyperplasia of the prostate.[7] In about one-third of cases, the nodules can be detected on rectal examination, yet only 5% to 10% of these men have problems sufficient to warrant surgical intervention (Fig. 29-4).

BPH is characterized by formation of large discrete lesions in the periurethral region. As they enlarge, these nodules tend to compress the urethra and cause partial or almost complete obstruction of urine flow. The etiology of BPH is uncertain, but the increasing incidence with advancing age suggests the possibility of an imbalance between male and female sex hormones. The nodules associated with BPH do not usually involve the posterior lobe of the prostate gland, which is a frequent site of prostatic cancer.

The resulting obstruction to urinary outflow can give rise to urinary tract infection, difficulty in voiding, hypertrophy, and eventually destructive changes of the bladder wall, hydroureter, and hydronephrosis. Hypertrophy and changes in bladder-wall structure develop in stages. At first, the exaggerated criss-cross fibers form trabeculations; then herniations or sacculations; finally diverticula develop as the herniations extend through the bladder wall (Fig. 29-5). These diverticula are readily infected, since urine is seldom completely emptied from them. Back pressure on the ureters promotes hydroureter and hydronephrosis, and, as a result, the kidney develops the physiological sequelae of atrophy—failure to concentrate urine, to retain sodium, and to remove metabolic acids from the blood. There is danger of eventual renal failure.

The symptoms of BPH are related to the compression of the urethra with accompanying bladder distention and hypertrophy, urinary tract infection, and renal disease. The typical picture includes outflow obstruction with a decreased urinary stream. As the obstruction increases, there may be acute retention with overdistention of the bladder. The presence of residual urine in the bladder causes urinary frequency and a constant desire to empty the bladder, which becomes worse at night. With marked bladder distention, there may be overflow

Figure 29–4. Benign nodular hyperplasia of the prostate.

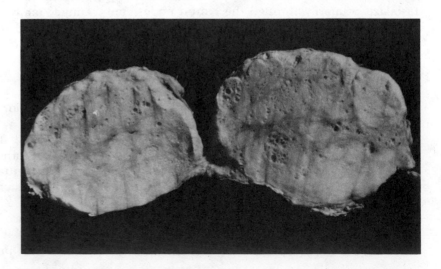

incontinence whenever there is the slightest increase in intra-abdominal pressure. Uremia, which occurs in the late stages of the disease, is discussed in Chapter 27.

Severe urinary obstruction usually is surgically treated. There are several surgical approaches. The preference of the surgeon, the severity of the disease, and the location of the nodules are usually determining factors in the type of procedure to be done. Prostate surgery for BPH does not usually cause loss of sexual function, since much of the gland remains. An occasional side effect of the surgery is retrograde ejaculation (into the bladder). When this happens, sensual pleasure will remain, but the man will be sterile.

Cancer of the Prostate

Next to cancer of the lung, prostatic cancer is the most frequent type of male cancer. About 57,000 new cases are diagnosed annually in the United States and more than 20,000 men die of the disease each year. In men under age 40, it rarely is fatal, whereas it is the third highest cause of male cancer deaths in the 55-to-74-year age group.[8] The cause is largely unknown, although tumor growth is strikingly influenced by sex hormones, being inhibited by estrogen and stimulated by testosterone. Prostatic cancers, like most cancers, are divided into four stages: stage A(I), occult cancer in which the cells are well differentiated; stage B(II), confined within the prostatic capsule; stage C(III), extracapsular extension; and stage D(IV), demonstrable metastasis.

More than half of all prostatic cancers are discovered while still localized to the prostate; studies indicate that 68% of these patients are alive 5 years following treatment.[8] In more advanced disease, metastasis can occur by way of the lymphatics, involving the vesical, sacral/external iliacs, and lumbar lymph nodes. The cancer may also spread through the vertebral veins. Venous metastasis accounts for the high frequency of pelvic, femoral head, and lumbar spine involvement, and spread to the skin, viscera, and bone marrow is also common.

Treatment methods include surgery, radiation therapy, and hormone therapy. Total removal of the prostate gland, seminal vesicles, and cuff of the bladder—a radical prostatectomy—is effective for localized lesions in healthy men without evidence of metastasis. In this operation, the nerve and muscle tissue surrounding the prostatic capsule is interrupted, which generally renders the patient impotent. Estrogen in the form of diethylstilbestrol (DES) may be administered to inhibit tumor growth. The

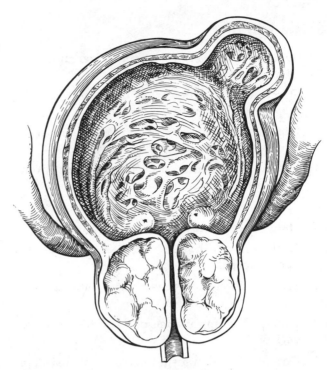

Figure 29–5. Destructive changes of the bladder wall with development of diverticulum due to benign prostatic hypertrophy.

hormone blocks release of the pituitary gonadotropins that stimulate testosterone production. This treatment can shrink the tumor and thereby reduce pain, and may be effective for several years. Estrogen is not without side effects, however, as fluid retention, gynecomastia, testicular atrophy, impotence, and a feminine skin appearance may develop. Castration (removal of the testes) offers another means of ending testosterone production. Radiotherapy by both external therapy and interstitial irradiation has been employed, although it has not been as effective as surgical or hormonal treatment. This therapy is helpful in reducing the pain associated with osseous metastasis.

In summary, the prostate is a firm glandular structure that surrounds the urethra. Inflammation of the prostate occurs as either an acute or a chronic process. Chronic prostatitis is probably the most common cause of relapsing urinary tract infections in the male. Benign prostatic hypertrophy is a common disorder of men over age 50. Because the prostate encircles the urethra, this condition tends to cause obstruction of urinary outflow from the bladder. Cancer of the prostate is the most frequent type of cancer of the male genitourinary system and is the third highest cause of male cancer deaths in men 55 to 74 years of age.

:Study Guide

After you have studied this chapter, you should be able to meet the following objectives:

: : Describe three structural disorders to which the male genitourinary system is subject.

: : Explain the relationship that may exist between circumcision and balanoposthitis.

: : Explain the potential significance of condyloma acuminatum and penile leukoplakia.

: : List the signs of penile cancer.

: : State the cause of cryptorchidism.

: : Differentiate hydrocele, hematocele, and spermatocele.

: : State the potential risk associated with testicular torsion.

: : Explain the importance of early treatment for varicocele.

: : Describe the manifestations of dermatosis, epididymitis, and orchitis.

: : Relate environmental factors to scrotal cancer.

: : State a general classification of testicular tumors with reference to their frequency.

: : State the clinical manifestations of prostatitis.

: : Describe the physical dysfunction related to the presence of benign prostatic hypertrophy.

: : State the treatment measures for prostatic cancer.

:References

1. Robbins SL, Cotran R: Pathologic Basis of Disease, pp 1220, 1222. Philadelphia, WB Saunders, 1979
2. Rubin P (ed): Clinical Oncology, ed 5, pp 150, 152. Rochester, American Cancer Society, 1978
3. Facts About Testicular Cancer, pp 7, 9. American Cancer Society, 1978
4. Robbins SL, Cotran R: Pathologic Basis of Disease, p 123. Philadelphia, WB Saunders, 1979
5. Meares EM: Prostatitis, a review. Med Clin North Am 2:3, 1975
6. Blandy J: Urology, p 923. London, Blackwell Scientific Publications, 1976
7. Harbitz TB, Haugen OA: Histology of the prostate in elderly men. A study in an autopsy series. Acta Pathol Microbiol Scand 80:756, 1972
8. Facts on Prostate Cancer, pp 3, 10. American Cancer Society, 1978

:Suggested Readings

Basso–Alise A: The prostate in the elderly male. Hosp Pract 12(10):117–123, 1977

Cohen S: Patient assessment: Examination of the male genitalia. Programmed instruction. Am J Nurs 79(4):689–712, 1979

Conklin M, Klint K, Morway A et al: Should health teaching include self-examination of the testes? Am J Nurs 78(12):207, 1978

Duckett JW: Epispadias. Urol Clin North Am 5(1): 107–126, 1978

Dwoskin JY: Hypospadias. Urol Clin North Am 5(1): 95–106, 1978

Gault PA: The prostate. Coping with dangerous and distressing complications. Nursing '77 7(4):34–38, 1977

Hoppmann HJ, Fraley EE: Squamous cell carcinoma of the penis. J Urol 120(10):393–398, 1978

Javadpour N: The National Cancer Institute experience with testicular cancer. J Urol 120(12):651–659, 1978

Kochen M, McCurdy S: Circumcision and the risk of cancer of the penis. American Diseases of Children 134:484–486, 1980

McKenzie DJ: Peyronie's disease. J Med Assoc Ga 67: 426–427, 1978

Murray BLS, Wilcox LJ: Testicular self-exam. Am J Nurs 78(12):2074–2075, 1978

Prostate Ca: Focus on early Dx and prognostic accuracy. Hosp Pract 14(9):129–131, 1979

Raifer J, Walsh P: Testicular descent. Urol Clin North Am 5(1):233–235, 1978

Tobiason SJ: Benign prostatic hypertrophy. Am J Nurs 79(2):286–290, 1979

Wilson JD: The pathogenesis of benign prostatic hyperplasia. Am J Med 68(5):745–756, 1980

30

Debbie Lynn Cook

Structure and Function of the Female Reproductive System

The female genitourinary system consists of the internal paired ovaries, the uterine tubes, the uterus, the vagina and the external mons pubis, the labia majora, the labia minora, the clitoris, the urethra, the perineal body, and the anus. Although the female urinary structures are anatomically separate from the genital structures, their anatomic proximity provides a means for cross-contamination and shared symptomatology between the two systems (Fig. 30-1). This chapter focuses on the internal and external genitalia. It includes a discussion of hormonal and physical changes that occur throughout the life cycle in response to the gonadotropic hormones. The reader is referred to a specialty text for a discussion of pregnancy.

:The Internal Genitalia

The Ovaries

The ovaries are flat, almond-shaped structures measuring 4 to 5 cm in length and weighing approximately 2 to 3 g. They are located on either side of the uterus below the fimbriated ends of the two oviducts or fallopian tubes. The ovaries are attached to the posterior surface of the broad ligament and to the uterus by the ovarian ligament.

The ovaries, like the male testes, have a dual function in that they store the female germ cells or ova, and produce the female sex hormones estrogen and progesterone. Unlike the male gonads, which produce sperm throughout the man's reproductive life, the female gonads contain a fixed number of ova at birth which diminish throughout the woman's life.

Structurally, the mature ovary is composed of an inner medulla which contains supportive connective tissue and an outer cortex of germinal epithelium. The germinal epithelium contains the primary oocytes that are present at birth and that become the graafian follicles under the influence of the pituitary and ovarian hormones. A graafian follicle is a fully developed follicle. Usually one follicle matures during each cycle throughout the reproductive years. The extruded ovum is engulfed by the fallopian tube fimbriae and propelled toward the uterus.

The Fallopian Tubes

The fallopian or uterine tubes are slender cylindrical structures attached bilaterally to the uterus and supported by the upper folds of the broad ligament. The end of the fallopian tube that is near the ovary forms a funnel-shaped opening with fringed projections

Figure 30–1. Female reproductive system as seen in the sagittal section. (From Chaffee EE, Greisheimer EM: Basic Physiology and Anatomy, 3rd ed. Philadelphia, JB Lippincott, 1974)

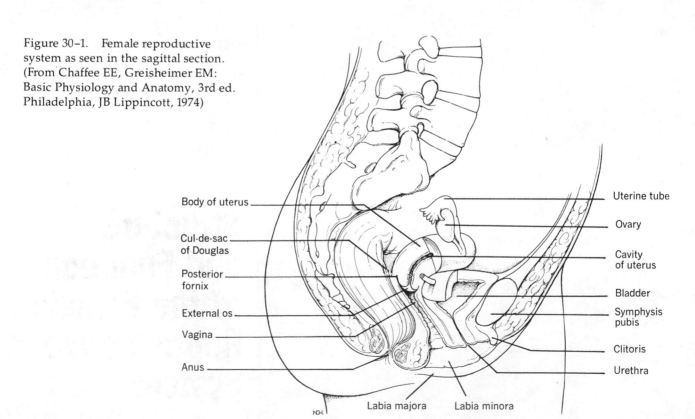

called fimbriae (Fig. 30-2). The fallopian tubes are formed of smooth muscle and lined with a ciliated mucus-producing epithelial layer. The beating of the cilia, along with the contractile movements of the smooth muscle, propel the nonmobile ova toward the uterus. If coitus has been recent, the ovum may encounter a sperm in the fallopian tube and fertilization may occur. The fallopian tube is the normal site of fertilization. Besides providing a passageway for ova and sperm, the fallopian tubes also provide for drainage of tubal secretions into the uterus. Infection and inflammation may disrupt fallopian tube patency and impair their function.

The Uterus

The uterus is a thick-walled muscular organ. This pear-shaped, hollow structure is located between the bladder and the rectum. The uterus can be divided into three parts: the top, called the fundus, the lower constricted part, called the cervix, and the portion between the fundus and the cervix, called the body of the uterus. The uterus is supported on both sides principally by the broad and round ligaments.

In most women, the uterus is found in a forward-lying or anteverted position, in which the uterine fundus and body rest on top of the urinary bladder. The uterus may assume other positions such as anteflexion, retroflexion, or retroversion without causing problems. Uterine position may change in response to many factors.

The wall of the uterus is composed of three layers: the perimetrium, the myometrium, and the endometrium. The *perimetrium* is the outer serous covering which is derived from the abdominal peritoneum. This outer layer merges with the peritoneum that covers the broad ligaments. Anteriorly, the perimetrium is reflected over the bladder wall, forming the vesicouterine pouch, and posteriorly it extends to form the *cul-de-sac* or *pouch of Douglas*. Because of the proximity of the perimetrium to the urinary bladder, infection of this organ often causes uterine symptoms, particularly during pregnancy.

The middle muscle layer, the *myometrium*, forms the major portion of the uterine wall. The myometrium has the amazing capacity to change in length during pregnancy and labor. The *endometrium* is the inner layer of the uterus, continuous with the lining of the fallopian tubes and vagina. The endometrium is made up of a basal and a superficial layer. The superficial layer is shed during menstruation and regenerated by cells of the basal layer. Ciliated cells promote movement of tubal–uterine secretions out of the uterine cavity into the vagina.

The Cervix

The round cervix is the neck of the uterus that projects into the vagina. The cervix is composed of a connective tissue matrix of glands and muscular tissue elements, forming a firm, fibrous structure that becomes soft and pliable under the influence of

Figure 30–2.   Schematic drawing of female reproductive organs, showing path of the oocyte as it moves from the ovary into the fallopian (uterine) tube; path of sperm is also shown, as is the usual site of fertilization. (From Chaffee EE, Lytle IM: Basic Physiology and Anatomy, 4th ed. Philadelphia, JB Lippincott, 1980)

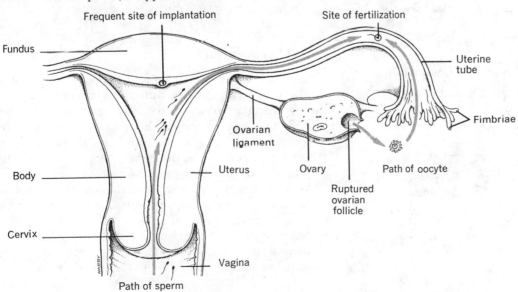

hormones produced during pregnancy. Glandular tissue provides a rich supply of protective mucus that changes in character and quantity during the menstrual cycle as well as during pregnancy. The cervix is richly supplied with blood from the uterine artery, and can be a site of significant blood loss during delivery.

The opening of the cervix, the *os*, forms a pathway between the uterus and the vagina. The vaginal opening is called the external os and the uterine opening, the internal os. The space between these two openings is the endocervical canal. Endocervical secretions protect the uterus from infection, alter receptivity to sperm, and form a mucoid "plug" during pregnancy. The endocervical canal provides a route for menstrual discharge and sperm entrance. Pelvic infection may ascend or descend through the cervix.

The Vagina

The vagina is a fibromuscular tube lined with mucus-secreting squamous epithelial cells. This structure connects the internal and external genitalia and is located behind the urinary bladder and

urethra. The vagina is about 7.5 to 10 cm in length and functions as a route for discharge of menses and other secretions. It also serves as an organ of sexual fulfillment and reproduction.

The membranous vaginal wall forms two longitudinal folds and several transverse folds or rugae. Vaginal tissue is usually moist, with a pH maintained within the bacteriostatic level of 4 to 6. The vaginal epithelial cells store glycogen under the influence of estrogen. Both pH and keratinization of these cells are likewise influenced by estrogen levels. During a routine "Pap" smear, the estrogen level can be measured by examining the cellular structure and configuration. This test is known as the maturation index.

:The External Genitalia

The external genitalia are located at the base of the pelvis in the perineal area and include the mons pubis, labia majora, labia minora, clitoris, and perineal body. The urethra and anus, while not genital structures, are usually considered in a discussion of the external genitalia. The external genitalia, also known collectively as the vulva, are diagrammed in Figure 30-3.

The Mons Pubis

The mons pubis is a rounded eminence located anterior to the symphysis pubis of the bony pelvis. The mons is a fat pad covered with skin and hair. The amount of fat and hair of the mons pubis usually increases under the hormonal stimulus of puberty, and its color deepens. The skin which is abundant in sebaceous glands, may become infected due to changes in dietary habits, normal variations, or poor hygiene. The mons pubis is the site of pubic lice infestation.

The Labia Majora

The labia majora are analogous to the male scrotum. These structures are the outermost lips of the vulva, beginning anteriorly at the base of the mons pubis and ending posteriorly at the anus. The labia majora are composed of folds of skin and fat and become covered with hair at the onset of puberty. Prior to puberty, the labia majora have a skin covering similar to that covering the abdomen. With sufficient hormonal stimulation, the labia of a mature woman close over the urethral and vaginal openings; this can change following childbirth or surgery. The labia majora are rich in sebaceous glands. They are subject to the same types of problems as the mons pubis.

Figure 30–3.   External genitalia of the female. (From Chaffee EE, Lytle IM: Basic Physiology and Anatomy, 4th ed. Philadelphia, JB Lippincott, 1980)

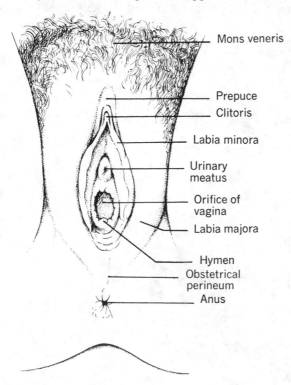

Mons veneris

Prepuce
Clitoris

Labia minora

Urinary meatus

Orifice of vagina

Labia majora

Hymen
Obstetrical perineum
Anus

The Labia Minora

The labia minora are located between the labia majora. These delicate cutaneous structures are smaller than the labia majora, and are made up of skin, fat, and some erectile tissue. Unlike the skin of the labia majora, the labia minora are hairless and usually light pink in color. The edges may be ragged or smooth and may protrude from the labia majora. The labia minora begin anteriorly at the hood of the clitoris and end posteriorly at the base of the vagina. The area between them is called the vestibule. Within the vestibule are located the urethral and vaginal openings (introitus), as well as the Bartholin's lubricating glands. During sexual arousal, the labia minora become distended with blood and enlarged; with resolution, the labia throb, then return to normal size. The sebaceous glands secrete odoriferous fluid, both in the presence and absence of sexual arousal.

The Clitoris

The clitoris is located below the clitoral hood or prepuce, which is formed by the joining of the two labia minora. The female clitoris is an erectile organ, rich in blood and nerve supply. It is analogous to the male penis, being a highly sensitive organ that becomes distended during sexual stimulation.

The Urethra

The urethra or urinary meatus is the external opening of the internal urinary bladder. The urethra is posterior to the clitoris and is usually closer to the vaginal opening than to the clitoris. The urethra, the vaginal opening, and the Bartholin glands lie within the vestibule.

The urethral opening is the site of the Skene's glands, which have a lubricating function. When infected, these glands or the meatus may become inflamed and painful. An isolated urethral infection is most commonly caused by the gonococci. Inflammation may occur secondary to trauma, increased sexual activity, or structural defects such as diverticula. Secretions indicating infections may be discharged during urination or gynecologic examination.

The Introitus and the Hymen

The vaginal orifice is commonly known as the introitus. The opening may be oval, circular, or sievelike, and may be partially or completely occluded. Occlu-

sion may occur because of the presence of an intact or partially intact hymen (Fig. 30-4). The hymen is composed of connective tissue. Contrary to a popular notion, an intact hymen may or may not indicate virginity, as this tissue can be stretched without tearing. At puberty, an intact hymen may require surgical intervention to permit discharge of menstrual fluids. The vaginal introitus is the opening between the external and internal genitalia.

The Bartholin Glands

Between the hymenal opening and the posterior joining of the labia minora are located the ducts of the Bartholin glands. These glands lubricate the vestibular area. Bacterial infection of the Bartholin ducts may cause bilateral or unilateral labial swelling and pain that may become so severe as to inhibit ambulation. Purulent discharge is suggestive of gonococcal infection, and a culture of the discharge is necessary to rule it out. Infection may progress to abscess formation, which requires excision and drainage.

The Perineal Body

The perineal body is that tissue located posterior to the vaginal opening and anterior to the anus. The perineal body is composed of fibrous connective tissue and is the site of insertion of several perineal muscles. During childbirth, it is sometimes necessary to make an incision, called an episiotomy, in this tissue.

The Anus

The anus is the external opening of the rectum. Defecation occurs under conscious control of the external rectal sphincter when the innervation is intact. The

Figure 30–4.   Variations of the hymen. From left to right: virginal, nondilated; septate, septum may or may not stretch; cribriform; parous, at least one full-term delivery. (From Pierson EC, D'Antonio WV: Female and Male. Philadelphia, JB Lippincott, 1974)

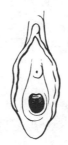
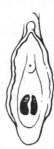
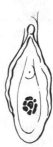
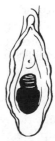

anus is darkly pigmented and surrounded by hair which may be sparse or abundant. Anal fissure, rectovaginal fistula, or hemorrhoids may provide a site for inflammation and infection, and all may necessitate surgical intervention.

:Oogenesis and Ovulation

Oogenesis is the process of generation of ova that begins at the sixth week of fetal life. These primitive germ cells will ultimately provide the 100,000 to 400,000 primordial follicles that are present at birth in a female infant.

By three months, the fetal ovaries are developed, and descend to their permanent pelvic position with the aid of the ligamentous gubernaculum. Remnants of the primitive genital system provide lateral supporting attachments to the uterus, and in the mature female, these supporting structures evolve into the round and suspensory ligaments.

The newborn's ovaries are smooth, pale, and elongated. They become shorter, thicker, and heavier before the onset of menarche, which is initiated under the influence of the pituitary. The hormonal stimulus for this development is believed to be follicular rather than systemic estrogen.

Beginning at puberty, a cyclic rise in pituitary follicle-stimulating hormone (FSH) and luteinizing hormone (LH) stimulates the development of several graafian follicles. Only the most mature graafian follicle will develop fully, while the others will continue to produce hormones but will atrophy or become atretic. In the mature graafian follicle, FSH stimulates the development of cell layers as the follicle ripens. The outermost cells (the theca externa) and the inner cells (the theca interna) provide connective, vascular, and lymph tissue support. Next, granulosa cells surround and support the ovum and the follicle. The ovum becomes suspended on a stalk of granulosa within the fluid-filled atrium of the follicle. Follicular cells provide this fluid. A space called the zona pellucida develops around the ovum, and the first layer of granulosa around the zona becomes the corona radiata. As a follicle ripens ovarian estrogen is released. The estrogen exerts a negative feedback on pituitary FSH, which inhibits multiple follicular development and predominance of LH. As estrogen suppresses FSH, LH predominates and the follicle bursts. Normally, the ovum is then transported through the fallopian tube toward the uterus. The process of follicular rupture is called ovulation (see Fig. 30-5).

The site of rupture becomes hemorrhagic. Leakage of this blood onto the peritoneal surface is believed by some to cause the "mittelschmerz" (middle-pain, or intermenstrual pain) of ovulation. Estrogen levels drop slightly at this time and may cause midcycle bleeding. The hemorrhagic site is invaded by yellow lipochrome-bearing thecal cells which form a mass called the corpus luteum. Progesterone secretion begins in this structure. If fertilization does not occur, the corpeus luteum atrophies and is replaced with white scar tissue, the corpus albicans. In the event of fertilization, the corpus luteum remains functional for three months and provides hormonal support for pregnancy.

:Menopause

Menopause is the cessation of menstrual cycles. It is as much a process as is menstruation—not an event. At first the process takes the form of less frequent and lighter menses, to culminate in total cessation of menses. This process, also known as the climacteric, may go on for one to several years. The usual age of a menopausal woman is 45 to 50 years. However, with improved nutrition, menopause may occur later in life, so a woman may have a longer reproductive period. A woman who has not menstruated for a full year is said to have completed menopause.

Menopause is due to the gradual cessation of ovarian function and resultant diminished levels of estrogen. Though estrogens derived from the adrenal cortex continue to circulate in a woman's body, they are insufficient to maintain the secondary sexual characteristics in the same manner as ovarian estrogens. As a result, breast tissue, body hair, skin elasticity, and subcutaneous fat decrease as the ovaries and uterus diminish in size and the cervix and vagina become pale and friable. The woman may find intercourse painful and traumatic, though some type of vaginal lubrication may be helpful.

Systemically, a woman may experience significant vasomotor instability secondary to the decrease in estrogens and the relative increase in pituitary FSH. This instability may give rise to "hot flashes," palpitations, dizziness, and headaches as the blood vessels dilate. A woman may feel anxious or depressed about these uncontrollable and unpredictable events.

Societal mores influence behaviors. A society that emphasizes youthfulness, fitness, and vigor does not look favorably upon aging as a positive process, and menopause is regarded as a hallmark of advancing age. A woman who focuses her energy on

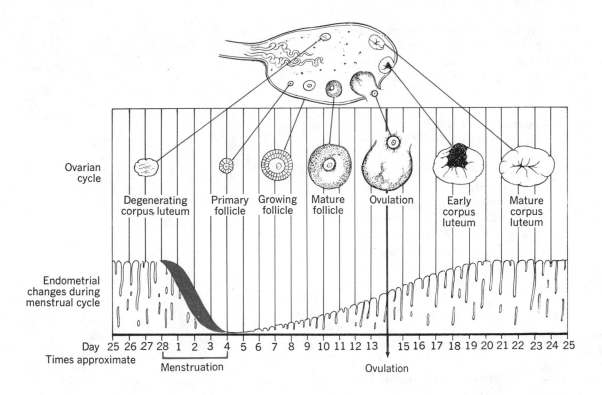

Correlation of Hormonal Activities with Ovarian and Uterine Changes

Phase	Menstrual	Follicular	Ovulation	Luteal	Premenstrual
Days 1 2 3 4 5 6 7 8	9 10 11 12 13 14	15 16 17 18 19 20	21 22 23 24 25	26 27 28 1 2	
Ovary	Degenerating corpus luteum; Beginning follicular development	Growth and maturation of follicle	Ovulation	Active corpus luteum	Degenerating corpus luteum
Estrogen production	Low	Increasing	High	Declining, then a secondary rise	Decreasing
Progesterone production	None	None	Low	Increasing	Decreasing
FSH production	Increasing	High, then declining	Low	Low	Increasing
LH production	Low	Low, then increasing	High	High	Decreasing
Endometrium	Degeneration and shedding of superficial layer. Coiled arteries dilate, then constrict again	Reorganization and proliferation of superficial layer	Continued growth	Active secretion and glandular dilatation; highly vascular; edematous	Vasoconstriction of coiled arteries; beginning degeneration

Figure 30–5. Schematic diagram of an ovarian cycle and the corresponding changes in the endometrium. (From Chaffee EE, Lytle IM: Basic Physiology and Anatomy, 4th ed. Philadelphia, JB Lippincott, 1980)

"beauty and youth" may feel frustrated or depressed by the natural aging process. On the other hand, a woman who values her attributes other than physical may welcome advancing age as a time when she may more fully develop as a person.

In summary, the female genitourinary system consists of the ovaries, the paired uterine or fallopian tubes, the uterus, the vagina, and the external genitalia. The genitourinary system in the female serves both sexual and reproductive functions. All of the primordial follicles that will develop into ova are present in the ovaries of a female at birth. Beginning at puberty, the gonadotropic hormones are secreted in a cyclic manner and the menstrual cycle is established. The reproductive period ceases with menopause at which time there is a gradual cessation of ovarian function and diminished levels of estrogen.

:Study Guide

After you have studied this chapter, you should be able to meet the following objectives:

: :   Describe the anatomy of the ovaries.

: :   Explain the function of the fallopian tubes.

: :   Describe the anatomical features of the uterine wall.

: :   State the function of endocervical secretions.

: :   Describe the anatomical relationships of the vagina, the external genitalia, and the mons pubis.

: :   Describe the anatomy of the labia minora with reference to the labia majora.

: :   State the function of the Bartholin glands, with reference to potential physiological dysfunction.

: :   Describe the normal changes that occur during the menstrual cycle.

: :   Describe the physiology of normal menopause.

:Suggested Readings

Martin LL: Health Care of Women. Philadelphia, JB Lippincott, 1978

Sloane E: Biology of Women. New York, JW Wiley, 1980

31

Stephanie MacLaughlin
Debbie Lynn Cook

Alterations in Structure and Function of the Female Reproductive System

Disorders of the female genitourinary system may have widespread effects on both physical and psychological function. These conditions bear close relationships to sexuality and reproductive function. The reproductive structures are located very close to other pelvic structures, so disorders of the reproductive system are likely to exert their effects on other pelvic organs.

The discussion in this chapter has been divided into three parts: (1) benign conditions of the female genitourinary system, (2) neoplasms, and (3) disorders of the breast.

:Benign Conditions

Benign conditions of the female genitourinary system are generally indicated by disturbances in function and structure. This section of the chapter focuses on menstrual disorders, structural defects, inflammatory conditions, abnormal benign growths of uterine tissue, and benign ovarian disorders.

Menstrual Disorders

As discussed in Chapter 30, menstruation is a normal physiological process that begins at the time of menarche and continues until menopause. This process has from time immemorial been laden with superstitions and taboos that often serve to psychologically distort the significance of the event. While pregnancy is usually a positively reinforced period of time in a woman's life, menstruation is often viewed negatively. As a result, many women do not seek treatment for menstrual irregularities, yet some of them represent more serious underlying problems.

Dysfunctional menstrual cycles
Although abnormal uterine bleeding can occur for many reasons, such as abortion, blood dyscrasias, and neoplasms, the most frequent cause is what is commonly referred to as dysfunctional menstrual cycles or bleeding. Dysfunctional menstrual cycles occur when the hormonal support of the normal cyclic endometrial changes is altered. There is evidence to suggest that deprivation of estrogen causes retrogression of a previously built-up endometrium, and bleeding. A lack of progesterone can cause abnormal menstrual bleeding, in that in its absence estrogen induces development of a much thicker endometrial layer with a richer blood supply. Progesterone causes vasoconstriction and myometrial contractions that normally occur at the time of men-

struation and that help to control the amount of blood lost. Both types of hormone deficiency are associated with absence of ovulation, hence the term *anovulatory bleeding*. Dysfunctional cycles may take the form of *amenorrhea* (absence of menstruation), *oligomenorrhea* (scanty menstruation), *menorrhagia* (excessive menstruation) or *metrorrhagia* (bleeding between periods). *Menometrorrhagia* is heavy bleeding both during and between menstrual periods. Dysfunctional menstrual cycles can originate as a primary disorder of the ovaries or as a secondary defect in ovarian function related to hypothalamic-pituitary stimulation. The latter can be initiated by emotional stress, marked variation in weight (sudden gain or loss), or by nonspecific endocrine or metabolic disturbances.

Dysmenorrhea and premenstrual tension
Dysmenorrhea is pain or discomfort with menstruation. Although not usually a serious medical disorder, dysmenorrhea causes some degree of monthly disability for a significant number of women. There are two forms of dysmenorrhea—primary and secondary.

Primary dysmenorrhea begins at the time of menarche or within several years of its onset. It is not associated with physical abnormality or pathology. The pain may be spasmotic or congestive in nature. Spasmotic dysmenorrhea, as the name implies, refers to spasmotic pain in the lower abdomen or back that is relieved with menses. Spasmotic dysmenorrhea diminishes following pregnancy, with use of oral contraceptives, and with the passage of the years. *Congestive dysmenorrhea* causes back, abdominal, and leg pains and is associated with premenstrual tension.

Premenstrual tension is a marked exaggeration in the physical, mental, and emotional tension that accompanies the hormonal and metabolic changes associated with the premenstrual phase of the normal menstrual cycle. There may be difficulty in concentrating, depression, irritability, and emotional lability as well as headaches, insomnia, and breast swelling and discomfort. There are often abdominal, back, pelvic, and leg pains as well as overt edema. Migraine–prone persons may have headaches at this time. Unlike the symptoms associated with spasmotic dysmenorrhea, which are seen in younger women, premenstrual tension and congestive dysmenorrhea tend to worsen with age and are relieved only with menopause.

Secondary dysmenorrhea is dysmenorrhea experienced by a woman whose menses previously were painless. The triggering event may be cervical stenosis related to surgical procedures such as cervical conization or cauterization, infections, childbirth, or stenosis due to oral contraceptive use.

Treatment of dysmenorrhea is directed at symptom control. Diuretics may be prescribed for relief of the edema. Analgesic agents such as aspirin and acetaminophen (Tylenol) may relieve uterine cramping and back pain. Indomethacin (Indocin) and ibuprofen (Motrin), which are prostaglandin inhibitors, may be prescribed to treat primary dysmenorrhea. These drugs are taken several days before the start of menses. Ovulation may be suppressed and primary dysmenorrhea treated by any of the oral contraceptive drugs. Relief of secondary dysmenorrhea is dependent upon identifying the cause of the problem.

Toxic shock syndrome

In recent years toxic shock syndrome has become recognized as a life-threatening event. It is characterized by extreme hypotension. Although some cases have been reported in men and children, by far the greatest number of cases occur in menstruating women. In one study of 37 cases reported during a 5-year-period in Wisconsin, 35 occurred in menstruating women, and 10 of these women had at least one recurrent episode during subsequent menstrual periods.[1] The majority of these women were tampon users. *Staphylococcus aureus* was the organism most frequently cultured from the cervix and vagina.[2]

Toxic shock syndrome is characterized by high fever, headache, confusion, diffuse skin rash and conjunctivitis, sore throat, vomiting, watery diarrhea, and shock. There is frequently desquamation (peeling) of the skin of the hands and feet during convalescence. Other types of shock are discussed in greater detail in Chapter 14.

Structural Defects

The uterus and the pelvic structures are maintained in proper position by the uterosacral ligaments, the round ligaments, and the cardinal ligaments. The two cardinal ligaments maintain the cervix at its normal level. The uterosacral ligaments hold the uterus in a forward position (Fig. 31-1). The vagina is encased in the semirigid structure of the strong investing fascia. The muscular floor of the pelvis supports the uterus and the vagina.

There are often variations in the position of the uterus, some of which are innocuous and some of which may be due to weakness and relaxation of the pelvic floor and perineum, giving rise to various disorders.

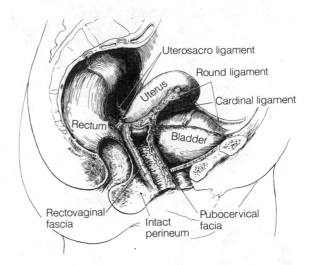

Figure 31–1.   Normal support of the uterus and vagina. (Mattingly RF: TeLinde's Operative Gynecology, 5th ed, p 487. Philadelphia, JB Lippincott, 1977)

Variations and disorders of uterine position

Normally the uterus is flexed about 45° anteriorly with the cervix positioned posteriorly and downward. When the woman is standing, the angle of the uterus is such that it lies practically horizontal, resting loosely on the bladder. There are many minor variations in the axis of the uterus in relation to the cervix that are considered normal, and certain physiologic displacements that arise during pregnancy. Usually none of these cause symptoms. The displacements to which attention should be directed include anteflexion, anteversion, retroflexion, and retroversion. Retroversion is the most common of them.[3]

Retroversion describes the condition in which the uterus is tilted posteriorly while the cervix remains tilted forward. Simple retroversion of the uterus is an asymptomatic disorder, found in 20% of normal women. It is a congenital condition due to the shortness of the anterior vaginal wall and the relaxed uterosacral ligaments; these force the uterus to fall back into the cul-de-sac of Douglas.

Should treatment of retroversion be required, a Smith-Hodge pessary ring may be placed to force the uterus into a more anteverted position (Fig. 31-2). This treatment may be prescribed for infertility problems in which all laboratory studies have given negative results and retroversion seems to be the only problem. It is hoped that the cervical canal will then be able to receive the ejaculate, and conception will follow.

Retroversion can also follow certain diseases such as endometriosis or pelvic inflammatory dis-

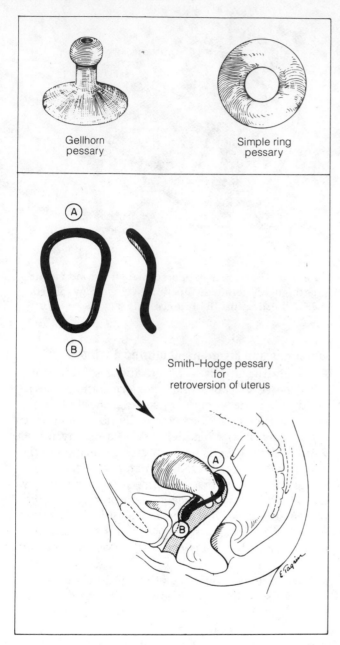

Figure 31–2. Smith–Hodge pessary that is used to treat retroversion of the uterus. Gellhorn and simple ring pessaries are used to treat uterine prolapse. (From Green TH, Jr: Gynecology: Essentials of Clinical Practice, 3rd ed. Boston, Little, Brown & Co., 1972)

ease, which produces fibrous tissue adherence with retraction of the fundus posteriorly. Large fibroids may also cause the uterus to move into a posterior position. Surgical treatment may be required to correct the retroversion.

Disorders of pelvic relaxation

In the female anatomy, nature is faced with the problems of supporting the pelvic viscera against the force of gravity and increases in intra-abdominal pressure associated with coughing, sneezing, laughing, and so on, while at the same time allowing for urination, defecation, and normal reproductive tract function (in particular, the delivery of a baby).

Three supporting structures are provided for the abdominal pelvic organs: the ilia, the peritoneum, and the pelvic diaphragm (Fig. 31-3). The iliac bones provide support for parts of the digestive tract, and the peritoneum holds the pelvic viscera in place. The main support for the viscera is, however, the pelvic diaphragm, made up of muscles and connective tissue that stretch across the bones of the pelvic outlet (Fig. 31-3). There is an inherent weakness in the pelvic diaphragm because of the openings that must exist for the urethra, the rectum, and the vagina. During pregnancy and childbirth, the muscles of the pelvic diaphragm may become stretched and strained. After numerous pregnancies, the organs may begin to slide out of, or prolapse from, the pelvis.

Relaxation of the pelvic outlet usually comes about because of overstretching of the perineal supporting tissues during pregnancy and childbirth. Although the tissues may be stretched only during these times, there may be no difficulty until later in life, such as the fifth or sixth decade, when there is further loss of elasticity and muscle tone. Even in a woman who has not borne children, the combination of aging and postmenopausal changes may give rise to problems related to relaxation of the pelvic support structures. The three most common conditions associated with this relaxation are cystocele, rectocele, and uterine prolapse. They may occur separately or in association with one another.

Cystocele. Cystocele is a herniation of the bladder into the vagina. It occurs when the normal muscle support for the bladder is weakened, so that the bladder sags below the uterus. The vaginal wall stretches and bulges downward by force of gravity and the pressure due to coughing, lifting, straining at stool, and so on. Finally the bladder herniates through the anterior vaginal wall, and a cystocele forms (Fig. 31-4).

The symptoms include an annoying bearing-down sensation, difficulty in emptying the bladder, urinary frequency and urgency, and cystitis.

Rectocele and enterocele. Rectocele is the herniation of the rectum into the vagina. It occurs when the posterior vaginal wall and underlying rectum bulge forward, ultimately protruding through the introitus as the pelvic floor and perineal muscles become weakened. The symptoms include discomfort due to the protrusion of the rectum and difficulty in defecation (Fig. 31-4).

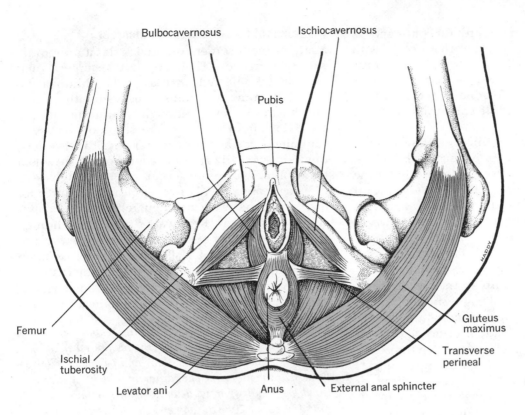

Figure 31–3.   Muscles of the pelvic floor (female perineum).
(From Chaffee EE, Lytle IM: Basic Physiology and Anatomy,
4th ed. Philadelphia, JB Lippincott, 1980)

The area between the uterosacral ligaments just posterior to the cervix may become weakened, with formation of a hernial sac into which the small bowel falls when the woman is standing. This defect, an *enterocele*, may extend into the rectovaginal septum. It may be congenital or acquired through birth trauma.

Uterine prolapse.   Uterine prolapse is the bulging of the uterus into the vagina. Prolapse is ranked as *first*, *second*, or *third degree* depending upon how far the uterine protrudes through the introitus.

The symptoms are due to irritation of the exposed mucous membranes of the cervix and vagina and the discomfort of the protruding mass. Often prolapse is accompanied by perineal relaxation, cystocele, or rectocele. A pessary (Fig. 31-2) may be inserted to hold the uterus in place, and may stave off surgical intervention in women who want to have children, and in older women for whom the surgery might pose risk.

Figure 31–4.   Diagram showing relaxation of pelvic support structures with descent of the uterus, as well as cystocele and rectocele. (Mattingly RF: TeLinde's Operative Gynecology, 5th ed, p 488. Philadelphia, JB Lippincott, 1977)

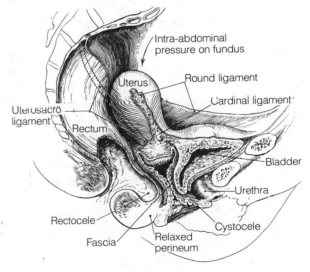

Stress incontinence. Urinary stress incontinence is the involuntary leaking of urine that occurs with coughing, sneezing, walking, lifting, and similar stresses. It usually occurs when the woman is standing, regardless of how much or how little urine is in the bladder. It is a source of embarrassment and discomfort.

Most often stress incontinence follows injury to the supporting musculature during childbirth. There is then less pelvic support anteriorly for the bladder neck and urethra. Clinically significant stress incontinence is rare in childless women, although it can occur secondarily to congenital weakness of the involved structures, poor sphincter tone, or poor innervation of the pelvic floor. The disorder is quite common in multiparous women.

Diagnosis is more complex than with other problems of pelvic support. Diagnostic procedures include pelvic and neurologic examination, cystoscopy and urethroscopy, residual urine determinations, and intravenous pyelography. Urethroscopy provides a means for measuring the degree of anatomic derangement, and usually serves as a means of confirming the diagnosis. Through urethroscopy, it has been shown that women with stress incontinence have permanent genitourinary tract changes that are analogous to those occurring in continent women during the first stages of voiding. These changes include (1) loss of the posterior urethra vesicle angle (PUV), which is normally about 90°; (2) descent and funneling of the bladder neck; and (3) backward and downward rotation of the bladder neck. This means that in women with stress incontinence, the bladder and urethra are already in an anatomic position for the first stage of voiding, so that any activity such as coughing, sneezing, or laughing increases the downward pressure on the bladder and is sufficient to force the urine to escape involuntarily.

Two types of urinary stress incontinence have been identified: Type I, in which the defect involves only a loss of the PUV angle, and Type II, in which the defect involves the loss of the PUV angle plus a downward and backward rotational descent of the urethra and bladder neck with a change in the axis of the urethra. Nonsurgical measures may offer relief in mild cases of stress incontinence. These measures include pelvic exercises, use of pessaries, and weight reduction. Pelvic (Kegel) exercises involve the alternate tensing and relaxing of the gluteal muscles and the muscles of the pelvic floor, which is done by attempting to stop the urinary stream while voiding.

Treatment of pelvic relaxation disorders
Many of the disorders of pelvic relaxation require surgical correction. These are elective surgeries and are usually deferred until after the childbearing years. Often the symptoms associated with the disorders are not severe enough to warrant surgical correction. In other cases, the stress of surgery is contraindicated because of other physical disorders; this is particularly true of older women in whom many of these disorders occur.

There are a number of surgical procedures for the conditions resulting from relaxation of pelvic support structures. Removal of the uterus through the vagina (vaginal hysterectomy) with appropriate repair of the vaginal wall (colporrhaphy) is often done in uterine prolapse accompanied by cystocele or rectocele. A vesicourethral suspension may be done to alleviate symptoms of stress incontinence.

In summary, structural defects of the female genitourinary system frequently occur as the result of weaknesses and relaxation of the pelvic floor and perineum. Retroversion of the uterus is a condition in which the uterus is tilted posteriorly; it is usually asymptomatic, and is found in about 20% of women. Cystocele and rectocele involve herniation of the bladder and rectum into the vagina. Uterine prolapse occurs when the uterus bulges into the vagina. Stress incontinence is the involuntary leaking of urine that occurs with coughing, sneezing, and other activities. Pelvic relaxation disorders frequently result from overstretching of the perineal supporting muscles during pregnancy and childbirth. The loss of elasticity of these structures, which is a normal accompaniment of aging, contributes to these problems.

Inflammations

Inflammations, including infections of the lower genitourinary tract (vulva, vagina, and cervix), are relatively common since this area is readily accessible to infectious organisms, and the moisture and warmth of these tissues provide an excellent environment for growth of pathogens.

The upper genitourinary tract (uterus, fallopian tubes, and ovaries) is less accessible to infectious organisms because a natural barrier is provided by the mouth of the cervix. Although infections of the upper genitourinary tract are less common, their sequelae are much more severe because of their proximity to the peritoneal cavity.

Vulvitis
Vulvitis, or inflammation of the vulva, is not a specific disease. It can develop consequent to local and

systemic disorders. For example, a monilial infection is frequently seen in diabetics. Vulvitis may be secondary to more serious vulvar diseases such as carcinoma and Paget's disease. A third example is the irritating drainage associated with vaginitis, which causes vulvar inflammation. Vulvitis may also be a component of a venereal disease or a local dermatitis. And finally, vulvar itching may be due to the atrophy that is a normal part of the aging process.

Treatment of vulvitis focuses on measures to relieve the irritation, such as keeping the area clean and dry. Harsh soaps and irritating agents should be avoided. Tight-fitting pantyhose and panty girdles provide a favorable environment for growth of microorganisms, and should not be worn. Hydrocortisone cream may give immediate relief of symptoms.

Bartholin cyst

A Bartholin cyst is not a true cyst; rather, it is an infection of the Bartholin gland due to a clogged duct. The obstruction most commonly follows a gonorrheal infection, but it also occurs with atrophic vaginitis. The cyst can attain the size of an orange (Fig. 31-5). These cysts are extremely tender and painful when acutely inflamed. Treatment consists of administration of appropriate antibiotics and excision of the intact cyst. If this is impossible due to edema and cellulitis, incision and drainage of the cyst are performed.

Vaginitis

Vaginitis is inflammation of the vagina, and is characterized by vaginal discharge, burning, itching, redness, and swelling of the vaginal tissues. There is often pain on urination and with sexual intercourse. Vaginitis may be caused by chemical irritants, foreign bodies, or infectious agents. The most frequent cause is infection due to Trichomonas (a flagellate), Monilia (a yeast or fungus infection), or Hemophilus (gram-negative bacillus). These infections are summarized in Table 31-1.

Normally, Döderlein's bacilli, a part of the normal flora of the estrogen-stimulated vaginal epithelium, produce lactic acid, which serves to maintain a low pH in the vaginal tissues. This low pH and the thick vaginal epithelium protect the vagina from invading organisms. However, if the normal vaginal physiology is disturbed by chemicals, antibiotics, douching, and so on, the defenses against pathogens decrease.

Every woman has a normal vaginal discharge during the menstrual cycle, but it should not cause

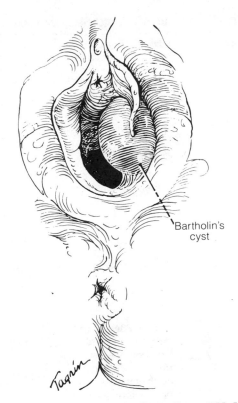

Figure 31–5. Bartholin's cyst. (From Green TH, Jr: Gynecology: Essentials of Clinical Practice, 3rd ed. Boston, Little, Brown & Co., 1977)

itching or burning, or have an unpleasant odor. Should these symptoms occur, they are suggestive of inflammation or infection.

Trichomoniasis. Trichomonas is a genus of one-celled protozoa, the trichomonads, which normally inhabit the vagina in small numbers and are innocuous. A change in the normal environment of the vagina may, however, foster an overgrowth of the organisms, resulting in symptomatic trichomoniasis. Trichomonads are harbored in the male urethra and prostate and can therefore be transmitted sexually. Symptoms of a trichomonal vaginitis include a profuse, thin, frothy, malodorous, and irritating discharge which ranges in color from yellow to yellow-gray to yellow-green. There is substantial vulvovaginal itching and burning. Diagnosis is made microscopically. Metronidazole (Flagyl) is given orally. If the woman is pregnant, Flagyl suppositories are used (after the first trimester) because of concern that the medication in oral form may be harmful to the fetus. Treatment is also

Table 31-1 Vaginal Infections: Symptoms and Treatment

Inflammation	Causative Organism	Symptoms	Precipitating Factors	Treatment
Trichomonas vaginitis	*Trichomonas vaginalis* (protozoan flagellate)	Copious, foul-smelling, profuse, yellow, frothy vaginal discharge; burning, itching, swelling, redness	Fatigue Pregnancy Systemic illness Transmitted sexually	Furazolidone-nifuroxime (Tricofuron); metronidazole (Flagyl) should not be used in early pregnancy; sexual partner should be treated
Monilial vaginitis	*Candida albicans* (fungus or yeast)	Mild to moderate thick white, cheesy, odorless discharge; burning, itching, swelling, redness	Oral contraceptives Pregnancy Antibiotic therapy Diabetes	Nystatin (Mycostatin); effective control of diabetes
Hemophilus vaginitis	*Hemophilus vaginalis* (gram-negative bacillus)	Foul-smelling (fishy), whitish-gray discharge; minimal inflammation	Transmitted sexually	Sulfathiazole, sulfacetamide, and benzolysulfanilamide (triple sulfa cream); ampicillin; metronidazole (Flagyl)
Atrophic vaginitis	Estrogen deficiency; inflammation and irritation due to thinned vaginal epithelium; secondary bacterial infection may exist	Vaginal discharge; bleeding; pruritus	Surgical removal of ovaries Menopause	Estrogen cream or suppositories; oral estrogen

indicated for the woman's sexual partner, since the organism is harbored asymptomatically in the man and reinfection is likely if he goes untreated.

Moniliasis or candidiasis.   Candidiasis, yeast infection, thrush, and moniliasis are all names for the vaginal inflammation caused by the fungus *Candida albicans*. These organisms are often present in healthy people. When the balanced relationship with other organisms is upset, clinically evident vaginitis may develop. Causes for the overgrowth of *Candida albicans* include (1) antibiotic therapy, which suppresses the normal bacterial flora; (2) high hormone levels due to pregnancy or use of an oral contraceptive, which cause an increase in vaginal glycogen stores and thus predispose to an overgrowth; and (3) diabetes mellitus, which increases the sugar levels in the vaginal mucosa and thus is a predisposing factor in overgrowth of the organisms. Symptoms include a thick, cheesy, odorless vaginal discharge with intense inflammation and burning. The diagnosis is confirmed microscopically. Fungicidal creams, ointments, and tablets such as miconidazole, nystatin, and candicidin are effective in treating moniliasis.

Hemophilus vaginitis.   This type of inflammation of the vagina is caused by the hemophilus bacterium.

Prior to 1955, when the organism was isolated, a vaginal discharge that did not show evidence of trichomonads or monilia was termed nonspecific vaginitis. It is now known that most cases of nonspecific vaginitis are caused by the hemophilus bacillus. The symptoms of hemophilus vaginitis include a profuse, grayish discharge that has an intense fishy odor. Burning, itching, and erythema are absent because the bacteria have only minimal inflammatory potential. Diagnosis is determined microscopically by the presence of "clue cells"— epithelial cells containing numerous bacilli. The most successful treatment of hemophilus vaginitis is with oral ampicillin, although intravaginal sulfonamide creams and suppositories can be used. Both sexual partners should be treated, because it is spread sexually.

Atrophic vaginitis.   Atrophic vaginitis is an inflammation of the vagina that occurs after menopause or removal of the ovaries and their estrogen supply. Estrogen deficiency inhibits growth of the vaginal epithelium, rendering these tissues more susceptible to infection and irritation. Furthermore, Döderlein's bacilli disappear, so that vaginal secretions become less acid. Symptoms of atrophic vaginitis include itching, burning, and painful intercourse.

These symptoms can usually be reversed with low doses of estrogen or local application of estrogen creams or vaginal suppositories.

Prevention and treatment

The treatment of vaginal infections centers around use of appropriate anti-infectives. Measures to promote healing and prevent reinfection include attention to hygiene, maintenance of a normal vaginal flora and healthy vaginal mucosa, and avoidance of contact with organisms known to cause vaginal infections. Many feminine deodorants and douches are irritating, and alter the normal vaginal flora. Tight clothing prevents dissipation of body heat and evaporation of skin moisture and thus promotes favorable conditions for the growth of pathogens as well as causing irritation. Nylon and other synthetic undergarments, pantyhose, and swimsuits tend to hold body moisture next to the skin and to harbor infectious organisms, even after they have been washed. Cotton undergarments that withstand hot water, and bleach (a fungicide) may be preferable for women who are bothered with such infections. Swimsuits and other garments that do not withstand hot water should be hung in the sunlight to dry.

Cervicitis

Acute cervicitis is due to Trichomonas and Candida and other organisms. *Chronic* cervicitis often affects parous women and follows long-term infection due to laceration of the cervix during childbirth. The bacteria become deeply embedded in the cervical glands and the surrounding stroma of the cervix, setting up an irritating alkaline vaginal drainage. The cervix becomes boggy and inflamed, somewhat resembling the picture of cervical cancer. Yellow-orange nodules, called nabothian cysts, and polyps may form in the cervical area.

Untreated cervicitis may extend to include development of pelvic cellulitis, giving rise to back pain, painful intercourse, and dysmenorrhea. Diagnosis of cervicitis is based on vaginal examination, colposcopy, cytologic smears, and biopsy. Cervicitis often resembles cancer of the cervix; it is important that this more serious disorder be ruled out prior to treatment. Treatment usually involves cryosurgery or cauterization, which causes the tissues to slough and thus leads to eradication of the infection.

Pelvic inflammatory disease

Pelvic inflammatory disease (PID) is an inflammation of the upper reproductive tract involving the uterus (endometritis), the fallopian tubes (salpingitis), and the ovaries (oophoritis). The most common cause of PID is untreated gonorrhea; the

organisms ascend through the endocervical canal to the endometrial cavity and then to the tubes and ovaries. The endocervical canal is slightly dilated during menstruation, thus bacteria can gain entrance to the uterus and other pelvic structures. Once inside the uterus, the gonococci multiply rapidly in the favorable environment of the sloughing endometrium.

Symptoms of PID include vaginal discharge followed by fever and abdominal pain during or just after a menstrual period. There is bilateral pelvic tenderness and an exquisitely painful cervix. Fever (102° to 103°F) and an elevated white blood cell count (20,000 to 30,000 per cu mm) are seen, even though the woman may not appear acutely ill. Treatment generally involves hospitalization with administration of antibiotics intravenously. Bed rest in Fowler's position (head and knees elevated) facilitates pelvic drainage.

Acute postabortal or puerperal infection accounts for some 15 to 20% of all cases of pelvic inflammatory disease. This type of PID differs from gonorrheal infection in its course, complications, and clinical manifestations, all of which are more serious and may be life threatening. This is because the gravid (pregnant) or postpartal uterus is extremely susceptible to infection, and the site of placental attachment with its rich vascular channels offers little protection against bacterial invasion, affording direct tissue penetration. Thus it is not uncommon for diffuse cellulitis (inflammation) and peritonitis to develop. Postabortal or puerperal PID is most often due to a mixed bacterial invasion, frequently by gram-negative bacteria (e.g., *E. coli*, Pseudomonas, Proteus, and Klebsiella). These highly virulent pathogens liberate their toxins in massive quantities, and absorption of the endotoxins results in generalized vasoconstriction, with pale, cold, and clammy skin, even though marked fever is present. Hemodynamic changes may eventually give rise to endotoxic shock with progressive renal, cardiac, hepatic, and pulmonary failure—possibly death. Clinically, there is high fever, rapid pulse, and shaking chills; the woman appears extremely ill. Pelvic pain is extreme and there is a purulent discharge from the cervix. The treatment of endotoxic (septic) shock is discussed in Chapter 14.

In summary, infection and inflammation can affect the female genitourinary tract. Vulvitis is an inflammation of the vulva, usually localized, sometimes developing as a secondary disorder in systemic diseases, such as diabetes and vulvar cancer. Vaginitis is an inflammation of the vagina caused by chemical irritants, the presence of foreign bodies, or infectious agents. The most frequent types of vaginal infection are trichomonas, monilial, and hemophilus vaginitis. Atrophic vaginitis results from an estrogen deficiency and occurs after menopause or removal of the ovaries. Cervicitis can occur as a primary infection with vaginitis, or secondarily from long-term infection following laceration of the cervix during childbirth. Pelvic inflammatory disease is a serious infection of the upper genitourinary system. It can result from a gonorrheal infection or occurs acutely following childbirth or abortion. Acute postabortal puerperal infections exert serious and widespread effects which can culminate in septic shock.

Benign Growths and Aberrant Tissue

In endometriosis, tissue closely resembling endometrial tissue occurs aberrantly—outside the uterus; in *adenomyosis*, islands of endometrial and stromal tissue are found inside the myometrium. In either case, the aberrant tissue undergoes cyclic proliferative and secretory changes similar to those of the normal endometrium. A *leiomyoma* is a benign tumor of smooth muscle of the uterine wall.

Endometriosis

Endometriosis is the condition in which functional endometrial tissue is found in ectopic sites outside the uterus. The site may be the ovaries, the broad ligaments, the pouch of Douglas (cul-de-sac), the pelvis, the vagina, the vulva, the perineum. Rarely, endometrial implants have been found in the nostrils, umbilicus, lungs, and limbs.

The cause of endometriosis is not known. There appears to have been an increase in incidence in the developed western countries during the past 4 to 5 decades. It is more frequent in women who have postponed childbearing and is consistent with the western trend of postponing childbearing and limiting family size. There are several theories that attempt to account for endometriosis. One theory suggests that menstrual blood containing fragments of endometrium is forced upward through the fallopian tubes into the peritoneal cavity. Another postulates that there are dormant, immature cellular elements that are spread over a wide area, persisting into adult life, and the ensuing metaplasia accounts for the endometrial tissue. Yet another theory suggests that the endometrial tissue may metastasize through the lymphatics or the vascular system.

The gross pathologic changes that occur in endometriosis differ as their location and duration. In the ovary, the endometrial tissue may form cysts that rupture, causing peritonitis and adhesions. Elsewhere in the pelvis, the tissue may take the form

of small lesions, called "mulberry spots," which are surrounded by scar tissue, and which cause intermittent bleeding into the gastrointestinal tract or urinary tract at the time of menses. If extensive, this fibrotic tissue may occasionally mimic carcinoma, and can cause bowel obstruction.

Endometriosis may be difficult to diagnosis because its symptoms mimic those of other pelvic disorders. Furthermore, the severity of symptoms does not always reflect the extent of the disease. The most frequent symptoms are infertility, abnormal bleeding, and pain prior to and during menstruation or during intercourse. Accurate diagnosis can be accomplished only through laparoscopy.

Treatment centers on three aspects: (1) pain relief, (2) hormone therapy, and (3) surgery. In young unmarried women, simple observation and analgesics may be the sole treatment. The use of hormones to induce physiologic amenorrhea is based on the observation that pregnancy affords temporary relief by inducing atrophy of the endometrial tissue. This is accomplished through administration of estrogen or progesterone preparations, which inhibit the pituitary gonadotropins and suppress ovulation. Surgical treatment involves total hysterectomy (removal of the uterus) and bilateral salpingo-oophorectomy (removal of the fallopian tubes and ovaries).

Adenomyosis

Adenomyosis is the condition in which endometrial glands and stroma are found within the myometrium interspersed between the smooth muscle fibers. In contrast to endometriosis, which is usually a problem of young, infertile women, adenomyosis is generally found in multiparous women who are in their late thirties or forties. It is thought that events associated with repeated pregnancies, deliveries, and uterine involution may cause the endometrium to be displaced throughout the myometrium. Adenomyosis has also been associated with vigorous and deep curettage (surgical scraping of the uterine cavity). Adenomyosis is associated with fibroids, endometrial polyps, and endometrial carcinoma.

The two common symptoms of adenomyosis are menorrhagia and dysmenorrhea which become progressively more severe. An enlarged uterus is common, too. There may also be dyspareunia, metrorrhagia, and a sensation of pelvic pressure or diffuse pelvic and lower abdominal pain.

For younger women who desire to preserve their childbearing potential, surgical resection of the affected areas with preservation of the uterus is a feasible treatment modality. For the older woman who has completed her family and has severe symptoms, total hysterectomy (with preservation of the ovaries if she is premenopausal) is the treatment preferred.

Leiomyomas

Leiomyomas are benign neoplasms of smooth muscle origin. They are also known as myomas or, colloquially, as "fibroids." They are the most common form of pelvic tumor and are believed to occur in one out of every four or five women above the age of 35. They are seen more often and their rate of growth is more rapid in black women than in white women. Leiomyomas usually develop in the corpus of the uterus; they may be submucosal, subserosal, or intramural (Fig. 31-6). *Intramural* fibroids are embedded within the myometrium. They are the most common form of fibroids, taking the form of a symmetrical enlargement of the nonpregnant uterus. *Subserosal* tumors are located beneath the surface of the uterus. They are recognized as irregular projections on the uterine surface; they may become pedunculated, displacing or impinging upon other genitourinary structures and causing hydroureter or bladder problems. Submucosal fibroids displace endometrial tissue and are more likely to cause bleeding, necrosis, and infection than either of the other types.

Leiomyomas may be manifested as follows: they may be asymptomatic and be discovered during a routine pelvic examination, or they may cause bleeding, particularly at the time of the menstrual period. Their rate of growth is variable, with often a rapid increase in size during pregnancy. These tumors may outgrow their blood supply, become infarcted, and undergo degenerative changes. Most fibroids regress with menopause, but if bleeding or other problems persist, hysterectomy may be required. Malignant transformations are rare.

Benign Ovarian Disorders

The ovaries have a dual function: they produce germ cells or ova, and they synthesize the female sex hormones. Therefore, disorders of the ovaries frequently cause menstrual and fertility problems. Benign conditions of the ovaries can present as primary lesions of the ovarian structures or as secondary disorders related to hypothalamic, pituitary, or adrenal dysfunction. Included in the latter group are functioning ovarian tumors, benign ovarian cysts, and the Stein-Leventhal syndrome.

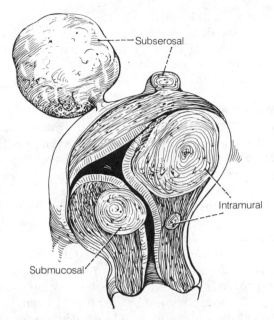

Figure 31–6.   Diagram of submucosal, intramural, and subserosal leiomyomas. (From Green TH, Jr: Gynecology: Essentials of Clinical Practice, 3rd ed. Boston, Little, Brown & Co., 1977)

Functioning ovarian tumors

Functioning ovarian tumors are of three types: estrogen-secreting, androgen-secreting, and mixed estrogen-androgen secreting. These tumors may be either benign or malignant. One such tumor, the *granulosa cell* tumor, is associated with *excess estrogen production*. When it develops during the reproductive period, the persistent and uncontrolled production of estrogen interferes with the normal menstrual cycle, causing irregular and excessive bleeding or amenorrhea and fertility problems. When it develops after menopause, it causes postmenopausal bleeding, stimulation of the glandular tissues of the breast, and other signs of renewed estrogen production. *Androgen-secreting tumors* inhibit ovulation and estrogen production. They tend to cause hirsutism and development of masculine characteristics, such as baldness, acne, oily skin, breast atrophy, and deepening of the voice.

Benign ovarian cysts

Cysts are the most common form of ovarian tumor. Many are benign. A follicular cyst is one that is due to occlusion of the duct of the follicle. Each month several follicles begin to develop and are blighted at various stages of development. These follicles may form cavities that fill with fluid, producing a cyst.

There may be bleeding into the cyst. This causes considerable discomfort, a dull aching sensation on the affected side. The cyst may become twisted, or may rupture into the intra-abdominal cavity. These cysts usually regress spontaneously.

Stein-Leventhal syndrome

Ovarian dysfunction associated with infrequent or absent menses in obese infertile women was first reported in the 1930s by Stein and Leventhal, for whom the syndrome was named. It is relatively rare and is sometimes called *polycystic ovarian disease*. However, the word "ovarian" is misleading in that the hypothalamic-pituitary hormones and the adrenal gland may be involved.

The syndrome is characterized by hirsutism, obesity, and infertility. It is usually recognized at puberty or soon after as the genitalia develop and the menses become irregular or are absent. There is bilateral ovarian enlargement. The condition is usually successfully treated by bilateral wedge resection of the ovaries. In other cases, fertility has been achieved by administration of the hypothalamic-pituitary stimulating drug clomiphene (Clomid). This drug is used with utmost caution because it can induce extreme enlargement of the ovaries.

In summary, there are a number of benign conditions other than structural changes and infections that affect the female genitourinary system. Endometriosis and adenomyosis are disorders of displaced endometrial tissue. In endometriosis the displaced tissue is located outside the uterus and in adenomyosis it is located within the uterine wall. Leiomyomas are benign smooth muscle tumors. They are often called fibroids when they are located in the uterine wall. Ovarian tumors are frequently functional, producing either female or male sex hormones. Benign ovarian cysts can result from accumulation of fluid within a follicle. The Stein-Leventhal syndrome is sometimes called polycystic ovarian disease. It is characterized by hirsutism, obesity, and infertility.

:Cancer

Significant changes in the frequencies of common gynecologic cancers have occurred in the United States between 1970 and 1980. Endometrial cancer is now the most commonly reported gynecologic cancer, with ovarian cancer reported second. Cervical cancer now ranks third, having ranked first until 1970. Clear-cell adenocarcinoma of the vagina, which was practically unheard of until the late 1960s,

has been reported with increasing frequency, most often associated with in utero exposure to diethylstilbestrol. Demographic changes, namely an increased survival rate of elderly women, have brought about increases in the incidence of some forms of cancer, while advances in chemotherapy and radiation therapy have shown improvement in cure rates of some gynecologic cancers.

Carcinoma of the Vulva

Carcinoma of the vulva accounts for about 5% of all malignancies of the female genitourinary system. This type of cancer is seen most frequently in women who are over age 60.

Over 95% of cancers of the vulva are squamous cell carcinomas.[3] The initial lesion often appears as an inconspicuous thickening of the skin, a small raised area or lump, or an ulceration that fails to heal. These lesions often resemble eczema or dermatitis, and may produce few symptoms other than pruritus, local discomfort, and exudation. Therefore, the symptoms are frequently treated with various home remedies before medical attention is sought. The lesion often becomes secondarily infected, and this causes pain and discomfort. Gradually the malignant lesion spreads superficially or as a deep furrow involving all of one labial side. Because there are many lymph channels around the vulva, the cancer metastasizes freely to the regional lymph nodes. It seems to make little difference whether the tumor is well differentiated or undifferentiated; lymph node metastases can occur in either case. The most common extension is to the superficial inguinal and femoral regions.

Early diagnosis is important in treatment of vulvar carcinoma. Because the lesion is often mistaken for other conditions, such as dermatitis, biopsy and treatment are often delayed. The five-year survival rate for women whose lesions are less than 3 cm in diameter is 60% to 80% following surgical treatment.[4] The five-year survival rate for those whose lesions are larger is only 10% following surgical treatment.

Carcinoma of the Vagina

Vaginal cancers are extremely rare. They account for about 1% of malignancies of the female reproductive system. About 90% of these are squamous cell carcinomas.[5]

A second type of vaginal cancer, adenocarcinoma, has been recently associated with maternal use of diethylstilbestrol (DES) to prevent abortion; this was common practice during a period of time which began in the 1940s.

In the late 1960s, eight cases of vaginal adenocarcinoma were reported in adolescents.[6] Investigation disclosed that the mothers of seven of the eight girls took DES, a nonsteroidal synthetic estrogen, during pregnancy.[7] A tumor registry of clear-cell adenocarcinoma of the genital tract in young women was established, and by 1979 close to 400 cases had been reported. About 60% of these women had definite prenatal exposure to DES. At the time of banning of DES, an estimated four million American women had taken the drug.

The incidence of clear-cell adenocarcinoma of the vagina is quite low, approximately 0.1% in young women who were exposed in utero to maternal synthetic estrogen. Although only a small percentage of estrogen-exposed girls actually develop clear-cell adenocarcinoma, 75 to 90% of them do develop benign adenosis of the vagina, or have a congenital anomaly of the cervix or vagina. Physicians emphasize that in these cases the incidence of other carcinomas is greatly increased. Thus the really significant damage stemming from DES exposure may be not vaginal adenocarcinoma, but rather another form of carcinoma, arising when the woman reaches middle age.

Although most women with vaginal adenocarcinoma have abnormal bleeding, 20% are asymptomatic, with the cancer being discovered during a routine pelvic examination. The tumor is most often detected on the upper anterior wall of the vagina, although it may be found at any cervical or vaginal site. Any DES-exposed girl should be encouraged to have semiannual gynecological examinations beginning at age 14, or at menarche. Examination should include careful inspection of the cervix and the vagina.

Treatment of vaginal adenocarcinoma must take into consideration the size, location, and spread of the lesion, and the patient's age. Radical surgery and radiation are both curative. In upper vaginal involvement, radical surgery includes a radical hysterectomy, pelvic lymph node dissection, and placement of a graft from the buttock to the area from which the vagina was excised. The ovaries are usually preserved unless they are diseased. Extensive lesions and those located in the middle or lower vaginal area are usually treated by radiation therapy. The prognosis depends on the stage of the disease, involvement of lymph nodes, and on the degree of mitotic activity of the tumor. The overall five-year survival rate is 30 to 60%.

Cancer of the Cervix

Fortunately, cervical cancer is the most readily detected and the most easily curable of all of the female reproductive system cancers—if detected early—the cure rate being 80 to 90%.[8] At present, however, because these measures are not being followed universally, the cure rate is only about 60%. Obviously there is a need for more widespread screening.

Cervical cancer is more frequent in women who have had many sexual experiences before age 20, who have had multiple sex partners, and who have had several or more children. All of these factors contribute to cervical lacerations and chronic cervicitis. It is more frequent, too, when the male sex partner is uncircumsised, although the reasons for this are not clear. A relationship between herpes virus II and cancer of the cervix has been suggested.[9] In one study, 23% of women with herpes II infection had either cervical dysplasia or cancer of the cervix.[10] Since this virus is spread by sexual contact, its association with cervical cancer provides a tempting hypothesis to explain the possible relationship between sexual practices and cervical cancer.

One of the most important advances in the early diagnosis and treatment of cancer of the cervix was made possible by the observation that this cancer arises from precursor cell changes, which begin with development of atypical cervical cells, with progression to cancer in situ and finally to invasive cancer of the cervix. Atypical cells differ from normal cervical squamous epithelium. There are changes in the nuclear and cytoplasmic parts of the cell, and more variation in cell size and shape (dysplasia). Cancer in situ is localized to the immediate area, whereas invasive cancer of the cervix is a cancer that spreads beyond the epithelial layer of the cervix. A system of grading and specific terminology has been devised to describe the dysplastic changes of cancer precursors.[11] This system involves use of the term cervical intraepithelial neoplasia (CIN). The CIN system grades according to changes in the epithelial thickness of the cervix: grade I involves one-third of the epithelial layer; grade II, one-third to two-thirds; and grade III, two-thirds to full thickness changes.

The atypical cellular changes that precede frank neoplasia can be recognized by a number of direct and microscopic techniques, including the Papanicolaou (Pap) smear. The precursor lesions can exist in a reversible form, which sometimes regresses spontaneously, or they may progress and undergo malignant change. Cancers of the cervix have a long latent period; the natural history of the disease indicates an average latent period of 8 to 30 years before it becomes invasive.[12] After the pre-invasive period, growth is rapid and, if untreated, death follows within 2 to 5 years.

Diagnosis: the Pap smear

The Pap smear was discussed in Chapter 7. The purpose of the Pap smear, or test, is to diagnose and detect the presence of any abnormal cells on the surface of the cervix. This test detects both precancerous and cancerous lesions. Although some clinicians suggest that the Pap test need not be done annually if there have been several normal tests in succession, other clinicians maintain that an annual test is the safest procedure to follow. If the woman has had a herpes infection, is a "DES daughter," or has a strong family history of cervical cancer, it has been suggested that yearly Pap smears be done.[13] There are several methods for classifying the Pap smear. One method divides the results into five classes:

Class I: Normal, or no abnormal cells
Class II: Atypical cells below the level of neoplasia
Class III: Contains abnormal cells typical of dysplasia
Class IV: Contains cells consistent with cancer in situ
Class V: Abnormal cells consistent with invasive squamous cell carcinoma

If the Pap smear shows precancerous or cancerous cells, a colposcopy is usually done. This is a vaginal examination with the colposcope, an instrument that affords a well-lighted and magnified stereoscopic view of the cervix. During colposcopy, staining of the cervical tissue with an iodine solution (Schiller's test) or other preparations may be done, and a biopsy, or removal of a tissue sample, may be made to evaluate changes in the layer structure of the tissue that covers the cervix.

Treatment

Early treatment of cervical cancer involves removal of the lesion by one of various techniques. If the biopsy reveals severe dysplasia, a conization is often performed. For this procedure, the woman is hospitalized and given a general anesthetic; a cone-shaped section of tissue is removed from the cervical opening. Many physicians, trained in the use of the colposcope, express the belief that conization is too radical a procedure. These physicians suggest that the scarring associated with this procedure can interfere with the ability to conceive and bear children, and they recommend the use of electrocautery,

cryosurgery, or laser beam. Cancer in situ is treated by conization, local excision, or hysterectomy. Depending upon the stage of involvement, invasive cancer of the cervix is treated with surgery (hysterectomy) and radiation.

Endometrial Cancer

Endometrial cancer is now becoming more common. There are two possible reasons for this increase in incidence. One is that endometrial cancer is primarily a disease of older women (peak age 55 to 65), with the increase in incidence reflecting a demographic shift, that is, an increase in the elderly population. A second factor is the circumstantial evidence that excessive estrogen stimulation causes endometrial cancer. Recently there has been a sharp rise in endometrial cancer reported in middle-aged women who have received estrogen therapy for menopausal symptoms. In fact, the majority of women who develop endometrial cancer have a history of circumstances that is consistent with exposure to abnormal hormone levels. These women often are obese or have diabetes and other evidence of endocrine disturbances, are hypertensive, have the Stein-Leventhal syndrome, or have a history of previous use of sequential birth control pills. Some are mothers who took DES during pregnancy; others took estrogen for menopausal symptoms, are nulliparous and infertile, or have had menstrual irregularities and ovulation failure, or have had breast cancer and have been treated with hormone therapy.

As with cervical cancer, it is believed that precancerous abnormalities in the endometrium precede endometrial cancer. These precancerous changes include endometrial hyperplasia or an abnormal pattern of growth in the cells that line the uterus. These cellular changes may be spontaneous or they may be linked to excessive exposure to exogenous estrogens. Hyperplasia often causes abnormal bleeding and spotting, and is usually diagnosed upon dilatation and curettage (D and C), which consists of dilating the cervix and scraping the uterine cavity.

The major initial symptom of endometrial cancer is abnormal painless bleeding. *Any postmenopausal bleeding is abnormal*, and may indicate endometrial cancer or its precursor stages. Because bleeding is such an early warning sign of the disease and because endometrial cancer tends to be rather slow-growing, particularly in its early stages, the chances of cure are good if prompt medical attention is sought. Later signs of uterine cancer include cramping, pelvic discomfort, postcoital bleeding, lower abdominal pressure, and enlarged lymph nodes. Although the Pap test is useful in detecting endometrial cancer, it is negative in approximately 25% of women with endometrial cancer.[14] Endometrial smears, obtained by direct aspiration of the uterine cavity, are far more accurate, with abnormal findings reported in 95 to 100% of women with endometrial cancer.[15] Endometrial biopsy, which can be done in the physician's office, is another method of diagnosis as is the D and C.

Early endometrial cancer is treated by total abdominal hysterectomy, with removal of the ovaries and fallopian tubes. If the cancer has reached advanced stages, where it is quite invasive, internal radiation by multiple small intrauterine radium or radioactive cobalt sources followed by surgery may be used. Metastatic disease is often treated with massive doses of the progestins.

Ovarian Cancer

Ovarian cancer is the third most common cause of cancer of the female genitourinary system. In 1979, it was estimated that ovarian cancer accounted for 24% of all female genitourinary cancers and 47% of all gynecological cancer deaths.[15] The incidence of ovarian cancer increases with age, being greatest in the 50- to 59-year age group. Ovarian cancer is difficult to diagnose, and 60% to 70% of women have metastatic disease prior to the time of diagnosis. Unfortunately, there are no screening or other early methods of detection for this form of cancer.

Cancers of the ovary are frequently asymptomatic, or the symptoms are so vague that the woman rarely consults her physician until the disease is far advanced. These vague discomforts include abdominal distress, flatulence, and bloating (especially after ingesting food). These gastrointestinal manifestations may precede other symptoms by months. Many women will take antacids or bicarbonate of soda for a time prior to consulting a physician. The physician may also dismiss the woman's complaints as being due to other conditions, causing a further delay in diagnosis and treatment. It is not fully understood why the initial symptoms of ovarian cancer are manifested by gastrointestinal disturbances. It is thought that biochemical changes in the peritoneal fluids may irritate the bowel, or that pain originating in the ovary may be referred to the abdomen and be interpreted as a gastrointestinal disturbance.

Cancer of the ovary is complex because of the diversity of tissue types originating in the ovary. As a result, there are a number of different types of ovarian cancers. These different cancers display various degrees of virulence depending on the type of tumor that is involved. A well-differentiated cancer of the ovary may have produced symptoms for many months and still be found operable at the time of surgery. On the other hand, a poorly differentiated tumor may have been clinically evident for only a few days, but found to be widespread and inoperable. There is often no correlation between the duration of symptoms and the extent of the disease.

Clinically evident ascites (fluid in the peritoneal cavity) is seen in about one-fourth of women with malignant ovarian tumors. This ascitic fluid is often aspirated for cytologic examination prior to surgery as a means of confirming the diagnosis of ovarian cancer. The treatment of ovarian cancer consists of surgical removal of the ovaries, fallopian tubes, and uterus. Radiation therapy and chemotherapy are used in conjunction with surgery.

The most hopeful prospect for early detection of ovarian cancer involves immunology. Immunologic diagnosis of subclinical ovarian cancer by means of identification of tumor-associated antigens in the serum awaits the methodology for isolating these antigens.

In summary, significant changes in the frequency of the various gynecologic cancers has occurred during the past 10 years. There has been an increased incidence of endometrial cancer. This form of cancer affects older women, and is associated with excessive estrogen stimulation of the endometrium, either from hormone therapy or as the result of endogenously produced estrogens. Vaginal cancer, which was practically unheard of before the 1960s, has been reported with increasing frequency, most often associated with in utero exposure to diethylstilbestrol. Cervical cancer is the most easily detected of the gynecologic cancers. It follows a predictable course of development involving precursor cell changes that can be identified through the Pap smear. If detected early, almost all cases of cervical cancer can be cured. Ovarian cancer, which produces few early symptoms, is the third leading cause of cancer deaths in women. At present, there are no screening tests for ovarian cancer.

:The Breast

Although anatomically separate, the breasts are functionally related to the female genitourinary system in that they respond to the cyclic changes in sex hormones and produce milk for infant nourishment. The breast also has importance because of sexual function and cosmetic appearance. Breast cancer

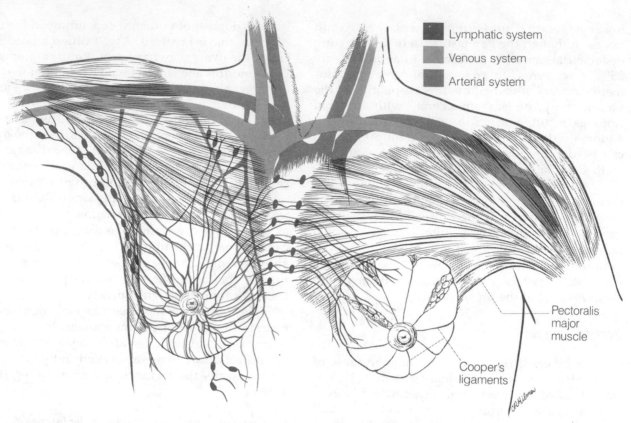

Figure 31–7. Diagram of the breasts showing the shared nerve, vascular and lymphatic supply, as well as the pectoral muscles.

represents one-fifth of all female malignancies. This high rate of breast cancer has drawn even greater attention to the importance of the breast throughout the lifespan.

Overall Structure

The breast or mammary tissue is located between the third and seventh ribs of the anterior chest wall, supported by the pectoral muscles and superficial fascia. Breasts are specialized glandular structures that have an abundant shared nerve, vascular, and lymphatic supply (Fig. 31-7). What we commonly call breasts are actually two parts of a single anatomical breast. It is this continuous nature of breast tissue that is important in both health and illness.

Structurally, the breast consists of fat, fibrous connective tissue, and glandular tissue. The superficial fibrous connective tissue is attached to the skin, a fact that is important in the visual observation of skin movement over the breast during breast self-examination. The breast mass is supported by the fascia of the pectoralis major and minor muscles and by the fibrous connective tissue of the breast. Fibrous tissue ligaments, called Cooper's ligaments,

extend from the outer boundaries of the breast to the nipple area in a radial fashion, like the spokes on a wheel (Fig. 31-7). These ligaments further support the breast and form septa that divide the breast into 15 to 25 lobes. Each lobe consists of grapelike lobules, or alveoli or glands, which are interconnected by ducts. The alveoli are lined with secretory cells capable of producing milk or fluid under the proper hormonal conditions (Fig. 31-8). The route of descent of milk and other breast secretions is from alveoli to duct, to intralobar duct, to lactiferous duct and reservoir, to nipple. Breast milk is produced secondary to complex hormonal changes associated with pregnancy. Fluid is produced and reabsorbed during the menstrual cycle. The breast responds to the cyclic changes in the menstrual cycle with fullness and discomfort.

The nipple is made up of epithelial, glandular, erectile, and nervous tissue. Areolar tissue surrounds the nipple and is recognized as the darker smooth skin between the nipple and the breast. The small bumps or projections on the areolar surface are Montgomery's tubercles, sebaceous glands that keep the nipple area soft and elastic. At puberty and dur-

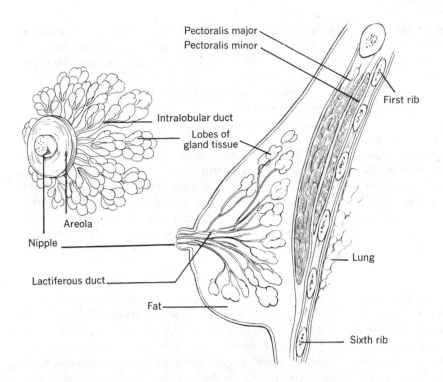

Figure 31–8.   Diagram of the breast showing the glandular tissue and ducts of the mammary glands. (From Chaffee EE, Lytle IM: Basic Physiology and Anatomy, 4th ed. Philadelphia, JB Lippincott, 1980)

ing pregnancy, increased levels of estrogen and progesterone cause the areola and nipple to become darker and more prominent and Montgomery's glands to become more active. The erectile tissue of the nipple is responsive to psychological and tactile stimuli, which contributes to the sexual function of the breast.

There are many individual variations in breast size and shape. The shape and texture vary with hormonal, genetic, nutritional, and endocrine factors, as well as with muscle tone, age, and pregnancy. A well-developed set of pectoralis muscles will support the breast mass higher on the chest wall. Poor posture, significant weight loss, and lack of support may cause the breast to droop.

Development

Men and women alike are born with rudimentary breast tissue, the ducts lined with epithelium. In women, the pituitary release of FSH, LH, and prolactin at puberty stimulates the ovary to produce and release estrogen. This estrogen stimulates the growth and proliferation of the ductile system. With the onset of ovulatory cycles, progesterone release stimulates the growth and development of ductile and alveolar secretory epithelium. By adolescence the breasts have developed characteristic fat deposition and contours.

Pregnancy

During pregnancy the breast is significantly altered by increased levels of both estrogen and progesterone. Estrogen stimulates increased vascularity of the breast as well as growth and extension of the ductile structures, causing "heaviness" of the breast. Progesterone causes marked budding and growth of the alveolar structures. The alveolar epithelium assumes a secretory state in preparation for lactation. The progesterone-induced changes that occur during pregnancy may confer some protection against cancer. Cellular changes that occur within the alveolar lining are thought to change the susceptibility of these cells to estrogen-mediated changes later in life.

Lactation

During lactation, milk is *secreted* by alveolar cells, which are under the influence of the anterior pituitary hormone prolactin. Milk *ejection* from the ductile system occurs in response to the release of posterior pituitary oxytocin. The stimulus for milk ejection occurs with the suckling of the infant. Suckling produces feedback to the hypothalamus, stimulating the release of oxytocin from the posterior pituitary. Oxytocin in turn causes contractile ejection of milk from the alveoli. A woman may have breast leakage for three months to a year after termination of breast feeding as breast tissue and hormones regress to the nonlactating state. Overzealous breast stimulation with or without pregnancy can likewise cause breast leakage.

Changes with Menopause

At onset of menopause, the levels of estrogen and progesterone are gradually reduced and the breasts regress secondary to the loss of glandular tissue. The lobular-alveolar structures disappear, leaving fat, connective tissue, and ducts. The breast generally becomes pendulous with the decrease in tissue mass.

Diseases of the Breast

Most breast disease may be described as being either benign or malignant. Breast tissue is never static; the breast is constantly responding to changes in hormonal, nutritional, psychological, and environmental stimuli which cause continual cellular changes. In light of this, strict adherence to a dichotomy of benign–malignant disease may not always be appropriate. However, this dichotomy is useful for the sake of simplicity and clarity.

Benign conditions

Benign breast conditions are nonprogressive. The specific conditions discussed in this chapter are mastitis, galactorrhea, ductal ectasia, intraductal papilloma, fibroadenoma, and fibrocystic disease.

Mastitis. Mastitis is an inflammation of the breast. It most frequently occurs during lactation, but may also result from other conditions.

In the lactating woman, inflammation results from an ascending infection that travels from the nipple to the ductile structures. The offending organisms originate from either the suckling infant's nasopharynx or the hands of the mother. During the early weeks of nursing, the breast is particularly vulnerable to bacterial invasion because of minor cracks and fissures that occur with vigorous suckling. Infection and inflammation cause obstruction of the ductile system, and the breast area becomes hard, inflamed, and tender if not treated early. Without treatment, the area becomes walled off and may abscess, requiring incision and drainage. Mastitis is not confined to the postpartum period, however; it can occur as a result of hormonal fluctuations, tumors, trauma, or skin infection. Cyclic inflammation of the breast occurs most frequently in adolescents who commonly have a fluctuating hormone level. Tumors may cause mastitis secondary to skin in-

volvement or lymphatic obstruction. Local trauma or infection may develop into mastitis because of ductal blockage of trapped blood, cellular debris, or extension of superficial inflammation.

Treatment for mastitis symptoms may include application of heat or cold, excision, aspiration, mild analgesia, and antibiotics.

Galactorrhea. Galactorrhea is the secretion of breast milk in a nonlactating breast. Galactorrhea may result from vigorous lovemaking, exogenous hormones, or internal hormonal imbalance. A pituitary tumor may produce large amounts of prolactin and cause galactorrhea. Galactorrhea occurs in both men and women and is usually benign.

Ductal ectasia. Ductal ectasia presents in older women as a spontaneous, intermittent, usually unilateral grayish-green nipple discharge. Palpation of the breast increases discharge. Ectasia occurs during or after menopause and is symptomatically associated with burning, itching, pain, and a pulling sensation of the nipple and areola. The disease results in inflammation of the ducts with subsequent thickening. Treatment requires removal of the involved ductal mass.

Intraductal papilloma. Intraductal papillomas are benign epithelial tissue tumors that range in size from 2 to 5 cm. Papillomas usually present with a bloody nipple discharge. The tumor may be palpated in the areolar area. The papilloma is probed via the nipple, and the involved duct thus removed.

Fibroadenoma. Fibroadenoma is seen in younger, premenopausal women. The clinical findings include a firm, rubbery, sharply defined round mass. On palpation the mass "slides" between the fingers and is easily movable. These masses are usually singular, with only 15% being multiple or bilateral. Fibroadenoma is asymptomatic and usually found by accident. Treatment involves simple excision.

Fibrocystic disease. Fibrocystic breast disease is a condition typified by the development of fibrosis and cystic tissue formation. It is the single most common disorder of the breast and accounts for over one-half of surgical procedures on the female breast.[16] The term "fibrocystic disease" has become a catch-all for breast irregularities that occur bilaterally, change cyclically, and in younger women are accompanied by dull aching pain and heaviness. Some clinicians believe that the term is overused and that the breast changes representative of the disorder are nothing more than the result of years of wear and tear. On the other hand, some clinicians believe that fibrocystic disease is a part of a continuum of breast pathology related to cancer.

Fibrocystic disease usually presents as nodular ("shotty"), granular breast masses that are more prominent and painful during the luteal or progesterone-dominant portion of the menstrual cycle. Discomfort ranges from heaviness to exquisite tenderness, depending upon the degree of vascular engorgement and cystic distention.

Treatment for fibrocystic breast disease is usually symptomatic. Aspirin, mild analgesics, and local heat or cold may be recommended. Some physicians attempt to aspirate prominent or persistent cysts and send any fluid obtained to the laboratory for cytologic analysis.

There is controversy regarding the relationship between fibrocystic disease and cancer of the breast. It appears that the catch-all term of fibrocystic disease encompasses several different disorders, some of which have a greater tendency to undergo malignant changes. Suffice it to say that any mass or lump on the breast should be viewed as possible carcinoma, and malignancy ruled out, before the conservative measures used to treat fibrocystic disease are employed.

Cancer

Cancer of the breast is the leading cause of death in women 40 to 44 years of age. One in eleven women in the U.S. will have breast cancer in her lifetime. Breast cancer strikes 109,000 American women every year and kills almost 36,000 women annually.[17]

Almost all breast cancers (90%) are found by women themselves, often through breast self-examination. Cancer may present clinically as a mass, a puckering, nipple retraction, or an unusual discharge. Some women identify cancer when only a thickening or subtle change in breast contour is noted. The various symptoms as well as the self-discovery rate of cancer support the need for regular, systematic self-examination.

Self breast examination (SBE) should be done routinely by everyone at risk. In the premenopausal woman, examination should be done 5 to 7 days after the cessation of menses. This time is most appropriate in relation to the cyclic breast changes in response to hormone levels. In postmenopausal women and in men, examination should be done at the same time, on the same day of every month. A woman can choose a day relative to her past menstrual history. Examination may conveniently be done in the shower or bath or at bedtime. The most important thing is to devise a regular, systematic, convenient, and consistent method of examination.

Risk of breast cancer

Women most at risk for breast cancer are menopausal; nulliparous; those who have had their first child after age 34; those who have a family history of breast cancer (particularly mothers and sisters); those who have had previous breast disease; those who have been exposed to radiation or carcinogenic agents; and those who work in a high-stress job and eat a high-fat diet.

Menopause and aging cause significant hormonally induced structural changes that are of even greater importance in relation to cancer risk if the woman has not borne a child before the age of 34. Pregnancy induces hormonal changes that cause apparently protective cellular changes as a result of estrogen opposition. First birth after age 34 does not confer this protection because of structural changes already existing in the breast after many years of estrogen dominance. Familial predisposition to cancer may be dietary, socioeconomic, genetic, or demographic. Stress and diet are capable of increasing endogenous estrogen levels by adrenal- and fat tissue-mediated biosynthesis. Prolonged, uninterrupted high-dose exposure to estrogens may induce cellular change that predisposes to breast cancer. Finally, extremely high doses of ionizing radiation can cause cancer. Individual risk is dependent upon accumulation of risk over time.

Paget's disease.   Paget's disease accounts for 2% to 3% of all breast cancers. The disease presents as an eczemoid lesion localized to the nipple and areola. Paget's disease is locally treated, but may indicate systemic disease. Systematic breast examination is therefore done in cases of Paget's disease, including mammogram and possibly biopsy.

Male breast cancer.   The number of men at risk for developing breast cancer is insignificant in relation to the risk to the female population. Seven hundred new cases of male cancer are discovered annually and 300 of these patients die annually. The man at risk is older, widowed, or divorced, and may have a history of estrogen use or endocrine imbalance. A man with a history of orchitis, orchiectomy, transsexuality, or Klinefelter's syndrome is also at risk.

Treatment of breast cancer

At present, the methods for treatment of breast cancer are controversial. Treatment may include surgery, chemotherapy, radiation, diet, or a combination of these therapies. There is considerable controversy regarding the value of a radical mastectomy as compared to simple excision of the tumor.

In summary, the breasts are functionally related to the genitourinary system in that they respond to cyclic stimulation by the female sex hormones and they provide nourishment for the infant. The breasts are subject to both benign and malignant disease. Mastitis is inflammation of the breast, occurring most frequently during lactation. Galactorrhea is an abnormal secretion of milk that may occur as a symptom of increased prolactin secretion. Both ductal ectasia and intraductal papilloma cause abnormal drainage from the nipple. Fibroadenoma and fibrocystic disease are characterized by abnormal masses in the breast which are benign. By far the most important disease of the breast is breast cancer, which is the leading cause of death in women. At present, breast self-examination affords a woman the best protection against breast cancer. It provides the means for early detection of breast cancer and in many cases allows for early treatment and cure.

:Study Guide

After you have studied this chapter, you should be able to meet the following objectives:

: : Relate the menstrual cycle to endocrine function.

: : Compare the symptoms of primary dysmenorrhea with those of secondary dysmenorrhea.

: : List the symptoms of toxic shock syndrome which the health professional should be able to recognize.

: : Describe the condition of uterine retroversion and its treatment.

: : Describe three types of dysfunction that may result from pelvic relaxation.

: : State the underlying problem related to stress incontinence.

: : Name three types of vaginitis and describe the treatment of each.

: : State measures to prevent vaginal infections which a health professional should convey to a client.

: : State the triad of organs involved in PID.

: : Describe the pathology involved in endometriosis on the basis of its location.

: : State the symptoms by which the health professional would be able to identify adenomyosis.

: : Compare intramural and subserosal leiomyomas.

: : State the underlying cause of functioning ovarian tumors.

: : Differentiate benign ovarian cyst from the Stein-Leventhal syndrome.

: : State one important prophylactic measure related to vulvar carcinoma.

: : Relate the association between use of diethylstilbestrol and vaginal carcinoma.

: : State a possible relationship between sexual practices and cervical cancer.

: : State the purpose of the "Pap" smear.

: : State the single most important factor in early detection of endometrial cancer.

: : State one reason why an ovarian cancer may be difficult to detect in an early stage.

: : Describe the anatomy of the female breast.

: : Describe the influence of hormones on breast development.

: : Explain the effects of estrogen and progesterone on the breast that occur during pregnancy.

: : Name and describe four or more benign disorders of the female breast.

: : Explain the importance of breast self-examination.

: : List some contributory factors in the development of breast cancer.

:References

1. Davis JP, Chesney PJ, Wand PJ, LaVenture M: Toxic shock syndrome. N Engl J Med 303(25):1429–1435, 1980
2. Shands KN et al: Toxic shock syndrome in menstruating women. N Engl J Med 303(25):1436–1442, 1980
3. Green TH: Gynecology, 3rd ed, pp 511, 539. Boston, Little, Brown and Company, 1977
4. McGowan L: Ovarian cancer: Improving survival. Hospital Medicine 15(10):6, 1979
5. Nolan T: Other neoplasms of the female genital tract. In Rubin P (ed): Clinical Oncology, 5th ed, p 127. Rochester, New York, The University of Rochester, 1978
6. Herbst AL, Alfelder H, Poskanzer D: Adenocarcinoma of the vagina: Association of maternal stilbestrol therapy with tumor appearance in young women. N Engl J Med 284(16):873–881, 1971
7. Welch WR et al: Pathology of prenatal diethylstilbestrol exposure. Pathol Annu 13 (Part 1):201, 1978
8. Facts on Uterine Cancer. American Cancer Society, 1978
9. Wilbanks GD: The role of herpes virus in cancer of the cervix. Obstet Gynecol Annu 5:305–329, 1976
10. Nahimias AJ, Roizman B: Infections with herpes simplex I and II. N Engl J Med 289:667, 719, 781, 1973

11. Richart RM: Cervical intraepithelial neoplasia. Pathol Annu 8:301–328, 1973
12. Behrman SJ: The annual Pap smear: Justifiable. Hosp Pract 16(3):10, 1981
13. Cancer Facts and Figures 1981, p 16. American Cancer Society, 1981
14. Greene TH: Gynecology, p 454. Boston, Little, Brown and Company, 1977
15. Barber HRK: Ovarian Cancer, p 4. American Cancer Society, 1978
16. Robbins SL, Cotran RS: Pathologic Basis of Disease. 2nd ed, p 1310. Philadelphia, WB Saunders, 1979
17. Facts on Breast Cancer. American Cancer Society, 1978

:Suggested Readings

Books

Barber HK: Ovarian Carcinoma Etiology, Diagnosis and Treatment. Masson Publishing, 1978
Barber HK, Fields DH, Kaufman SA: Quick Reference to OB–GYN Procedures. Philadelphia, JB Lippincott, 1979
Burke L, Mathews B: Colposcopy in Clinical Practice. Philadelphia, FA Davis, 1978
DiSala PJ, Creasman WT: Clinical Gynecologic Oncology. London, CV Mosby Company, 1981
Garrey MM, Govan ADT, Hodge C, Callander R: Gynaecology Illustrated. New York, Churchill Livingstone, 1978
Gray LA: Endometrial Carcinoma and Its Treatment. Springfield, Illinois, Charles C Thomas, 1977
Gusberg SB, Frick HC: Gynecologic Cancer. Baltimore, Williams and Wilkins, 1978
Hafez ESE, Evans TN: The Human Vagina. New York, North–Holland Publishing, 1978
Kistner RW: Gynecology, Principles and Practice. Chicago, Year Book Medical Publishers, 1979
Kobayashi M: Ultrasonography in Obstetrics and Gynecology. New York, Igaku–Shoin, 1980
Martin LL: Health Care of Women. Philadelphia, JB Lippincott, 1978
McGowan L: Gynecologic Oncology. New York, Appleton–Century–Crofts, 1978
Parsons L, Sonmers S: Gynecology. Philadelphia, WB Saunders, 1978
Pritchard J, MacDonald PC: Williams Obstetrics. New York, Appleton–Century–Crofts, 1976
Sloane E: Biology of Women. New York, John Wiley and Sons, 1980

Periodicals

Allen WM, Wolf RB: Ovarian resection in the Stein–Leventhal syndrome. Obstet Gynecol 33:569–573, 1969
Ballard P: Menstrual disorders in adolescence. Comprehensive Pediatric Nursing 2:21–33, 1978
Benedict J: Update on toxic shock syndrome. Perinatal Press 83–85, 1980

Briggs RM: High prevalence of cervical dysplasia in STD clinic patients warrants routine cytologic screening. Am J Public Health 70:1212–1214, 1980
Cervical cancer screening: The Pap smear. Consensus Development Conference Summaries 3:27–31, 1970
Cooperman AM, Esselstyn CB: Breast cancer: An overview. Surg Clin North Am 58(4):659, 1978
Crile G: Axioms on cysts and benign tumors of the breast. Hospital Medicine 13(5):56, 1977
The feminine condition: Diagnostic challenge to the physician. Emergency Medicine 11:214–218, 1979
Gelms J: Vulvar carcinoma: Pre-, intra- and post-operative care. Point View 17:14–16, 1980
Gever LN: From arthritis pain to dysmenorrhea: A new indication for prostaglandin inhibitors. Nursing 80, 101:81, 1981
Gollober M: Cervical cancer screening. Nurse Pract 4:17–18, 1979
Greenblatt RB: Estrogen replacement therapy? Yes. Patient Care 13:23–25, 1979
Jick H et al: The epidemic of endometrial cancer: A commentary. Am J Public Health 70:264–267, 1980
Kapp D, Schwartz P: Gynecologic oncology: Cancer update II. Conn Med 44(9):557, 1980
A late treatment for dysmenorrhea prostaglandin inhibitors. Emergency Medicine 12:138, 1980
Latinis B: Women's health care update. Nurse Pract 4:36–37, 1979
McCann J: New fine needle aspiration use: Pelvic diagnosis. Medical News and International Report 5(4), 1981
McGowan L: Ovarian cancer: Improving survival. Hospital Medicine 15:6–7, 1979
McGuire LS: Chronic vaginitis masking serious affective disorders. JOGN Nursing, 7:13–16, 1978
More on DES-related cancer. Nurses' Drug Alert 3:139, 1979
Prilook ME (ed): Hysterectomy: For whom, when, how? Patient Care 14:16–17+, 1980
Reed B, Singer A, Coppleson M: Sperm basic proteins in cervical cancer: Correlation with social class. Lancet 2:60, 1978
Ruzek SK: Emergent modes of utilization: Gynecological self-help. Nursing Dimensions 7:73–77, 1979
Roberts SJ: Dysmenorrhea. Nurse Pract 5:9–10, 1980
Sacks SR (ed): Put colposcopy to work for you? Patient Care 13:124–130, 1979
Schwartz P, Kapp P: Gynecologic oncology: Cancer update. Conn Med 44(8), 1980
Singer A: Further evidence for high risk male and female groups in the development of cervical cancer. Obstet Gynecol Surv 34:867–878, 1979
Singer A, Reed B, Coppleson M: A hypothesis: The role of high risk male in the etiology of cervical cancer. Am J Obstet Gynecol 126:110, 1976
Townsend DE, Rickert RM, Marks E, Nelson J: Invasive cancer following outpatient evaluation and therapy for cervical disease. Obstet Gynecol 57(2):145–149, 1981

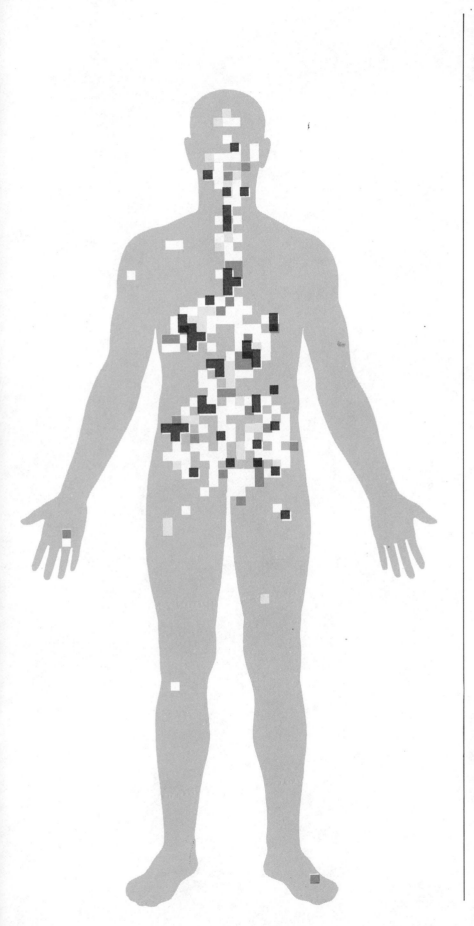

Alterations in Endocrine Function, Metabolism, and Nutrition

Body function is dependent upon energy from metabolism of carbohydrates, proteins, and fats that are derived from foodstuffs consumed in the daily diet. While it is the cardiorespiratory system that provides the oxygen needed for cell metabolism, it is the gastrointestinal tract in concert with the endocrine system that regulates the supply and utilization of metabolic fuels. The gastrointestinal tract provides the means whereby nutrients, vitamins, and minerals needed for growth, cell replacement, and body metabolism gain access to the confines of the body's internal environment. Within these confines, the endocrine system acts in regulating metabolism and is involved in all of the other integrative aspects of life including growth, sex differentiation, and adaptation to an ever-changing external environment. This unit is divided into three main parts: 1) control and alterations in function of the endocrine system, 2) control of metabolism and diabetes mellitus, and 3) control of gastrointestinal function and alterations in gastrointestinal, hepatobiliary, and pancreatic function.

32

Control of Endocrine Function

The endocrine system is involved in all of the integrative aspects of life, including growth, sex differentiation, metabolism, and adaptation to an ever-changing environment. This chapter focuses on general aspects of endocrine function, organization of the endocrine system, hormone receptors and hormone actions, and regulation of hormone levels.

:Overview of the Endocrine System

Hormones are generally thought of as *chemical messengers* that are transported in body fluids. Although the endocrine system was once thought to consist solely of what has come to be termed the *classic endocrine system*, which consists of discrete *endocrine glands*, it is now known that there are a number of other chemical messengers that modulate body processes.

Hormones of the classic endocrine system are synthesized by endocrine glands, secreted into the *bloodstream*, and then transported to distant sites, or *"target cells,"* where they exert their action. The *neuromediators*, such as acetylcholine and the catecholamines (epinephrine, norepinephrine, and dopamine), are also chemical mediators that are *synthesized by nerve cells* and *released from nerve endings*.

A number of hormonal peptides have now been identified; these *peptides* are produced by what is sometimes referred to as the *diffuse endocrine system*. Unlike the well-defined glands of the classic endocrine system, the diffuse endocrine system is dispersed throughout various organs and cells and is intermingled with nonendocrine cells.[1] There is still a great deal of mystery surrounding these hormonal peptides. A number of them have been found in both brain and peripheral tissues and their wide range of actions suggests that they act locally in a number of ways, depending on the tissues that they serve. Perhaps the most interesting of these peptides are the recently publicized endorphins and enkephalins.

The *endorphins* and *enkephalins* are endogenous morphine-like peptides that are found in many areas of the body including the pituitary gland, other areas of the brain, the gastrointestinal tract, and the blood. There is evidence that these peptides are derived from a larger prohormone *beta-lipotrophin*. Beta-endorphin corresponds to the 61-91 amino acid sequence of this molecule and is reported to be 5 to 10 times as potent as morphine.[2] Enkephalin corresponds to amino acid sequence 61-65. The endorphins, which are mainly distributed in the central nervous system, are thought to be involved in the perception of pain and the emotions. The enkephalins have been found throughout the gastrointestinal tract, particularly in the antrum of the stomach and the upper duodenum. Thus, like opiates which are used in the treatment of diarrhea, it seems likely that the enkephalins may be involved in controlling gastrointestinal motility as well as pain.

Indirect evidence of the *morphine-like activity (morphomimetic)* of the endorphins and enkephalins can be demonstrated in the laboratory using bioassay techniques. One method utilizes the guinea pig ileum to compare the action of endorphins with that of morphine. A substance is defined as morphomimetic if it (1) causes reduction in the amplitude of induced muscle contraction of the guinea pig ileum, and (2) if the effect can be reversed or prevented by the morphine antagonist, naloxone.[2] At present, the research related to the endorphins and enkephalins is still in the early stages and the effect that these peptides exert on the overall function of the body in still speculative.

Another group of chemical messengers are the *prostaglandins*, which modulate the action of hormones and neuromediators. The prostaglandins are liberated from the *membrane phospholipids* of many different types of cells in response to stimulation by hormones, neuromediators, immunologic reactions, and physical and chemical agents. There are several different prostaglandins and, although they are similar, there are subtle differences that are related to the tissues from which they arise. The actions of the prostaglandins differ with the tissue of origin. They are known to cause contraction of the uterus and gastrointestinal tract smooth muscle, and to produce dilatation of the bronchiole and vascular smooth muscle. They inhibit the secretion of gastric acid, control platelet aggregation, and mediate many inflammatory responses.

Function of Hormones

Hormones *do not initiate reactions*; rather they are *modulators of body and cellular responses*. Most hormones are *present in the blood at all times*—but in greater or lesser amounts depending on the needs of the body. Hormones can produce either a *generalized* or a *localized effect*. For example, antidiuretic hormone (ADH) acts selectively on the distal tubules and collecting ducts of the kidney, whereas epinephrine affects the function of many body systems. Table 32-1 lists the major functions and sources of body hormones.

Table 32-1 Functional Classification of Hormones

Function	Hormone	Major Source
Control of water and electrolyte metabolism	aldosterone	adrenal cortex
	antidiuretic hormone (ADH)	posterior pituitary
	calcitonin	C cells, thyroid
	parathyroid hormone	parathyroid
	angiotensin	kidney
Control of gastrointestinal function	cholecystokinin	gastrointestinal tract
	secretion	gastrointestinal tract
Regulation of energy, metabolism, and growth	glucagon	A cells, pancreatic islets
	insulin	B cells, pancreatic islets
	growth hormone	anterior pituitary
	somatomedin	liver?
	somatostatin	hypothalamus, CNS, pancreatic islets
	thyroid hormones	thyroid gland
Neurotransmitters	dopamine	CNS
	epinephrine	adrenal medulla
	norepinephrine	adrenal medulla and CNS
Reproductive function	chorionic gonadotropins	placenta
	estrogens	ovary
	oxytocin	posterior pituitary
	progesterone	ovary
	prolactin	anterior pituitary
	testosterone	testes
Stress and control of inflammation	glucocorticoids	adrenal cortex
Tropic hormones (regulation of other hormone levels)	adrenocorticotropic hormone (ACTH)	anterior pituitary
	follicle stimulating hormone (FSH)	anterior pituitary
	luteinizing hormone (LH)	anterior pituitary
	thyroid stimulating hormone (TSH)	anterior pituitary

Rate of Hormone Reaction

Hormones react at different rates. The neurotransmitters, such as epinephrine, have a reaction time of milliseconds. Thyroid hormone, on the other hand, requires days for its effect to occur. Hormones are continually being metabolized, or inactivated, and removed from the body. The *half-life* of a hormone is the time that it takes for the body to reduce the concentration of the hormone by one-half.

Hormone Receptors

Hormones exert their action by *binding to specific receptor sites* that are located on the surfaces of the target cells. The structure of these receptors varies in a manner that allows target cells to respond to one hormone and not to others. For example, receptors on the thyroid are specific for the thyroid-stimulating hormone, while receptors on the gonads respond to the gonadotropic hormones.

The response of a target cell to the action of a hormone will vary with the number of receptors that are present and with the affinity of these receptors

for hormone binding. There are a *number* of factors that influence the number of receptors that are present on target cells and their *affinity* for hormone binding (Fig. 32-1).

The number of hormone receptors on a cell may be altered for any of several reasons. Antibodies may destroy the receptor proteins. Obesity has been shown to cause a decrease in the number of insulin receptors that are present on fat cells, and it is speculated that this may influence impaired glucose tolerance in the obese noninsulin dependent diabetic. On the other hand, it has been shown that the oral hypoglycemic drugs, the sulfonylureas, cause an increase in the number of insulin receptors on body cells.

The affinity of receptors for binding of hormones is also affected by a number of conditions. For example, the pH of the body fluids plays an important role in the affinity of insulin receptors. In ketoacidosis, the lowering of the pH from 7.4 to 7.0 decreases insulin binding by about one-half.[3]

There are two ways in which hormone–receptor interactions go about the process of modulating cell activity. One type of response occurs with the pep-

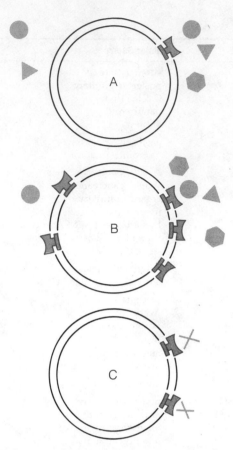

Figure 32–1. (*A*) Diagram showing the role of cell-surface receptors in mediating the action of hormones. Hormone action is affected by the number of receptors that are present (*B*) and by the affinity of these receptors for hormone binding (C).

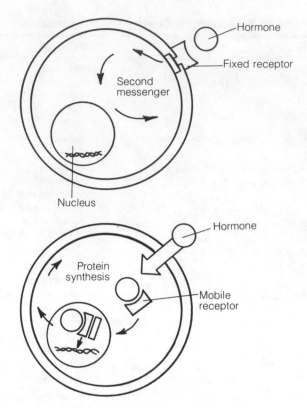

Figure 32–2. Diagram of the two types of hormone–receptor interactions.

tide hormones, which circulate in the blood in their free state. These hormones interact with *fixed membrane receptors* in a manner that incites the release of a *second messenger* (usually cyclic AMP), which in turn activates a series of enzyme reactions that serve to alter cell function (Fig. 32-2). Glucagon, for example, incites glycogen breakdown by way of the second messenger system. Table 32-2 lists hormones that act by the two types of receptors.

A second type of receptor mechanism is involved in mediating the action of hormones, such as the steroids and the thyroid hormones, which are transported in body fluids attached to carrier proteins (Fig. 32-2). These hormones, being lipid soluble, pass freely through the cell membrane and then attach to an intracellular "mobile" receptor in the cytoplasm of the cell. This hormone–receptor complex moves through the cytoplasm, becomes activated, and enters the nucleus where it causes

Table 32–2 Hormone–Receptor Interactions

Fixed Messenger Interactions

Glucagon

Insulin

Epinephrine

Parathyroid hormone

Thyroid-stimulating hormone

Adrenocorticotropic hormone

Follicle-stimulating hormone

Luteinizing hormone

Antidiuretic hormone

Secretin

Mobile Hormone–Receptor–Nuclear Interactions

Estrogen

Testosterone

Progesterone

Adrenal cortical hormones

Thyroid hormone

activation of repression of gene activity with subsequent production of messenger RNA and protein synthesis.

Control of Hormone Levels

Hormone secretion varies widely over a 24-hour period. Some hormones, such as growth hormone and adrenocorticotropic hormone (ACTH), have diurnal fluctuations that vary with the sleep–awakening cycle. Others, such as the female sex hormones, are secreted in a complicated cyclic manner. Levels of hormones like insulin and antidiuretic hormone (ADH) are regulated by the amount of organic and inorganic substances present in the body.

Levels of many of the hormones are regulated by feedback mechanisms that involve the hypotha-

Figure 32–3.   Diagram of the hypothalamus and the anterior and posterior pituitary. Hypothalamus releasing or inhibiting hormones are transported to the anterior pituitary via the portal vessels. ADH and oxytocin are produced by nerve cells in the supraoptic and paraventricular nuclei of the hypothalamus and then transported through the nerve axon to the posterior pituitary where they are released into the circulation. (From Chaffee EE, Greisheimer EM: Basic Physiology and Anatomy, 3rd ed. Philadelphia, JB Lippincott, 1974)

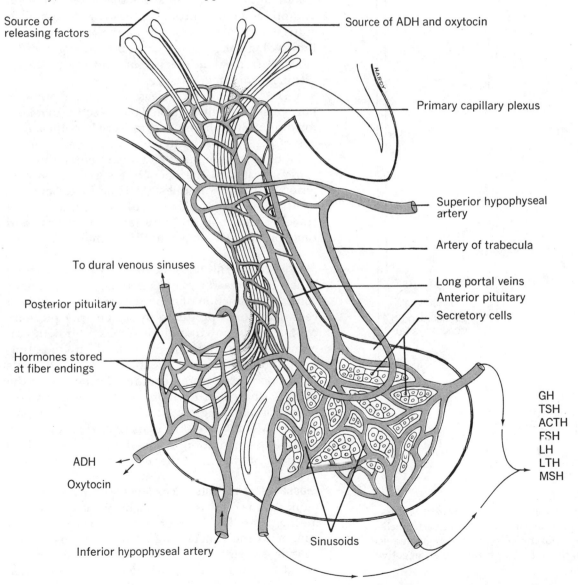

Source of releasing factors

Source of ADH and oxytocin

Primary capillary plexus

Superior hypophyseal artery

Artery of trabecula

To dural venous sinuses

Long portal veins

Posterior pituitary

Anterior pituitary

Secretory cells

Hormones stored at fiber endings

GH
TSH
ACTH
FSH
LH
LTH
MSH

ADH

Oxytocin

Inferior hypophyseal artery

Sinusoids

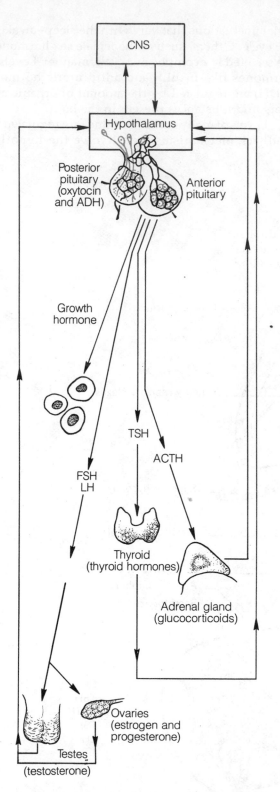

Figure 32–4. Control of hormone production by hypothalamic–pituitary–target cell feedback mechanism. Hormone levels from the target glands regulate release of hormones from the anterior pituitary via a negative feedback system.

lamic–pituitary–target cell system. Other hormones are regulated by blood levels of organic and inorganic substances.

Hypothalamic-pituitary regulation

Because the integration of body function relies on input from both the nervous system and the endocrine system, it seems logical that input from the nervous system would participate in regulation of hormone levels. In this respect, the hypothalamus and the pituitary (hypophysis) act as an integrative link between the central nervous system and the many endocrine-mediated functions of the body. These two structures are connected by the hypophyseal portal system, which begins in the hypothalamus and drains into the anterior pituitary gland, and by the nerve axons that connect the supraoptic and paraventricular nuclei of the hypothalamus with the posterior pituitary gland (Fig. 32-3). Embryologically, the anterior pituitary gland developed from glandular tissue and the posterior pituitary from neural tissue.

The synthesis and release of anterior pituitary hormones is largely regulated by the action of releasing or inhibiting hormones from the hypothalamus. It is at the level of the hypothalamus that emotion, pain, body temperature, and other neural input are communicated to the endocrine system. The posterior pituitary hormones, ADH and oxytocin, are synthesized in the cell bodies of the nerve axons that travel to the posterior pituitary. The release and function of ADH are discussed in Chapter 22.

Anterior pituitary gland. The pituitary gland has been called the "master gland" because its hormones control the function of a number of target glands or cells. Hormones produced by the anterior pituitary control body growth and metabolism (growth hormone), function of the thyroid gland (thyroid-stimulating hormone), glucocorticoid hormone levels (adrenocorticotropic hormone), function of the gonads (follicle-stimulating and luteinizing hormone), and breast growth and milk production (prolactin). Melanocyte-stimulating hormone, which controls pigmentation of the skin, is produced by the pars intermedia of the pituitary.

Feedback mechanisms. The level of many of the hormones in the body is regulated by negative feedback mechanisms. The function of this type of system is similar to the functioning of the thermostat in a heating system. In the endocrine system, sensors detect a change in the hormone level and adjust hormone secretion so that body levels are maintained within an appropriate range; i.e., when the sensors detect a decrease in hormone levels, they initiate changes that cause an increase in hormone production, and when hormone levels rise above the set-point of the system, the sensors cause hormone production and release to decrease. For example, an increase in thyroid hormone is detected by sensors in the hypothalamus or anterior pituitary gland, and this causes a reduction in the secretion of thyroid-stimulating hormone with a subsequent decrease in the output of thyroid hormone from the thyroid gland. The feedback loops for the hypothalamic–pituitary feedback mechanisms are illustrated in Figure 32-4. Exogenous forms of hormones (given as drug preparations) can influence the normal feedback control of hormone production and. release. One of the most common examples of this influence occurs with administration of the adrenal cortical hormones, which cause suppression of the hypothalamic–pituitary–target cell system that regulates the production of these hormones.

In summary, the endocrine system acts as a communications system that uses chemical messengers, or hormones, for transmission of information from cell to cell and from organ to organ. Hormones act at the level of the cell membrane, which has surface receptors that are specific for the different types of hormones. Many of the endocrine glands are under the regulatory control of other parts of the endocrine system. The hypothalamus and the pituitary gland form a complex integrative network that joins the nervous system and the endocrine system, and it is this central network that controls the output from many of the other glands in the body.

:Study Guide

After you have studied this chapter, you should be able to meet the following objectives:

: : Compare the classic endocrine system with the diffuse endocrine system.

: : Describe the role of the endorphins and the enkephalins as it is currently understood.

: : State the function of the prostaglandins.

: : State a general description of hormone function.

: : Explain the variations that may occur in the number of hormone receptors on a cell.

: : Describe the mechanisms of hormone-receptor interactions.

: : Explain how the negative feedback mechanisms regulate hormone levels.

:References

1. Polak JM, Path MRC, Bloom SR: Neuropeptides of the gut: A newly discovered major control system. World J Surg 3:393–406, 1979
2. Guillemin R: Beta-lipotropin and endorphins: Implications of current knowledge. Hosp Pract 13(11):54, 1978
3. Kahn CR: Probing receptor activity in cell control. Patient Care 13(1):84, 1979

33

Alterations in Endocrine Function

Disorders of endocrine function are generally characterized by a disturbance in hormone production or by an alteration in the body's response to a particular hormone. In addition to discussing the general aspects of endocrine dysfunction, this chapter focuses on disorders of growth hormone, adrenal corticosteroid hormones, and thyroid hormone. Content related to other endocrine disorders has been integrated into other sections of the book, and the reader is referred to the index for rapid location of this material.

:General Aspects of Altered Endocrine Function

Disturbances of endocrine function can usually be divided into two categories: hypofunction and hyperfunction.

Hypofunction of an endocrine gland can occur for a variety of reasons. Congenital defects can result in absence or impaired development of the gland or the absence of an enzyme needed for hormone synthesis. Destruction of the gland may occur due to disruption in blood flow, infection or inflammation, autoimmune responses, or neoplastic growth. There may be a decline in function with aging, or the gland may atrophy as the result of drug therapy or for unknown reasons. Some endocrine-deficient states are associated with receptor defects: hormone receptors may be absent; the receptor binding of hormones may be defective; or the cellular responsiveness to the hormone may be impaired. It is suspected that in some cases a gland may produce a biologically inactive hormone, or that an active hormone may be destroyed by circulating antibodies before it can exert its action.

Hyperfunction is generally associated with excessive hormone production. This can result from excess stimulation and hyperplasia of the endocrine gland or from a hormone-producing tumor of the gland. Sometimes an ectopic tumor will produce too much hormone, for example, certain bronchogenic tumors which produce hormones such as antidiuretic hormone (ADH) and adrenocorticotropic hormone (ACTH).

Endocrine disorders can generally be divided into two groups—primary disorders and secondary disorders. *Primary defects* in endocrine function originate within the target gland responsible for producing the hormone. In *secondary disorders* of endocrine function, the target gland is essentially normal, but its function is altered by defective levels of stimulating hormones or releasing factors from the hypothalamic–pituitary system. For example, adrenalectomy produces a *primary deficiency* of adrenal corticosteroid hormones. Removal or destruction of the pituitary gland, on the other hand, eliminates ACTH stimulation of the adrenal cortex and brings about a *secondary deficiency*.

There are a number of techniques for assessing endocrine function and hormone levels. One technique *measures the effect of a hormone* on body function. Measurement of blood glucose, for example, reflects insulin levels and is an *indirect method* of assessing insulin availability. Another technique, the *bioassay*, measures the effect of a hormone on animal function. A bioassay can be done using the intact animal or a portion of tissue from the animal. At one time, female rats or male frogs were used to test women's urine for the presence of human chorionic gonadotropin, which is produced by the placenta during pregnancy. Today, the most widely used technique for measuring hormone levels is the *radioimmunoassay*. This method uses a radiolabeled form of the hormone and a hormone antibody that has been prepared by injecting an appropriate animal with a purified form of the hormone. The unlabeled hormone in the sample being tested competes with the radiolabeled hormone for attachment to the binding sites of the antibody. Measurement of the radiolabeled hormone–antibody complex then provides a means of arriving at a measure of hormone level in the sample. Since hormone binding is competitive, the amount of radiolabeled hormone–antibody complex that is formed will decrease as the amount of unlabeled hormone in the sample is increased.

:Growth Hormone

Growth hormone (GH), sometimes called somatotropin, is a single peptide that contains 191 amino acids. It induces growth of all tissues that are capable of growing, enhances protein synthesis in all cells of the body, increases the mobilization and utilization of fatty acids, and decreases glucose utilization. The secretion of GH fluctuates over a 24-hour period. Its levels are normally increased (1) during deep sleep, (2) in hypoglycemia and starvation, (3) with increases in blood levels of amino acids (particularly arginine), and (4) following trauma, excitement, and heavy exercise.

Growth hormone exerts an indirect effect on skeletal growth by stimulating the production of several small proteins collectively called *somato-medin*. Although the source of somatomedin is uncertain, it is thought to be produced in the liver and to a lesser extent in the kidney and skeletal muscle. Somatomedin is required for growth of cartilage and bone, and without its presence, growth of the long bones will not occur.

Growth hormone exerts many effects on metabolism and, contrary to what has been believed in the past, GH is produced throughout life. Growth hormone facilitates protein synthesis; it enhances the transport of amino acids through the cell membrane in a manner similar to that involved in insulin-mediated transport of glucose. Growth hormone also decreases the breakdown of cell proteins, and enhances RNA synthesis and influences the ribosomes to produce larger amounts of proteins. As a function of its protein-sparing effect, GH causes increased lipolysis and mobilization of fatty acids from adipose tissue. Under the influence of GH, fat is utilized for energy in preference to glucose and amino acids. Lastly, GH causes decreased utilization of carbohydrates and enhances glycogen storage. In the presence of increased growth hormone levels, the peripheral utilization of glucose is reduced and insulin resistance is increased.

Growth Hormone Deficiency

A deficiency of growth hormone during childhood leads to dwarfism. In many instances, this deficiency is accompanied by a deficiency in all of the anterior pituitary hormones, so that all parts of the body nevertheless develop proportionally. Because of deficient gonadotropin levels, however, persons with this condition do not develop sexually. In situations of selective GH deficiency (in which levels of the other anterior pituitary hormones are unaffected), sexual maturity does occur and such persons have been known to reproduce. In a rare condition, called Laron dwarfism, GH levels are actually high but there is a hereditary defect in somatomedin production.

Growth Hormone Excess

Growth hormone excess occurring prior to puberty and before fusion of the epiphyses of the long bones has occurred results in gigantism. When GH excess occurs in adulthood or after the epiphyses of the long bones have fused, a condition known as acromegaly develops.

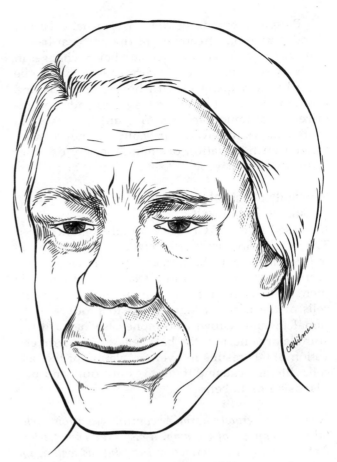

Figure 33–1. Drawing of a person with acromegaly showing protrusion of the jaw, slanting forehead, and increased size of the nose.

Acromegaly

Acromegaly is characterized by enlargement of the small bones in the hands and feet and in the membranous bones of the face and skull. As a result, there is a pronounced enlargement of the hands and feet, a broad and bulbous nose, a protruding lower jaw, and a slanting forehead (Fig. 33-1). The teeth become splayed, causing a disturbed bite, with difficulty in chewing. There is also enlargement of cartilaginous structures in the larynx and respiratory tract, resulting in a deepening of the voice and tendency to develop bronchitis. Vertebral changes often lead to kyphosis or a hunched back.

The pituitary gland is located in the pituitary fossa, or sella turcica ("Turkish saddle"), which lies directly below the optic nerve. Almost all persons with acromegaly have a recognizable adenohypophyseal tumor.[1] Enlargement of the pituitary gland eventually causes erosion of the surrounding bone and, because of its location, this leads to visual complications due to compression of the optic nerve.

Present methods of diagnosis usually permit identification and treatment of the problem before damage to vision has occurred and before changes in the bony structures become permanent. This can be done by measuring growth hormone levels and through the use of skull x-ray studies and computerized axial tomography (CAT scan). Pituitary tumors can be removed surgically or they can be treated with radiation or chemotherapy or other forms of drug therapy.

Metabolic effects of increased growth hormone levels

Increased levels of GH have a diabetogenic effect. The increase in *mobilization of fatty acids* predisposes to *ketoacidosis* and the *decrease in the peripheral utilization of glucose* tends to *elevate blood sugar*. The increase in blood sugar, in turn, stimulates the beta cells of the islets of Langerhans to produce additional insulin. Growth hormone also has a direct stimulatory effect on the beta cells.[2] Long-term elevation of GH results in overstimulation of the beta cells, literally causing them to "burn out" and predisposing to diabetes.

In summary, growth hormone controls growth in skeletal tissue capable of growing. It also exerts an effect on metabolism, and is secreted in the adult as well as the child. Its metabolic effects include an increase in protein synthesis, a decrease in the peripheral utilization of carbohydrate, and increased mobilization and utilization of fatty acids. A deficiency of growth hormone in the child causes dwarfism. An excess of growth hormone in the child leads to gigantism, and in the adult it causes a condition known as acromegaly.

:Thyroid Disorders

The thyroid gland is a shield-shaped structure located immediately below the larynx in the anterior middle portion of the neck. The thyroid gland is composed of a large number of tiny sac-like structures called follicles (Fig. 33-2). These are the functional cells of the thyroid. Each follicle is formed by a single layer of epithelial (follicular) cells and is filled with a secretory substance called colloid, which consists largely of a glycoprotein–iodine complex, thyroglobulin.

Production of Thyroid Hormone

The thyroglobulin that fills the thyroid follicles is a large glycoprotein molecule that contains 140 tyrosine amino acids. In the process of thyroid synthesis, iodine is attached to these tyrosine amino

Figure 33–2.   Diagram of the thyroid gland and the follicular structure. (From Chaffee EE, Lytle IM: Basic Physiology and Anatomy, 4th ed. Philadelphia, JB Lippincott, 1980)

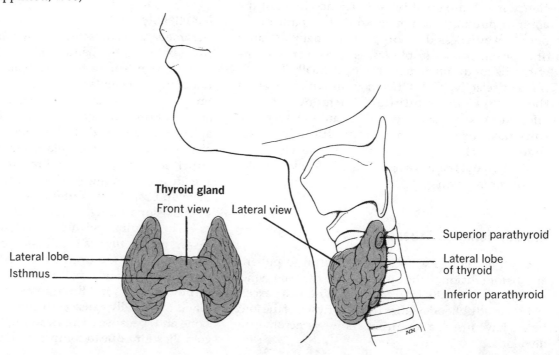

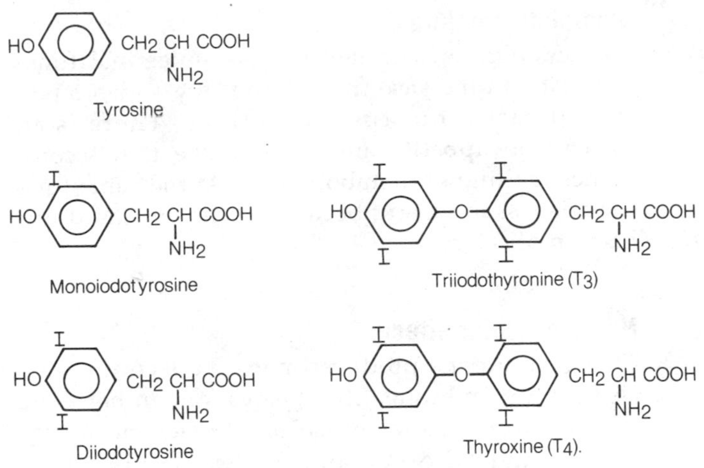

HO⟨◯⟩ CH2 CH COOH
              |
              NH2

Tyrosine

HO⟨◯⟩ CH2 CH COOH
              |
              NH2

Monoiodotyrosine

HO⟨◯⟩—O—⟨◯⟩ CH2 CH COOH
                        |
                        NH2

Triiodothyronine (T3)

HO⟨◯⟩ CH2 CH COOH
              |
              NH2

Diiodotyrosine

HO⟨◯⟩—O—⟨◯⟩ CH2 CH COOH
                        |
                        NH2

Thyroxine (T4).

Figure 33–3.   Chemistry of thyroid hormone production.

acids. Both thyroglobin and iodide (I^-) are secreted into the colloid of the follicle by the follicular cells.

The thyroid is remarkably efficient in its utilization of iodine. A daily absorption of 100 to 200 μg of dietary iodine is sufficient to form normal quantities of thyroid hormone. In the process of removal of iodine from the blood and its storage for future use, iodine is pumped into the follicular cells against a concentration gradient. As a result, the concentration of iodide within the normal thyroid gland is about 40 times that in the blood. Once inside the follicle, most of the iodide is oxidized by the enzyme peroxidase in a reaction that facilitates combination with a tyrosine molecule to form *monoiodotyrosine* and then *diiodotyrosine* (Fig. 33-3). In time, two diiodotyrosine residues become coupled to form *thyroxine* (T_4); or a monoiodotyrosine and a diiodotyrosine become coupled to form *triiodothyronine* (T_3). Only T_4 (90%) and T_3 (10%) are secreted into the circulation. Thyroid hormones are bound to thyroid-binding globulin and other plasma proteins for transport in the blood. There is evidence that T_3 is the active form of the hormone, and that T_4 is converted to T_3 before it becomes active.

Regulation of Thyroid Function

The secretion of thyroid hormone is regulated by the *hypothalamic–pituitary–thyroid* feedback system (Fig. 33-4). In this system, *thyrotrophin-releasing hormone* (TRH), which is produced by the hypothalamus, controls the release of *thyroid-stimulating hormone* (TSH) from the anterior pituitary gland. TSH increases the overall activity of the thyroid gland by (1) increasing the thyroglobin breakdown and release of thyroid hormone from follicles into

the blood stream, (2) activating the iodide pump, (3) increasing the oxidation of iodide and coupling of iodide to tyrosine, and (4) increasing the number of follicle cells and the size of the follicles. The effect of TSH on the release of thyroid hormones occurs within about 30 minutes, while the other effects require days or weeks. Increased levels of thyroid hormone act in the feedback mechanism by inhibiting TRH. High levels of iodides cause a temporary decrease in thyroid activity that lasts for several weeks, probably through a direct inhibition of TSH on the thyroid. Lugol's solution, which is an iodide preparation, is sometimes given to hyperthyroid patients in preparation for surgery as a means of de-

Figure 33–4.   Diagram of the hypothalamic–pituitary–thyroid feedback system which regulates body levels of thyroid hormone.

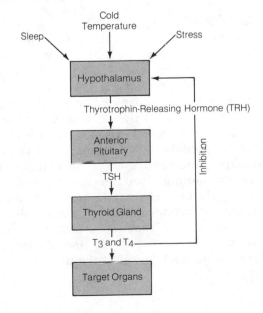

creasing thyroid function. Cold exposure is one of the strongest stimuli for increased thyroid hormone production and is probably mediated through TRH from the hypothalamus.

Actions of Thyroid Hormone

There are no major organs in the body that are not affected by altered levels of thyroid hormone. Thyroid hormone has two major effects: (1) it increases metabolism and (2) it is necessary for growth and development in children, including mental development and attainment of sexual maturity.

Metabolic rate

Thyroid hormone increases the metabolism of all body tissues except the retina, spleen, testes, and lung. The basal metabolic rate (BMR) can increase by 60 to 100% above normal when large amounts of thyroxine are secreted.[3] As a result of this higher metabolism, there is an increase in the rate of glucose, fat, and protein utilization. Lipids are mobilized from adipose tissue, and the catabolism of cholesterol by the liver is increased. As a result, blood levels of cholesterol are decreased in hyperthyroidism and increased in hypothyroidism. Muscle proteins are broken down and used as fuel, probably accounting for some of the muscle fatigue that occurs with hyperthyroidism. The absorption of glucose from the gastrointestinal tract is increased. Since vitamins are essential parts of metabolic enzymes and coenzymes, an increase in metabolic rate causes a more rapid utilization of vitamins and tends to cause vitamin deficiency.

Cardiovascular function

Cardiovascular and respiratory functions are strongly affected by thyroid function. With an increase in metabolism, there is a rise in oxygen consumption and production of metabolic endproducts with an accompanying increase in vasodilatation. Blood flow to the skin, in particular, is augmented as a means of dissipating body heat that results from the higher metabolism. Blood volume, cardiac output, and ventilation are all increased as a means of maintaining blood flow and oxygen delivery to body tissues. Heart rate and cardiac contractility are enhanced as a means of maintaining the needed cardiac output. Blood pressure, on the other hand, is apt to change very little, since the increase in vasodilatation tends to offset the increase in cardiac output.

Gastrointestinal tract

Thyroid hormone enhances gastrointestinal function with an increase in both motility and production of gastrointestinal secretions. There is an increase in appetite and food intake that accompanies the higher metabolic rate. At the same time there is loss in weight because of the increased utilization of calories.

Neuromuscular effects

Thyroid hormone produces marked effects on muscle function and tone. Slight elevations in hormone levels cause skeletal muscles to react more vigorously, and a drop in hormone levels causes muscles to react more sluggishly. In the hyperthyroid state, a fine muscle tremor is present. The cause of this tremor is unknown, but it may represent an increased sensitivity of the neural synapses in the spinal cord that control muscle tone.

In the infant, thyroid hormone is necessary for normal brain development. The hormone enhances cerebration; in the hyperstate, it causes extreme nervousness, anxiety, and difficulty in sleeping.

Evidence suggests that there is a strong interaction between thyroid hormone and the sympathetic nervous system. As will be discussed later, many of the signs and symptoms of hyperthyroidism suggest overactivity of the sympathetic division of the autonomic nervous system, for example, tachycardia, palpitations, and sweating. In addition, tremor, restlessness, anxiety, and diarrhea may reflect autonomic nervous system imbalances. Drugs that block sympathetic activity have proved to be valuable adjuncts in the treatment of hyperthyroidism because of their ability to relieve some of these undesirable symptoms.

Alterations in Thyroid Function

An alteration in thyroid function can represent either a hypofunctional or a hyperfunctional state. The manifestations of these two altered states are summarized in Table 33-1. Disorders of the thyroid may represent a congenital defect in thyroid development or they may develop later in life, with a gradual or a sudden onset.

Goiter is an increase in the size of the thyroid gland. It can occur in hypothyroid, euthyroid, and hyperthyroid states and gives little indication of the type of thyroid abnormality that is present when considered apart from other manifestations.

Table 33-1   Manifestations of Hypothyroid and Hyperthyroid State

Level of Organization	Hypostate	Hyperstate
Basal metabolic rate	decreased	increased
Sensitivity to catecholamines	decreased	increased
General features	myxedematous features deep voice impaired growth (child)	exophthalmos lid lag decreased blinking
Blood cholesterol levels	increased	decreased
General behavior	mental retardation (infant) mental and physical sluggishness somnolent	restless, irritable, anxious hyperkinetic wakeful
Cardiovascular function	decreased cardiac output bradycardia	increased cardiac output tachycardia and palpitations
Gastrointestinal function	constipation decreased appetite	diarrhea increased appetite
Respiratory function	hypoventilation	dyspnea
Muscle tone and reflexes	decreased	increased, with tremor and fibrillatory twitching
Temperature tolerance	cold intolerance	heat intolerance
Skin and hair	decreased sweating coarse and dry skin and hair	increased sweating thin and silky skin and hair
Weight	gain	loss

Tests of thyroid function

There are various tests that aid in diagnosing thyroid disorders. *Direct measures* of T_3, T_4, TSH, and thyroid-binding globulin have been made through *radioimmunoassay methods.* The *resin uptake test* for T_3 and T_4 measures the unsaturated binding sites of the thyroid hormones. The *TSH stimulating test* differentiates primary and secondary thyroid disorders. The *radioactive iodine uptake test* measures the ability of the thyroid gland to remove and concentrate iodine from the blood. The *thyroid scan* detects thyroid nodules and active thyroid tissue. *Protein-bound iodine* (PBI) measures the organic iodine that is bound to plasma proteins. This test is easily influenced by medications that contain iodine and by conditions that affect binding of thyroid hormone; therefore, it is not used as frequently as it was in the past. The *basal metabolic rate* (BMR) is an indirect measure of thyroid function, and it too has been largely replaced by more accurate and quantitative tests.

Hyperthyroidism

Hyperthyroidism, or *thyrotoxicosis,* results from excessive delivery of thyroid hormone to the peripheral tissue. It is seen most frequently in women 20 to 40 years of age. It is commonly associated with hyperplasia of the thyroid gland, multinodular goiter, and adenoma of the thyroid. Occasionally it develops as the result of ingestion of an overdose of thyroid hormone. When the condition is accompanied by exophthalmos (bulging of the eyeballs) and goiter, it is called Graves' disease. Thyroid crisis or storm is an acutely exaggerated manifestation of the hyperthyroid state.

Many of the manifestations of hyperthyroidism are related to the increase in oxygen consumption and increased utilization of metabolic fuels associated with the *hypermetabolic state* as well as the *increase in sympathetic nervous system activity* that occurs. The fact that many of the signs and symptoms of hyperthyroidism resemble those of excessive sympathetic activity suggests that the thyroid hormone may heighten sensitivity of the body to the catecholamines or that thyroid hormone itself may act as a pseudocatecholamine. With the hypermetabolic state, there are frequent complaints of nervousness, irritability, and fatigability. Weight loss is common despite a large appetite. Other manifestations include tachycardia, palpitations, shortness of breath, excessive sweating, and heat intolerance. The person appears restless and has a fine muscle tremor. Even in persons without exophthalmos there is an abnormal retraction of the eyelids and infrequent blinking so that they appear to be staring. The hair and skin are usually thin and have a silky appearance. The signs and symptoms of hyperthyroidism are summarized in Table 33-1.

Thyroid storm (crisis) is an extreme and life-threatening form of thyrotoxicosis, rarely seen today because of improved diagnosis and treatment methods. When it does occur, it is seen most often in undiagnosed cases or in persons with hyperthyroidism who have not been adequately treated. It is often precipitated by stress, such as an infection (usually respiratory), by diabetic ketoacidosis, by physical or emotional trauma, or in some situations by palpation of the hyperactive thyroid gland. Thyroid storm is manifested by a very high fever, extreme cardiovascular effects (tachycardia, congestive failure, and angina), and severe central nervous system effects (agitation, restlessness, and delirium). The mortality is high.

Graves' disease is a state of *hyperthyroidism*, *goiter*, and *exophthalmos*. The cause of Graves' disease

Figure 33–5. Woman with Graves' disease. Note the exophthalmos and enlarged thyroid gland. (From Chaffee EE, Lytle IM: Basic Physiology and Anatomy, 4th ed. Philadelphia, JB Lippincott, 1980)

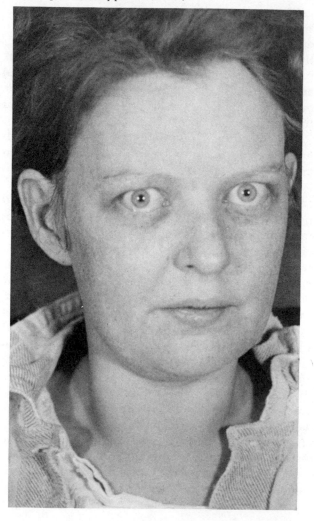

and the development of the exophthalmos, which results from edema and cellular infiltration of the orbital structures and muscle, is poorly understood. Current evidence suggests that it is an immune disorder characterized by abnormal stimulation of the thyroid gland by thyroid-stimulating antibodies that act through the normal TSH receptors. The exophthalmos is thought to result from an exophthalmos-producing factor whose action is enhanced by antibodies. The ophthalmopathy of Graves' disease can cause severe eye problems, including paralysis of the extraocular muscles, involvement of the optic nerve with some visual loss, and corneal ulceration because the lids do not close over the protruding eyeball. The exophthalmos usually tends to stabilize following treatment of the hyperthyroidism. Unfortunately, not all of the ocular changes are reversible. Figure 33-5 depicts a woman with Graves' disease.

Treatment of hyperthyroidism is directed toward reducing the level of thyroid hormone. This can be accomplished through *surgical removal* of part or all of the thyroid gland, through *eradication* of the gland with *radioactive iodine*, or through the use of drugs that decrease thyroid function and thereby the effect of the thyroid hormone on the peripheral tissues. The beta-adrenergic blocking drug *propranolol* is often administered to block the effects of the hyperthyroid state on sympathetic nervous system function. It is given in conjunction with other antithyroid drugs such as *propylthiouracil* and *methimazole*. These drugs prevent the thyroid gland from converting iodine to its organic (hormonal) form in the thyroid and block the conversion of T_4 to T_3 in the tissues. *Lugol's solution* (iodide) may be given to depress the thyroid gland in preparation for surgery. Unfortunately, this action is short-lived, and in a few weeks the symptoms reappear and may be intensified.

Hypothyroidism

Hypothyroidism can occur as a congenital or an acquired defect. When there is no thyroid function at birth, the condition is called *cretinism*. When the condition occurs later in life it is called *myxedema*. Presently the term *cretin* hardly seems appropriate for describing the normally developing infant in whom replacement thyroid hormone therapy was instituted shortly after birth.

Congenital hypothyroidism. Congenital hypothyroidism is perhaps one of the most common causes of preventable mental retardation. It affects about 1 out of 5000 infants. Hypothyroidism in the infant may result from a congenital lack of the thyroid gland, or from abnormal biosynthesis of thyroid hormone or deficient TSH secretion. With congenital lack of the thryoid gland, the infant usually appears normal and functions normally at birth because hormones have been supplied in utero by the mother.

Thyroid hormone is essential for normal brain development and growth, almost half of which occurs during the first 6 months of life. If untreated, congenital hypothyroidism causes mental retardation and impairment of growth. In hypothyroid infants treated before 3 months of age, 70% will have an IQ higher than 85. If, however, treatment is delayed to between 3 months and 7 months, 85% of these infants will have definite retardation.[4]

Fortunately, neonatal screening tests have been instituted to detect congenital hypothyroidism during early infancy. Screening is usually done in the hospital nursery between the first and the fifth days of life. In this test, a drop of blood is taken from the infant's heel, and analyzed for T_4 and TSH. In 1977, the cost of the screening test was but 60¢ per infant (testing for TSH added slightly to this cost).[5] Clearly, the cost of detecting congenital hypothyroidism is far less than the cost of institutionalization would be, were mental retardation to occur because of a delay in diagnosis and treatment.

Acquired hypothyroidism (myxedema). Hypothyroidism in the adult may be mild, with only a few signs and symptoms, or may be a life-threatening condition called myxedema coma. It can occur as the result of destruction of the thyroid (*primary hypothyroidism*) or as a *secondary* disorder due to impaired hypothalamic–pituitary feedback stimulation of the thyroid gland. Primary hypothyroidism is much more common than secondary hypothyroidism. It can develop after thyroidectomy; due to destruction of the thyroid gland with radioactive iodine; or as a result of ingestion of goitrogens (thiocyanate, lithium, para-aminosalicylic acid, and iodine preparations), which are capable of suppressing thyroid function. Destruction of the gland may be the end result of chronic thyroiditis, such as Hashimoto's (autoimmune) thyroiditis. In many cases, the decrease in function is due to atrophy of the gland for reasons unknown. Iodine deficiency elicits a compensatory increase in the size of the gland (goiter) and may cause hypothyroidism.

Myxedema affects almost every organ system in the body. The manifestations of the disorder are largely related to two factors: (1) the *hypometabolic state* resulting from the hormone deficiency and (2) accumulation of a *mucopolysaccharide substance in the interstitial spaces*. This substance attracts water and causes a *nonpitting mucus-type of edema* that is characteristic of myxedema. Although the myxedema is obvious in the face and other superficial parts, it also affects many of the body organs and is responsible for many of the manifestations of the severe hypothyroid state.

The hypometabolic state associated with myxedema is characterized by a gradual onset of fatigue, tendency to gain weight despite a loss in appetite, and cold intolerance. As the condition progresses, the skin becomes dry and rough and acquires a pale yellowish cast that is due primarily to carotene deposition. Gastrointestinal motility is decreased, giving rise to constipation, flatulence, and abdominal distention. Nervous system involvement is manifested in mental dullness, lethargy, and impaired memory.

As a result of fluid accumulation, the face takes on a characteristic puffy look, especially around the eyes. The tongue is enlarged, and the voice is hoarse and husky. Myxedematous fluid can collect in the interstitial spaces of almost any organ system. Pericardial or pleural effusion may develop. Mucopolysaccharide deposits in the heart cause generalized cardiac dilatation, bradycardia, and other signs of altered cardiac function. The signs and symptoms of hypothyroidism are summarized in Table 33-1.

Hypothyroidism is treated by replacement therapy with purified thyroid hormones obtained from domestic animals such as cows, pigs, and sheep, or with synthetic preparations.

Myxedema coma is a life-threatening end-stage expression of hypothyroidism. It is characterized by coma, hypothermia, cardiovascular collapse, hypoventilation, and severe metabolic disorders that include hyponatremia, hypoglycemia, and lactic acidosis. It occurs most often in the elderly and is seldom seen in persons under age 50.[6] The fact that it occurs more frequently in winter months suggests that cold exposure may be a precipitating factor. The severely hypothyroid person is unable to metabolize sedatives, analgesics, and anesthetic drugs, and these agents may precipitate coma.

In summary, thyroid hormones play a role in metabolism of almost all body cells and are necessary for normal physical and mental growth in the infant and small child. Alterations in thyroid function can present as either a hyperstate or a hypostate. Hyperthyroidism causes an increase in metabolic rate and alterations in body function that are similar to those produced by enhanced sympathetic nervous system activity. Graves' disease is characterized by the triad of hyperthyroidism, goiter, and exophthalmos. Hypothyroidism can occur as either a congenital or an acquired defect. When it is

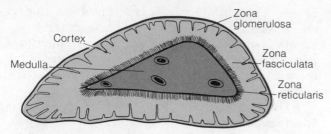

Figure 33–6. Diagram of the adrenal gland showing the medulla and the three layers of the cortex. The zona glomerulosa is the outer layer of the cortex and is primarily responsible for mineralocorticoid production. The middle layer, the zona fasciculata, and the inner layer, the zona reticularis, produce the glucocorticoids and the adrenal sex hormones.

Figure 33–7. Predominant biosynthetic pathways of the adrenal cortex. Critical enzymes in the biosynthetic process include 3-beta-dehydrogenase and 11-, 17-, and 21-hydroxylase. A deficiency in one of these enzymes blocks the synthesis of hormones that are dependent upon that enzyme and routes the precursors into alternate pathways. An absolute 3-beta-dehydrogenase deficiency is a potentially lethal defect.

present at birth, it is called cretinism; when it occurs later in life, it is termed myxedema. Congenital hypothyroidism leads to mental retardation and impaired physical growth unless treatment is initiated during the first months of life. Hypothyroidism leads to a decrease in metabolic rate and an accumulation of a mucopolysaccharide substance within the intercellular spaces; this substance attracts water and causes a mucus-type of edema called myxedema.

:Alterations in Adrenal Function

The adrenal glands are small, bilateral structures that weigh about 5 g each and lie retroperitoneally at the apex of each kidney (Fig. 33-6). The medulla or inner

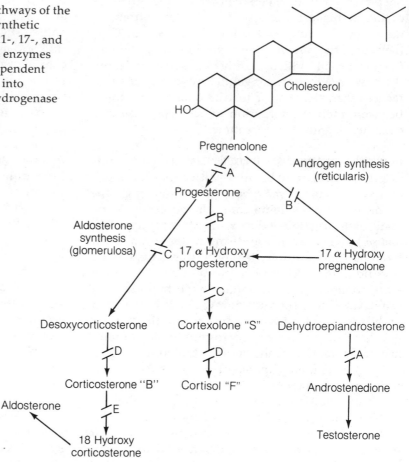

portion of the gland secretes epinephrine and nor-epinephrine and is an extension of the sympathetic nervous system. The cortex forms the bulk of the adrenal gland and is responsible for secreting three types of hormones: the glucocorticoids, the miner-alocorticoids, and the adrenal sex hormones. Since the sympathetic nervous system secretes cate-cholamines, adrenal medullary function is not essential for life, but adrenal cortical function is. Total loss of adrenal cortical function is fatal in 3 to 10 days if untreated.[7] This section of the chapter describes the synthesis and function of the adrenal cortical hormones and the effects of adrenal cortical insufficiency and excess.

Biosynthesis of Adrenal Cortical Hormones

More than 30 hormones are produced by the adrenal gland. Of these hormones, *aldosterone* is the principal *mineralocorticoid*, cortisol (hydrocortisone) the major glucocorticoid, and androgens the chief sex hormones. All of the adrenal cortical hormones have a similar structure in that all are steroids and are synthesized from acetate and cholesterol; thus, the glucocorticoid drugs are often called steroids. Each of the steps involved in the synthesis of the various hormones requires a specific enzyme (Fig. 33-7).

The adrenogenital syndrome
(a defect in biosynthesis)
The adrenogenital syndrome describes a congenital condition due to an autosomal recessive trait, in which there is a deficiency of one of the specific enzymes (11-, 17-, or 21-hydroxylase) required for normal biosynthesis of the adrenal cortical hormones. The lowered levels of cortisol associated with the defect lead to increased ACTH levels, adrenal hyperplasia, and excess adrenal androgen. These three deficiencies are characterized by some degree of virilism; hence the term adrenogenital syndrome. In a female infant, the increased androgens may cause pseudohermaphroditism; a male infant may be born with a slightly enlarged penis. A salt-losing condition causing impaired synthesis of mineralo-corticoids is seen when the deficiency of 21-hydroxylase is total or nearly so. Its manifestations reflect the degree of deficiency and the person's age at the time it is recognized.

Actions of the Adrenal Cortical Hormones
Adrenal sex hormones
The adrenal sex hormones are synthesized primarily by the zona reticularis and the zona fasciculata of the cortex (Fig. 33-6). These sex hormones probably ex-ert little effect on normal sexual function. There is evidence, however, that the adrenal sex hormones contribute to the pubertal growth of body hair, particularly pubic and axillary hair in women. They may also play a role in steroid hormone economy of the pregnant woman and the fetal–placental unit.[8]

The mineralocorticoids
The mineralocorticoids play an essential role in regulating potassium and sodium levels and water balance. They are produced in the zona glomerulosa, the outer layer of cells of the adrenal cortex. Aldosterone is regulated by the renin–angiotensin mechanism and by blood levels of potassium. The adrenocorticotropic hormone (ACTH) is relatively unimportant in the day-to-day regulation of aldosterone. Increased levels of aldosterone promote sodium retention by the distal tubules of the kidney while increasing urinary losses of potassium. The influence of aldosterone on fluid and electrolyte balance is discussed in Chapter 22.

Figure 33–8.   Diagram showing the hypothalamic-pituitary–adrenal (HPA) feedback system that regulates glucocorticoid (cortisol) levels. Cortisol release is regulated by ACTH. Stress exerts its effects on cortisol release through the HLA system and the corticotrophin-releasing factor (CRF) which controls the release of ACTH from the anterior pituitary gland. Increased cortisol levels incite a negative feedback inhibition of ACTH release. Pharmacologic doses of synthetic steroids inhibit ACTH release by way of the hypothalamic CRF. (Modified from Tepperman J: Metabolic and Endocrine Physiology, 4th ed, p 173. Chicago, Year Book Medical Publishers, Inc., 1980)

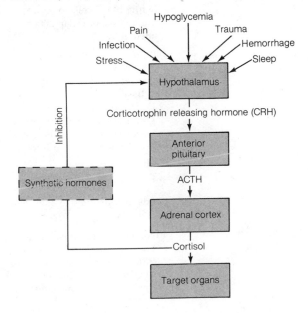

The glucocorticoids

The glucocorticoid hormones are synthesized in the zona fasciculata and the zona reticularis. The blood levels of these hormones are regulated by negative feedback mechanisms of the hypothalamic–pituitary–adrenal (HPA) system (Fig. 33-8). In this system, cortisol levels increase as ACTH levels rise. There is considerable diurnal variation in ACTH levels, which reach their peak in the early evening hours and decline from late evening and through the night. As will be discussed later, one of the earliest signs of Cushing's syndrome is loss of this diurnal variation. Increased plasma cortisol levels act in a negative feedback manner on receptors in the hypothalamus to decrease corticotropin-releasing factor, and on the anterior pituitary to decrease ACTH. Stimulation of hypothalamic receptors and the release of cortisone releasing factor (CRF) serve to integrate neural influences with the function of the adrenal cortex.

The glucocorticoids perform a necessary function in response to stress, and are essential for survival. When produced as part of the stress response, these hormones aid in *regulating the metabolic functions* of the body and in *controlling the inflammatory response*. The actions of cortisol are summarized in Table 33-2. The reader will note that many of the actions attributed to cortisol result from administration of pharmacological preparations of the hormone.

Metabolic effects. Cortisol stimulates glucose production by the liver, promotes protein breakdown, and causes mobilization of fatty acids. As body proteins are broken down, amino acids are mobilized and transported to the liver, where they are used in the production of glucose. The mobilization of fatty acids serves to convert cell metabolism from utilization of glucose for energy to utilization of fatty acids instead.

As glucose production by the liver rises and peripheral glucose utilization falls, there is moderate insulin resistance. In diabetics and persons who are diabetes-prone, this has the effect of raising the blood sugar.

Psychic effects. The glucocorticoid hormones appear to be involved either directly or indirectly in emotional disturbances. Receptors for these hormones have been identified in brain tissue, which suggests that they play a role in regulation of behavior.[9] It has been noted that persons treated with adrenal cortical hormones have displayed behavior ranging from mildly aberrant to psychotic.

Anti-inflammatory effects. Large quantities of cortisol are required for an effective anti-inflammatory action. This is achieved by administration of pharmacologic doses of synthetic cortisol. The increased cortisol blocks inflammation at an early stage by decreasing capillary permeability and stabilizing the lysosomal membranes so that inflammatory mediators are not released. Cortisol suppresses the immune response by reducing antibody and cell-mediated immunity. With this lessened inflammation comes a reduction in fever. During the healing phase, cortisol suppresses fibroblast activity and thereby lessens scar formation. A recently described

Table 33–2   Actions of Cortisol

Major Influence	Effect on Body
Glucose metabolism	Stimulates gluconeogenesis
	Decreases glucose utilization by the tissues
Protein metabolism	Increases breakdown of proteins
	Increases plasma protein levels
Fat metabolism	Increases mobilization of fatty acids
	Increases utilization of fatty acids
Anti-inflammatory action (pharmacologic levels)	Stabilizes lysosomal membranes of the inflammatory cells, preventing the release of inflammatory mediators
	Decreases capillary permeability to prevent inflammatory edema
	Depresses phagocytosis by white blood cells to reduce the release of inflammatory mediators
	Suppresses the immune response
	Causes atrophy of lymphoid tissue
	Decreases eosinophils
	Decreases antibody formation
	Decreases the development of cell-mediated immunity
	Reduces fever
	Inhibits fibroblast activity
Psychic effect	Tends to contribute to emotional stability
Permissive effect	Facilitates the response of the tissues to humoral and neural influences, such as that of the catecholamines, during trauma and extreme stress

attribute of cortisol is its ability to inhibit prostaglandin synthesis, which may account in large part for its anti-inflammatory actions.[10]

Suppression of adrenal function

A highly significant aspect of long-term therapy with pharmacologic preparations of the adrenal cortical hormones is adrenal insufficiency upon withdrawal of the drugs. The deficiency is due to suppression of the hypothalamic–pituitary–adrenal axis. Chronic suppression causes atrophy of the entire system; and abrupt withdrawal of drugs can cause acute adrenal insufficiency. Furthermore, recovery to a state of normal adrenal function may be prolonged, requiring up to 12 months.[11]

Tests of Adrenal Cortical Function

There are a number of diagnostic tests by which adrenal cortical function and the hypothalamic–pituitary axis may be evaluated. Blood levels of cortisol and ACTH can be measured using radioimmunoassay methods. A *24-hour urine specimen* measures the excretion of *17-ketosteroids*, *17-ketogenic steroids*, and *17-hydroxycorticosteroids*. These metabolic end products of the adrenal hormones and the male androgens provide information about alterations in the biosynthesis of the adrenal cortical hormones. *Suppression and stimulation tests* afford a means of assessing the state of the *hypothalamic–pituitary–adrenal feedback system*. For example, a test dose of ACTH may be given to assess the response of the adrenal cortex to pituitary stimulation. Similarly, administration of dexamethasone (a synthetic glucocorticoid drug) provides a means of measuring negative feedback suppression of ACTH. Adrenal tumors and ectopic ACTH-producing tumors are generally unresponsive to ACTH suppression by dexamethasone. Metyrapone (Metopirone) blocks the final step in cortisol synthesis, producing 11-dehydroxycortisol which does not inhibit ACTH. This test measures the ability of the pituitary to release ACTH.

Glucocorticoid Hormone Excess (Cushing's Syndrome)

Cushing's syndrome is characterized by a chronic elevation in glucocorticoid (and adrenal androgen) hormones. Because the condition is most frequently caused by increased ACTH production, the mineralocorticoids are usually not involved in the syndrome.

Cushing's syndrome can result from either overproduction of hormones by the body or from long-term therapy with one of the potent pharmacologic preparations of glucocorticoids (*iatrogenic Cushing's syndrome*).* There are three important forms of Cushing's syndrome that are due to excess glucocorticoids production by the body. One is a *pituitary form* which results from excess production of ACTH by a tumor of the pituitary gland; it accounts for about two-thirds of the disease cases and, because this form of the disease was the one originally described by Cushing, it is called Cushing's disease. The other forms of excess glucocorticoid levels are referred to as Cushing's syndrome.† The second form is the *adrenal form*, caused by an adrenal tumor. The third is the *ectopic* Cushing's, due to an ACTH-producing tumor such as occurs in some bronchogenic cancers.

The major manifestations of Cushing's syndrome represent an exaggeration of the normal effects of cortisol. Altered *fat metabolism* causes a peculiar deposition of fat characterized by a protruding abdomen, subclavicular fat pads or "buffalo hump" on the back, and a round, plethoric "moon face." There is muscle weakness and the extremities are thin due to *protein breakdown* and muscle wasting. In advanced cases, the skin over the forearms and legs becomes thin, having the appearance of parchment. Purple striae (stretch marks), from stretching of the catabolically weakened skin and subcutaneous tissues, are distributed on the abdomen and hips. *Osteoporosis* results from destruction of bone proteins and alterations in calcium metabolism. With osteoporosis there may be back pain, compression fractures of the vertebrae, and rib fractures. As calcium is mobilized from bone, renal calculi may develop. Derangements in glucose metabolism are found in some 90% of patients, with clinically overt *diabetes mellitus* occurring in about 20%.[12] The glucocorticoids possess mineralocorticoid properties; this causes hypokalemia due to excess potassium excretion and hypertension resulting from sodium retention. There is *inhibition of the inflammatory and immune responses* with an increased susceptibility to infection. Cortisol increases gastric acid secretion, and this may provoke gastric ulceration and bleeding. An accompanying *increase in androgen* levels causes hirsutism, mild acne, and menstrual irregularities in women.

---

*Iatrogenic = physician-induced.

†In this text the term Cushing's syndrome designates both Cushing's disease and Cushing's syndrome.

Excess levels of the glucocorticoids may give rise to extreme emotional lability, ranging from mild euphoria and absence of normal fatigue to grossly psychotic behavior. The manifestations of glucocorticoid excess are summarized in Table 33-3.

Diagnosis of Cushing's syndrome depends upon the finding of elevated levels of cortisol. As was mentioned, one of the prominent features of Cushing's syndrome is loss of the diurnal pattern of cortisol secretion. Therefore, cortisol determinations are often made on three blood samples: one taken in the morning, one in late afternoon or early evening, and a third specimen drawn the following morning after a midnight dose of dexamethasone. Measurement of plasma ACTH, 24-hour urinary 17-ketosteroids, 17-ketogenic steroids, and 17-hydroxycorticosteroids, and suppression or stimulation tests of the hypothalamic–pituitary–adrenal system are often made. Skull x-ray films and intravenous pyelograms, which outline the shadows of the kidneys and adrenal glands, may be done. Computerized tomograms (CT) afford a means for locating adrenal or pituitary tumors.

The *treatment of Cushing's syndrome*, whether by surgery, irradiation, or drugs, is largely determined by the etiology. Adrenalectomy may be done if an adrenal tumor is present. With the recent development of the transsphenoidal approach for removal of a pituitary tumor using microsurgical techniques, surgical treatment today is far more efficient than in the past. In children and in adults with mild clinical symptoms, cobalt radiation is often the preferred method for treating pituitary Cushing's. One drawback of radiation therapy is the long time lag (18 months in some cases) before complete remission occurs.[13] Adrenolytic agents are administered in persons with inoperable tumors, in those whose tumors have not been fully treated, and in those in whom irradiation has not yet taken effect. Two such agents are cyproheptadine and O,p'-dichlorodiphenyldichloroethane.

Adrenal Insufficiency

There are two forms of adrenal insufficiency: primary and secondary. Primary adrenal insufficiency, or Addison's disease, is due to destruction of the

Table 33–3 Manifestations of Adrenal Cortical Insufficiency and Excess

Parameter	Adrenal Cortical Insufficiency	Glucocorticoid Excess
Electrolytes	Hyponatremia* Hyperkalemia*	Hypokalemia
Fluids	Dehydration* (elevated BUN, others)	Edema
Blood pressure	Hypotension* Shock* Orthostatic hypotension	Hypertension
Musculoskeletal	Muscle weakness* Fatigue*	Muscle wasting Fatigue
Hair and skin	Skin pigmentation Loss of hair (axillary and pubic)	Easy bruisability Hirsutism, acne, and striae (abdomen and thighs)
Inflammatory response	Low resistance to trauma, infection, and stress	Decrease in eosinophils Lymphocytopenia
Gastrointestinal	Nausea, vomiting* Abdominal pain*	Possible gastrointestinal bleeding
Glucose metabolism	Hypoglycemia*	Impaired glucose tolerance Glycosuria Elevated blood sugar
Emotional	Depression and irritability	Emotional lability to psychosis
Other	Menstrual irregularity Decreased axillary and pubic hair in women	Oligomenorrhea Impotence in the male Centripetal obesity (moon face and buffalo hump)

*Present in acute adrenal insufficiency

adrenal gland. Secondary adrenal insufficiency is due to a disorder of the hypothalamic–pituitary–adrenal system.

Primary adrenal insufficiency (Addison's disease)

In 1855, Thomas Addison, an English physician, provided the first detailed clinical description of primary adrenal insufficiency. Addison's disease is a relatively rare disorder in which there is destruction of all layers of the adrenal cortex. Most often the underlying problem is idiopathic adrenal atrophy, which probably has an autoimmune basis. Tuberculosis is an infrequent cause, as is amyloidosis, or a fungal infection (particularly histoplasmosis). Adrenalectomy, sometimes done palliatively in cancer, is an obvious cause of primary adrenal insufficiency.

Addison's disease, like insulin-dependent diabetes mellitus, is a *chronic metabolic disorder that requires lifetime hormone replacement therapy*. The adrenal cortex has a large reserve capacity, and the manifestations of adrenal insufficiency do not usually become apparent until about 90% of the gland has been destroyed.[14] These manifestations are primarily related to (1) hyperpigmentation due to elevated ACTH levels, (2) mineralocorticoid deficiency, and (3) glucocorticoid deficiency. Although lack of the adrenal androgens exerts few effects in men because the testes produce these hormones, women will have sparse axillary and pubic hair. The manifestations of adrenal insufficiency are summarized in Table 33-3.

Hyperpigmentation. In Addison's disease, ACTH levels are elevated in response to the fall in cortisol. At this point it is of interest to note that the amino acid sequence of ACTH is strikingly similar to that of melanocyte-stimulating hormone (MSH); thus, *hyperpigmentation* is seen in about 98% of persons with Addison's disease and is *helpful in distinguishing the primary and secondary forms*. The skin looks bronzed or suntanned in both exposed and unexposed areas, and the normal creases and pressure points tend to become especially dark. The gums and oral mucous membranes may become bluish-black in color. This hyperpigmentation becomes more pronounced during periods of stress.

Mineralocorticoid deficiency. Mineralocorticoid deficiency causes increased urinary losses of sodium, chloride, and water along with decreased excretion of potassium. The result is hyponatremia, loss of extracellular fluid, decreased cardiac output, and hyperkalemia. There may be an abnormal appetite for salt. Orthostatic hypotension is common. Dehydration, weakness, and fatigue are often present as early symptoms. If sodium and water loss is extreme, cardiovascular collapse and shock will ensue.

Glucocorticoid deficiency. Because of a lack of glucocorticoids, the patient has poor tolerance to stress. This deficiency causes hypoglycemia, lethargy, weakness, fever, and gastrointestinal symptoms such as anorexia, nausea, vomiting, and weight loss.

Secondary adrenal insufficiency

Secondary adrenal insufficiency can occur as the result of hypopituitarism or because the pituitary gland has been surgically removed. However, a far more common cause than either of these is the rapid withdrawal of glucocorticoids that have been administered therapeutically. These drugs suppress the hypothalamic–pituitary–adrenal system, with resulting adrenal cortical atrophy and lack of cortisol. It is important to note that this suppression continues long after drug therapy has been discontinued, and could be critical during periods of stress or when surgery is done. It has been suggested that a person receiving pharmacologic doses of the glucocorticoids for more than 1 to 4 weeks may have suppression of the hypothalamic–pituitary–adrenal system for up to a year after the drugs have been discontinued.[15]

Acute Adrenal Crisis

Acute adrenal crisis is a life-threatening situation. In Addison's disease as the underlying problem, exposure to even a minor illness or stress can precipitate nausea, vomiting, muscular weakness, hypotension, dehydration, and vascular collapse. The onset of adrenal crisis may be sudden; or it may progress over a period of several days. Meningococcal septicemia (Waterhouse–Friderichsen syndrome) causes an acute fulminating form of adrenal insufficiency. The symptoms may also occur suddenly in children with salt-losing forms of the adrenogenital syndrome.

Adrenal insufficiency is *treated* with replacement glucocorticoid therapy. In acute adrenal insufficiency, cortisol is given intravenously followed by rapid infusion of saline and glucose. The day-to-day regulation of the chronic phase of Addison's is usually accomplished with oral cortisol, and higher doses are given during periods of stress. Because these patients are likely to have episodes of hyponatremia and hypoglycemia, they need to have a regular schedule for meals and exercise.

In summary, the adrenal cortex produces three types of hormones: mineralocorticoids, glucocorticoids, and adrenal sex hormones. The mineralocorticoids along with the renin-angiotensin mechanism aid in controlling body levels of sodium and potassium. The glucocorticoids have anti-inflammatory actions and aid in regulating glucose, protein, and fat metabolism during periods of stress. These hormones are under control of the hypothalamic–pituitary–adrenal system. The adrenal sex hormones exert little effect on the day-to-day control of body function, but probably contribute to the development of body hair in women. Cushing's syndrome exists when the glucocorticoid level is abnormally high. This syndrome may be due to pharmacologic doses of cortisol, to a pituitary or adrenal tumor, or to an ectopic tumor that produces ACTH. The clinical manifestations of Cushing's syndrome reflect the very high level of cortisol that is present. Chronic adrenal insufficiency is called Addison's disease. It can be caused by destruction of the adrenal gland or by dysfunction of the hypothalamic–pituitary–adrenal system. Adrenal insufficiency requires replacement therapy with cortical hormones. Acute adrenal insufficiency is a life-threatening situation.

:Study Guide

After you have studied this chapter, you should be able to meet the following objectives:

: : Compare endocrine hypofunction and endocrine hyperfunction.

: : Describe the radioimmunoassay method of measuring hormone levels.

: : State the general functions of growth hormone.

: : State the effects of a deficiency in growth hormone.

: : Describe the conditions predisposing to acromegaly.

: : Explain the potential relationship between growth hormone and diabetes.

: : Describe the synthesis of thyroid hormones.

: : Describe the hypothalamic–pituitary–thyroid feedback system.

: : Explain why blood cholesterol levels are decreased in hyperthyroidism.

: : State the relationship between cardiovascular function and thyroid function.

: : Describe the general effects of thyroid hormone on the muscular system.

: : Name three tests of thyroid function.

: : List the signs and symptoms of hyperthyroidism which the health professional should be able to recognize.

: : State the manifestations of thyroid storm.

: : State the triad of conditions that constitute Graves' disease.

: : Describe the effects of congenital hypothyroidism.

: : Describe the manifestations of the condition known as myxedema.

: : State the underlying cause of the adrenogenital syndrome.

: : State the role of the adrenal sex hormones and the mineralocorticoids.

: : Explain the regulation of the glucocorticoids by negative feedback mechanisms.

: : Explain the influence of cortisol on body metabolism.

: : Describe the action of cortisol on inflammation.

: : State the purpose of the 24-hour urine specimen with reference to adrenal cortical function.

: : State the underlying cause or causes of Cushing's syndrome.

: : Describe the clinical manifestations of Cushing's syndrome.

: : Explain the underlying pathology that is present in Addison's disease.

: : Compare the manifestations of Addison's disease with those of secondary adrenal insufficiency.

: : Describe the overall treatment of adrenal insufficiency.

:References

1. Daughaday WH, Cryer P: Growth hormone hypersecretion and acromegaly. Hosp Pract 13, No. 8:76, 1978
2. Guyton A: Textbook of Medical Physiology, 6th ed, p 924. Philadelphia, WB Saunders, 1981
3. Guyton A: Textbook of Medical Physiology, 6th ed, p 936. Philadelphia, WB Saunders, 1981
4. Klein AH et al: Improved prognosis in congenital hypothyroidism treated before age three months. J Pediatr 81:912, 1972
5. Fisher D: Screening for congenital hypothyroidism. Hosp Pract 12(12):77, 1977

6. Meek JC: Myxedema coma. Critical Care Quarterly 3:131, 1980

7. Robbins SL, Cotran RS: Pathologic Basis of Disease, 2nd ed, p 1399. Philadelphia, WB Saunders, 1979

8. Tepperman J: Metabolic and Endocrine Physiology, 4th ed, p 173. Chicago, Year Book Medical Publishers, 1980

9. McEwan BS: Influences of the adrenocortical hormone on pituitary and brain function. Monogr Endrocrinol 12:467–492, 1978

10. Tepperman J: Metabolic and Endocrine Physiology, 4th ed, p 189. Chicago, Year Book Medical Publishers, 1980

11. Tepperman J: Metabolic and Endocrine Physiology, 4th ed, p 187. Chicago, Year Book Medical Publishers, 1980

12. Robbins SL, Cotran RS: Pathologic Basis of Disease, 2nd ed, p 1395. Philadelphia, WB Saunders, 1979

13. Gold EM: Cushing's syndrome. Hosp Pract 14(6):75, 1979

14. Robbins SL, Cotran RS: Pathologic Basis of Disease, 2nd ed, p 1391. Philadelphia, WB Saunders, 1979

15. Axelrod L: Glucocorticoid therapy. Medicine 55(1):49, 1976

:Suggested Readings

Alterations in adrenal and thyroid function

Kern EB, Laws ER, Randall R, Westward WB: A transsphenoidal approach to the pituitary. Postgrad Med 63:97–108, 1978

Smith MJT, Selye H: Reducing the negative effects of stress. Am J Nurs 79(11):1953–1955, 1979

Sowers DK, Sowers JR: Pituitary emergencies. Critical Care Quarterly 3:45–54, 1980

Vinicor F, Cooper J: Early recognition of endocrine disorders. Hospital Medicine 15(9):38, 1979

Volpe R: The role of autoimmunity in hypoendocrine and hyperendocrine function. Ann Intern Med 87(1):86–99, 1977

Adrenal

Fredlund PN, Mecklenburg RS: Acute adrenal insufficiency: Diagnosis and management. Hospital Medicine 15(6):28–47, 1979

Hall RCW, Popkin MK, Stickney SK, Gardner ER: Presentation of the steroid psychoses. J Nerv Ment Dis 167(4):229, 1979

McEwen BS: Influences of adrenocorticol hormones on pituitary and brain function. Monogr Endocrinol 12:467, 1978

McFarlane J: Congenital adrenal hyperplasia. Am J Nurs 76(8):1290, 1976

Sanford SJ: Dysfunction of the adrenal gland: Physiologic considerations and nursing problems. Nurs Clin North Am 15(3):481, 1980

Schimke RN: Adrenal insufficiency. Critical Care Quarterly 3:19, 1980

Tzagournis M: Acute adrenal insufficiency. Heart Lung 7(4):603, 1978

Wachter–Shikora N: ACTH—A review of anatomy, physiology, and structure related to neuroendocrine effects. Journal of Neurosurgical Nursing 11(2):105, 1979

Wilson KS, Parker A: Adrenal suppression after short-term corticosteroid therapy. Lancet 1030, 1979

Thyroid

Carlson HE, Hershman JM: The hypothalamic–pituitary–thyroid axis. Med Clin North Am 59(5):1045, 1975

Dussault JH, Morissette J, Letarte J et al: Modification of a screening program for neonatal hypothyroidism. J Pediatr 92(2):274, 1978

Fisher DA: Thyroid function in the fetus and newborn. Med Clin North Am 59(5):1099, 1975

Fisher DA, Klein AH: Thyroid development and disorders of thyroid function in the newborn. N Engl J Med 304(12):702, 1981

Larsen PR: Tests of thyroid function. Med Clin North Am 59(5):1063, 1975

Lyon J, Spence DA: Congenital thyroid disease detected by screening program. Alaska Med 20(4):56, 1978

Mackin JF, Canary JJ, Pittman CS: Current concepts: Thyroid storm and its management. N Engl J Med 291(26):1396, 1974

Mazzaferri EL: Thyroid storm. Hospital Medicine 15(11):7, 1979

McKenzie JM, Zakarija M, Bonnyns M: Graves' disease. Med Clin North Am 59(5):1177, 1975

Meek JC: Myxedema coma. Cleve Clin Q 00:131–137, 1980

Oppenheimer JH, Surks MI: The peripheral action of the thyroid hormones. Med Clin North Am 59(5):1055, 1975

Safrit HF: Diagnosis and management of Graves' disease. Hospital Medicine 15(10):74, 1979

Sakamoto A, Salamoto G, Sugano H: History of cervical radiation and incidence of carcinoma of the pharynx, larynx and thyroid. Cancer 44:718, 1979

Spaulding SW, Noth RH: Thyroid–catecholamine interactions. Med Clin North Am 59(5):1123, 1975

Vagenakis AG, Braverman LE: Adverse effects of iodides on thyroid function. Med Clin North Am 59(5):1075, 1975

Verebey K, Volavka J, Clouet D: Endorphins in psychiatry: An overview and a hypothesis. Arch Gen Psychiatry 35:877, 1978

Vope R: Thyroiditis: Current views of pathogenesis. Med Clin North Am 59(5):1163, 1975

Wake MM, Brensinger JF: The nurse's role in hypothyroidism. Nurs Clin North Am 15(3):453, 1980

34

Control of Metabolism

All body activities require energy whether they involve an individual cell, a single organ, or the entire body. Metabolism is the organized process through which carbohydrates, fats, and proteins from ingested food are broken down, transformed, or otherwise converted into cellular energy. This chapter focuses on glucose, fat, and protein metabolism and the hormonal regulation of this process.

:Glucose, Fat, and Protein Metabolism

The process of metabolism is unique in that it not only allows for the continuous release of energy, but it couples this energy release with physiologic functioning. For example, the energy used for muscle contraction is derived largely from energy sources that are stored in the muscle cells. This energy is then released as the muscle contracts. Because most of our energy sources come from the three to four meals that we eat each day, the ability to store energy and control its release is important.

There are two phases of metabolism—anabolism and catabolism. *Anabolism* is the phase of metabolic storage and synthesis of cell constituents. Anabolism does not provide energy for the body, rather it requires energy. *Catabolism*, on the other hand, involves the breakdown of complex molecules into substances that can be used in the production of energy. The chemical intermediates for anabolism and catabolism are called *metabolites*, for example, lactic acid is one of the metabolites formed when glucose is broken down in the absence of oxygen.

Both anabolism and catabolism are catalyzed by *enzyme systems* that are located within body cells. A *substrate* is a substance upon which an enzyme acts. Enzyme systems selectively transform fuel substrates into cellular energy and facilitate the use of energy in the process of assembling molecules to form energy substrates and storage forms of energy.

Since body energy cannot be stored as heat, the cellular oxidative processes that release energy are flameless and have low temperature reactions. Instead of releasing only heat—as occurs when the same fuel is burned in the environment—the free energy that is released from the oxidation of foods is converted to chemical energy that can be stored. The body transforms carbohydrates, fats, and proteins into the intermediary compound, adenosine triphosphate (ATP). Adenosine triphosphate is often called the energy currency of the cell because almost all body cells use ATP as their energy source. The metabolic events involved in ATP formation allow cellular energy to be stored, used, and then replenished.

Glucose Metabolism

Glucose is an efficient fuel which, when metabolized in the presence of oxygen, breaks down to form carbon dioxide and water. Although many tissues and organ systems are able to use other forms of fuel, such as fatty acids and ketones, the brain and nervous system rely almost exclusively on glucose as a fuel source. The nervous system can neither store nor synthesize glucose, rather it relies on the minute-by-minute extraction of glucose from the blood as a means of meeting its energy needs. In the fed and early fasting state, the nervous system requires about 100 to 115 grams of glucose per day to meet its metabolic needs.[1,2]

The liver regulates the entry of glucose into the blood. Glucose ingested in the diet is transported from the gastrointestinal tract, via the portal vein, to the liver before it gains access to the circulatory system (Fig. 34-1). The liver both stores and synthesizes glucose. When blood sugar is increased, the liver removes glucose from the blood and stores it for future use. Conversely, the liver releases its glucose stores when blood sugar drops. In this way, the liver acts as a buffer system to regulate blood sugar levels. Generally speaking, it can be said that blood sugar levels reflect the difference between the amount of glucose that is released into the circulation by the liver, and the amount of glucose that is removed from the blood by body cells.

Excess glucose is stored in two forms: (1) it can be converted to fatty acids and then stored in *fat cells as triglycerides*, or (2) it can be stored in the *liver and skeletal muscle as glycogen*. Small amounts of glycogen are also stored in the skin and in some of the glandular tissues.

Glycogenolysis

Glycogenolysis, or the breakdown of glycogen, is controlled by the action of two hormones: *glucagon* and *epinephrine*. Epinephrine is more effective in stimulating glycogen breakdown in muscle. The liver, on the other hand, is more responsive to glucagon. The synthesis and degradation of glycogen is important because it helps maintain blood sugar levels during periods of fasting and strenuous exercise. Only the liver, in contrast to other tissues which store glycogen, is able to release its glucose stores into the blood for use by other tissues, such as the brain and nervous system. This is because glycogen breaks down to form a phosphorylated glucose molecule. Glucose is too large, in its phosphorylated form, to pass through the cell membrane. The liver, but not skeletal muscle, has the enzyme glucose-6-phosphatase that is needed to remove the phosphate group and to allow the glucose molecule to enter the blood stream.

Although they are rare, there are a number of genetic disorders in which glycogen breakdown is impaired. All of these disorders result in excessive accumulation of abnormal forms of glycogen. *Von Gierke's disease* involves a genetic *deficiency of glucose-6-phosphatase*. Children with this disease have stunted growth, liver enlargement, hypoglycemia, and hyperlipidemia due to mobilization of fatty acids. *McArdle's disease* is characterized by a deficiency in skeletal muscle glycogen, and as a result of this, the disease causes extreme muscle weakness.

Gluconeogenesis

The synthesis of glucose is referred to as *gluconeogenesis*, or the building of glucose from new sources. The process of gluconeogenesis converts amino acids, lactate, and glycerol into glucose. Most of the gluconeogenesis occurs in the liver. Although fatty acids can be used as fuel by many body cells, they cannot be converted to glucose.

Glucose produced through the process of gluconeogenesis is either stored in the liver as glycogen or it is released into the general circulation. During periods of food deprivation, or when the diet is low in carbohydrates, gluconeogenesis provides the glucose that is needed to meet the metabolic needs of the brain and other glucose-dependent tissues.

Several hormones stimulate gluconeogenesis, including *glucagon*, *glucocorticoid hormones* from the adrenal cortex, and *thyroid hormone*.

Alcohol ingestion interferes with the liver's ability to produce glucose. This is because the metabolism of alcohol competes for the use of the same hydrogen carrier, nicotinamide-adenine dinucleotide (NAD), that is needed for glucose production. Although probably not a frequent occurrence, alcohol-induced hypoglycemia can occur after a period of fasting. Because glucose stimulates insulin release, this tends to occur more readily when alcohol is drunk in combination with sugar-containing mixers.

Fat Metabolism

The average American diet provides 40% to 50% of calories in the form of fats. In contrast to glucose which yields only four calories per gram, each gram

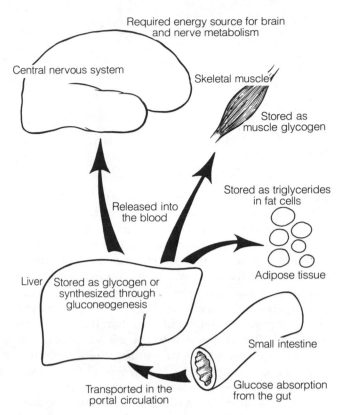

Figure 34–1. Regulation of blood glucose by the liver.

of fat yields nine calories. Additionally, another 30% to 50% of the carbohydrates that are consumed in the diet are converted to triglycerides for storage.

A *triglyceride* contains *three fatty acids* that are linked by a *glycerol* molecule (Fig. 34-2). Fatty acids and triglycerides can be derived from dietary sources, they can be synthesized in the body, or they can be mobilized from fat depots. Excess carbohydrate is converted to triglyceride and is then transported by lipoproteins in the blood to adipose cells for storage. *One gram of anhydrous (water-free) fat stores more than six times as much energy as one hydrated gram of glycogen.* One of the reasons that weight loss is greatest at the beginning of a fast or weight-loss program is that it is at this time that the body is using its glycogen stores. Later, when the body begins to use energy stored as triglycerides, water losses are decreased and weight loss tends to plateau.

The mobilization of fat for use in energy production is facilitated by the action of enzymes or lipases that break the triglycerides into three fatty acids and a glycerol molecule. Following triglyceride breakdown, both the fatty acids and the glycerol molecule leave the fat cell and enter the circulation. Once in the circulation, many of the fatty acids are trans-

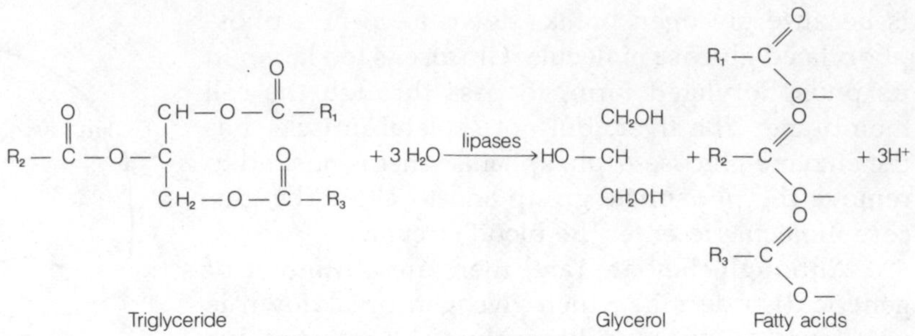

$$R_2 - C - O - C \begin{matrix} CH-O-C-R_1 \\ O \\ CH_2-O-C-R_3 \end{matrix} + 3\,H_2O \xrightarrow{\text{lipases}} \begin{matrix} CH_2OH \\ HO-CH \\ CH_2OH \end{matrix} + R_2-C + 3H^+$$

Figure 34–2.   Mobilization of fatty acids
from triglycerides.   Triglyceride   Glycerol   Fatty acids

ported to the liver where they are removed from the blood and are then either used by liver cells as a source of energy or are converted to ketones.

The efficient burning of fatty acids requires a balance between carbohydrate and fat metabolism. The ratio of fatty acid and carbohydrate utilization is altered in situations that favor fat breakdown, such as diabetes mellitus and fasting. In these situations, the liver produces more ketones than it can use; this excess is then released into the blood stream. Ketones can be an important source of energy, since even the brain adapts to the use of ketones during prolonged periods of starvation. A problem arises, however, when fat breakdown is accelerated and the production of ketones exceeds tissue utilization. Since ketone bodies are organic acids they cause

Figure 34–3.   Influence of the pancreatic hormones, insulin, and glucagon on the release of glucose into the blood by the liver.

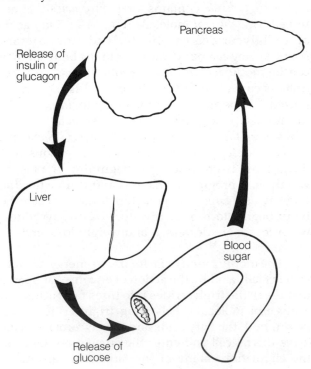

Pancreas

Release of
insulin or
glucagon

Liver

Blood
sugar

Release of
glucose

ketoacidosis when they are present in excess amounts. The activation of lipases and the subsequent mobilization of fatty acids is stimulated by epinephrine, glucocorticoid hormones, growth hormones, and glucagon.

Protein Metabolism

About three-fourths of body solids are proteins. Proteins are essential for the formation of all body structures, including genes, enzymes, contractile proteins in muscle, matrix of bone, and hemoglobin of red blood cells.

Amino acids are the building blocks of proteins. Unlike glucose and fatty acids, there is only a limited facility for the storage of excess amino acids in the body. Most of the stored amino acids are contained in body proteins. Amino acids in excess of those needed for protein synthesis are converted to fatty acids, ketone bodies, or glucose and are then stored or used as metabolic fuel. Each gram of protein yields four calories. Since fatty acids cannot be converted to glucose, the body must break down proteins and use the amino acids as a major source of substrate for gluconeogenesis during periods when metabolic needs exceed food intake. The liver has the enzymes and transfer mechanisms needed to deaminate and to convert the amino groups (NH_2) from the amino acid to urea. Thus the breakdown or degradation of proteins and amino acids occurs primarily in the liver, which is also the site of gluconeogenesis.

:Control of Metabolism

Metabolism is controlled by neural and endocrine influences. Neural stimuli influence the release of hormones that are concerned with metabolism. The autonomic nervous system has a direct effect on many metabolic functions through the release of *epinephrine* and *norepinephrine*.

While the respiratory and circulatory systems

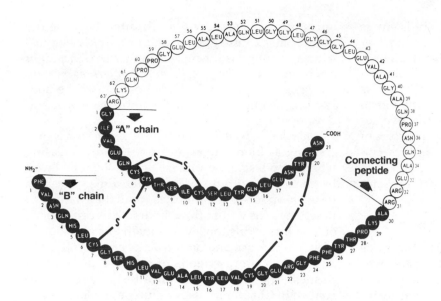

Figure 34–4.   Amino-acid sequence of porcine proinsulin showing the A chain, the B chain, and the C-peptide link. (From Shaw WN, Chance RE: Diabetes 17, No. 12:738, 1968)

combine efforts to furnish the body with oxygen needed for metabolic purposes, it is the liver, in concert with the pancreatic hormones insulin and glucagon, that controls the body's fuel supply (Fig. 34-3). Secretion of both insulin and glucagon is regulated by blood sugar levels. *Insulin* is released in response to an *increase in blood sugar levels* and *glucagon release* occurs when there is a *drop* in *blood sugar levels*. Both insulin and glucagon are transported from the pancreas, via the *portal circulation*, to the liver where they exert an almost instantaneous effect on blood glucose levels.

Insulin

Insulin is produced by the pancreatic cells in the islets of Langerhans. The active form of the hormone is composed of two polypeptide chains—an A chain and a B chain (Fig. 34-4). Before 1967, it was assumed that each chain was formed separately and then joined. It is now known that the chains emerge with the appropriate linkage required for biologic activity from a single chain called *proinsulin*. In converting proinsulin to insulin, enzymes in the beta cell cleave proinsulin at specific sites to form two substances, active *insulin* and a *C-peptide* chain (the link that served to join the A and B chains before they were separated). Both active insulin and the C-peptide chain are released simultaneously from the beta cell (Fig. 34-5). The C-peptide chains can be measured and this measurement can be used as a means to study beta-cell activity. For example, injected insulin in the mature-onset diabetic would provide few, if any, C-peptide chains, whereas insulin secreted by the beta cells would be accompanied by secretion of C-peptide chains.

Figure 34–5.   A scanning electron micrograph of a beta cell from the islets of Langerhans in the pancreas-secreting insulin. (Courtesy of Kenneth Siegesmund, Ph.D., Anatomy Department, Medical College of Wisconsin)

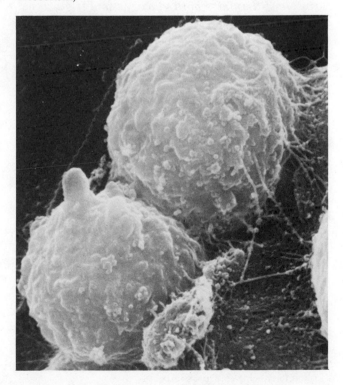

Insulin that is secreted by the beta cells enters the portal circulation and travels directly to the liver where about 50% of it is either utilized or degraded. Once it has been released into the general circulation, insulin has a half-life of about 15 minutes. This is because circulating insulin is rapidly bound to peripheral tissues or is destroyed by the liver or kidneys. There is much similarity in the structure of insulin among the different species; this has permitted use of insulin extracted from beef and pork sources to be used in treatment of human diabetes mellitus.

Actions of insulin

The actions of insulin are threefold: (1) it provides for glucose storage, (2) it prevents fat breakdown, and (3) it increases protein synthesis. Although there are several hormones that are known to increase blood sugar, *insulin is the only hormone that is currently known to have a direct effect in lowering blood sugar*. The actions of insulin are summarized in Table 34-1.

Insulin lowers blood sugar by *facilitating its transport into skeletal muscle and adipose tissue*. Although liver cells do not require insulin for glucose transport, a rise in insulin levels does cause an increase in hepatic uptake of glucose, presumably by increasing the intracellular trapping of glucose through the attachment of a phosphate group. Insulin also *decreases the breakdown of glucose and fat stores and stimulates both glycogen and triglyceride synthesis*. In relation to body proteins, insulin both *inhibits protein breakdown* and *increases protein synthesis*. When sufficient glucose and insulin are present, protein breakdown is inhibited because the body is able to use glucose and fatty acids as a fuel source. Insulin also increases the *active transport of amino acids into body cells and accelerates protein synthesis within the cell*. In the child and the adolescent, insulin is needed for normal growth and development.

Insulin is regulated by blood glucose levels, increasing as blood sugar levels rise and decreasing when blood sugar declines. Serum insulin levels begin to rise within minutes after a meal, reach a peak in about thirty minutes, and then return to baseline levels within three hours. Between periods of food intake, insulin levels remain low and sources of stored glucose and amino acids are mobilized to supply the energy needs of glucose-dependent tissues. The glucose tolerance test, which is described in Chapter 35, uses a glucose challenge as an indirect measure of the body's ability to secrete insulin and to remove glucose from the blood.

Glucagon

Glucagon is a small protein molecule that is produced by the pancreatic alpha cells of the islets of Langerhans. Like insulin, glucagon travels by way of the portal vein to the liver where it exerts its main action.

The actions of glucagon are diametrically opposed to those of insulin. Glucagon stimulates *glycogenolysis* and *gluconeogenesis*, increases *lipolysis*, and enhances the *breakdown of proteins*. The actions of glucagon are summarized in Table 34-2.

It has been suggested that abnormalities in glucagon secretion contribute to the elevation in blood sugar that is observed in diabetes mellitus. Unger suggests that it is the ratio of insulin to glucagon, rather than the absolute amount of either

Table 34-1   Actions of Insulin

Glucose

Increases glucose transport into skeletal muscle and adipose tissue

Increases glycogen synthesis

Decreases gluconeogenesis

Fats

Increases glucose transport into fat cells

Increases fatty acid transport into adipose cells

Increases triglyceride synthesis

Proteins

Increases active transport of amino acids into cells

Increases protein synthesis by accelerating translation of RNA by ribosomes and increase transcription of DNA in the nucleus to form increased amounts of RNA

Decreases protein breakdown by enhancing use of glucose and fatty acids as a fuel source

Table 34-2   Actions of Glucagon

Glucose

Promotes the breakdown of glycogen into glucose-6-phosphate

Increases gluconeogenesis

Fats

Enhances lipolysis in adipose tissue, liberating glycerol for use in gluconeogenesis

Proteins

Increases breakdown of proteins into amino acids for use in gluconeogenesis

Increases transport of amino acids in hepatic cells

Increases conversion of amino acids into glucose precursors

hormone, that determines blood sugar levels.[3] According to theory, glucagon secretion is unopposed in the diabetic because of the lack of insulin which therefore leads to increased production of glucose by the liver.

Catecholamines

The catecholamines, epinephrine and norepinephrine, help maintain blood sugar levels during periods of stress. The actions of epinephrine are summarized in Table 34-3. Epinephrine inhibits insulin release and promotes glycogenolysis by stimulating the conversion of muscle and liver glycogen to glucose. It is important to recall that muscle glycogen cannot be released into the blood; nevertheless, the mobilization of these stores for muscle use conserves blood sugar for use by other tissues such as the brain and the nervous system. During periods of exercise and other types of stress, epinephrine inhibits insulin release from the beta cells and thereby decreases the movement of glucose into muscle cells. The catecholamines also increase *lipase activity* and thereby cause *increased mobilization of fatty acids*; this also serves to conserve glucose. The blood sugar elevating effect of epinephrine is an important *homeostatic mechanism in hypoglycemia*.

Somatostatin

Somatostatin is also produced in the pancreas; it is secreted by the delta cells in the islets of Langerhans. Somatostatin inhibits the secretion of insulin, glucagon, and growth hormone. At present, the physiologic significance of somatostatin is largely unknown.

Growth Hormone and the Adrenal Cortical Hormones

Both growth hormone and the glucocorticoid hormones from the adrenal gland have the potential to elevate blood sugar.

Growth hormone

Increased growth hormone tends to cause a state of insulin insensitivity. Growth hormone decreases both the cellular utilization and the uptake of glucose; therefore, increased levels of growth hormone tend to cause an increase in blood glucose levels. In turn, this increase in blood sugar increases the stimulus for insulin secretion by the beta cells. Growth hormone also has a direct stimulatory effect on the beta cells, thus these two combined effects can literally cause the beta cells to "burn out." When this

Table 34-3 Actions of Epinephrine

Mobilizes glycogen stores
Decreases movement of glucose into body cells
Inhibits insulin release from beta cells
Mobilizes fatty acids from adipose tissue

occurs, as it can in persons with increased levels of growth hormone (acromegaly), diabetes develops. In persons who already have diabetes mellitus, an increase in growth hormone tends to cause problems in the control of blood sugar levels.

Adrenal cortical hormones

Cortisol and other adrenal cortical hormones stimulate gluconeogenesis by the liver, sometimes increasing the rate of hepatic glucose production six to tenfold. These hormones also cause a moderate decrease in tissue utilization of glucose. In predisposed persons, the prolonged elevation of the adrenal cortical hormones can lead to hyperglycemia and the development of diabetes mellitus.

In summary, glucose, fats, and proteins serve as fuel sources for cellular metabolism. These fuel sources are ingested during meals and are then stored for future use. When sufficient insulin is present, glucose enters liver or muscle cells and is stored as glycogen, or enters fat cells for storage as triglycerides. Glycogen provides for the short-term energy needs of the body. Storage forms of fat are mobilized during periods of food deprivation or in conditions such as diabetes mellitus in which glucose entry into body cells is impaired.

The brain relies almost exclusively on glucose as a fuel source, and when glucose stores have been depleted, the liver synthesizes glucose from amino acids, lactate, and glycerol in a process called gluconeogenesis. It is important to note that while glucose can be converted to fatty acids for storage, there is no pathway for converting fatty acids to glucose. Instead, fatty acids are used directly as a fuel source or are converted to ketones by the liver. When ketone production exceeds utilization, ketoacidosis develops.

:Study Guide

After you have studied this chapter, you should be able to meet the following objectives:

: : Differentiate anabolism and catabolism.

: : Name the compound that serves as the cellular energy source.

∶ ∶ Describe glucose regulation by the liver.

∶ ∶ Describe the role of glucagon in glycogenolysis.

∶ ∶ State the purpose of gluconeogenesis.

∶ ∶ Explain how fat is mobilized for use in energy production.

∶ ∶ Describe the role of the liver in protein metabolism.

∶ ∶ State the sequence of events in insulin production.

∶ ∶ Describe the actions of insulin with reference to glucose, fats, and proteins.

∶ ∶ Compare the actions of insulin with those of glucagon.

∶ ∶ Describe the role of epinephrine in glycogenolysis.

∶ ∶ Explain the relationship between growth hormone and diabetes mellitus.

∶ ∶ Explain the role of the adrenal cortical hormones in gluconeogenesis.

:References

1. Sauded C, Felig P: The metabolic events of starvation. Am J Med 60:117, 1976
2. Cahill CF Jr: Starvation in man. Clin Endocrinol Metab 5, No. 2:405, 1976
3. Unger RH: The esential role of glucagon in the pathogenesis of diabetes mellitus. Lancet 14, 1975

35

Diabetes Mellitus

Diabetes mellitus is a chronic alteration in health which currently affects over 10 million persons in the United States. Each year the incidence of diabetes increases by 6%; this is evidenced by the fact that 600,000 Americans are diagnosed annually as having the disease. If the present trend continues, the number of diabetics in the United States can be expected to double every 15 years. This means that every baby born today has a one-in-five chance of developing diabetes in its lifetime.[1]

Diabetes affects persons in all age groups and from all walks of life. Among both young and old, diabetes increases the risk of vascular problems, blindness, peripheral neuropathies, and kidney disease. Diabetes increases the risk of maternal complications during pregnancy, and infants of diabetic mothers have a greater than normal incidence of congenital anomalies; they are also more prone to develop neonatal complications, such as respiratory distress syndrome and hypoglycemia.

The term diabetes mellitus means the "running through of sugar." In spite of its recent increase, the disease did not have its origin in the twentieth century. Reports of the disorder can be traced back to the first century A.D. when Aretaeus the Cappadocian described the disorder as a chronic affection that was characterized by intense thirst and voluminous honey-sweet urine—"the melting down of flesh into urine."[2] It was the discovery of insulin by Banting and Best in 1921 that transformed the once-fatal disease into a chronic health problem.

Diabetes can be defined as an insulin deficiency state that interferes with carbohydrate, protein, and fat metabolism. The uncontrolled diabetic is unable to transport glucose into fat and muscle cells, and as a result there is increased breakdown of fat and protein. Diabetes is accompanied by a predisposition to vascular changes in both the vessels of the microcirculation and the macrocirculation. There are those who believe that the vascular disorders are a complication of diabetes and others who believe that diabetes is an accompaniment of vascular disorders.

:Types of Diabetes

Although diabetes mellitus is clearly a disorder of insulin availability, it is probable that diabetes is not a single disease. A classification system that divides diabetes into *insulin-dependent* and *noninsulin-dependent* was developed by an international workshop sponsored by the National Diabetes Data Group of NIH (Table 35-1). The system has been endorsed by the American Diabetes Association.

The group also proposed a classification of *gestational diabetes* (diabetes that develops during pregnancy), *impaired glucose tolerance* (abnormal glucose tolerance test without other signs of diabetes), and *diabetes caused by other conditions* (e.g., Cushing's disease).

Insulin-Dependent Diabetes Mellitus (IDDM)

Insulin-dependent diabetes is characterized by an absolute insulin deficiency state. This form of diabetes was formerly called juvenile diabetes, but the term has proved to be inaccurate because it can occur at any age. Persons with IDDM often experience marked alterations in blood sugar and are frequently referred to as "brittle diabetics." Because of their absolute lack of insulin, persons with this form of diabetes are particularly prone to develop ketoacidosis.

Noninsulin-Dependent Diabetes Mellitus (NIDDM)

This form of diabetes has been called maturity-onset diabetes, and is associated with a lack of insulin availability, rather than an absolute insulin deficiency. It has been reported that this relative insulin deficiency arises because (1) inadequate amounts of insulin are produced in relation to need, (2) insulin is destroyed before it can exert its effect, (3) insulin release is out of phase with food intake and blood sugar levels, or (4) there is a decrease in the number of insulin receptors on the cells. Individuals with NIDDM are usually older and frequently overweight, and have fewer problems with control than juvenile-onset diabetics. Often this form of diabetes can be controlled by diet alone. Noninsulin-dependent diabetes is said to be ketosis resistant, meaning that these diabetics do not readily develop ketoacidosis. Evidence suggests that it requires more insulin to transport glucose into fat cells than is required to prevent lipolysis. In the maturity-onset diabetic there is probably enough insulin to prevent the breakdown of adipose tissue but not enough to lower blood sugar by transporting glucose into fat cells.

:Etiology of Diabetes

Because diabetes is apparently not a single disorder, it is probable that it does not have a single cause. A number of etiologic factors, including inheritance,

Table 35–1   Classification of Diabetes and Glucose Intolerance States

Classification	Former Terminology	Characteristics
Diabetes Mellitus (DM)		
Type I		
Insulin-dependent diabetes mellitus (IDDM)	Juvenile-onset diabetes	Persons in this subclass are dependent upon injected insulin
		Ketosis prone
Type II		
Noninsulin-dependent diabetes mellitus (NIDDM) 1. Nonobese NIDDM 2. Obese NIDDM (60%–90%)	Adult-onset, maturity-onset diabetes	Persons in this subclass are not insulin dependent, but they may use insulin
		Not ketosis prone
		Frequently obese
Other Types		
Pancreatic disease	Secondary diabetes	Presence of diabetes and associated condition
Hormonal		
Drug or chemical induced insulin receptor abnormalities		
Certain genetic defects		
Other types		
Impaired Glucose Tolerance (IGT)		
Nonobese IGT	Asymptomatic, chemical, subclinical, borderline, latent diabetes	Based on nondiagnostic fasting glucose levels and glucose tolerance test between normal and diabetic
Obese IGT		
IGT associated with other conditions, which may be (1) pancreatic disease, (2) hormonal, (3) drug or chemical, (4) insulin-receptor abnormalities, or (5) genetic syndromes		
Gestational Diabetes Mellitus (GDM)	Gestational diabetes	Glucose intolerance that developed during pregnancy
		Increased risk of perinatal complications
		Increased risk of developing diabetes within five to ten years after parturition

Adapted from National Diabetes Data Group: Classification and diagnosis of diabetes mellitus and other categories of glucose intolerance. Diabetes 28:1042, 1979.

have been implicated in the development of diabetes. Inheritance is thought to be autosomal recessive, with variable penetrance of the genes that determine the expression of diabetes. Studies suggest that heredity plays a greater role in the development of maturity-onset diabetes than it does in the development of juvenile-onset diabetes.[3,4] Of particular interest is a new approach to the study of genetics that uses antigens detected from the cell surface of nucleated cells—histocompatibility antigens (HLA antigens, Chap. 5). Insulin-dependent diabetes is associated with an increased or decreased frequency of certain HLA types.

Although their role is not clearly understood, viruses and beta-cell toxins have also been suspected as causative factors in diabetes. It has been observed that the onset of insulin-dependent diabetes rises in later summer and winter; this corresponds with the prevalence of common viral infections in the community.[5,6] Mumps,[7] Coxsackievirus-group B, type A,[8] and congenital rubella[9,10] have been associated with development of insulin-dependent diabetes.

Fortunately, not all predisposed individuals—those with a family history of diabetes or known exposure to beta toxic agents—develop diabetes. This suggests that there are other environmental or risk factors which contribute to the development of clinical diabetes. A significant risk factor for development of diabetes in predisposed individuals is obesity. There is a hyperinsulinemia that has been demonstrated in obesity, suggesting that such individuals have an increased resistance to insulin (Fig. 35-1).

Failure of the beta cells to produce sufficient insulin is a primary cause of diabetes. Hypoglycemia can also result as a secondary disorder in the course of another disease. Secondary causes of carbohydrate intolerance include endocrine disorders: excess production of growth hormone, glucocorticoids, catecholamines, and glucagon. The diabetes that accompanies acromegaly (growth hormone) and Cushing's disease (glucocorticosteriod) is an example of glucose intolerance due to excess endocrine activity. Chronic pancreatitis or surgical removal of the pancreas reduces the number of functioning cells and causes hyperglycemia.

Several diuretics—the thiazides, furosemide, and ethacrynic acid—tend to elevate blood sugar. These diuretics increase potassium loss which is

Figure 35–1. The mean absolute insulin responses in thin and obese diabetic subjects during 3-hour (100 G) oral glucose tolerance curve. (From Bagdade JD, Biermann EL, Porter D: The significance of basal insulin levels in evaluation of the insulin response to glucose in diabetic and nondiabetic subjects. J Clin Invest 46, No. 10:1553, 1967)

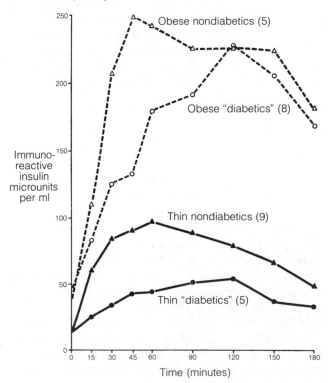

thought to impair insulin release. Other drugs known to cause hyperglycemia include the following: diazoxide, glucocorticosteroids, levodopa, oral contraceptives, sympathomimetics, phenothiazines, phenytoin, and total parenteral nutrition (hyperalimentation). Drug-related increases in blood sugar are usually reversed once the drug has been discontinued.

Diagnostic Tests

There are various tests that measure blood and urine glucose levels. These tests are used to screen for diabetes and to follow the progress of persons with known diabetes. Tests that measure insulin levels usually involve the use of radioimmunoassay techniques, and are not routinely used in the diagnosis of diabetes.

Blood tests

The glucose tolerance test. The glucose tolerance test is an important screening test for diabetes. The test measures the body's ability to store glucose by removing it from the blood. The test measures the blood sugar response to a given amount of concentrated glucose at selected intervals, usually ½, 1, 1½, 2, and 3 hours (urine glucose is also measured at these times). Insulin levels may be measured at these intervals. In the normal individual, blood sugars will return to normal within three hours after ingestion of a glucose load, in which case it can be assumed that sufficient insulin is present to allow glucose to leave the blood and to enter body cells. Since the diabetic lacks the ability to respond to an increase in blood glucose by releasing adequate insulin to facilitate storage, blood sugar levels not only rise above those observed in normal individuals, but remain elevated for longer periods of time (Fig. 35-2). The glucose tolerance test is a useful diagnostic measure for detecting subclinical forms of diabetes—the stage of the disease in which the fasting blood sugar may still be normal, and other obvious signs of diabetes are not yet detectable. A variation of the glucose tolerance test is the cortisone glucose tolerance test. The administration of cortisone challenges the body's ability to metabolize glucose. Another form of the glucose tolerance test is used for screening purposes; this form of the test involves sampling blood sugar two hours following a glucose challenge. Fasting blood sugars measure blood sugar levels after food has been withheld for a period of 8 to 12 hours.

Home blood glucose monitoring. Recent technological advances have provided the means for improving diabetes control through home monitoring of blood glucose levels. The system uses a drop of capillary blood obtained by pricking the finger with a special needle or small lancet. The drop of blood is placed on a reagent strip.

One method makes use of a glucose reflectance meter (Ames, Eyetone, or Bio-Dynamics Stattik) for reading the results of the test. In another method (Chemstrip bG) the results are obtained by comparing the color changes on the reagent strip with color blocks provided with the test strips. Home monitoring methods provide the diabetic with a means for adjusting insulin, food, and activity based on each day's glucose reading.

Glycosylated hemoglobin. This test measures the amount of glycosylated hemoglobin (hemoglobin into which glucose has been incorporated) that is present in the blood. Normally hemoglobin does not contain glucose when it is manufactured and released from the bone marrow. During its 120-day life span in the red blood cell, 5% to 10% of the hemoglobin normally becomes glycosylated.[11] Since glucose entry into the red blood cell is not insulin dependent, the rate at which glucose becomes attached to the hemoglobin molecule is dependent upon blood sugar. Glycosylation is essentially irreversible; hence the level of glycosylated hemoglobin that is present in the blood provides an index of blood sugar levels over the previous two months or more.

Urine tests

Two types of tests are used to measure glucose content in the urine, copper reduction and glucose oxidase tests. Clinitest utilizes a copper-reduction reagent that is responsive to a number of substances. Consequently, Clinitest may give false positive results. The glucose oxidase tests (Tes–Tape, Clinistix, and Diastix) contain an enzyme that specifically reacts with glucose. Certain substances interfere with color changes in the glucose oxidase tests and in some situations may produce a false negative result. The glucose oxidase tests are very sensitive to small amounts of glucose and are usually not recommended for use in children. The actual amount of glucose (mg% or mg/100 ml urine) represented by the results of the various tests, as 1+, 2+, 3+, and 4+, also varies. For example, a 2+ result with Clinitest is representative of ¾ mg% glucose; with Diastix it represents ½ mg% glucose; and with Tes-

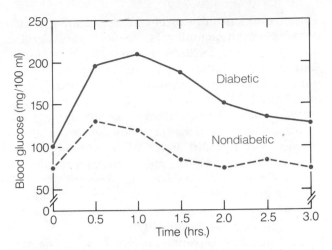

Figure 35–2. Results of a glucose tolerance test for diabetics and nondiabetics. Blood samples are usually taken at one-half hour intervals following ingestion of a glucose solution containing 1.75 gram of glucose per kg of body weight. The test may be modified for use as a screening tool.

Tape, ¼ mg%. Because many factors affect the accuracy of both types of urine tests, the reader is referred to other literature sources, including the package insert which comes with the urine testing reagent. The pharmacist is a valuable resource when the effect of a specific drug on urine testing methods is under consideration.

:Signs and Symptoms of Clinical Diabetes Mellitus

Diabetes mellitus may have a rapid or insidious onset. In IDDM, signs and symptoms are often acute and of sudden origin. On the other hand, NIDDM often develops more insidiously; its presence may be detected during a routine medical examination or when a patient seeks medical care for other reasons.

The most commonly identified signs and symptoms of diabetes are those which are often referred to as the three "polys"—*polyuria* (excessive urination), *polydipsia* (excessive thirst), and *polyphagia* (excessive hunger). These three symptoms are closely related to the hyperglycemia (elevated blood sugar) and glycosuria (sugar in the urine) that is present in diabetes. Glucose is a small, osmotically active molecule. When blood sugar is sufficiently elevated, the amount of glucose that is filtered by the glomeruli of the kidney will exceed the amount that can be reabsorbed by the renal tubules; this results in *glycosuria* and large accompanying losses of water in the urine.

Thirst results from intracellular dehydration which occurs as blood-sugar levels rise and water is pulled out of body cells, including those in the thirst center. Cellular dehydration also causes dryness of the mouth. This early symptom may be easily overlooked in NIDDM in which there is a gradual increase in blood sugar without accompanying signs of ketoacidosis. Polyphagia is usually not present in persons with NIDDM. In IDDM, it probably results from cellular starvation and depletion of cellular stores of carbohydrates, fats, and proteins.

Weight loss is a frequent occurrence in the uncontrolled insulin-dependent diabetic. The causes of weight loss are twofold. First, there is a loss of body fluids due to osmotic diuresis. Vomiting may exaggerate the fluid loss in ketoacidosis. Secondly, there is a loss of body tissue as the lack of insulin forces the body to use its fat stores and cellular proteins as sources of energy. In terms of weight loss there is often a marked difference between NIDDM and IDDM. Weight loss is an almost universal phenomenon in the uncontrolled insulin-dependent diabetic, whereas the individual with uncomplicated NIDDM often has problems with obesity.

There are other signs and symptoms related to hyperglycemia, including recurrent blurring of vision, fatigue, paresthesias, and increased incidence of yeast infections. In NIDDM, these are often the symptoms that prompt an individual to seek medical attention. Blurred vision occurs at a time when blood sugar levels are being brought under control. This is because there was a loss of water from the eye during the period of poor control, and then as blood sugar decreases with treatment water moves back into the lens, making it difficult to focus. Both hyperglycemia and glycosuria favor the growth of yeast organisms. Pruritus and vulvovaginitis due to candidial infections are frequent initial complaints in the woman with NIDDM.

In summary, the classical signs and symptoms of clinical diabetes mellitus include increases in thirst and urination, hunger in the presence of weight loss, dehydration, visual changes, fatigue, paresthesias, hyperglycemia, and glycosuria.

Acute Complications

The three major acute complications of diabetes are hypoglycemia, ketoacidosis, and hyperosmolar coma. It is important for the reader to recognize that *the body responds to acute changes in physiologic function with a series of predictable responses.* The acute complications of diabetes are no exception.

Hypoglycemia

Hypoglycemia, often called insulin reaction or insulin shock, occurs when blood sugar falls below 50 mg per 100 ml of blood (see Table 35-2). An insulin reaction is characterized by sudden onset and the rapidity with which it progresses. The signs and symptoms of hypoglycemia can be divided into two categories, those caused by *altered cerebral function* and those related to *activation of the autonomic nervous system*. Because the brain relies on blood glucose as its main energy source, hypoglycemia causes behaviors related to altered cerebral function. There is often headache, difficulty in problem solving, disturbed or altered behavior, coma, and convulsions. At the onset of the hypoglycemic episode, activation of the *parasympathetic nervous system* causes hunger. The intitial parasympathetic response is followed by activation of the *sympathetic nervous system*; this causes anxiety, sweating, and constriction of the skin vessels (the skin is cool and clammy). Although individual persons respond differently in insulin reaction, each person usually has the same pattern of response during each insulin reaction. For this reason, it is helpful if this response pattern can be identified during the early stages of treatment in the insulin-dependent diabetic.

Table 35-2   Signs and Symptoms of Insulin Reaction*

Onset—sudden

Laboratory findings
  Blood sugar less than 50 mg/100 ml

Impaired cerebral function (due to decreased glucose availability for brain metabolism)
  Feeling of vagueness
  Headache
  Difficulty in problem solving
  Slurred speech
  Impaired motor function
  Change in emotional behavior
  Convulsions
  Coma

Compensatory autonomic nervous system responses
  Parasympathetic responses
    Hunger
    Nausea
    Hypotension
    Bradycardia
  Sympathetic responses
    Anxiety
    Sweating
    Vasoconstriction of skin vessels (skin is pale and cool)
    Tachycardia

*There is a wide variation in manifestation of signs and symptoms among individuals, that is, not every diabetic will have all or even most of the symptoms.

The signs and symptoms of hypoglycemia are more variable in children and in the elderly. Elderly persons may not display the typical autonomic responses that are associated with hypoglycemia, but frequently develop signs of impaired function of the central nervous system, including mental confusion and bizarre behavior.

Many factors tend to precipitate insulin reaction in the insulin-dependent diabetic: error in insulin dose, failure to eat, increased exercise, decreased insulin needs following removal of a stress situation, change in insulin site. Alcohol tends to decrease liver gluconeogenesis, and the diabetic needs to be cautioned about its potential for causing hypoglycemia, especially if it is consumed in large amounts or on an empty stomach.

The most effective treatment of an insulin reaction is the immediate ingestion of a concentrated carbohydrate source, such as sugar, honey, candy, or orange juice. Alternative methods for elevating blood sugar may be required when the diabetic is unconscious or unable to swallow. Glucagon may be given intravenously, intramuscularly, or subcutaneously. The liver contains only a limited amount of glycogen (about 75 grams); glucagon will be ineffective in persons whose glycogen stores have been depleted. A small amount of honey or glucose gel (tubes of cake-decorating gel can be used for this purpose) can be inserted into the buccal pouch (under the tongue) in situations where swallowing is impaired. In situations of severe, life-threatening hypoglycemia, it may be necessary to administer glucose (20 to 50 ml of a 50% solution) intravenously.

Diabetic ketoacidosis

Ketoacidosis occurs when ketone production by the liver exceeds cellular utilization and renal excretion. In the insulin-dependent diabetic, insulin lack leads to mobilization of fatty acids and a subsequent increase in ketone production.

When compared with an insulin reaction, diabetic ketoacidosis is usually slower in onset and recovery is more prolonged. Blood sugar levels are elevated and urine sugar is greater than 2%. Plasma pH and bicarbonate are decreased and urine tests for acetone (Acetest or Ketostix) are positive. The signs and symptoms of ketoacidosis are summarized in Table 35–3.

There are two major metabolic derangements in diabetic ketoacidosis, *hyperglycemia* and *metabolic acidosis*. The hyperglycemia leads to osmotic diuresis, dehydration, and a critical loss of electrolytes. The metabolic acidosis is caused by the excess ketoacids that require buffering by the bicar-

Table 35–3 Signs and Symptoms of Diabetic Ketoacidosis

Onset—(1 to 24 hours)

Laboratory findings
  Blood sugar greater than 250 mg/100 ml
  Urine sugar greater than 2%
  Ketonemia and presence of ketones in the urine
  Decreased plasma pH (less than 7.3) and bicarbonate (less than 24 mEq)

Dehydration due to hyperglycemia
  Warm, dry skin
  Dry mucous membranes
  Tachycardia
  Weak, thready pulse
  Acute weight loss
  Hypotension

Ketoacidosis
  Anorexia, nausea, and vomiting
  Odor of ketones on the breath
  Depression of the central nervous system
    Lethargy and fatigue
    Stupor
    Coma
  Abdominal pain

Compensatory responses
  Rapid, deep respirations (Kussmaul breathing)

bonate ion; this leads to a marked decrease in serum bicarbonate levels. The breath has a characteristic fruity smell due to the presence of the volatile ketoacids. A number of signs and symptoms that occur in diabetic ketoacidosis are related to compensatory mechanisms. The heart rate increases as the body compensates for a decrease in blood volume, and the rate and depth of respiration increase (Kussmaul breathing) as the body attempts to prevent further decreases in pH. Metabolic acidosis and its treatment are discussed in Chapter 23.

Diabetic ketoacidosis is seen most frequently in the insulin-dependent diabetic. It can occur at the onset of the disease, often before the disease has been diagnosed. For example, a mother may bring a child into the hospital with reports of lethargy, vomiting, and abdominal pain, unaware that the child has diabetes. Stress tends to increase the release of gluconeogenic hormones and predisposes the person to the development of ketoacidosis. Consequently, the development of ketoacidosis is often preceded by physical or emotional stress, for example, infection, pregnancy, or extreme anxiety.

The treatment of diabetic ketoacidosis focuses on correcting the fluid and electrolyte imbalances and returning blood pH to normal. Usually this is accomplished through the administration of insulin

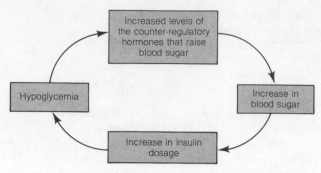

Figure 35–3. Events that occur with the Somogyi phenomenon.

and intravenous fluid and electrolyte replacement solutions. Frequent monitoring of laboratory tests of serum electrolytes is used as a guide for fluid and electrolyte replacement. Identification and treatment of the underlying cause, for example infection, is also important.

Somogyi phenomenon

The Somogyi phenomenon describes a cycle of insulin-induced post-hypoglycemic episodes. In 1924, Joslin and his associates noted that hypoglycemia was associated with alternate episodes of hyperglycemia.[12] It was not until 1959, however, that Somogyi presented the results of his 20 years of studies which confirmed the observation that "hypoglycemia begets hyperglycemia."[13] In a diabetic with the Somogyi mechanisms designed to elevate blood sugar, there is an increase in blood levels of catecholamines, glucagon, cortisol, and growth hormone. These hormones cause blood sugar to become elevated and cause some degree of insulin resistance. A vicious cycle begins when the increase in

Table 35–4   Signs and Symptoms of Hyperosmolar Coma

Onset—insidious; 24 hours to 2 weeks

Laboratory findings
    Blood sugar greater than 600 mg/100 ml
    Serum osmolarity 350 mOsm/kg or greater

Severe dehydration
    Dry skin and mucous membranes
    Extreme thirst

Neurologic manifestations
    Depressed sensorium
      lethargy to coma
    Neurologic deficits
      positive Babinski sign
      paresis or paralysis
      sensory impairment
      hyperthermia
      hemianopia
    Seizures

blood sugar and insulin resistance is treated with larger insulin doses. Often the hypoglycemic episode occurs during the night or at a time when it is not recognized, rendering this diagnosis of the phenomenon more difficult. Figure 35-3 illustrates the events that occur with the Somogyi phenomenon.

Hyperosmolar coma

Hyperosmolar, hyperglycemic nonketotic coma (HHNK) is characterized by a plasma osmolarity of 350 mOsm per liter or more, a blood sugar in excess of 600 mg per 100 ml of blood, absence of ketoacidosis, and depression of the sensorium.[14]

Hyperosmolar coma may occur in a variety of conditions including NIDDM, acute pancreatitis, severe infections, myocardial infarction, hyperthyroidism, and treatment with oral or parenteral hyperalimentation solutions. Two factors appear to contribute to the hyperglycemia that precipitates the condition; one is an increased resistance to the effects of insulin and the other is an excessive carbohydrate intake.

In hyperosmolar states, the increased serum osmolarity has the effect of pulling water out of body cells, including brain cells. The most prominent manifestations are dehydration, neurologic signs and symptoms, polyuria, and thirst (Table 35-4). One patient is reported to have consumed nine quarts of skim milk in a single day. The neurologic signs include grand mal seizures, hemiparesis, Babinski reflexes, aphasia, muscle fasciculations, hyperthermia, hemianopia, nystagmus, visual hallucinations, and others.[15] Blood glucose levels of 4800 mg per 100 ml of blood have been reported. The onset of hyperosmolar coma is often insidious, and because it occurs most frequently in older individuals, it may be mistaken for a stroke.

Treatment of hyperosmolar coma requires judicious medical observation and care. This is because water moves back into brain cells during treatment, posing a threat of cerebral edema. There are also extensive potassium losses that have occurred during the diuretic phase of the disorder and that require correction. Because of the problems encountered in the treatment, and the serious nature of the disease conditions that cause hyperosmolar coma, the prognosis for this disorder is less favorable than that of ketoacidosis; the mortality rate has been reported to be 40% to 70%.[15]

Chronic Complications

The chronic complications of diabetes include the neuropathies, nephropathies, and other vascular lesions. Interestingly, these disorders occur in the insulin-independent tissues of the body—those tissues that do not require insulin for glucose entry into the cell. This probably means that intracellular glucose concentrations in these tissues approach or equal those in the blood.

The interest among researchers in explaining the causes and development of chronic lesions in the diabetic has led to a number of theories. Several of these theories have been summarized for the reader in preparation for understanding specific chronic complications.

The polyol pathway

A polyol is an organic compound that contains three or more hydroxyl groups. The polyol pathway refers to the intracellular enzymes and mechanisms responsible for changing the number of hydroxyl units on a sugar. In the sorbitol pathway, glucose is transformed to sorbitol and then sorbitol is converted to fructose. The rate at which sorbitol can be converted to fructose and then metabolized is limited. Sorbitol is osmotically active, and it has been hypothesized that the presence of excess amounts may alter cell function in those tissues that use this pathway.

Formation of abnormal glycoproteins

Glycoproteins, or what might be termed sugar proteins, are normal components of the basement membrane in smaller blood vessels and capillaries. It has been suggested that the increased intracellular concentration of glucose, which is associated with diabetes, favors the formation of abnormal glycoproteins. These abnormal glycoproteins are thought to produce structural defects in the basement membrane of these vessels.

Problems with tissue oxygenation

Proponents of the tissue oxygenation theories suggest that many of the chronic complications of diabetes arise because of a decrease in oxygen delivery in the small vessels of the microcirculation. Among the factors believed to contribute to this inadequate oxygen delivery is a defect in red cell function which interferes with release of oxygen from the hemoglobin molecule. In support of this theory is the finding of a two to threefold increase in glycosylated hemoglobin ($HbA_{1a} + HbA_{1b} + HbA_{1c}$) in persons with diabetes. This hemoglobin has a glycoprotein substituted for valine in the beta chain, causing a high affinity for oxygen.[16] There is a reported decrease in red cell 2,3 DPG during the acidotic and recovery phases of diabetic ketoacidosis. The glycolytic intermediate 2,3 DPG decreases the hemoglobin affinity for oxygen. Both an increase in glycosylated hemoglobin and a decrease in 2,3 DPG tend to increase the hemoglobin's affinity for oxygen, and less oxygen is released for tissue use.

Peripheral neuropathies

Although it is known that the incidence of peripheral neuropathies is high among diabetics, it is difficult to document exactly how many diabetics are affected by these disorders. This is because of the diversity in clinical manifestations and because the condition is often far advanced before it is recognized.

Two types of pathologic changes have been observed in connection with diabetic peripheral neuropathies. The first is a thickening of the wall of the nutrient vessels that supply the nerve, leading to the assumption that vessel ischemia plays a major role in the development of these neural changes The second and more recent finding has been a segmental demyelinization process that affects the Schwann cell. This demyelinization process is accompanied by a slowing of nerve conduction. Recent research on the sorbitol pathway suggests that the formation and accumulation of sorbitol within nerve cells may lead to injury and impair nerve conduction.

Table 35–5   Classification of Diabetic Peripheral Neuropathies

Somatic

Polyneuropathies, bilateral sensory
  Paresthesias, including numbness and tingling
  Impaired pain, temperature, light touch, two point discrimination, and vibratory sensation
  Decreased ankle and knee-jerk reflexes

Mononeuropathies
  Involvement of a mixed nerve trunk that includes loss of sensation, pain, and motor weakness

Amyotrophia
  Associated with muscle weakness, wasting, and severe pain of muscles in the pelvic girdle and thigh

Autonomic

Impaired vasomotor function
  Postural hypotension

Impaired gastrointestinal function
  Gastric atony
  Diarrhea, often postprandial and nocturnal

Impaired genitourinary function
  Paralytic bladder
  Incomplete voiding
  Impotence
  Retrograde ejaculation

Cranial nerve involvement
  Extraocular nerve paralysis
  Impaired pupillary responses
  Impaired special senses

It now appears that the diabetic peripheral neuropathies are not a single entity. The clinical manifestations of these disorders vary with the location of the lesion(s). Although there are several methods for classifying the diabetic peripheral neuropathies, a simplified system divides them into somatic and autonomic disturbances (Table 35-5).

In addition to the actual discomforts that are associated with the loss of sensory or motor function, lesions in either the somatic or peripheral nervous system predispose the diabetic to additional complications. Loss of feeling, touch, and position sense increases the risk of falling. Impairment of temperature and pain sensation increases the risk of serious burns and injuries to the feet. Defects in vasomotor reflexes can lead to dizziness and syncope when the person moves from the supine to the standing position. Incomplete emptying of the bladder due to vesicle dysfunction predisposes the person to urinary stasis and bladder infections, and increases the risk of renal complications.

Nephropathies

The diabetic is predisposed to several types of renal disease, including pyelonephritis and nephropathies. Pyelonephritis occurs in the nondiabetic as well as in the diabetic and is discussed in Chapter 26. Nephropathies refer to chronic renal vascular complications and are a common cause of death in long-term diabetic patients.

The basement membrane of the glomerulus is composed of complex glycoproteins. It has been suggested that the increased intracellular concentration of glucose in the diabetic contributes to the formation of abnormal glycoproteins and glycoprotein linkage in the basement membrane of the glomerulus. Kimmelstiel–Wilson's disease involves the development of nodular lesions in the glomerular capillary of the kidney (Fig. 35-4). The accompanying arteriolar lesions impair blood flow. There is a progressive loss of kidney function and eventual renal failure. Kimmelstiel–Wilson lesions are thought to occur only in the diabetic. Diffuse glomerulosclerosis is a linear thickening of the glomerular membrane and is found in both diabetics and nondiabetics. Changes in the basement membrane in Kimmelstiel–Wilson's disease and diffuse glomerulosclerosis allow plasma proteins to escape in the urine, causing proteinuria, development of hypoproteinemia (decreased levels of plasma proteins), and edema.

Retinopathy

Diabetes is the leading cause of acquired blindness in the United States. Although the diabetic is at increased risk for developing cataracts and glaucoma, retinopathy is the most common pattern of disease in the eye. It has been estimated that at least 50% of diabetics show detectable signs of retinopathy 10 years following diagnosis.

There are two types of diabetic retinopathy: (1) background or nonproliferative, and (2) proliferative retinopathy (Fig. 35-5). Nonproliferative or background retinopathy is characterized by microaneurysms, or fusiform outpouchings, that protrude from one side of the capillary. These microaneurysms form weakened spots in the capillary wall that tend to leak fluid or to rupture, giving rise to retinal edema and hemorrhage. Hard waxy exudates form as pockets of protein, and lipids leak through the wall of the weakened capillary. Usually there is a constant reabsorption of old hemorrhages and exudate as new hemorrhages are being formed.

Proliferative retinopathy differs from background retinopathy in that new blood vessels (neovascularization) develop on the surface of the retina and extend into the area between the retina and vitreous. These new vessels, like the background microaneurysms, are very fragile and tend to rupture easily. When hemorrhage occurs, blood from these lesions flows into the vitreous, obstructing the flow of light from the lens to the retina. As the condition progresses, scar tissue and adhesions de-

Figure 35–4.   Diagram of the nodular lesions in the glomerular capillary of the nephron that are associated with diabetes mellitus.

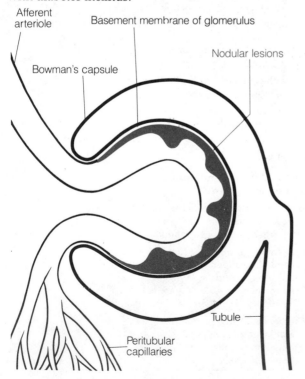

Afferent arteriole

Basement membrane of glomerulus

Nodular lesions

Bowman's capsule

Tubule

Peritubular capillaries

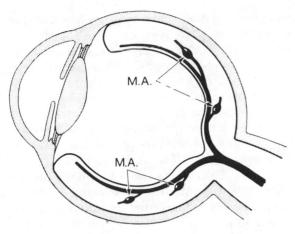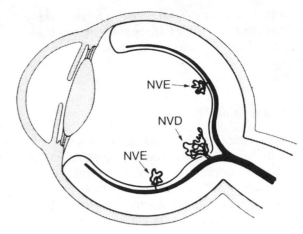

Figure 35–5.   Proliferative and nonproliferative lesions in retinopathy of the diabetic. *Background retinopathy*: In background diabetic retinopathy, the blood vessel changes are contained within the retina. The microaneurysms (MA) are shown schematically within the substance of the retina. *Proliferative retinopathy*: In proliferative diabetic retinopathy, new vessel formation breaks through the surface of the retina to grow into the vitreous cavity. When the vessels are near the optic nerve or disc area, they are termed neovascularization of the disc (NVD); when the new vessel formation occurs away from the disc elsewhere in the retina, it is referred to as neovascularization elsewhere (NVE). Copyright 1978 by the American Diabetes Association, Inc. Reprinted from Diabetes Forecast by permission.

velop between the vitreous and the retina. When the scar tissue contracts it can cause vitreous hemorrhage or retinal detachment. Fortunately, only about 3% to 10% of diabetics develop the proliferative type of diabetic retinopathy.

The retinal vessels can be viewed by means of an ophthalmoscope. This allows for early diagnosis and follow-up observation of retinal lesions. The intravenous injection of fluorescein dye provides a method for outlining the retinal vasculature and for detecting sites of obstruction and leakage. Normally, the retinal capillary endothelial cells are tightly joined so that the dye does not escape into the vitreous.

Methods used in the treatment of diabetic retinopathy include destruction and scarring of the proliferative lesions with photocoagulation. Removal and replacement of the vitreous with a clear replacement solution (vitrectomy) may be used in those situations where vitreal hemorrhage has caused blindness.

Vascular complications

There is little doubt that diabetes contributes to disease of both the micro- and macrocirculation. Diabetic involvement of the small vessels in the retina is an example of disease of the microcirculation. It is also known that diabetics are at risk for developing lesions of vessels in the macrocirculation, including the coronaries, cerebral vessels, and peripheral arteries.

Studies suggest that diabetes is an important risk factor in the development of heart disease, including coronary artery disease, and other forms of myocardial dysfunction.[17] Autonomic innervation of the heart may also become impaired in the diabetic. With impaired autonomic function the heart rate response to many stresses is less.

Vascular disorders also affect the cerebral circulation. There is evidence to suggest that cerebral artery atherosclerosis develops earlier and is more extensive in diabetics than in nondiabetics.

The effects of the disease on vessels in the lower extremities is evidenced by an increased frequency of peripheral vascular insufficiency and intermittent claudication in diabetics as compared with nondiabetics. Impairment of the peripheral vascular circulation may become severe enough to cause ulceration, infection, and eventually gangrene of the feet. The need to amputate portions of the lower extremities, because of complications arising from severe peripheral vascular disease, is a threat to many older diabetics.

There is much controversy about the cause(s) of vascular pathology in diabetes. Among the factors that are thought to contribute to the increased prevalence of atherosclerosis in diabetics are hypertension, hyperlipidemia, and increased platelet adhesiveness, other alterations in blood coagulation factors, and accumulation of sorbitol within the walls of the larger vessels.

Infection and Diabetes

While not specifically either an acute or a chronic complication, infections are common concerns of the diabetic. There are certain types of infections that occur with increased frequency in diabetics: soft tissue infections of the extremities, osteomyelitis, urinary tract infections and pyelonephritis, candidial infections of skin and mucous surfaces, and tuberculosis. At present, there is a question whether the problem seems more prevalent because the infections are more serious in diabetics.

There are several known causes for the suboptimal response to infection in the diabetic. One is the presence of chronic complications, such as vascular disease and neuropathies, and the other is the presence of hyperglycemia and altered neutrophil function. Sensory deficits may cause the diabetic to ignore minor trauma and infection, and vascular disease may impair circulation and delivery of blood cells and other substances needed to produce an adequate inflammatory response and effect healing. Pyelonephritis and urinary tract infections are relatively common in the diabetic, and it has been suggested that these infections may bear some relationship to the presence of a neurogenic bladder or nephrosclerotic changes in the kidney. Hyperglycemia and glycosuria may influence the growth of microorganisms and increase the severity of the infection. Recently, it has been shown that there is impaired chemotaxis and phagocytosis in neutrophils that have been exposed to increased concentrations of glucose.

:Treatment of Diabetes

The treatment plan for diabetes usually involves diet, exercise, and hypoglycemic agents. Weight loss and dietary management may be sufficient to control blood sugar levels in persons with NIDDM.

Diet

Diet therapy is usually individually prescribed to meet the specific need of each diabetic. For example, an obese noninsulin-dependent diabetic will have different dietary needs from a teenage insulin-dependent diabetic. There are three methods of dietary

control in treating diabetes: one is the free diet that prescribes that a given percentage of the diet be allocated to carbohydrates, proteins, and fats. The diabetic is free to select foods within this distribution. The second method is the weighed diet. With this form of diet control, the diabetic receives a list of food groups with the appropriate amounts of each food described by weight rather than by measurements. The third and most frequently used method is the exchange diet.[18] The exchange diet uses six exchange lists. Each exchange list contains designated amounts of foods that have about the same number of calories and an equal amount of carbohydrate, fat, and protein.

Exercise

Exercise has long been credited with improving glucose tolerance and decreasing blood lipid levels. So important is exercise in the management of diabetes that a planned program of regular exercise is usually considered to be an integral part of the therapeutic regimen for every diabetic.

During short-term exercise, the uptake of glucose into the exercising muscle increases 7 to 20-fold. Blood levels of insulin tend to regulate glucose release by the liver. In the nondiabetic, exercise is accompanied by an adrenergically induced decrease in insulin release from the beta cells and an increased breakdown of liver glycogen stores with release of glucose into the bloodstream. When exercise is prolonged for more than two hours, the exercising muscles obtain the greater amount of their energy from fatty acids, and glucose release from the liver is derived from gluconeogenesis.

In the diabetic, the beneficial effects of exercise are accompanied by an increased risk of hypoglycemia. The reasons for decrease in blood sugar levels during exercise in the insulin-dependent diabetic are twofold. First, there is an increased absorption of insulin from the subcutaneous injection site. This increased absorption is more pronounced when insulin is injected into the subcutaneous tissue of the exercised muscle, but it seems to occur even when insulin is injected into other body areas. Second, because the diabetic cannot decrease blood insulin levels, there is a decrease in glucose release by the liver.

Hypoglycemic Agents

There are two forms of hypoglycemic agents, the oral sulfonylureas and injectable insulin. Phenformin, a previously used oral hypoglycemic agent, was discontinued from general use in the United States in

1977 following a directive from the United States Department of Health, Education, and Welfare. This was due to a very toxic side-effect, lactic acidosis.

Sulfonylureas

The sulfonylureas are thought to cause release of insulin from the pancreas and to increase insulin binding and the number of insulin receptors. This means that these agents are effective only when some residual beta-cell function remains. They cannot be substituted for insulin in the insulin-dependent diabetic who has an absolute insulin deficiency. There are several sulfonylurea preparations available; these preparations differ in dose and duration of action (Table 35-6). Because the sulfonylureas increase the rate at which glucose is removed from the blood, it is important to recognize that these drugs can cause hypoglycemic reactions.

Insulin

Insulin-dependent diabetes requires treatment with insulin. Insulin is destroyed in the gastrointestinal tract and must be administered by injection. All insulin is measured in units, the international unit of insulin being defined as the amount of insulin required to lower the blood sugar of a fasting 2-kg rabbit from 120 to 145 mg/100 ml blood. Insulin preparations are categorized according to onset, peak, and duration of action. There are three principal types of insulin: short, intermediate, and long-acting (Table 35-7). Insulin is supplied in U40 and U100 (units per ml) strengths. Efforts are being made to phase out the use of the U40 strength and to encourage use of the U100 purified preparations which is endorsed by the American Diabetic Association. Insulin regimens using two to three daily injections of regular insulin or regular mixed with NPH or Lente insulin are growing in use. These regimens provide a blood glucose level that is within a more normal physiologic range than that provided by the one time a day injection.

In summary, diabetes mellitus is a chronic disease characterized by a state of insulin deficiency. This insulin deficiency can be absolute as in insulin-dependent diabetes mellitus or it can be relative as in noninsulin-dependent diabetes. The metabolic disturbances that are associated with diabetes affect almost every system in the body. The acute complications include diabetic keto-acidosis, hypoglycemia, and, in the noninsulin-dependent diabetic, nonketotic hyperosmolar ketoacidosis. The chronic complications of diabetes affect the non-insulin-dependent tissues, including the retina, blood vessels, kidney, and peripheral nervous system.

Table 35–6   Sulfonylurea Preparations: Half-life and Duration of Action

Sulfonylurea Preparations	Half-life (hours)	Duration of Action (hours)
Tolbutamide (Orinase)	4–6	6–12
Tolazamide (Tolinase)	7	10–14
Acetohexamide (Dymelor)	5–7	12–24
Chlorpropamide (Diabinese)	36	Up to 60 hours

Table 35–7   Insulin: Half-life and Duration of Action

Type of Preparation	Activity Peak (hours)	Duration (hours)
Rapid-acting		
Insulin injection (regular, crystalline zinc)	½–3	5–7
Insulin zinc suspension (prompt, Semilente)	1–4	12–16
Intermediate-acting		
Globin zinc insulin	6–10	12–18
Isophane insulin suspension (NPH)	8–12	18–24
Insulin zinc suspension (Lente)	8–12	18–24
Long-acting		
Protamine zinc insulin suspension (PZI)	8–16	24–36
Insulin zinc suspension extended (Ultralente)	8–16	24–36

:Study Guide

After you have studied this chapter, you should be able to meet the following objectives:

: : State a clinical description of diabetes mellitus.

: : List the distinguishing characteristics of IDDM and NIDDM.

: : Describe the suspected role of two environmental factors in the etiology of diabetes mellitus.

: : State the purpose of the glucose tolerance test.

: : State the advantages of home blood glucose monitoring.

: : Explain the purpose of measuring the level of glycosylated hemoglobin in the blood.

: : Name and describe two types of urinary tests for glucose.

: : Describe the three "polys" that characterize diabetes mellitus.

: : Describe the clinical manifestations of hypoglycemia which the health professional should be able to recognize.

: : Describe the significant derangements seen in diabetic ketoacidosis.

: : Explain how "hypoglycemia begets hyperglycemia."

: : Describe the clinical condition resulting from the hyperosmolar state.

: : Define *polyol*.

: : Describe the pathologic changes that may occur with diabetic peripheral neuropathies.

: : Describe the pathology underlying diabetic retinopathy.

: : Describe the vascular complications that may occur with diabetes mellitus.

: : Explain the relationship between diabetes mellitus and infection.

: : Explain why exercise is beneficial to diabetics.

: : State the presumed actions of the sulfonylureas.

: : Name and describe the three types of insulin.

:References

1. Every sixty seconds. Diabetes Forecast, No. 6, 1978, p 23.
2. Waif SO (ed): Diabetes Mellitus. Indianapolis, Eli Lilly, 1980
3. Tattersoll RB, Fajans SS: A difference between the inheritance of classical juvenile-onset and maturity-onset type of diabetes of young people. Diabetes 24:1, 1975
4. Cudworth AG, Woodrow JC: Evidence of HLA-linked genes in juvenile-onset diabetes. Br Med J 3:133, 1975
5. Gamble DR, Taylor KW: Seasonal incidence of diabetes mellitus. Br Med J 3:631, 1969
6. MacMillan DR, Kotoyan M, Zeidner D et al: Seasonal variation in the onset of diabetes in children. Pediatrics 59:113, 1977
7. Sulz HA, Hart BA, Zielezny M et al: Is mumps virus an etiologic factor in juvenile diabetes mellitus? Preliminary report. J Pediatr 86:654, 1975
8. Yoon JW, Onodera T, Jensen AB et al: Virus-induced diabetes mellitus, XI. Replication of Coxsackie B 3 virus in human pancreatic beta cell cultures. Diabetes 27:778, 1978
9. Johnson GM, Tudor RB: Diabetes mellitus and congenital rubella infection. Am J Dis Child 120:453, 1970
10. Plotkin SA, Kaye R: Diabetes mellitus and congenital rubella. Pediatrics 46:450, 1970
11. Diabetic control measured by glycosylated Hb level. Hosp Pract 12, No. 4:42, 1977
12. Joslin EP, Gray H, Root HL: Insulin in hospital and home. J Metabol Res 2:651, 1924
13. Somogyi M: Exacerbation of diabetes in excess insulin action. Am J Med 26:169, 1957
14. Whitehouse FW: Two minutes with diabetes: "My patient is not responding and is very dehydrated." Med Times 101:35, 1970
15. Podolsky S: Hyperosmolar nonketotic coma in the elderly diabetic. Med Clin North Am 62, No. 4:816, 1978
16. Ditzel J, Standl E: The problem of tissue oxygenation in diabetes mellitus. Acta Med Scand (Suppl 578):49, 1975
17. Sanderson JE: Diabetes and the heart. Chest Heart Stroke 3:35, 1978–79
18. American Diabetes Association: Exchange Lists for Meal Planning. New York, 1976

:Suggested Readings

Benson E, Metz R: Diabetic ketoacidosis. Hosp Med 15, No. 5:26, 1979

Bern M: Platelet functions in diabetes mellitus. Diabetes 27, No. 3:342, 1978

Boden G, Master R, Gordon S et al. Monitoring metabolic control in diabetic outpatients with glycosylated hemoglobin. Ann Intern Med 92, No. 3:357, 1980

Bruce GL: The Somogyi phenomenon: Insulin-induced posthypoglycemic hyperglycemia. Heart Lung 7, No. 3:463, 1978

Clement RS, Vourganti B: Fatal ketoacidosis: Major causes and approaches to their prevention. Diabetes Care 5, No. 1:314, 1978

Colwell JA, Halushka PV, Sarji KE et al: Platelet function and diabetes mellitus. Med Clin North Am 62, No. 4:753, 1978

Eliopoulos CE: Adult diabetes: Diagnosis and management of diabetes in the elderly. Am J Nurs 78, No. 11:884, 1978

Ellenberg M: Sexual functioning in diabetic patients. Ann Intern Med 92:331, 1980

Felts PW, Marshall WF: What's new in exercise. Diabetes Forecast 16, 17, 38, 1979

Flood TM: Diet and diabetes mellitus. Hosp Pract 14, No. 2:61, 1979

Gale EAM, Kurtz AB, Tattersall RB: In search of the Somogyi effect. Lancet 279, 1980

Graighead JE: Current views on the etiology of insulin dependent diabetes mellitus. N Engl J Med 299, No. 26:1439, 1978

Hamburger SC: Diagnosis and management of diabetic ketoacidosis—Selected aspects. Crit Care Quart 2:53, 1979

Hare JW, Rossini A: Diabetic comas: The overlap concept. Hosp Pract 14, No. 5:95, 1979

Harrison LC: Current concepts: Insulin resistance in obese diabetic patients. Consultant No. 2, 64, 1979

Holt WS, Wolf KP, Takach RJ: Diabetic retinopathy. J Maine Med Assoc 70, No. 11:9, 1979

Hosking DJ, Bennett B, Hampton JR et al: Diabetic autonomic neuropathy. Diabetes 27, No. 10:1043, 1978

Johnson DG: The pathogenesis of diabetes mellitus. Ariz Med 36, No. 10:766, 1979

Kilo C: The use of oral hypoglycemic agents. Hosp Pract 14, No. 3:103, 1979

Kiser D: The Somogyi effect. Am J Nurs 80, No. 2:236, 1980

Lundin DV: Reporting urine test results: Switching from + to %. Am J Nurs 78, No. 5:878, 1978

Michels DG: What role for vitrectomy in managing diabetic retinopathy? Hosp Pract 12, No. 9:73, 1977

Misbin RI: Insulin resistance in ketoacidosis. N Engl J Med 297, No. 16:893, 1977

Olefsky J: The insulin receptor: Its role in insulin resistance of obesity and diabetes. Diabetes 25, No. 12:1154, 1976

Palumbo PJ: How to treat maturity-onset diabetes mellitus. Geriatrics 23, No. 12:57, 1977

Perrin ED: Laser therapy for diabetic retinopathy. Am J Nurs 80, No. 4:664, 1980

Rubenstein P, Suciu–Foca N, Nicholson JF: Genetics of juvenile diabetes mellitus. N Engl J Med 297, No. 19:1036, 1977

Schade DS, Eaton RP: Pathogenesis of diabetic ketoacidosis: A reappraisal. Diabetes Care 3, No. 2:296, 1979

Skyler JS: Counterregulatory hormones, rebound hyperglycemia, and diabetic control. Diabetes Care 6, No. 2:526, 1979

Slater NL: Insulin reactions vs. ketoacidosis: Guidelines for diagnosis and intervention. Am J Nurs 78, No. 5:875, 1978

Tillerman DB, Miller ME, Pitchon HE: Infection and diabetes mellitus. West J Med 130, No. 6:515, 1979

Turkington RW: Depression masquerading as diabetic neuropathy. JAMA 243, No. 11:1147, 1980

Unger RH: The essential role of glucagon in the pathogenesis of diabetes mellitus. Lancet 14, 1975

Ventura E: Foot care in diabetes. Am J Nurs 78, No. 5:886, 1978

Viberti GC: Glucose-induced hyperkalaemia: A hazard for diabetics. Lancet 1:690, 1978

Vranic M, Berger M: Exercise and diabetes mellitus. Diabetes 78:147, 1979

Walesky ME: Diabetic ketoacidosis. Am J Nurs 78, No. 5:872, 1978

West K, Erdreich L, Stober J: A detailed study of risk factors for retinopathy and nephropathy in diabetes. Diabetes 29:501, 1980

Wimberley D: When a pregnant woman is diabetic: Intrapartal care. Am J Nurs 79, No. 3:451, 1979

Zinman B: Exercise and diabetic control. Primary Care 4, No. 4:637, 1977

36

Control of Gastrointestinal Function

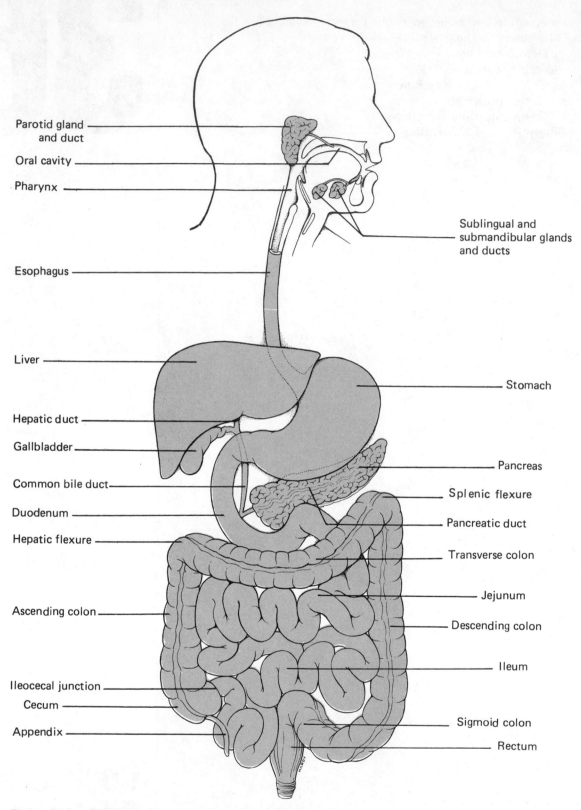

Figure 36–1.   Diagram of the digestive system. (From Chaffee EE, Lytle IM: Basic Physiology and Anatomy, 4th ed. Philadelphia, JB Lippincott, 1980)

The process of digestion and absorption of nutrients requires an intact and healthy gastrointestinal tract epithelial lining that is able to resist the effects of its own digestive secretions. It involves the movement of materials through the gastrointestinal tract at a rate that facilitates absorption, and it requires the presence of enzymes that are needed for digestion and absorption of nutrients. Structurally, the gastrointestinal tract is a long, hollow tube with its lumen inside the body and its wall acting as an interface between the internal and external environments. The wall does not normally allow harmful agents to enter the body, nor does it permit body fluids and other materials to escape.

The digestive system is truly an amazing structure. In this system, enzymes and hormones are produced, vitamins are synthesized and stored, and food is dismantled and then reassembled. Catalysts and reactants play a role, and some are recycled and used again. Finally, wastes are collected and eliminated in an efficient manner. No doubt a manmade industry, designed to accomplish similar achievements would require miles of space, elaborate equipment, and a huge expenditure of capital. While this chapter cannot cover gastrointestinal function in its entirety, it is designed to provide the reader with an overview that is deemed essential to an understanding of subsequent chapters.

Nutrients, vitamins, minerals, electrolytes, and water enter the body through the gastrointestinal tract. As a matter of semantics, it should be pointed out that the gastrointestinal tract is also referred to as the digestive tract, the alimentary canal, and, at times, the gut. The intestinal portion may also be called the bowel. For our purposes, the salivary glands, the liver, and the pancreas, which produce secretions that aid in digestion, are considered accessory structures.

:Organization and Structure of the Digestive System

In the digestive tract, food and other materials move slowly along its length as they are systematically broken down into ions and molecules that can be absorbed into the body itself. In the large intestine unabsorbed nutrients and wastes are collected for later elimination. What is important for the reader to recognize is that while the gastrointestinal tract is located within the body, it is really a long hollow tube, the lumen of which is an extension of the external environment. Thus, nutrients do not become part of the internal environment until they have passed through the intestinal wall and have entered the blood or lymph channels.

For simplicity and understanding, the digestive system can be divided into four parts (Fig. 36-1). The *upper part*—the mouth, esophagus, and stomach—acts as an intake source and "holding tank" in which

Figure 36–2. Schematic diagram of the transverse section of the digestive system. (From Thompson JS: Core Textbook of Anatomy. Philadelphia, JB Lippincott, 1977)

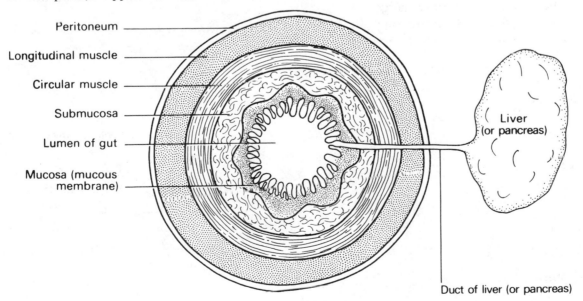

initial digestive processes begin. The *middle portion* consists of the small intestine—the duodenum, jejunum, and ileum. It is in the small intestine that the majority of digestive and absorptive processes occur. The *lower segment*—the cecum, colon, and rectum—serves as a storage channel for efficient elimination of waste. The *fourth part* consists of the accessory structures, the salivary glands, the liver, and the pancreas. These structures produce digestive secretions and help regulate the use and storage of nutrients.

The digestive tract, once it leaves the mouth, is essentially a five-layered tube (Fig. 36-2). The inner luminal layer, or *mucosa*, is so named because its cells produce mucus that lubricates and protects the inner surface of the alimentary canal. The epithelial cells in this layer have a rapid turnover rate, being replaced every four to five days. Approximately 250 grams of these cells are shed each day in the stool. Because of the regenerative capabilities of the mucosal layer, injury to this layer of tissue heals rapidly without leaving scar tissue. The *submucosal layer* is made up of connective tissue. This layer contains blood vessels, nerves, and structures responsible for secreting digestive enzymes. Movement in the gastrointestinal tract is facilitated by the *circular* and *longitudinal* smooth muscle layers. The fifth layer, the *peritoneum*, is loosely attached to the outer wall of the intestine.

The *peritoneum* is the largest serous membrane in the body, having a surface area which is about equal to that of the skin. The peritoneal membrane is composed of two layers, a thin layer of squamous cells resting on a layer of connective tissue. If the squamous layer becomes injured due to surgery or inflammation, there is danger that adhesions (fibrous scar-tissue bands) will form, causing sections of the viscera to heal together. Unfortunately, adhesions may alter the position and movement of the abdominal viscera.

The *peritoneal cavity* is potential space that is formed between what is called the *parietal* and the *visceral peritoneum*. The parietal peritoneum comes in contact with, and is loosely attached to, the abdominal wall, while the abdominal organs are in contact with the visceral peritoneum. Thompson compares the two layers of the peritoneum to a deflated balloon.[1] If you "make a fist" into the balloon, the outer surface can be equated with the parietal peritoneum, and the fist interface with the visceral peritoneum (Fig. 36-3). In this case, the area within the balloon would approximate the peritoneal cavity. The connective tissue layer of the peritoneum forms both the parietal and visceral peritoneum, while the smooth squamous-cell layer of the membrane lines the cavity. The adjacent membrane layers within the peritoneal cavity are separated by a thin layer of serous fluid. This fluid prevents friction between continuously moving abdominal structures. In certain pathologic states the fluid in the potential space of the peritoneal cavity is increased, causing ascites.* The *mesentery* is a double fold of peritoneum which encloses and supports the abdominal organs (Fig. 36-4). The mesentery is no more than 20 cm to 25 cm deep, about 15 cm long in the small intestine, and 7 cm long in the large intestine.

Movement in the Gastrointestinal Tract

Smooth muscle controls movement in the gastrointestinal tract. These movements are both tonic and rhythmic. The *tonic movements* are continuous

---

*The reader is referred to Chapter 38 for a discussion of edema fluid.

Figure 36–3.   Comparison of the peritoneal cavity to a balloon. (From Thompson JS: Core Textbook of Anatomy. Philadelphia, JB Lippincott, 1977)

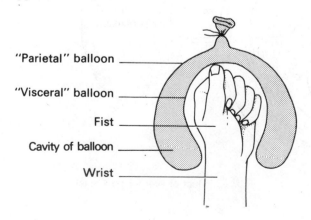

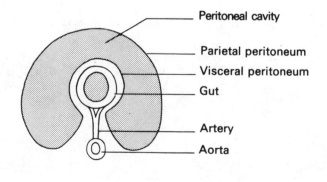

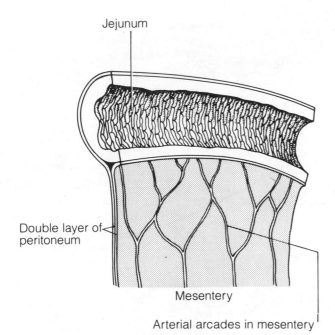

Figure 36–4.   Diagram showing the attachment of the mesentery to the portions of the small bowel. (From Thompson JS: Core Textbook of Anatomy. Philadelphia, JB Lippincott, 1977)

movements that last for long periods of time—minutes or even hours. Tonic contractions *occur* at *sphincters*. The rhythmic movements consist of intermittent contractions that are responsible for mixing and moving food along the digestive tract. *Peristaltic movements* are *rhythmic propulsive* movements that occur when the smooth muscle layer constricts, forming a contractile band that forces the intraluminal contents forward. During peristalsis the segment of intestine that lies distal or ahead of the contracted portion relaxes, so that the contents move forward with ease. Normal peristalsis always moves from the direction of the mouth toward the anus.

The activity of gastrointestinal smooth muscle is controlled by local, humoral and neural influences. The rhythmic movements of the digestive tract are self-perpetuating much like the activity of the heart. These movements are integrated by an *intramural network* that lies within the wall of the gut and extends its entire length. This network has two layers of nerve fibers, a *submucosal network* (*Meissner's plexus*), and a second layer that lies between the *circular* and *longitudinal layers* of smooth muscle (the *myenteric* or *Auerbach's plexus*). The intramural network is responsible for many of the locally controlled movements that occur in the digestive tract. The afferent fibers of this system are located largely

within the submucosal network, and the motor fibers within the myenteric plexus (Fig. 36-5). For example, stretching the bowel or the presence of chemical irritants in the lumen of the bowel can increase peristalsis via the submucosal network.

The intrinsic tonic and rhythmic activity of the digestive tract can be modified by the autonomic nervous system (Fig. 36-6). The *parasympathetic* fibers originate in the *vagus* and in the *sacral portion* of the spinal cord. The postganglionic fibers of this system are part of the *myenteric plexus*. The *sympathetic* fibers originate in the *thoracic* and *upper lum-*

Figure 36–5.   Schematic diagram showing the submucosal and myenteric neural network or plexus.

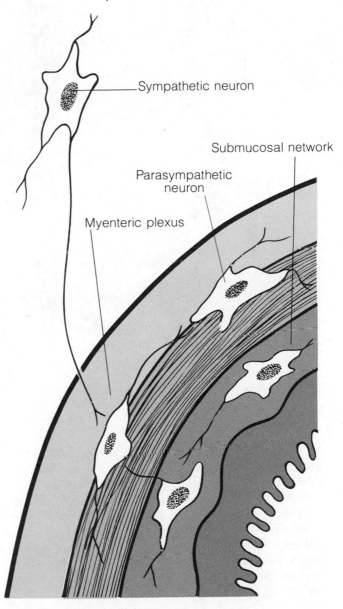

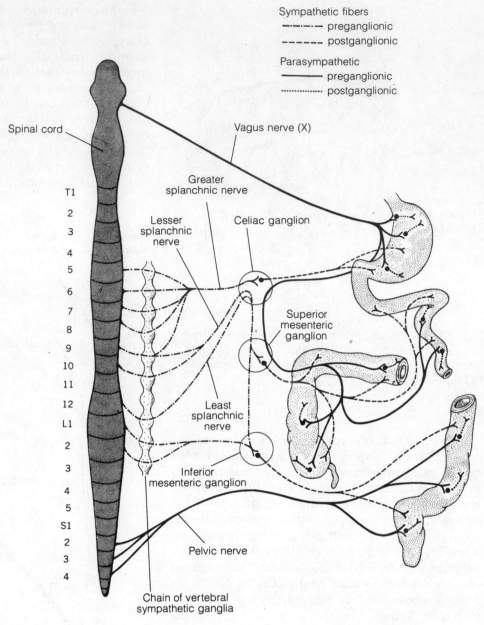

Figure 36–6.   Diagram showing the autonomic innervation of the gastrointestinal tract. (Drawing by Edith Tagrin reproduced from *Human Design* by William S. Beck, © 1971 by Harcourt Brace Jovanovich, Inc. by permission of the publisher.)

bar portions of the spinal cord. The fibers then pass to the mesenteric and celiac ganglia which are a collection of nerves. The postganglionic fibers of the sympathetic nervous system then travel with the blood vessels to all parts of the gut. Generally, the parasympathetic nervous system increases gastrointestinal activity, while the sympathetic nervous system slows its activity. In fact, strong sympathetic stimulation can actually block movements in the digestive tract.

As might be expected, the storage function of the *colon* dictates that movements within this section of the gut are different from those in the small intestine. Basically, movements in the colon are of two types. First, there are the segmental mixing movements, called *haustrations*, so named because they occur within the sacculations called haustra. These movements produce a local digging type of action which ensures that all portions of the fecal mass are exposed to the intestinal surface. Second, there are the *propulsive mass movements* which may occur several times a day. Defecation is normally initiated by the mass movements.

Defecation

Defecation is controlled by the action of two sphincters, the *internal* and *external sphincters*. The internal sphincter is controlled by the autonomic nervous system, and the external sphincter is under the conscious control of the cerebral cortex.

The defecation reflex is integrated in the sacral segment of the spinal cord. In this reflex arc, afferent fibers from the rectum communicate with nerves in the sacral cord and with parasympathetic efferent fibers that move back to the bowel (Fig. 36-6). The efferent signals from this reflex cause increased activity to occur along the entire length of the large bowel. Other actions associated with defecation, such as abdominal pushing movements, are simultaneously integrated in the spinal cord. To prevent involuntary defecation from occurring, the external anal sphincter is under the conscious control of the cortex. Thus, as efferent impulses arrive at the sacral cord, signaling the presence of a distended rectum, messages are transmitted to the cortex. If defecation is inappropriate, the cortex initiates impulses that constrict the external sphincter and inhibit efferent parasympathetic activity. Normally, the afferent impulses in this reflex loop fatigue easily and the urge to defecate soon dies out. At a more convenient time, contraction of the abdominal muscles compresses the contents in the large bowel reinitiating afferent impulses to the cord.

Secretory Function

Secretions in the digestive tract fall into three main categories: (1) hormones that regulate gastrointestinal function and growth, (2) secretions that facilitate digestion and absorption, and (3) mucus that serves to protect the mucosal surface from the action of its own digestive secretions and enzymes. This discussion focuses primarily on secretions produced in the mouth and alimentary canal.

Control of secretory function

The secretory activity of the gut is influenced by local, humoral, and neural influences. Neural control of gastrointestinal secretory activity is mediated through the autonomic nervous system. As with mobility, the parasympathetic nerves increase secretory activity, while sympathetic activity has an inhibitory action. Many of the local influences, including pH, osmolality, and chyme, consistently act as stimuli for neural and humoral mechanisms.

Gastrointestinal hormones

The gastrointestinal tract is the largest endocrine organ in the body. It produces hormones that pass from the portal circulation into the general circulation, and then back to the digestive tract where they exert their action. Among the hormones produced by the gastrointestinal tract are *gastrin*, *secretin*, *cholecystokinin*, and *enteroglucagon*. These hormones influence mobility and the secretion of electrolytes, enzymes, and other hormones. It has been observed that gastrin also influences growth of the exocrine pancreas and the mucosa of the stomach and small intestine. It is reported that removal of the stomach tissue that produces gastrin results in atrophy of these tissues. This atrophy can be reversed by administration of exogenous gastrin.

Gastrointestinal secretions

The secretions of the gastrointestinal tract include saliva, bile, and pancreatic and intestinal secretions.

Water. *Water* is an important constituent of gastrointestinal secretions. Each day about 7000 ml of fluid are secreted into the digestive tract (Table 36-1). All but 50 ml to 200 ml of this fluid is reabsorbed.

Saliva. *Saliva* is secreted in the mouth. The salivary glands consist of the parotid, submaxillary, sublingual, and buccal glands. Saliva has three functions. The first of these is protection and lubrication. Saliva is rich in mucus, which serves to protect the oral mucosa and to coat the food as it passes through the mouth, pharynx, and esophagus. The sublingual and buccal glands produce only mucous types of secretions. The second function is its protective antimicrobial action. The saliva not only cleanses the mouth but contains the enzyme lysosome, which has an antibacterial action. Thirdly, saliva contains ptyalin and amylase which initiate the digestion of dietary starches. Of particular interest is the high potassium content in saliva—two to thirty times that of plasma depending on the rate of secretion. Secretions from the salivary glands are primarily regulated by the autonomic nervous system. Parasympa-

Table 36-1   Secretions of the Gastrointestinal Tract

Secretions	Amount (daily)
Salivary	1200 ml
Gastric	2000 ml
Pancreatic	1200 ml
Biliary	700 ml
Intestinal	2000 ml
Total	7100 ml

thetic stimulation decreases flow. The dry mouth that accompanies anxiety attests to the effects of sympathetic activity on salivary secretions.

Mumps or *parotitis* is an infection of the parotid glands. Although most of us associate mumps with the contagious viral form of the disease, inflammation of parotid glands can occur in the seriously ill person who does not receive adequate oral hygiene and who is unable to take oral fluids. The drug potassium iodide increases the secretory activity of salivary glands, including the parotid glands. In a small percentage of persons, parotid swelling may occur in the course of treatment with this drug.

Gastric secretions. The gastric mucosa secretes mucus, hydrochloric acid, pepsin, and intrinsic factor. The function of the stomach is to store foods and fluids temporarily to allow for consumption of food in three meals per day. The churning action of the stomach breaks the food down into smaller particles while hydrochloric acid and pepsin begin the digestive process. Intrinsic factor is required for absorption of vitamin B_{12}, the lack of which causes pernicious anemia. Both parasympathetic stimulation via the vagus, and gastrin increase gastric secretions. It has long been known that histamine increases gastric-acid secretions. Recent research and clinical use of the histamine-H_2 receptor antagonist cimetidine suggest that histamine may be the final common pathway for gastric-acid production. Gastric-acid secretion and its relationship to peptic ulcer is discussed in Chapter 37.

Intestinal secretions. The *small intestine* both secretes digestive juices and receives secretions from the liver and pancreas. There is a concentration of mucus-producing glands in the duodenum at the site where the contents from stomach and secretions from the liver and pancreas enter. These glands, called *Brunner's glands*, serve to protect the duodenum from the acid content in the gastric chyme and from the action of the digestive enzymes. The activity of Brunner's glands is strongly influenced by autonomic factors. For example, sympathetic stimulation causes a marked decrease in mucus production, leaving this area more susceptible to irritation. Interestingly, 50% of peptic ulcers occur at this site.

In addition to mucus, the intestinal mucosa produces two other types of secretions. The first is a secretion of a serous type of fluid (pH 6.5 to 7.5) by specialized cells (crypts of Lieberkühn) in the intestinal mucosal layer. This fluid, which is produced at the rate of 2000 ml per day, acts as a diluent for absorption. The second type consists of surface enzymes that aid absorption. These enzymes are the peptidases—enzymes that separate amino acids—and the disaccharidases—that split sugars.

The *large intestine* usually secretes only mucus. As with other parts of the digestive tract, autonomic nervous system activity has a strong influence on mucus production by the bowel. During intense parasympthetic stimulation, mucus secretion may increase to the point where the stool contains large amounts of obvious mucus. Although the bowel normally does not secrete water or electrolytes, these substances are lost in large quantities when the bowel becomes irritated or inflamed.

Digestion and Absorption

Digestion is the process of dismantling foods into their constituent parts which are small enough to be absorbed. Digestion requires hydrolysis, enzyme cleavage, and fat emulsification. Hydrolysis is the breakdown of a compound that involves a chemical

Figure 36–7. The mucous membrane of the small intestine. Note the numerous villi on a circular fold. (Chaffee EE, Lytle IM: Basic Physiology and Anatomy, 4th ed. Philadelphia, JB Lippincott, 1980)

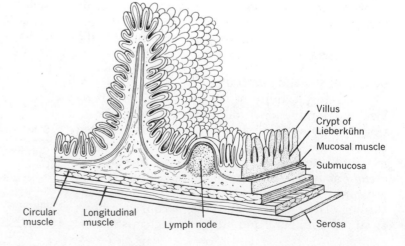

Villus
Crypt of Lieberkühn
Mucosal muscle
Submucosa
Serosa
Circular muscle
Longitudinal muscle
Lymph node

reaction with water. The importance of hydrolysis to digestion is evidenced by the amount of water (about eight liters) that is secreted into the gastrointestinal tract daily.

Absorption occurs mainly in the small intestine. The stomach is a poor absorptive structure, and only a few lipid-soluble substances, including alcohol, are absorbed from the stomach. The absorptive function of the large intestine focuses mainly on water reabsorption.

The mucosal surface of the small intestine is designed to facilitate absorption (Fig. 36-7). The mucosal folds, the villi and microvilli in the small intestine, increase its absorptive capacity 600-fold, for a total surface area of about 250 square meters.

Absorption for the intestine is accomplished by active transport and diffusion. A number of substances require a specific transport carrier or system. For example, vitamin B_{12} is not absorbed in the absence of intrinsic factor. Transport of amino acid and glucose occurs only in the presence of sodium. Water is absorbed passively, obeying the usual laws of osmosis.

In summary, the gastrointestinal tract is a long, hollow tube that extends from the mouth to the anus. In addition to the secretions of the esophagus, stomach, and small and large intestine, the gastrointestinal system relies on secretions of the salivary glands, the pancreas, and the liver which are considered accessory organs. The lumen of the gastrointestinal tract is actually not part of the internal environment of the body, and food must be digested and absorbed before it can be utilized.

:Study Guide

After you have studied this chapter, you should be able to meet the following objectives:

: : Describe the physiological function of the four parts of the digestive system.

: : Describe the physiology of peristalsis.

: : Describe the action of the internal and external sphincters in control of defecation.

: : Describe the role of gastrointestinal hormones in the process of digestion.

: : Explain the protective function of saliva.

: : Describe the function of the gastric secretions in the process of digestion.

: : Name the secretions of the small and the large intestine.

: : State a clinical definition of digestion.

:Reference

1. Thompson JS: Core Textbook of Anatomy, p 292. Philadelphia, JB Lippincott, 1977

:Suggested Readings

Chaffee EE, Lytle IM: Basic Physiology and Anatomy, 4th ed, pp 416, 430, 458. Philadelphia, JB Lippincott, 1980

Guyton AC: Textbook of Medical Physiology, 6th ed, pp 784, 801, 816, 827. Philadelphia, WB Saunders, 1981

Johnson LR: Gastrointestinal Physiology. St. Louis, CV Mosby, 1977

37

Alterations in integrity of gastrointestinal tract wall
  Esophagus
    Dysphagia
    Esophagitis
    Hiatal hernia
    Esophageal diverticulum
    Carcinoma of esophagus
  Stomach
    Acute gastritis
    Chronic gastritis
    Tests for gastric acid production
    Gastric and peptic ulcers
    Complications of peptic ulcer
    Treatment of peptic ulcer
    Cancer of the stomach
  Small and large intestine
    Inflammatory bowel disease
    Diverticular disease
    Appendicitis
    Colorectal cancer
    Peritonitis
Alterations in digestion and absorption of nutrients
    Absorption of carbohydrates
    Fat absorption
    Protein adsorption
  Malabsorption
    Malabsorption syndrome
Alterations in motility of gastrointestinal tract
  Diarrhea
    Large-volume diarrhea
    Small-volume diarrhea
    Treatment
  Constipation
  Intestinal obstruction

Alterations in Gastrointestinal Function

Gastrointestinal disorders are not cited as the leading cause of death in the United States, nor do they receive the same publicity as heart disease and cancer. Yet, according to government reports, digestive diseases rank third in the total economic burden of illness, causing considerable human suffering, personal expenditures for treatment, lost working hours, and a drain on the nation's economy. It has been estimated that 20 million Americans, one out of every nine persons in the United States, have digestive disease.[1] What is even more important is the fact that proper nutrition or a change in health practices could prevent or minimize many of these disorders. This chapter discusses three types of gastrointestinal disorders: (1) disorders that result in alterations in the integrity of the gastrointestinal tract, (2) alterations in the digestive and absorptive functions of the gastrointestinal tract, and (3) altered motility of the gastrointestinal tract.

Manifestations of gastrointestinal tract disorders

There are several signs and symptoms that are common to many types of gastrointestinal disorders. These include anorexia, nausea, vomiting, and gastrointestinal bleeding. Because they occur with so many of the disorders, they are discussed separately as an introduction to the content that follows.

Anorexia.   Anorexia is a loss of appetite. There are a number of factors that influence appetite. One of these factors is hunger, which is stimulated by contractions of the empty stomach. The desire for food intake is also regulated by the hypothalamus and other associated centers in the brain. Smell plays an important role, as evidenced by the fact that appetite can be stimulated or suppressed by the smell of food. Loss of appetite is associated with emotional situations, such as fear, depression, frustration, and anxiety. Many drugs and disease states cause anorexia. In uremia, for example, the accumulation of nitrogenous wastes in the blood contributes to the development of anorexia. Anorexia is often a forerunner of nausea, and most conditions that cause nausea and vomiting also produce anorexia.

Anorexia nervosa is an extreme disorder of food aversion. It usually occurs in young women. Although it is thought to have an emotional component, the exact cause is largely unknown. It results in severe weight loss and malnutrition, in amenorrhea, and in psychological disturbances that focus around a fear of becoming fat and a morbid refusal to eat.

Nausea.   Nausea is an ill-defined and unpleasant sensation. It is basically a conscious recognition of stimulation of the medullary vomiting center. Nausea is usually preceded by anorexia, and stimuli such as foods and drugs that cause anorexia in small doses will usually produce nausea when given in larger doses. A common cause of nausea is distention of the duodenum, or lower small intestinal tract. Nausea is frequently accompanied by autonomic responses such as watery salivation, vasoconstriction with pallor, sweating, and tachycardia.

Vomiting.   Vomiting is the sudden and forceful oral expulsion of the contents of the stomach. It is usually, but not always, preceded by nausea. The contents that are vomited are called *vomitus*.

The act of vomiting is integrated by the *vomiting center*, which is located in the dorsal portion of the reticular formation of the medulla near the sensory nucleus of the vagus. The act of vomiting consists of taking a deep breath, closing the airways, and producing a strong, forceful contraction of the diaphragm and abdominal muscles along with relaxation of the gastroesophageal sphincter. Respiration ceases during the act of vomiting. Vomiting may be accompanied by dizziness, light-headedness, a decrease in blood pressure, and bradycardia.

The vomiting center may be stimulated directly, or by impulses from the chemoreceptor trigger zone or afferent neurons of the autonomic nervous system. Many chemicals and drugs incite nausea and vomiting. These agents exert their effect by stimulating the medullary *chemoreceptor trigger zone*, which relays impulses to the vomiting center. The phenothiazine derivatives, such as chlorpromazine (Thorazine) and prochlorperazine (Compazine), depress vomiting caused by stimulation of the chemoreceptor trigger zone. *Hypoxemia* exerts a direct effect on the vomiting center in terms of producing nausea and vomiting. This direct effect probably accounts for the vomiting that occurs during periods of decreased cardiac output, shock, environmental hypoxia, and brain ischemia caused by increased intracranial pressure. Inflammation of any of the intra-abdominal organs, including the liver, gall bladder, or urinary tract, can cause vomiting because of stimulation of *visceral afferent pathways* that communicate with the vomiting center. Distention or irritation of the gastrointestinal tract also causes vomiting through stimulation of visceral afferent neurons.

Gastrointestinal bleeding.   Bleeding from the gastrointestinal tract can be evidenced by blood that appears in either the vomitus or feces. It can result from disease or trauma to the gastrointestinal structures, as a result of primary diseases of the blood vessels (i.e., esophageal varices or hemorrhoids) or because of disorders in blood clotting.

Hematemesis.   The presence of blood in the stomach is usually irritating and causes vomiting. Hematemesis refers to blood in the vomitus. It may be bright red or have a "coffee ground" appearance because of the action of the digestive enzymes.

Melena.   Blood that appears in the stool may range in color from a bright red to a tarry black. Bright-red blood usually indicates that the bleeding is from the lower bowel. When it coats the stool, it is often the result of bleeding hemorrhoids. The word *melena* means black and refers to the passage of black and "tarry" stools. These stools have a characteristic odor that is not easily forgotten. The presence of tarry stools usually indicates that the source of bleeding is above the level of the ileocecal valve, although this is not always the case. With hypermotility of the gastrointestinal tract, there may be bright-red blood in the stools, even though the bleeding is from the upper gastrointestinal tract. Melena can occur when there is entrance of as little as 100 ml of blood into the gastrointestinal tract.[2] Furthermore, tarry stools have been shown to continue for as long as 3 to 5 days following administration of 1000 ml to 2000 ml of blood into the gastrointestinal tract, indicating that melena is not necessarily a good sign of continued bleeding.[3] *Occult* (hidden) blood that can only be detected by chemical means, may persist for 2 weeks to 3 weeks.[2]

Blood urea nitrogen (BUN) is frequently elevated following hematemesis or melena. This results from breakdown of the blood by the digestive enzymes and the absorption of the nitrogenous end products into the blood. The BUN usually reaches a peak within 24 hours following the gastrointestinal hemorrhage. It does not appear when the bleeding is in the colon, since digestion does not take place at this level of the digestive system. There is also an elevation in body temperature that usually follows gastrointestinal hemorrhage. This also occurs within 24 hours and may last for a few days to a few weeks.

:Alterations in the Integrity of the Gastrointestinal Tract Wall

Characteristic of the gastrointestinal tract is the mucous membrane that lines its entire length from mouth to anus. This mucosal layer varies somewhat in structure, depending on its location and function. In the upper part of the digestive tract (mouth and esophagus) the mucus produced by the goblet cells acts as a lubricant to facilitate passage of food particles. In the stomach and small intestine, the mucous membrane is required to withstand the corrosive effects of hydrochloric acid and digestive enzymes. The mucosal layer in the small intestine is designed to facilitate absorption of nutrients.

The mucus-producing cells of the epithelial layer of the gastrointestinal tract have a rapid turnover rate of about 4 to 5 days. During periods of irritation or injury, this turnover rate is increased and the cells are shed at a more rapid rate. When this occurs, the rate of replacement does not always keep pace with the rate of cell loss, and the area becomes denuded, reddened, and swollen. Fortunately, the mucosal surface heals rapidly and the area usually regenerates within a few days once the irritating stimulus has been removed. Cell regeneration is impaired, however, when the injury is extensive or prolonged. Radiation, anticancer drugs, and other factors that impair growth of rapidly proliferating cells interfere with regeneration of the gastrointestinal mucosal lining. Treatment with anticancer agents frequently causes such side effects as stomatitis, anorexia, nausea, vomiting, and diarrhea.

Smooth muscle of the gastrointestinal tract heals by scar tissue replacement. Thus, when the injury extends into the smooth muscle layer, there is impaired regeneration of both the muscularis and mucosal layers; this renders the area more susceptible to future irritation and injury.

The Esophagus

The esophagus is a tube that connects the oropharynx with the stomach. It lies posterior to the trachea and larynx and extends through the mediastinum, intersecting the diaphragm at the level of the 11th thoracic vertebra. The esophagus functions primarily as a conduit for passage of food from the pharynx to the stomach, and the structures of its walls are designed for this purpose; the smooth muscle layers provide the peristaltic movements needed to move food along its length, while the epithelial layer secretes mucus, which protects its surface and aids in lubricating food.

Dysphagia
The act of swallowing is dependent upon the coordinated action of the tongue and pharynx. These structures are innervated by the 5th, 9th, 10th, and 12th cranial nerves. *Dysphagia* refers to difficulty in

deglutition (the act of swallowing). It can result from altered nerve function or from narrowing of the esophagus. Lesions of the central nervous system, such as a stroke, often involve the cranial nerves that control deglutition. Cancer of the esophagus and stenosis due to scarring reduce the size of the esophageal lumen and make swallowing difficult.

Esophagitis

Esophagitis refers to inflammation of the esophagus. Causative agents include chemical injury (lye, ammonia, and other caustic substances), infections, and trauma from repeated ingestion of irritating foods, such as hot liquids and spicy foods. The most common cause of esophagitis is the reflux of gastric secretions into the esophagus as the result of a hiatus hernia. Symptoms associated with esophagitis include heartburn and pain. The pain is usually located in the epigastric or retrosternal area and often radiates to the throat, shoulder, or back. As with inflammation of the mucosal layer in other parts of the gastrointestinal tract, esophagitis causes hyperemia, edema, and erosion of the luminal surface. When the damage is severe or prolonged, scarring occurs and the wall of the esophagus becomes thickened and fibrotic; this leads to difficulty in swallowing.

Hiatal hernia

A hiatal or diaphragmatic hernia is the herniation of the stomach through the diaphragm into the thorax. Since intra-abdominal pressure is greater than thoracic pressure, the main problem associated with a hiatus hernia is reflux of gastric secretions into the esophagus.

There are two types of hiatal hernias. The more common one is the sliding type in which the esophagogastric junction "slides" into the thoracic cavity when the person lies down, then moves back into the abdomen when the person assumes the upright position. The "rolling" or paraesophageal hernia is the condition in which the gastroesophageal junction remains in its normal anatomic position while the curvature of the stomach herniates through the diaphragmatic opening (Fig. 37-1).

Conditions that predispose to the development of a hiatal hernia and reflux of gastric contents into the esophagus include (1) congenital or acquired weakness of the hiatal muscle, (2) conditions that increase intra-abdominal pressure (*e.g.*, obesity, pregnancy, tight-fitting clothes, and ascites), or (3) a congenital or acquired shortening of the esophagus. The latter can occur when there is extensive scarring of the esophagus or can result from reflex spasms.

The signs and symptoms of a hiatal hernia are related to the reflux of gastric contents into the esophagus. The most common manifestation is pain and heartburn, which occurs about ½ hour to 1 hour following a meal. Heartburn is aggravated by any bodily position, such as the recumbent position, that increases the reflux. Often the heartburn occurs during the night. Because of its location, the pain may be confused with angina. Swelling or stenosis caused by scar tissue may cause dysphagia.

The treatment of a hiatal hernia generally focuses on conservative measures. These measures include avoidance of positions and conditions that increase gastric reflux. Frequent, small feedings are

Figure 37–1. Diagram showing normal position of the esophagus and stomach and positional changes that occur with a sliding and paraesophageal hernia. (From Brunner LS, Suddarth DS: Textbook of Medical Surgical Nursing, 3rd ed. Philadelphia, JB Lippincott, 1975)

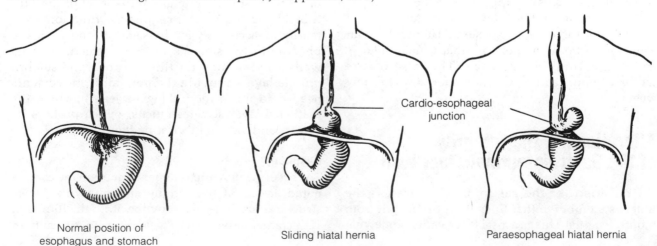

Normal position of
esophagus and stomach

Sliding hiatal hernia

Paraesophageal hiatal hernia

Cardio-esophageal
junction

preferred to large meals because they prevent gastric distention. It is recommended that meals be eaten sitting up and that the recumbent position be avoided for several hours following a meal. Bending for long periods should be avoided, since it tends to increase intra-abdominal pressure and cause gastric reflux. Sleeping with several pillows helps to prevent reflux during the night. When esophagitis occurs, it may be necessary to institute treatment measures, such as use of antacids, to decrease gastric secretions. Surgical treatment may become necessary when there is persistent gastric reflux that is causing damage to the esophageal wall and that cannot be controlled by conservative means.

Esophageal diverticulum

A diverticulum of the esophagus is an outpouching of the esophageal wall caused by a weakness of the muscularis layer. An esophageal diverticulum tends to retain food. Complaints that the food "stops" before it reaches the stomach are very common, as are reports of gurgling, belching, coughing, and foul-smelling breath. Additionally, the trapped food may cause esophagitis and ulceration. Since the condition is usually progressive, correction of the defect requires surgical intervention.

Carcinoma of the esophagus

Carcinoma of the esophagus accounts for 2% of all cancer deaths in the United States. This disease is common in men over age 60.[4] It is reported that environmental factors contribute to the development of esophageal cancers. These environmental factors include (1) alterations in function that cause food or drink to remain in the esophagus for prolonged periods of time, (2) reflux esophagitis, and (3) continued exposure to irritants such as alcohol and tobacco. The incidence of esophageal cancer among heavy drinkers is 25 times greater than that of nondrinkers. In contrast to cancer of the lung, esophageal cancer is seen more frequently among pipe and cigar smokers than cigarette smokers. Unfortunately, the outlook for persons with cancer of the esophagus is particularly grim, the 5-year survival rate being only about 4%.[5] This is because the tumor has usually spread to other areas before symptoms develop.

The Stomach

The stomach is a large reservoir for the digestive tract; it lies in the upper abdomen, anterior to the pancreas, splenic vessels, and left kidney. Anteriorly, the stomach is bounded by the anterior ab-

dominal wall and the left inferior lobe of the liver. While in the stomach, food is churned and mixed with hydrochloric acid and pepsin before being released into the small intestine.

Acute gastritis

Acute gastritis is a transient irritation of the gastric mucosa which is caused by local irritants such as bacterial endotoxins, caffeine, alcohol, and aspirin. Normally, the stomach lining is impermeable to the acid it secretes, a property that allows the stomach to contain acid and pepsin without having its wall digested. It is becoming increasingly evident that the production of prostaglandins is an important factor in protecting the gastrointestinal mucosa against the injurious effects of irritating luminal agents. The mechanism by which this works is unknown. Drugs such as aspirin and indomethacin inhibit prostaglandin production. Occult bleeding due to gastric irritation occurs in about 70% of persons who take aspirin on a regular basis (*e.g.*, as a treatment for arthritis).[6] Alcohol is also known to disrupt the mucosal barrier, and when aspirin and alcohol are taken in combination, as they often are, there is increased risk of gastric irritation.

The complaints of persons with acute gastritis vary. Often, persons with aspirin-related gastritis are totally unaware of the condition or may complain only of heartburn or sour stomach. Gastritis associated with excessive alcohol consumption is a different situation: it often causes a transient gastric distress, which may lead to vomiting and in more severe situations, to bleeding and hematemesis. Gastritis due to infectious organisms, such as the staphylococcus endotoxins, usually has an abrupt and violent onset, with gastric distress and vomiting, following the ingestion of a contaminated food source by about 5 hours. Acute gastritis is usually a self-limiting disorder; complete regeneration and healing usually occur within several days.

Chronic gastritis

Chronic gastritis is a separate entity from that of acute gastritis. This condition is characterized by progressive and irreversible atrophy of the glandular epithelium of the stomach. Atrophy of the epithelial layer involves the pepsin-producing chief cells and the acid-producing parietal cells. The parietal cells also produce intrinsic factor, which is required for vitamin B_{12} absorption. This means that both achlorhydria (lack of hydrochloric acid) and pernicious anemia occur when there is extensive atrophy of the gastric mucosa.

There appear to be two forms of chronic gastritis. The most common form is referred to as *simple atrophic gastritis*. Simple atrophic gastritis is seen most frequently in elderly persons and in heavy drinkers or cigarette smokers. A second form of the disorder, *autoimmune atrophic gastritis*, is thought to be caused by antibodies that destroy gastric mucosal cells. With the simple form of the disease there is usually only moderate impairment of acid and pepsin secretion, while vitamin B_{12} absorption remains impaired. This retention of acid production in a mucosal surface that has impaired defenses predisposes to peptic ulcer formation. Persons with autoimmune gastritis usually have severe impairment of acid and pepsin secretion, and about 20% of such persons have pernicious anemia.

The signs and symptoms of chronic gastritis are rather vague. Often the disorder produces no discernible symptoms. Symptoms, when they do occur, range from mild distress to complaints similar to those of peptic ulcer. In contrast to gastric ulcer pain, the discomfort associated with atrophic gastritis is not relieved by antacid therapy, nor does true gastritis pain occur during the night.

The clinical significance of atrophic gastritis resides not in its symptoms, but in its ability to produce more serious disorders—namely, pernicious anemia. While chronic gastritis can occur without impairment of vitamin B_{12} absorption, pernicious anemia develops only in its presence. When pernicious anemia is present, there is an accompanying histamine-fast lack of hydrochloric acid.

Atrophic gastritis also predisposes to gastric ulcer, anemia, and cancer of the stomach. It has been estimated that 50% of persons with gastric ulcers have an associated chronic gastritis. A second problem that frequently occurs with chronic gastritis is a recurrent iron deficiency anemia. The cause of this anemia is unclear, although there is evidence to suggest that a minimum level of hydrochloric acid is required for iron absorption. A more serious outcome is cancer of the stomach. Approximately 10% of persons with atrophic gastritis eventually develop gastric carcinoma.[6]

Tests for gastric acid production

A laboratory procedure called gastric analysis is done to assess the hydrochloric acid content of gastric secretions. This procedure involves the withdrawal of samples of gastric secretions through a tube that has been inserted into the stomach. Histamine or its analog may be administered subcutaneously during the sampling procedure for the purpose of stimulating acid production. When pernicious anemia is present, such stimulation fails to increase acid levels. In this case, the observed

achlorhydria is said to be histamine-fast. A second means for assessing hydrochloric acid secretion is a method called *tubeless gastric analysis*. Tubeless gastric analysis is a screening test that involves the use of a cation resin dye. An acid pH of less than 3.5 is required so that the dye can be released and absorbed in the small intestine. The presence of dye in the urine is interpreted to mean that there is sufficient hydrochloric acid in the stomach to maintain a pH that favors dye absorption.

Gastric and peptic ulcers

Gastric and peptic ulcers, with their remissions and exacerbations, represent a chronic health problem. At present, 10% of the population has or will develop a peptic ulcer. As a health problem, ulcer disease accounts for 10% of hospital admissions. In terms of location, duodenal ulcers are 5 to 10 times more common than gastric ulcers. Ulcers in the duodenum occur at any age and are frequently seen in early adulthood. Interestingly, duodenal ulcers seem to have a seasonal trend, with a higher incidence of recurrence in the spring and fall. Gastric ulcers, on the other hand, tend to affect the older age group with peak incidence in the sixth and seventh decades. Both types of ulcers affect men 3 to 4 times as frequently as they do women.

At present, there is considerable confusion regarding the terms *peptic ulcer* and *gastric ulcer*. A peptic ulcer can occur in any area of the gastrointestinal tract that is exposed to acid–pepsin secretions. For example, ulcerations in the esophagus due to reflux of gastric secretions would be classified as a peptic ulcer. Peptic ulcers also occur in the stomach, in the duodenum, at the surgical junction where the stomach has been resected and joined to the jejunum (gastrojejunostomy), and in a Meckel's diverticulum that contains misplaced gastric tissue. A gastric ulcer, as the word implies, is descriptive of an ulcer of the stomach. Unlike peptic ulcers, gastric ulcers can occur in the absence of hydrochloric acid (*i.e.*, gastric ulcers associated with chronic gastritis). The remaining discussion of ulcers focuses on peptic ulcer, although the reader is reminded that not all stomach ulcers are peptic ulcers.

A peptic ulcer represents a break in the continuity of the mucosal layer. Generally speaking, it can be said that peptic-ulcer formation reflects (1) an imbalance between acid–pepsin production or (2) an inability of the affected mucosal layer to resist the destructive action of these digestive agents. Evidence suggests that hydrochloric acid is an important causative agent in duodenal ulcers, whereas decreased tissue resistance plays a greater role in the development of gastric ulcers. Simple as this sounds, only in rare cases can ulcer development be traced to a single cause. It is more likely that both factors contribute to the development of a peptic ulcer. Nevertheless, it seems helpful, in terms of understanding ulcer development, to view these differences in causation in terms of the function that the mucosal surface affords the stomach and the duodenum.

Increased acid–pepsin production. Hydrochloric acid production is influenced by several factors, including neural and hormonal stimulation. The hormone gastrin, which is produced in the antrum of the stomach, is a potent stimulus for hydrochloric acid secretion. Increased levels of gastric acid have also been attributed to (1) increased numbers of acid–pepsin producing cells in the stomach, (2) increased sensitivity of the parietal cells to food and other stimuli (*e.g.,* both alcohol and caffeine are potent stimulators of hydrochloric acid secretion), (3) excessive vagal stimulation, and (4) impaired inhibition of gastric secretions as food moves into the intestine.

The intractable peptic ulcers observed in the *Zollinger–Ellison syndrome* are caused by a gastrin-secreting tumor of the pancreas. In persons with this disorder, gastric-acid secretion reaches such levels that ulceration becomes inevitable.

Normally, gastrin secretion is inhibited as food moves into the intestine. It has been postulated that this reflex inhibition of gastrin may be impaired in certain types of ulcers. For example, *Cushing's ulcer* is a special type of stress ulcer that occurs in association with severe brain injury or neurosurgery. It results from increased central stimulation of the vagus nerve, which is unresponsive to reflex mechanisms that normally control gastric secretions.

Resistance of the mucosal surface. The defenses of the mucosal surface are dependent upon an adequate blood flow and an intact mucosal barrier. It can be assumed that any disruption in the mucosal barrier decreases these defenses and renders the mucosal surface more susceptible to the destructive effects of the hydrogen ion.

It has been suggested that a fundamental abnormality in persons with gastric ulcers is an increased permeability of the epithelial layer of the stomach to hydrogen ions which causes injury to the mucosal surface and decreases its resistance to further injury. It also is possible that a chronically diseased mucosal membrane is unable to secrete sufficient mucus to form an effective barrier. Bile is known to disrupt the mucosal barrier, and reflux of bile from the intestine into the stomach has been implicated in gastric ulcer. In addition to bile, a number of drugs are recognized as "barrier breakers." Both aspirin and alcohol are known to damage this barrier.

The duodenum, which acts as a passageway for digestive enzymes and acid-laden chyme, is a frequent site of peptic ulcers. Brunner's glands, which are located between the pylorus and the site where bile and pancreatic enzymes enter the duodenum, produce a large amount of viscid mucus, which serves to protect this area. The activity of these glands is inhibited by sympathetic stimulation; this may help to explain why anxiety and stress contribute to duodenal ulcer development.

Ischemia or decreased blood flow impairs mucus secretion and tends to make the mucosal surface less resistant to the destructive effects of hydrochloric acid. *Curling's ulcer* is a stress ulcer that occurs following severe burns, trauma, or sepsis and is thought to result from local ischemia.

Of recent interest is the relationship between the incidence of duodenal ulcers and blood types. It has been observed that persons with duodenal ulcers have a higher-than-normal frequency of blood group O when compared with an ulcer-free population. As a means of further explanation, it should be pointed out that about 75% of the general population secrete a water-soluble substance, similar to their blood type, into their saliva and gastric secretions. Persons with type-O blood and certain other persons with a particular red cell antigen (Lewis a) are "non-secretors" of a primary-blood-group antigen in their saliva. For reasons that are unclear, these persons appear to be more susceptible to duodenal ulcers than are persons who secrete primary-blood-group antigens.

The clinical manifestations of uncomplicated peptic ulcer focus on discomfort and pain. The pain, which is described as burning, gnawing, or cramp-like, is usually rhythmic in nature and frequently occurs when the stomach is empty—between meals and at 1 o'clock or 2 o'clock in the morning. Characteristically, the pain is relieved by food or antacids. A peptic ulcer can affect one or all of the layers of the duodenum or stomach. The ulcer may penetrate only the mucosal surface or it may extend into the smooth muscle layers. Occasionally, an ulcer will penetrate the outer wall of the stomach or duodenum. Healing of the muscularis layer involves replacement with scar tissue; although there is regeneration of the mucosal layers that cover the scarred muscle layer, the regeneration is often less than perfect, which contributes to repeated episodes of ulceration and complications.

Complications of peptic ulcer

Complications of peptic ulcer include hemorrhage, obstruction, and perforation. *Hemorrhage* occurs in 10% to 15% of persons with ulcers. Evidence of bleeding may consist of hematemesis or melena. Bleeding may be sudden, severe, and may occur without warning, or it may be insidious, producing only occult (hidden) blood in the stool. *Obstruction* is caused by edema, spasm, or contraction of scar tissue; it occurs when there is impairment of free passage of luminal contents through the pylorus or adjacent areas. *Perforation* occurs when the ulcer erodes all the layers of the wall of the stomach or duodenum. With perforation, gastrointestinal contents enter the peritoneum and cause peritonitis, or penetrate adjacent structures such as the pancreas. Peritonitis is discussed as a separate topic at the end of this chapter.

Treatment of peptic ulcer

Treatment of peptic ulcer focuses on measures to (1) decrease or neutralize the hydrochloric acid, (2) increase the resistance of the mucosal layer, and (3) promote healing.

Conservative treatment measures include (1) efforts to relieve stress and anxiety, (2) dietary management, (3) antacids, and (4) other medications that act to decrease gastric-acid secretion.

Although in the past the conservative treatment of peptic ulcers has usually included use of a bland diet, there is at present considerable controversy as to its value. Most physicians would agree that coffee and alcoholic beverages should be avoided. Most physicians would agree, too, that the use of food as an antacid should also be avoided, because such feedings are generally accompanied by a rebound increase in gastric-acid secretion. The value of the hourly milk-and-cream regimen, which has been used for years, has also come under question. There is evidence that the calcium in milk may actually increase gastric-acid secretion. The use of milk and cream is also associated with an increased risk of developing the milk-alkali syndrome.

Medications used in the treatment of peptic ulcers include the selective use of antacids, anticholinergic drugs, cimetidine, and sedatives or tranquilizers (Table 37-1). Anticholinergic drugs are less effective inhibitors of gastric-acid secretions than antacids and cimetidine and, therefore, they are usually used in combination with other methods of treatment. Sedatives and tranquilizers are individualized forms of treatment that are used for persons in which stress is a large contributing factor.

Antacids, either self-prescribed or physician-prescribed, represent a large business in the United States; approximately 110 million dollars are spent each year for these medications.[7] There are essentially four types of antacids that are used to relieve gastric acidity: sodium bicarbonate, calcium carbonate, aluminum hydroxide, and magnesium hydroxide. Because sodium bicarbonate is water-soluble, it leaves the stomach rapidly and produces a very transient effect. It contains large amounts of sodium and tends to cause metabolic alkalosis. It is mainly used as a home remedy. *Calcium preparations* are constipating and may cause hypercalcemia and the milk-alkali syndrome. There is also evidence that oral calcium preparations increase gastric-acid secretion after their buffering effect has been utilized. *Magnesium hydroxide* is a potent antacid that acts as a laxative. Approximately 5% to 10% of the magnesium in this preparation is absorbed into the intestine; therefore, magnesium hydroxide should not be used in persons with renal failure since magnesium must be excreted through the kidneys. *Aluminum hydroxide* reacts with hydrochloric acid to form aluminum chloride. It combines with phosphate in the intestine and is often used for treating the hyperphosphatemia that occurs with renal failure. The adsorptive effects of aluminum hydroxide may affect absorption of other substances, such as bile salts and tetracycline. Many antacids contain a *combination of ingredients*, such as magnesium aluminum hydroxide.

Cimetidine is a histamine-2 antagonist that blocks the secretion of hydrochloric acid regardless of the stimulus for its secretion, suggesting that histamine is the "final common mediator" of gastric-acid secretion. In 1977, when the drug was released for clinical use by the Food and Drug Administration, only two indications for its use were approved: short-term use in treatment of duodenal ulcer, and hypersecretion of gastric acid, such as occurs with the Zollinger–Ellison syndrome. There is evidence that the drug is now being used for more diverse purposes.[8] Recently, there has been a reported reduction in liver blood flow that accompanies treatment with the drug, and decreased metabolism of drugs (propranolol) by the liver following its use.[9] Since the drug is new, it is likely that other problems may become apparent as its use is continued.

When the conservative management of peptic ulcer is ineffective, surgical intervention is often needed. There are three types of surgical procedures that are done: (1) subtotal gastrectomy, in which 75% to 80% of the stomach is removed and the remaining portion attached to the jejunum, (2) truncal vagotomy and drainage, in which the vagus

Table 37–1 Drugs Used in Treatment of Peptic Ulcer

Drug	Mechanisms of Action
Anticholinergics	Blocks vagal stimulation of gastric acid secretion
	Decreases gastric motility allowing antacids to remain in the stomach
Antacids	
Calcium carbonate	Neutralizes the gastric acid, but may cause rebound gastric acid secretion
	Can cause hypercalcemia associated with the milk-alkali syndrome
	Has a constipating effect
Magnesium hydroxide	Neutralizes gastric acid
	About 5% to 10% is absorbed in the intestine and may cause an increase in blood magnesium levels in persons with renal failure
	Has a laxative effect
Aluminum hydroxide	Neutralizes gastric acid
	Binds with phosphate in the intestine and may be used to treat hyperphosphatemia in renal failure
	May also bind with other substances and drugs, increasing their excretion in the stool
Histamine-2 antagonists (cimetidine)	Blocks histamine-2 receptors, inhibiting gastric acid secretion. Approved by F.D.A. for short-term use in treatment of duodenal ulcers and for ulcers caused by hypersecretion of gastric acid
Sedatives and tranquilizers	Relieves anxiety and tension in persons in whom this is a problem

nerve trunks are cut and the outlet of the stomach enlarged, and (3) truncal vagotomy and antrectomy, in which the vagus nerve trunks are cut and the distal 50% of the stomach is removed.

One of the complications following surgery for peptic ulcers is the *dumping syndrome*. It occurs to some extent in about 20% of persons who have this type of operation. It is believed to be caused by the rapid entry of hyperosmolar liquids into the intestine and is characterized by nausea, vomiting, diarrhea, diaphoresis, palpitations, tachycardia, lightheadedness, and flushing which occurs either while eating or shortly after. It is often followed (in about 2 hours) by an episode of hypoglycemia, resulting from the rapid absorption of glucose which acts as a stimulus for insulin release by the beta cells of the pancreas. Treatment consists of limiting the diet to small, frequent feedings, which are taken without liquids and which are low in simple sugars (these are the most osmotically active parts of the diet). Symptoms usually diminish with time.

Cancer of the stomach

Cancer of the stomach strikes approximately 23,000 persons each year and causes about 15,000 deaths. Although its incidence has decreased about 40% in the last 25 years, it remains the seventh leading cause of death in the United States.[5] Among the factors that increase the risk of gastric cancer are a genetic predisposition, carcinogenic factors in the diet (*e.g.*, nitrates, smoked foods), atrophic gastritis, and gastric polyps. Fifty percent of gastric cancers occur in the pyloric region or adjacent to the antrum. When compared with a benign ulcer, which has smooth margins and is concentrically shaped, gastric cancers tend to be larger, are irregularly shaped, have irregular margins, and are usually located in the greater curvature of the stomach.

Unfortunately, stomach cancers are often asymptomatic until late in their course. Symptoms, when they do occur, are usually vague and include indigestion, anorexia, weight loss, vague epigastric pain, vomiting, and an abdominal mass. Diagnosis of gastric cancer is accomplished by means of a variety of techniques, including barium x-ray studies, gastroscopy studies with biopsy, and cytological studies (Pap smear) of gastric secretions. Cytological studies can prove particularly useful as a routine screening test in persons with atrophic gastritis or gastric polyps.

Surgery in the form of subtotal gastrectomy is usually the treatment of choice. Radiation and chemotherapy have not proved particularly useful as primary treatment modalities in stomach cancer. When these methods are used, it is usually for palliative purposes or to control metastatic spread of the disease.

The Small and Large Intestine

There are many similarities in conditions that disrupt the integrity of the small and large bowel. The wall of both the small and large intestines consist of five layers (Fig. 36-2): an outer serosal layer; a muscularis layer, which is divided into a layer of circular and one of longitudinal muscle fibers; a submucosal layer; and an inner mucosal layer, which lines the lumen of the intestine. Among the conditions that predispose to disruption of the integrity of the intestine are inflammatory bowel disease, diverticulitis, appendicitis, and cancer of the colon and rectum.

Inflammatory bowel disease

Inflammatory bowel disease, which includes Crohn's disease and ulcerative colitis, affects over 100,000 persons in the United States.[10] There is evidence to suggest that the incidence of ulcerative colitis, which is an inflammatory disorder of the rectum and colon, has reached a plateau, whereas Crohn's disease, which can affect either the large or small bowel, has increased steadily over the past 15 years.

The causes of both Crohn's disease and ulcerative colitis are largely unknown. The diseases appear to have a familial occurrence that suggests a hereditary predisposition. One of the common beliefs is that hereditary factors increase the susceptibility to other etiological factors, such as immune responses and viral infections. There is a special susceptibility among the Jewish population for both Crohn's disease and ulcerative colitis. Although psychogenic factors may contribute to the severity and onset of both conditions, it seems unlikely that they are the primary cause.

Crohn's disease.　Crohn's disease (regional enteritis) is a recurrent granulomatous type of inflammatory response that can affect any area of the gastrointestinal tract. It is a slowly progressive, relentless, and often disabling disease. The disease usually strikes in early adulthood and affects both men and women equally. Its lesions are observed most frequently in the terminal ileum or ileocecal area of the bowel. The ileum is involved in about 80% of the cases. The colon is the second most frequent site of involvement and the condition may be confused with ulcerative colitis. Crohn's disease is a multisystem disease that is often accompanied by other manifestations, such as arthritis, gall stones, skin disorders, iritis, and keratitis.

A characteristic feature of Crohn's disease is the sharply demarcated granulomatous lesions that occur and that are surrounded by normal-appearing mucosal tissue. When the lesions are multiple, they are often referred to as skip lesions because they are interspersed between what appear to be normal segments of the bowel. All layers of the bowel are involved in regional enteritis, with the submucosal layer being affected to the greatest extent. The surface of the inflamed bowel usually has a characteristic "cobblestone" appearance resulting from the fissures and crevices that develop and surround areas of submucosal edema. There is usually a relative sparing of the smooth muscle layers of the bowel with marked inflammatory and fibrotic changes of the subserosal layer. The bowel wall, after a time, often becomes thickened and inflexible; its appearance has been likened to a lead pipe or rubber hose. The adjacent mesentery may become inflamed and the regional lymph nodes and channels enlarged. Fistulas are tubelike passages from a normal cavity or abscess that extend to a free surface of the body or another body cavity. In Crohn's disease, the inflammatory lesions may extend and penetrate the entire wall of the gut, causing abscess formation and the development of fistulous tracts. The characteristics of Crohn's disease are summarized in Table 37-2.

The *clinical course* of Crohn's disease is variable; often there are periods of exacerbations and remissions, with symptoms being related to the location of the lesions. The principal symptoms include intermittent diarrhea, colicky pain (usually in the lower right quadrant), weight loss, malaise, and low-grade fever. Perianal abscesses and fistula formation are common. Their occurrence is largely due to the severity of the diarrhea, which produces ulceration of the perianal skin. As the disease progresses, there may be bleeding and malabsorption. Complications include intestinal obstruction, abdominal abscess formation, and fistula formation. The overall mortality rate is about 18%. The majority of persons with

Table 37-2 Differentiating Characteristics of Crohn's Disease and Ulcerative Colitis

Characteristic	Crohn's Disease	Ulcerative Colitis
Type of inflammation	Granulomatous	Ulcerative and exudative
Type of lesion	Cobblestone	Crypt abscesses and pseudopolypi
Level of involvement	Primarily submucosal	Primarily mucosal
Extent of involvement	Skip lesions	Continuous
Areas of involvement	Primarily ileum Secondarily colon	Primarily rectum and left colon
Diarrhea	Common	Common
Rectal bleeding	Rare	Common
Fistulas	Common	Rare
Strictures	Common	Rare
Perianal abscesses	Common	Rare
Toxic megacolon	Rare	Common
Development of cancer	Rare	Relatively common

Crohn's disease eventually develop complications that require surgery.

Diagnosis is usually made following x-ray studies of the gastrointestinal tract, using barium as a radiopaque contrast medium. Proctosigmoidoscopy is often done to visualize the bowel and to obtain a biopsy.

Treatment methods focus on maintenance of adequate nutrition, measures to promote healing, and prevention and treatment of complications. Nutritional deficiencies are common in Crohn's disease due to diarrhea, steatorrhea, and other malabsorption problems. A nutritious diet that is high in calories, vitamins, and proteins is recommended. Fats often aggravate the diarrhea, and it is generally recommended that they be avoided. Elemental diets, which are nutritionally balanced, yet are residue-free and bulk-free, may be given for a period of time during the acute phase of the illness. These diets are largely absorbed in the jejunum and allow the inflamed bowel to rest. Total parenteral nutrition (parenteral hyperalimentation) consists of intravenous administration of hypertonic glucose solutions to which amino acids and fats may be added. This form of nutritional therapy may be needed when food cannot be absorbed from the intestine. Because of the hypertonicity of these solutions, they must be administered through a large-diameter central vein.

In addition to nutritional therapy, salicylazosulfapyridine (Azulfidine) and the adrenocorticosteroid hormones are frequently prescribed to treat the acute disease. Surgery is usually reserved for treatment of complications.

Ulcerative colitis. Ulcerative colitis is a nonspecific inflammatory condition of the colon. It usually begins in the rectum and spreads to the left colon. It may involve the entire colon. Like Crohn's disease, the chronic form of the disease is often associated with systemic manifestations such as migratory polyarthritis, ankylosing spondylitis, uveitis, inflammatory liver disease, and various skin manifestations. There are many similarities etween ulcerative colitis and Crohn's disease and, at present, it is questioned whether the two disorders might represent different manifestations of the same disease.

With ulcerative colitis, the inflammatory process tends to be confluent and continuous rather than skipping areas, as it does in Crohn's disease. Ulcerative colitis affects primarily the mucosal layer, although it can extend into the submucosal layer. Characteristic of the disease are the lesions that form in the crypts of Lieberkühn (see Fig. 36-7) in the base of the mucosal layer. The inflammatory process causes pinpoint mucosal hemorrhages to occur, which in time suppurate and develop into *crypt abscesses*. These inflammatory lesions become necrotic, and ulcerate. Although the ulcerations are usually superficial, they often extend, causing large, denuded areas. As a result of the inflammatory process, the mucosal layer often develops tongue-like projections that resemble polpys and are therefore called *pseudopolyps*. Because ulcerative colitis affects the mucosal layer, bleeding is an almost constant manifestation and bloody diarrhea is the most common complaint during the acute phase of the disease. With repeated episodes of colitis, there is thickening of the bowel wall. The pathologic features of Crohn's disease and ulcerative colitis are summarized in Table 37-2.

Ulcerative colitis usually follows a course of remissions and exacerbations. The severity of the disease varies from mild to fulminating. Accordingly, the disease has been divided into three types, depending on its severity: acute fulminating, chronic intermittent, and mild chronic. About 15% to 20% of persons with ulcerative colitis present with the *fulminating form* of the disease. This form presents with an acute episode of bloody diarrhea, fever, and acute abdominal pain. This is the most serious form of the disease and it has been reported that as many as 35% of persons with severe attacks may die.[11] About 60% have a *mild* form of the disease, in which bleeding and diarrhea are mild and systemic signs are absent. This form of the disease can usually be managed by conservative means. The remainder of the persons with chronic ulcerative colitis have a *chronic*, continuous form, which continues after the initial attack. As compared with the milder form, usually more of the colon surface is involved and the presence of systemic signs and complications is greater.

Diarrhea, which is the characteristic manifestation of ulcerative colitis, will vary according to the severity of the disease. There may be up to 30 to 40 bowel movements a day. Typically, the stools contain blood and mucus. Nocturnal diarrhea is usually present when daytime symptoms are severe. There may be mild abdominal cramping and incontinence of stools. Anorexia, weakness, and fatigability are common.

Diagnostic measures include colonoscopic examination, often with biopsy. Colon x-ray studies may be done using barium as a radiopaque contrast medium.

Measures used in *treating* ulcerative colitis vary with the severity of the disease. Hospitalization is required for persons with the acute, fulminating form of the disease. Sulfasalazine (an antimicrobial agent) may be used for both short-course and long-term therapy. The adrenocorticosteroid hormones are selectively used to lessen the inflammatory response. These drugs can be given by enema or in the form of a suppository. Surgical treatment (removal of the rectum and entire colon) with creation of an ileostomy may be required for those persons who do not respond to conservative methods of treatment.

Complications. *Toxic megacolon* is an acute, life-threatening complication of ulcerative colitis. It is characterized by dilatation of the colon and signs of systemic toxicity. It results from extension of the inflammatory response, with involvement of neural and vascular components of the bowel. Contributing factors include use of laxatives, narcotics and anticholinergic drugs, and the presence of hypokalemia.

Cancer of the colon is one of the feared complications of ulcerative colitis. The risk of developing cancer among persons who have had the disease for 15 years is about 5% to 10%, and after 25 years the risk becomes 40% to 50%.[6]

Diverticular disease

Diverticulosis describes a condition in which there is herniation of the mucosal layer of the colon through the muscularis layer. Diverticular disease is very common in the United States. It is thought to affect about 50% of persons over age 60.[12] While the disorder is very prevalent in the developed countries of the world, it is almost nonexistent in many of the African nations and other underdeveloped countries. This suggests that dietary factors (lack of fiber content), a decrease in physical activity, poor bowel habits (in which the urge to defecate is neglected), along with the effects of aging, contribute to the development of the disease.

Most diverticula occur in the sigmoid colon. In the colon, the longitudinal muscle does not form a continuous layer, as it does in the small bowel. Instead there are three separate longitudinal bands of muscle called the taeniae coli (Fig. 37-2). It is between these muscles, in the area where the blood vessels pierce the circular muscle layer to bring blood to the mucosal layer, that diverticula develop. An increase in intraluminal pressure provides the force for creating these herniations. The increase in pressure is thought to be related to the volume of the colonic contents. The more scanty the contents, the more vigorous the contractions and the greater the pressure. When the vigorous contractions continue over time, there is hypertrophy of both the circular and longitudinal muscle layers. In many cases, the haustra may become so thick from the hypertrophy that they are approximated during contractions, causing a marked increase in the pressure within the isolated segment. According to the laws of physics, the pressure within a tube increases as its diameter decreases. The sigmoid colon, which is the segment most vulnerable to the development of diverticula, is the segment of the colon with the narrowest diameter.

The vast majority of persons with diverticular disease remain asymptomatic. The disease is often found when x-ray studies are done for other purposes. When symptoms do occur, they are often

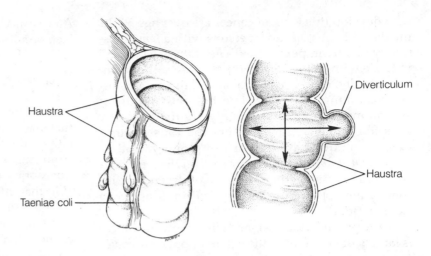

Figure 37–2. A portion of the sigmoid colon, showing the haustra and taeniae coli on the left. On the right is a longitudinal section of the colon showing the changes that occur in diverticular disease. There is hypertrophy of the muscle wall which causes the haustra to approximate during contractions of the colon. This causes a marked increase in pressure within that segment of the colon which contributes to diverticulum formation.

attributed to irritable bowel syndrome or other causes. There is often ill-defined lower abdominal discomfort; a change in bowel habits, such as diarrhea and constipation; bloating; and flatulence. One of the most common complaints is pain in the lower left quadrant. When it is accompanied by other symptoms, it is often referred to as *left-sided appendicitis*. This left-sided appendicitis is often accompanied by nausea and vomiting, tenderness in the lower left quadrant, a slight fever, and elevation in white blood cell count. These symptoms usually last for several days, unless complications occur, and are usually caused by localized inflammation of the diverticula, with perforation and development of a small localized abscess. Complications include perforation with peritonitis, hemorrhage, and bowel obstruction.

The usual treatment for diverticular disease is to prevent symptoms and complications. It includes increasing the bulk in the diet and bowel retraining so that the person has at least one bowel movement a day. Surgical treatment is reserved for complications.

Appendicitis

Acute appendicitis is extremely common. It is seen most frequently in the 5-year to 30-year age group but can occur at any age. The appendix becomes inflamed, swollen, and gangrenous, and it eventually perforates if not treated. Although the cause of appendicitis is not known, it is thought to be related to intraluminal obstruction due to a fecalith (hard piece of stool) or twisting.

Appendicitis usually has an abrupt onset, with pain referred to the epigastric or periumbilical area. This pain is due to stretching of the appendix during the early inflammatory process. At about the same time that the pain appears, there are one or two episodes of nausea. Initially the pain is vague, but

over a period of 2 hours to 12 hours it gradually increases and may become colicky in nature. When the inflammatory process has extended to involve the serosal layer of the appendix and the peritoneum, the pain becomes localized to the lower right quadrant. There is usually an elevation in temperature and a white blood cell count of over 10,000 per mm^3 with 75% or more polymorphonuclear cells. Palpation of the abdomen usually reveals a deep tenderness in the lower right quadrant which is confined to a small area about the size of the finger tip. It is usually located at about the site of the inflamed appendix. Many times the person with appendicitis will be able to place his finger directly over the tender area. Rebound tenderness, pain that occurs when pressure is applied to the area and then released, and spasm of the overlying abdominal muscles are common. Treatment consists of surgical removal of the appendix. Complications include peritonitis, localized periappendiceal abscess formation, and septicemia.

Colorectal cancer

More than 100,000 new cases of colon and rectal cancer are diagnosed each year, the same number as lung cancer. Although the outlook for cure is better with this cancer than with most other cancers, the 5-year survival rate is less than 50%. The main drawback to successful treatment is the fact that most lesions do not produce symptoms until late in the course of the disease.

Almost all cancers of the colon and rectum are carcinomas. Of these, about 16% occur in the cecum and ascending colon, 8% in the transverse and splenic flexures, 6% in the descending colon, 20% in the sigmoid colon, and 50% in the rectum.[4]

The cause of cancer of the colon and rectum is largely unknown. Its incidence increases with age, as evidenced by the fact that two-thirds of persons who develop this form of cancer are over age 50. Its incidence is increased in persons with a *family history of cancer*, in persons with *ulcerative colitis*, and in those with *familial multiple polyposis* of the colon.

Usually, cancer of the colon and rectum is present for a long period of time before it produces symptoms. *Bleeding* is a highly significant early symptom and it is usually the one that causes people to seek medical care. Other symptoms include a *change in bowel habits*, either diarrhea or constipation, and sometimes a sense of urgency or incomplete emptying of the bowel. Pain is usually a late symptom.

The prognosis for persons with colorectal cancer is largely dependent on the extent of bowel involvement and on the presence of metastasis at the time of diagnosis. This form of cancer can be divided into four categories, according to the classification system by Duke. The type-A tumor is limited to invasion of the mucosal and submucosal layers of the colon and has a 5-year survival rate of almost 100%. Type-B tumor involves the entire wall of the colon and has a 5-year survival rate of about 55% to 65%. With type-C tumor, there is invasion of the serosal layer, with involvement of the regional lymph nodes. The 5-year survival rate is approximately 25%. Type-D colorectal cancer involves far-advanced metastasis.[6]

Among the methods used in diagnosis of colorectal cancers are tests for occult blood and digital rectal examination, usually done during routine physical examinations; x-ray studies using barium (barium enema); and colonoscopy. Digital rectal examinations are most helpful in detecting neoplasms of the rectum.

Detection of blood in the stools. Almost all cancers of the colon amd rectum bleed intermittently even though the amount of blood is small and usually not apparent in the stools. It is therefore feasible to screen for colorectal cancers using commercially prepared tests for occult blood (Hemoccult) which are now available. This method utilizes a guaiac-impregnated filter paper. The technique involves preparing two slides per day from different portions of the same stool for 3 days to 4 days while the patient follows a high-fiber meatless diet. While the diet is not particularly appealing, this method of screening has been shown to be a relatively reliable and inexpensive method for screening of colorectal cancer. The routine test for occult blood is usually unreliable due to a high number of false-positive and false-negative tests when done on random stool samples and when patient is eating an unmodified diet. The American Cancer Society has endorsed the use of Hemoccult slides as a means of routine screening for colorectal cancer.[13]

Colonoscopy. Colonoscopy provides a means for direct visualization of the rectum and colon. The colonoscope consists of a flexible 4-cm glass bundle that has some 250,000 glass fibers with a lens at either end to focus and magnify the image.[14] Light from an external source is transmitted by the fiberoptic viewing bundle. Instruments are available that afford direct examination of the sigmoid colon or the entire colon. This method is used for screening persons at high risk for developing cancer of the colon (*e.g.*, those with ulcerative colitis) and for those with symptoms. Colonoscopy is also useful for obtaining a biopsy and for removing polyps. While this method is one of the most accurate for detecting early colorectal cancers, it is not suitable for mass screening since it is expensive and time consuming and must be done by a person who is highly trained in the use of the instrument.

Treatment. The only recognized treatment for cancer of the colon and rectum is surgical removal. Preoperative radiation may be used and has in some cases demonstrated increased 5-year survival rates. Postoperative adjuvant therapy with fluorouracil (5 FU) has had some success. Both radiation and chemotherapy are palliative treatment methods.

Peritonitis

Peritonitis represents an inflammatory response of the serous membrane that lines the abdominal cavity and covers the visceral organs. It can be caused by either bacterial invasion or chemical irritation. Most commonly, enteric bacteria enter the peritoneum because of a defect in the wall of one of the abdominal organs. The most common causes of peritonitis are perforated peptic ulcer, ruptured appendix, perforated diverticulum, gangrenous bowel, pelvic inflammatory disease, and gangrenous gall bladder. Other causes are abdominal trauma and wounds. Generalized peritonitis, while no longer the overwhelming problem it once was, is still a leading cause of death following abdominal surgery.

The peritoneum has several characteristics that either increase its vulnerability to or protect it against the effects of peritonitis. One weakness of the peritoneal cavity is that it is a large, unbroken space that favors the dissemination of contaminants. For the same reason, it has a large surface that permits rapid absorption of bacterial toxins into the blood. On the other hand, the peritoneum is particularly well adapted for producing an inflammatory response as a means of controlling infection. It tends, for example, to exude a thick, sticky, and fibrinous substance that adheres to other structures, such as the mesentery and omentum, and that serves to seal off the perforated viscus and aid in localizing the process. Localization is further enhanced by sympathetic stimulation that inhibits peristalsis. Although the paralytic ileus that occurs tends to give rise to associated problems, it does inhibit the movement of contaminants throughout the peritoneal cavity.

One of the most important manifestations of peritonitis is the translocation of extracellular fluid into the peritoneal cavity (through weeping of serous fluid from the inflamed peritoneum) and into the bowel as a result of bowel obstruction. Nausea and vomiting cause further losses of fluid. The fluid loss may then encourage development of hypovolemia and shock.

The onset of peritonitis may be acute, as in a ruptured appendix, or it may have a more gradual onset, as occurs in progressive inflammatory disease. Pain and tenderness are common symptoms. The pain is usually more intense over the inflamed area. The person with peritonitis usually lies very still because any movement aggravates the pain. Breathing is often shallow, in order to prevent movement of the abdominal muscles. The abdomen is usually rigid and sometimes described as boardlike, due to reflex muscle guarding. Vomiting is common. There is fever, elevation in white blood cell count, tachycardia, and frequently hypotension. Hiccoughs may develop because of irritation of the phrenic nerve. Paralytic ileus occurs shortly after the onset of widespread peritonitis and is accompanied by abdominal distention. Peritonitis that progresses and is untreated leads to toxemia and shock.

Treatment measures for peritonitis are directed toward (1) preventing the extension of the inflammatory response, (2) minimizing the effects of paralytic ileus and abdominal distention, and (3) correcting the fluid and electrolyte imbalances that develop. Surgical intervention may be needed to remove an acutely inflamed appendix or to close the opening in a perforated peptic ulcer. Oral fluids are forbidden. Nasogastric suction, which entails the insertion of a tube (placed through the nose) into the stomach or intestine, is employed to decompress the bowel and relieve the abdominal distention. Fluid and electrolyte replacement is essential. These fluids are prescribed on the basis of frequent blood chemistry determinations. Antibiotics are given to combat infection. Narcotics are often needed for pain relief.

A potential complication of peritonitis is abscess formation. Should it occur, the most desirable area for drainage is in the pelvis rather than in the area under the diaphragm. Therefore, the head of the bed is usually elevated about 60° to 70° (semi-Fowler's position) to encourage drainage of inflammatory exudate from the flank area into the pelvis.

In summary, the gastrointestinal tract is a five-layered tube that consists of an inner mucosal layer, a submucosal layer, a layer of circular and longitudinal smooth muscle, and an outer serosal layer. Disruption of the integrity of its wall can occur at any level, due to numerous pathological processes, including injury to the mucosal barrier, inflammation, structural changes, and neoplasms. The manifestations of alterations in the integrity of the digestive system depend on the process involved, the extent of the injury, and the area of the gastrointestinal tract that is involved.

:Alterations in Digestion and Absorption of Nutrients

The small intestine is involved primarily in the digestion and absorption of nutrients. The intestinal mucosa is impermeable to most large molecules. Therefore, most proteins, fats, and carbohydrates must be broken down into smaller particles before they can be absorbed. While some digestion of carbohydrates and proteins begins in the stomach, the major digestion takes place in the small intestine. The hydrolysis of fats to free fatty acids and monoglycerides takes place entirely in the small intestine. The liver, with its production of bile, and the pancreas, which supplies a number of digestive enzymes, also play important roles in digestion.

The distinguishing characteristic of the small intestine is its large surface area, which in the adult is estimated to be about 4500 square meters. Anatomic features that contribute to this enlarged surface area are the circular folds that extend into the lumen of the intestine, and the villi, which are fingerlike projections of mucous membrane, which number as many as 25,000, that line the entire small intestine. Each villus is covered with cells called enterocytes that contribute to the absorptive and digestive functions of the small bowel and goblet cells that provide mucus. The crypts of Lieberkühn are glandular structures that open into the spaces between the villi. The enterocytes have a life span of about 4 to 5 days and it is believed that replacement cells differentiate from cells that are located

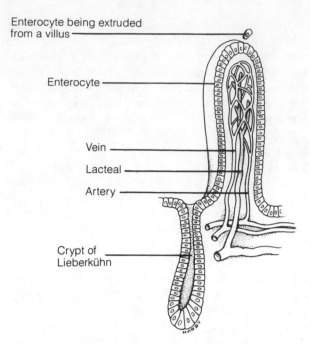

Enterocyte being extruded from a villus

Enterocyte

Vein

Lacteal

Artery

Crypt of Lieberkühn

Figure 37–3. Diagram of a single villus from the small intestine. (From Chaffee EE, Lytle IM: Basic Physiology and Anatomy, 4th ed. Philadelphia, JB Lippincott, 1980)

in the area of the crypts. The maturing enterocytes migrate up the villus and are eventually extruded from the tip.

Each villus is equipped with an artery, vein, and lymph vessel (lacteal), which brings blood to the surface of the intestine and which transports the nutrients and other materials that have passed into the blood from the lumen of the intestine (Fig. 37-3). Fats rely largely on the lymphatics for absorption. This means that a decrease in blood flow to the gut, which is caused by atherosclerosis or heart failure, may impair absorption of nutrients. Another cause of malabsorption is lymphatic obstruction due to lymphoma.

The enterocytes secrete a number of proteins, including enzymes that aid in the digestion of carbohydrates and proteins. These enzymes are called *brush border enzymes* because they adhere to the border of the villus structures. In this way they have access to the carbohydrates and protein molecules as they come in contact with the absorptive surface of the intestine. This mechanism of secretion places the enzymes where they are needed and eliminates the need to produce enough enzymes to mix with the entire contents that fill the lumen of the small bowel. The digested molecules either diffuse through the membrane or are actively transported across the mucosal surface to enter the blood or, in the case of

fatty acids, the lacteal. These molecules are then transported via the portal vein or lymphatics into the systemic circulation.

Absorption of carbohydrates

Carbohydrates must be broken down into monosaccharides, or single sugars, before they can be absorbed from the small intestine. The average daily intake of carbohydrate in the American diet is about 350 gm to 400 gm. Starch makes up about 50% of this total, sucrose (table sugar) about 30%, lactose (milk sugar) about 6%, and maltose about 1.5%.[15] Digestion of starch begins in the mouth with the action of amylase. Pancreatic secretions also contain an amylase. As a result of the action of amylase, starch is broken down into several disaccharides, including maltose, isomaltose, and α-dextrins. It is the brush border enzymes that convert the disaccharides into monosaccharides that can be absorbed (Table 37-3). Sucrose yields glucose and fructose, lactose is converted to glucose and galactose, and maltose is changed to glucose. When the disaccharides are not broken down to monosaccharides, they cannot be absorbed but remain as osmotically active particles in the contents of the digestive system, causing diarrhea.

Fructose is transported across the intestinal mucosa by facilitated diffusion, which does not require energy expenditure. In this case, fructose moves along a concentration gradient. Glucose and galactose, on the other hand, are transported via a sodium-dependent carrier system that utilizes ATP as an energy source (Fig. 37-4). Water absorption from the intestine is linked to absorption of osmotically active particles, such as glucose and sodium. It follows that an important consideration in facilitating the transport of water across the intestine (and decreasing diarrhea) following temporary disruption in bowel function is to include both sodium and glucose in the fluids that are taken. A number of carbonated soft drinks can be used for this purpose.

Lactase deficiency. The most common disaccharidase deficiency involves lactase. Although human infants have a high concentration of lactase following birth, this concentration falls rapidly in the first 4 to 5 years of life and may reach low levels in adolescence and adult life. It has been estimated that 3% to 19% of the adult white population, 70% of American blacks, and 90% of native Americans are deficient in lactase.[16] With a lactase deficiency, there is intolerance to milk, which is manifested in bloating, flatulence, cramping abdominal pain, and diarrhea.

Table 37-3   Enzymes Used in Digestion of Carbohydrates

Dietary Carbohydrates	Enzyme	Monosaccharides Produced
Lactose	Lactase	Glucose and galactose
Sucrose	Sucrase	Fructose and glucose
Starch	Amylase	
↓ Maltose and maltotriose	Maltase	Glucose and glucose
↓ α-Dextrins	Isomaltase	Glucose and glucose

These symptoms are usually relieved by avoiding lactose (milk) in the diet.

The fact that lactase availability declines following childhood and may be rather limited in the adult may help to explain why milk is sometimes poorly tolerated following gastrointestinal tract "flu" or other disorders. One can assume that with a limited ability to produce lactase, any disruption in the regeneration of intestinal mucosa might reduce lactase levels to a point where a temporary deficiency could occur.

Fat absorption

The average adult eats about 60 gm to 100 gm of fat daily, principally as triglycerides containing long-chain fatty acids. These triglycerides are broken down by pancreatic lipase. Bile salts act as a carrier system for the fatty acids and fat-soluble vitamins A, D, E, and K by forming micelles, which transport these substances to the surface of intestinal villi where they are absorbed. The major site of fat absorption is the upper jejunum. Medium-chain triglycerides, with fatty acids of lengths C-6 to C-10, are absorbed better than longer chains of fatty acids because they are more completely hydrolyzed by pancreatic lipase and they form micelles more easily. Because they are easily absorbed, medium-chain tri-glycerides are often used in the treatment of persons with malabsorption syndrome. The absorption of vitamins A, D, E, and K, which are fat-soluble vitamins, requires bile salts.

Fat that is not absorbed in the intestine is excreted in the stool. *Steatorrhea* is the term used to describe fatty stools. It usually indicates that there are 6.0 gm or more fat in a 24-hour stool sample. Normally, a chemical test is done on a 72-hour stool collection during which time the diet is restricted to 80 gm to 100 gm of fat per day.

Protein adsorption

Proteins are broken down by pancreatic enzymes, such as trypsin, chymotrypsin, carboxypeptidase, and elastase. The amino acids are liberated either intramurally or on the surface of the villi by brush border enzymes that degrade proteins into one, two, and three amino acid particles. These amino acids are transported across the mucosal membrane in a sodium-linked process that utilizes ATP as an energy source.

Malabsorption

Malabsorption is the failure to transport dietary constituents, such as fats, carbohydrates, proteins, vitamins, and minerals, from the lumen of the intes-

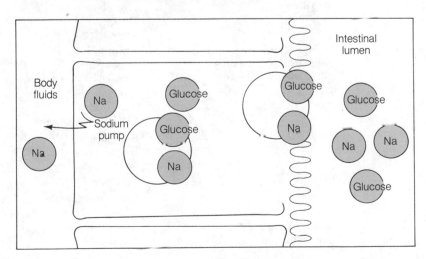

Figure 37–4.   Diagram of the hypothetical sodium-dependent transport system for glucose. The concentration of glucose builds up within the intestinal cell until a diffusion gradient develops, causing glucose to move into the body fluids. Sodium is transported out of the cell by the energy-dependent (ATP) sodium pump. This creates the gradient needed to operate the transport system.

tine to the body fluids. It can selectively affect a single constituent, such as vitamin B_{12} or lactose, or its effects can extend to all of the substances that are absorbed in a specific segment of the intestine. Malabsorption can occur because of a primary defect in the intestinal wall itself or because of impaired digestion such as occurs with deficiency of liver bile or pancreatic digestive enzymes. In selected cases, absorption of fats may be impaired due to obstruction of lymph flow from the intestine. Liver and pancreatic disorders are discussed in Chapter 38.

Malabsorption syndrome

Malabsorption refers to impaired absorptive function. The term *syndrome* indicates a constellation of symptoms arising from multiple causes. Thus, the *malabsorption syndrome* can be caused by celiac disease, tropical sprue, Crohn's disease, resection of large segments of the small bowel, or other conditions that decrease the surface area or function of the small intestine. *Celiac disease* is a condition in which there is an intolerance to dietary gluten and which results in the loss of villi from the small intestine. The effects of celiac disease are reversed by elimination of gluten from the diet. In tropical sprue, the changes that occur in the villi resemble those seen in celiac disease. The cause of this disorder is unclear, though administration of folic acid is known to be helpful in treatment.

The chief symptom of malabsorption syndrome is steatorrhea. The fat content causes bulky, yellow-gray, malodorous stools that float in the toilet and

Table 37–4   Site of Absorption and Requirements for Absorption of Dietary Constituents

Dietary Constituent	Site Absorption	Requirements	Manifestations
Water and electrolytes	Mainly small bowel	Osmotic gradient	Diarrhea Dehydration Cramps
Fat	Upper jejunum	Pancreatic lipase Bile salts Functioning lymphatic channels	Weight loss Steatorrhea Fat-soluble vitamin deficiency
Carbohydrates			
Starch	Small intestine	Amylase Maltase Isomaltase α-Dextrins	Diarrhea Flatulence Abdominal discomfort
Sucrose	Small intestine	Sucrase	
Lactose	Small intestine	Lactase	
Maltose	Small intestine	Maltase	
Fructose	Small intestine	—	
Protein	Small intestine	Pancreatic enzymes (trypsin, chymotrypsin, elastin, etc.)	Loss in muscle mass Weakness Edema
Vitamins			
A	Upper jejunum	Bile salts	Night blindness Dry eyes Corneal irritation
Folic acid	Duodenum and jejunum	Absorptive; may be impaired by some drugs (*i.e.*, anticonvulsants)	Cheilosis Glossitis Megaloblastic anemia
B-12	Ileum	Intrinsic factor	Glossitis Neuropathy Megaloblastic anemia
D	Upper jejunum	Bile salts	Bone pain Fractures Tetany
E	Upper jejunum	Bile salts	Uncertain
K	Upper jejunum	Bile salts	Easy bruising and bleeding
Calcium	Duodenum	Vitamin D and parathyroid hormone	Bone pain Fractures Tetany
Iron	Duodenum	Normal pH (hydrochloric secretion)	Iron deficiency anemia Glossitis

that make flushing of the toilet difficult. There is often weakness, weight loss, anorexia, and abdominal distention. Along with loss of fat in the stools, there is failure to absorb the fat-soluble vitamins. This can lead to easy bruising and bleeding (vitamin K deficiency), bone pain, predisposition to develop fractures and tetany (vitamin D and calcium deficiency), macroblastic anemia, and glossitis (folic acid deficiency). There may be neuropathy, atrophy of the skin, and peripheral edema. Table 37-4 describes the signs and symptoms of impaired absorption of dietary constituents.

In summary, the digestion and absorption of foodstuffs takes place in the small intestine. Here proteins, fats, carbohydrates, and other components of the diet are broken down into molecules that can be transported from the intestinal lumen into the body fluids. Malabsorption results when this transport system becomes impaired. It can involve a single dietary constituent or extend to involve all of the substances that are absorbed in a particular part of the small intestine. Malabsorption can result from disease of the small bowel, from disorders that impair digestion, or (in some cases) obstruct the lymph flow by which fats are transported to the general circulation.

:Alterations in Motility of the Gastrointestinal Tract

The movement of contents through the gastrointestinal tract is controlled by neurons that are located in the submucosal and myenteric plexuses of the gut. The axons from the cell bodies in the myenteric plexus innervate both the circular and longitudinal smooth muscle layers of the gut. These neurons receive impulses from local receptors that are located in the mucosal and muscle layers of the gut, and extrinsic input from the parasympathetic and sympathetic nervous systems. As a general rule, the parasympathetic nervous system tends to increase the motility of the bowel, whereas sympathetic stimulation tends to slow its activity.

The colon, which has sphincters at both ends—the ileocecal sphincter which separates it from the small intestine, and the anal sphincter which prevents movement of feces to the outside of the body—acts as a reservoir for fecal material. Normally, about 400 ml of water, 55 mEq of sodium, 30 mEq of chloride, and 15 mEq of bicarbonate are absorbed each day in the colon. At the same time, about 5 mEq of potassium are secreted into the lumen of the colon. The amount of water and electrolytes that remain in the stool reflect the absorption or secretion that oc-

curs in the colon. The average adult ingesting a "typical" American diet evacuates about 200 gm to 300 gm of stool each day.

Diarrhea

The usual definition of diarrhea is excessively frequent passage of unformed stools. The complaint of diarrhea is a general one and can be related to a number of factors, pathologic and otherwise. Diarrhea is usually divided into two types: large-volume and small-volume. Large-volume diarrhea results from an increase in the water content of the stool, and small-volume diarrhea from an increase in the propulsive activity of the bowel. Some of the common causes of small- and large-volume diarrhea are summarized in Table 37-5. *Often diarrhea is a combination of these two types.*

Large-volume diarrhea
Large-volume diarrhea can be classified as either secretory or osmotic, according to the cause of the increased water content in the feces. Water is either pulled into the colon along an osmotic gradient or is secreted into the bowel by the mucosal cells. This form of diarrhea is usually a painless, watery type of diarrhea without blood or pus in the stools.

In *osmotic diarrhea*, water is pulled into the bowel by the hyperosmotic nature of its contents. It occurs when there is failure to absorb osmotically active particles. In lactase deficiency, the lactose that is present in milk cannot be broken down and absorbed. Magnesium salts, which are contained in

Table 37-5　Causes of Large- and Small-Volume Diarrhea

Large-Volume Diarrhea

Osmotic Diarrhea
　Saline cathartics
　Dumping syndrome
　Lactose deficiency

Secretory Diarrhea
　Failure to absorb bile salts
　Fat malabsorption
　Chronic laxative abuse
　Carcinoid syndrome
　Zollinger–Ellison syndrome
　Fecal impaction
　Acute infectious diarrhea

Small-Volume Diarrhea

Inflammatory bowel disease
　Crohn's disease
　Ulcerative colitis

Infectious disease
　Shigellosis
　Salmonellosis

Irritable colon

milk of magnesia and many antacids, are poorly absorbed, and cause diarrhea when taken in sufficient quantities. Another cause of osmotic diarrhea is decreased transit time which interferes with absorption. This happens in the dumping syndrome, which was discussed earlier in relation to the surgical treatment of peptic ulcer. Osmotic diarrhea disappears with fasting.

Secretory diarrhea occurs when the secretory processes of the bowel are increased. Most acute infectious diarrheas are of this type. This type of diarrhea also occurs when excess bile salts or fatty acids are present in the gut contents as they enter the colon. This often happens with disease processes of the ileum, since bile salts are absorbed here. It may also occur when there is bacterial overgrowth in the small bowel, which also interferes with bile absorption. Some tumors, such as Zollinger–Ellison syndrome and carcinoid syndrome, cause increased secretory activity of the bowel.

Fecal impaction (the retention of hard, dried stool in the rectum and colon) stimulates increased secretory activity of the portion of the bowel that is proximal to the impaction. In this case the watery stool flows around the fecal mass and represents the body's attempt to break up the mass so that it can be evacuated. This cause should be considered in any elderly or immobilized person who develops watery diarrhea. Digital examination of the rectum is done to assess the fecal mass. In some cases, the mass may need to be removed manually with a gloved finger.

Small-volume diarrhea

Small-volume diarrhea is usually evidenced by frequency and urgency, and colicky-abdominal pains. This form of diarrhea is commonly associated with intrinsic disease of the colon, such as ulcerative colitis or Crohn's disease. It is usually accompanied by tenesmus (painful straining at stool), fecal soiling of clothing, and awakening during the night with the urge to defecate.

Treatment

Diarrhea causes loss of fluid and electrolytes from the body. This can be particularly serious in infants and small children, in persons with other illness, in the elderly, and even in previously healthy persons if it continues for any length of time. Fluid and electrolyte corrections are, therefore, considered to be a primary therapeutic goal in the treatment of diarrhea. Some oral electrolyte replacement solutions, such as Gatorade (which contains 21 mEq sodium, 17 mEq chloride, 2.5 mEq potassium, and 6.8 mEq phosphate in a 5% glucose solution), can be given as a replacement solution in situations of uncomplicated diarrhea that can be treated at home. Restricting oral foods and fluids may be helpful in acute diarrhea, since this decreases peristalsis. When intake is resumed following diarrhea, the diet should consist of bland foods that will not stimulate gastrointestinal motility. Cold liquids that move rapidly from the stomach to the small intestine and stimulate peristalsis should be avoided.

Drugs used in the treatment of diarrhea include camphorated tincture of opium (paregoric), diphenoxylate (Lomotil), and loperamide (Imodium) which are opium-like drugs. Adsorbents, such as kaolin and pectin, are able to adsorb undesirable constituents from solutions. These ingredients are included in many over-the-counter antidiarrheal preparations because they adsorb toxins responsible for certain types of diarrhea.

Constipation

Constipation can be defined as the infrequent passage of stools. The difficulty in defining the term constipation arises from the many individual variations of a function that is normal. In other words, what might be considered normal for one person (2 or 3 bowel movements per week) might well be considered evidence of constipation by another.

Some common causes of constipation are failure to respond to the urge to defecate, inadequate fiber in the diet, inadequate fluid intake, weakness of the abdominal muscles, inactivity, and bedrest, pregnancy, hemorrhoids, and gastrointestinal disease. Drugs such as narcotics, belladonna derivatives, diuretics, calcium, iron, and aluminum hydroxide, and phosphate gels tend to cause constipation. The sudden onset of constipation may indicate serious disease (*e.g.,* one sign of cancer of the colon and rectum is a change in bowel habits).

Treatment of constipation is usually directed toward relieving the cause. A conscious effort should be made to respond to the defecation urge. A time should be set aside after a meal, when mass movements in the colon are most apt to occur, for a bowel movement. An adequate fluid intake and bulk in the diet should be encouraged. Moderate exercise is essential, and persons on bedrest benefit from passive and active exercises. Laxatives and enemas should be used judiciously. They should not be used on a regular basis to treat simple constipation, as they interfere with the defecation reflex and may actually damage the rectal mucosa.

Intestinal Obstruction

Intestinal obstruction designates an impairment of movement of intestinal contents in a cephalocaudal direction. The causes of intestinal obstruction can be categorized under two headings: *mechanical* and *reflex paralytic (adynamic)*.

Mechanical obstruction can result from a number of conditions, either intrinsic or extrinsic, which encroach on the patency of the bowel lumen. These conditions include adhesions of the peritoneum, hernias, twisting of the bowel (volvulus), telescoping of the bowel (intussusception), fecal impaction, strictures, and tumors. There are three types of mechanical obstruction: simple, strangulated, and closed. With a *simple* obstruction, there is no alteration in blood supply. The term *strangulated* implies that there has been impairment of blood flow. When the bowel is obstructed on both ends, it is called a *closed* obstruction.

Reflex paralysis usually affects the small bowel. Because the ileum has the narrowest lumen, it is the most prone to obstruction. *Paralytic ileus* is seen most commonly following abdominal surgery or trauma. It occurs early in the course of peritonitis and can result from chemical irritation due to bile, bacterial toxins, electrolyte imbalances as in hypokalemia, and vascular insufficiency.

The major effects of both types of intestinal obstruction are *intestinal distention* and *loss of fluids and electrolytes*. Gases and fluids accumulate within the area. About 7 liters to 8 liters of electrolyte-rich extracellular fluid moves into the small bowel each day and normally most of this is reabsorbed. Intestinal obstruction interferes with this reabsorption process and a small amount of this extracellular fluid remains in the bowel or is lost in the vomitus. A loss of 7 liters to 8 liters, which represents about half of the extracellular fluid volume of an average adult, can occur in 24 hours or less following acute intestinal obstruction.

If untreated, the distention due to bowel obstruction tends to perpetuate itself by causing atony of the bowel, and further distention. Distention is further aggravated by the accumulation of gases. About 70% of these gases are estimated to be due to swallowed air. As the process continues the distention moves proximally involving additional segments of bowel.

Either form of obstruction may eventually lead to strangulation, gangrenous changes, and ultimately perforation of the bowel. The increased pressure within the intestine tends to compromise mucosal blood flow, leading to necrosis and exudation of blood into the luminal fluids. This promotes rapid growth of bacteria within the obstructed bowel. Anaerobes grow rapidly in this favorable environment and produce a lethal endotoxin.

The manifestations of intestinal obstruction depend on the degree of obstruction and its duration. With acute obstruction, the onset is usually sudden and dramatic. With chronic conditions, the onset is often more gradual. The cardinal symptoms of intestinal obstruction are pain, absolute constipation, abdominal distention, and vomiting. These symptoms are common to intestinal obstruction due to either mechanical obstruction or paralytic ileus. Electrolyte imbalances are also common to both.

With *mechanical obstruction*, there is development of hyperperistalsis as the body attempts to move the contents of the intestine around the occluded area. This causes severe *colicky pain*, in contrast to the *continuous pain* and *silent abdomen* that are seen with paralytic ileus. With mechanical obstruction, there is also borborygmus (rumbling sounds made by propulsion of gas in the intestine), audible high-pitched peristalsis, and peristaltic rushes. Visible peristalsis may appear along the course of the distended intestine. There is extreme restlessness and conscious awareness of intestinal movements. Weakness, perspiration, and anxiety are obvious. As the condition progresses, the vomitus may become fecal in nature and the peristaltic movements may decrease, then disappear as the bowel fatigues.

Should *strangulation* occur, the symptoms change. The character of the pain shifts from the intermittent colicky pain caused by the hyperperistaltic movements of the intestine to a severe, unrelenting pain that is made worse by movement. Signs of *peritoneal irritation*, such as rigidity of the abdomen, become apparent. If bowel sounds had been present, they disappear because of the peritoneal irritation. Strangulation increases the risk of mortality by about 25%.

Diagnosis of intestinal obstruction is usually based on history and physical findings. Abdominal x-ray studies will reveal a gas-filled bowel

Treatment consists of decompression of the bowel through nasogastric suction and correction of fluid and electrolyte imbalances. Strangulation and complete bowel obstruction require surgical intervention.

In summary, motility of the contents through the gastrointestinal tract relies on the activity of the myenteric plexus, which is located between the circular and longi-

tudinal smooth muscle layers. Alterations in gastro-
intestinal motility can be evidenced by diarrhea, by
constipation, or in acute situations by intestinal
obstruction.

:Study Guide

After you have studied this chapter, you should be able to meet the following objectives:

:: Describe four manifestations of gastrointestinal disorders.

:: Explain the significance of melena.

:: Describe the symptoms of hiatal hernia which the health professional should be able to recognize.

:: Explain why chronic gastritis is a more serious disorder than acute gastritis.

:: Distinguish between gastric ulcer and peptic ulcer.

:: State the factors that may influence hydrochloric acid production.

:: Explain the conditions under which Cushing's ulcer and Curling's ulcer might occur.

:: Describe the overall goals in treatment of peptic ulcer.

:: Describe the symptoms and treatment of the dumping syndrome.

:: Describe the underlying pathology found in Crohn's disease.

:: Summarize the pathology involved in ulcerative colitis.

:: Characterize toxic magacolon.

:: Explain why diverticular disease may be linked to environmental factors.

:: Explain what is meant by the phrase *left-sided appendicitis*.

:: Describe the symptoms of acute appendicitis.

:: State the significant symptoms of colorectal cancer.

:: Describe the Hemoccult test for occult blood.

:: List five causes of peritonitis.

:: Describe the chief symptoms of peritonitis.

:: Explain how the villi are adapted to their function.

:: Trace absorption of carbohydrates from the small intestine.

:: Describe the possible result of a lactase deficiency.

:: State the function of micelles in fat absorption.

:: Describe the symptoms that may be associated with the presence of the malabsorption syndrome.

:: Compare osmotic diarrhea, secretory diarrhea, and small-volume diarrhea.

:: Explain why a failure to respond to the defecation urge may result in constipation.

:: Explain why intestinal obstruction may ultimately result in strangulation.

:References

1. Report of the Congress of the United States. National Commission on Digestive Disease, Vol 1. Findings and Long-range Plans. National Institute of Health, Public Health Service, 1979. DHEW Publication No. (NIH) 79–1878
2. McBryde CM: Signs and Symptoms, p 400. Philadelphia, JB Lippincott, 1970
3. Schiff L, Stevens RJ, Shapiro N, Goodman S: Observation of oral administration of citrated blood in man. Am J Med Sci 203:409, 1942
4. Morton JH: Alimentary tract cancer. In Rubin P (ed): Clinical Oncology, ed 5, pp 85, 93. New York, American Cancer Society, 1978
5. Facts About Stomach and Esophageal Cancer, p 13. New York, American Cancer Society, 1978
6. Robbins SL, Cotran RS: Pathologic Basis of Disease, pp 133, 935, 986, 998. Philadelphia, WB Saunders, 1979
7. Isenberg JI: Peptic ulcer medical treatment. In Beeson PB, McDermott W, Wyngaarden JB (eds): Cecil Textbook of Medicine, ed 15, p 1513. Philadelphia, WB Saunders, 1979
8. Scade RR, Donaldson RM Jr: How physicians use cimetidine. N Engl J Med 304(21):1283, 1981
9. Freely J, Wilkinson GR, Wood JJA: Reduction in liver blood flow and propranolol metabolism by cimetidine. N Engl J Med 304(12):692–695, 1981
10. Report of the Congress of the United States. National Commission on Digestive Diseases, Vol 4 Epidemiology and Impact. National Institute of Health, Public Health Service, 1979. DHEW Publication No. (NIH) 79–1887
11. Janowitz HD: Chronic inflammatory disease of the intestine. In Beeson PB, McDermott W, Wyngarden JB (eds): Cecil Textbook of Medicine, ed 15, p 1570. Philadelphia, WB Saunders, 1979
12. Griffen WO: Management of diverticular disease of the colon. Hospital Medicine 14(11):108, 1978
13. Miller SF: Colorectal cancer: Are the goals of early detection achieved? CA 27(6):338–343, 1977

14. Overholt BF: Colonoscopy. New York, American Cancer Society, 1975
15. Castro GA: Digestion and absorption of specific nutrients. In Johnson LR (ed): Gastrointestinal Physiology, p 122. St. Louis, CV Mosby, 1977
16. Kosek MS: Medical genetics. In Krupp MA, Chatton MJ (eds): Current Medical Diagnosis and Treatment, p 1009. Los Altos, Lange Medical Publications, 1980

:Suggested Readings

Alpers D, Avioli LV: Inflammatory bowel disease (ulcerative colitis). Arch Intern Med 138:286, 1978

Bauer CL: Managing upper G.I. bleeding. Consultant 20:35, 1980

Bayless TM: Malabsorption in the elderly. Hosp Pract 14, No. 8:57–63, 1979

Belinsky I: Fiberoptic advances: Visualizing the pancreatic and biliary ducts. Am J Nurs 76, No. 6:936, 1976

Brady PG: Small intestinal syndromes: A guide to diagnosis. Hospital Medicine 15, No. 5:41, 1979

Borthistle BK: Managing lower G.I. bleeding in the elderly patient. Consultant 20, No. 10:230, 1980

Code CF: Prostaglandins and gastric ulcer. Hosp Pract 15, No. 7:62, 1970

Cohen S: Pathogenesis of coffee-induced gastrointestinal symptoms. N Engl J Med 303, No. 3:122, 1980

Fazio VW: Early diagnosis of anorectal and colon carcinoma. Hospital Medicine 15, No. 1:66–85, 1979

Fromm D: Stress ulcer. Hospital Medicine 14, No. 11:58, 1978

Goldstein F: Inflammatory bowel disease—better prospects. Consultant 20, No. 12:68, 1980

Greenburg JL: Constipation—"congestive bowel failure." Consultant 20, No. 11:94, 1980

Griggs BA, Hoppe MC: Nasogastric tube feeding. Am J Nurs 79:481, 1979

Gryboski JD, Spiro HM: Alimentary tract. Prognosis in children with Crohn's disease. Gastroenterology 74, No. 5:807, 1978

Korelitz BI: Ulcerative colitis. Hospital Medicine 14, No. 3:8, 1978

Kraft SC: Spotting early clues to Crohn's disease. Consultant 19, No. 3:165, 1979

Lanza FL, Royer GL, Nelson RS: Endoscopic evaluation of the effects of aspirin, buffered aspirin and enteric-coated aspirin on gastric and duodenal mucosa. N Engl J Med 303, No. 3:136, 1980

Law DH: Current concepts in nutrition. Total parenteral nutrition. N Engl J Med 297, No. 20:1104, 1977

Levitt MD: Intestinal gas production—recent advances in flatology. N Engl J Med 302, No. 26:1474, 1980

Lindner AE: Comparing ulcerative colitis and Crohn's disease. Consultant 18, No. 6:93, 1978

McCarthy DM: Peptic ulcer: Antacids or cimetidine? Hosp Pract 14, No. 12:52, 1979

Mendeloff AI: Dietary fiber and gastrointestinal diseases. Med Clin North Am 62, No. 1:165, 1978

Menguy R: Gastric mucosal injury from common drugs. Postgrad Med 63, No. 4:82, 1978

Moertel CG: Gastrointestinal cancer. Treatment with fluorouracil–nitrosourea combinations. JAMA 235, No. 19:2135, 1976

Mungas JE, Moossa AR, Block GE: Treatment of toxic megacolon. Surg Clin North Am 56, No. 1:95, 1976

Myers RT: Esophageal bleeding. Hospital Medicine 14, No. 2:80, 1978

Nagamachi Y, Nakamura T: Role of gastric mucosal pepsin in the pathogenesis of acute stress ulceration. World J Surg 3:215, 1979

Ross JR, Moore VA: Axioms on malabsorption. Hospital Medicine 11, No. 2:98, 1975

Roth JLA: Complications of colonic diverticulitis. Postgrad Med 60, No. 6:115, 1975

Rubin M, Battle WM, Snape WJ, Cohen S: The esophagus and dysphagia. Hospital Medicine 15, No. 2:6, 1979

Sachar DB: Differentiating types of diarrhea. Consultant 20, No. 3:29, 1980

Samborsky V: Drug therapy for peptic ulcer. Am J Nurs 78:2064, 1978

Shils ME: Guidelines for total parenteral nutrition. JAMA 220, No. 13:1721, 1972

Silverstein FE: Peptic ulcer: An overview of diagnosis. Hosp Pract 14, No. 2:78, 1979

Strickland RG: Acute and chronic gastritis. Hospital Medicine 15, No. 9:26, 1977

38

Alterations in Function of the Liver, the Gall Bladder, and the Exocrine Pancreas

The liver, the gall bladder, and the exocrine pancreas are classified as accessory organs of the gastrointestinal tract. In addition to producing digestive secretions, both the liver and the pancreas have other important functions. The exocrine pancreas, for example, supplies the insulin and glucagon needed in cell metabolism, while the liver synthesizes glucose, plasma proteins, and blood-clotting factors and is responsible for the degradation and elimination of drugs and hormones, among other functions. This chapter discusses disorders of the liver, the biliary tract and gall bladder, and the exocrine pancreas.

:The Liver

The liver is the largest organ in the body, weighing about 1.3 kg, or 3 lb, in the adult. It is located below the diaphragm and occupies much of the right hy-

Figure 38–1.   Superior posterior view (*top*) and inferior view (*bottom*) of the liver. (Chaffee EE, Lytle IM: Basic Physiology and Anatomy, 4th ed. Philadelphia, JB Lippincott, 1980)

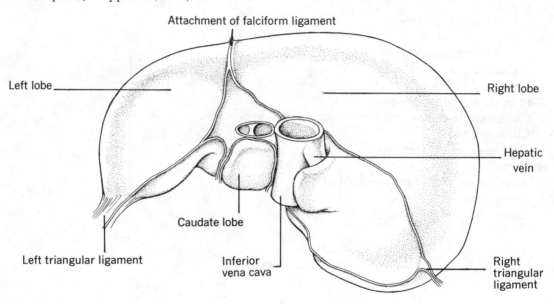

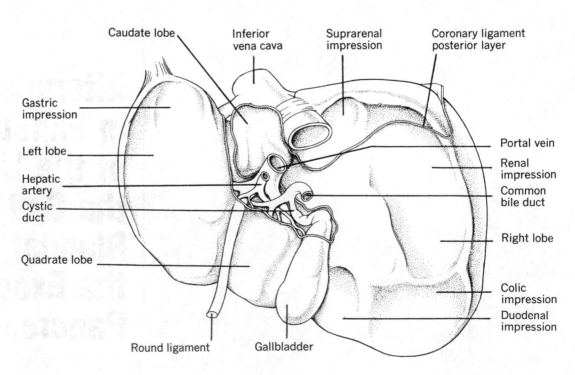

pochondrium. The falciform ligament, which extends from the peritoneal surface of the anterior abdominal wall between the umbilicus and diaphragm, divides the liver into two lobes, a large right lobe and a small left lobe (Fig. 38-1). There are two additional lobes on the visceral surface of the liver, the caudate and quadrate lobes. Except for that portion which is in the epigastric area, the liver is contained within the rib cage and in healthy persons cannot normally be palpated. The liver is surrounded by a tough fibroelastic capsule called Glisson's capsule.

The liver is unique among the abdominal organs in having a dual blood supply—the hepatic artery and the portal vein. About 400 ml of blood enters the liver through the hepatic artery and another 1000 ml enters by way of the valveless portal vein, which carries blood from the stomach, the small and large intestine, the pancreas, and the spleen (Fig. 38-2). Although the blood from the portal vein is incompletely saturated with oxygen, it supplies about 50% to 60% of the oxygen needs of the liver.[1] The venous outflow from the liver is carried by the valveless hepatic veins, which empty into the inferior vena cava just below the level of the diaphragm. The pressure difference between the he-

Figure 38–2.   The portal circulation. Blood from the gastrointestinal tract, spleen, and pancreas travels to the liver by way of the portal vein before moving into the vena cava for return to the heart. (Chaffee EE, Lytle IM: Basic Physiology and Anatomy, 4th ed. Philadelphia, JB Lippincott, 1980)

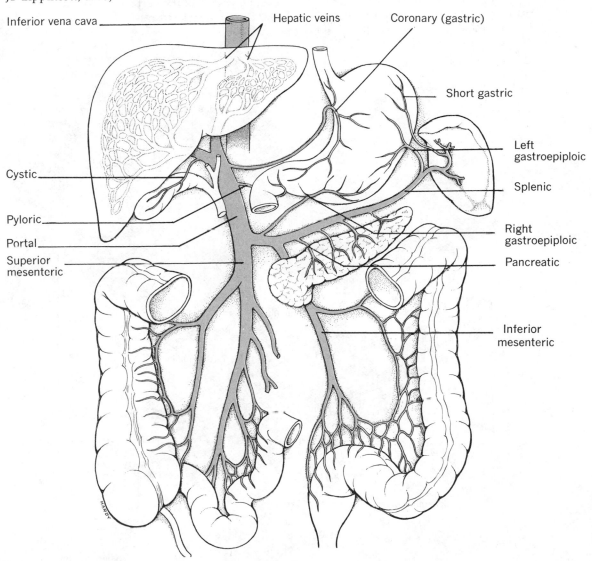

Inferior vena cava

Hepatic veins

Coronary (gastric)

Short gastric

Left gastroepiploic

Splenic

Cystic

Pyloric

Portal

Superior mesenteric

Right gastroepiploic

Pancreatic

Inferior mesenteric

patic vein and the portal vein is normally such that the liver stores about 200 ml to 400 ml of blood. This blood can be shifted back into the general circulation during periods of hypotension and shock. In congestive heart failure, in which there is an increase in the pressure within the vena cava, blood backs up and accumulates in the liver.

The lobules are the functional units of the liver. Each lobule is a cyclindrical structure that measures about 0.8 mm to 2 mm in diameter and is several millimeters in length. There are about 50,000 to 100,000 lobules in each of the two lobes. Each lobule is composed of cellular plates of hepatic cells arranged in spoke-like fashion and encircling a central vein (Fig. 38-3). The central vein opens into the hepatic vein and then into the vena cava. The hepatic

plates are usually two cells thick and are separated by *canaliculi*, which empty into the bile ducts. As bile is produced by the hepatic cells, it flows first into the canaliculi, then into the terminal bile ducts, and eventually into the one large bile duct that drains each lobe. Also, in the septa that separate the lobules are the *smaller portal venules*, which receive blood from the portal veins. The venules empty into the flat sinusoids that lie between the hepatic plates. Branches from the *hepatic artery*, which supplies the septal tissues, are also found in the intralobular septa, and blood from these arterioles empties into the sinusoids.

The venous sinusoids are lined with two types of cells: the typical endothelial cells and the Kupffer cells. The Kupffer cells are reticuloendothelial cells

Figure 38–3.   A section of liver lobule showing the location of the hepatic veins, hepatic cells, liver sinusoids, and branches of the portal vein and hepatic artery. (Chaffee EE, Lytle IM: Basic Physiology and Anatomy, 4th ed. Philadelphia, JB Lippincott, 1980)

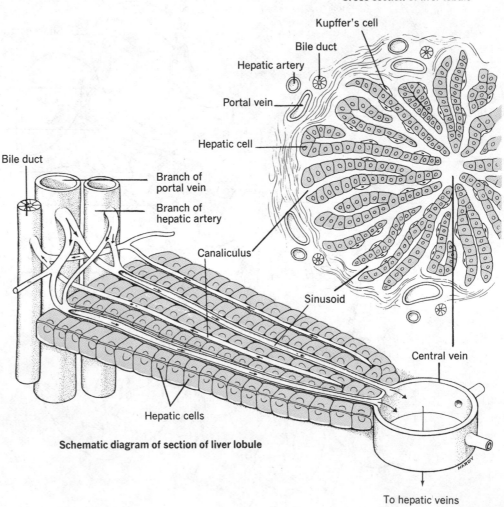

Cross section of liver lobule

Kupffer's cell

Bile duct

Hepatic artery

Portal vein

Hepatic cell

Bile duct

Branch of portal vein

Branch of hepatic artery

Canaliculus

Sinusoid

Central vein

Hepatic cells

Schematic diagram of section of liver lobule

To hepatic veins

which are capable of removing and phagocytizing old and defective blood cells, bacteria, and other foreign material from the portal blood as it flows through the sinusoid. This phagocytic action removes the colon bacilli and other harmful substances that filter into the blood from the intestine.

Functions of the Liver

The liver is one of the most versatile and active organs in the body. It produces bile; metabolizes hormones and drugs; synthesizes proteins, glucose, and clotting factors; stores vitamins and minerals; and converts fatty acids to ketones—and has other functions as well. In this process, the liver degrades excess nutrients and converts them into substances essential to the body. It builds carbohydrates from proteins, converts sugars to fats that can be stored, and interchanges protein molecules so that they can be used for a number of purposes. In its capacity for metabolizing drugs and hormones, the liver serves as an excretory organ. In this respect, the bile, which carries the end products of substances metabolized by the liver, is much like the urine, which carries the body wastes that are filtered by the kidneys. The functions of the liver are summarized in Table 38-1. The liver's role in carbohydrate, fat, and protein metabolism is discussed in Chapter 34. The discussion in this chapter focuses on the function of the liver in alcohol metabolism, production of bile, and removal of bilirubin.

Alcohol metabolism

More than 90% of alcohol that a person drinks is metabolized by the liver. The rest is excreted through the lungs, kidneys, and skin. As a substance, alcohol fits somewhere between a food and a drug. It supplies calories, but cannot be broken down or stored as protein, fat, or carbohydrate. As a food, alcohol yields 7.1 kilocalories per gram as compared with the 4.0 kilocalories produced by metabolism of an equal amount of carbohydrate. As a drug, it excites, hypnotizes, and then anesthetizes. (It is not a good anesthetic, however, because the euphoric stage lasts too long and the margin between the amount required for surgical anesthesia and that which will depress respiration is very narrow.[2])

Alcohol is readily absorbed from the gastrointestinal tract, being one of the few substances that can be absorbed from the stomach. The overall metabolism of alcohol requires six oxidative steps and uses three molecules of oxygen to produce two molecules of carbon dioxide. In the process, it translocates 12 hydrogen ions and utilizes vital cofactors, particularly nicotinamide-adenine dinucleotide

Table 38-1 Functions of the Liver and Manifestations of Altered Function

Function	Manifestations of Altered Function
Production of bile salts	Malabsorption of fat and fat-soluble vitamins
Elimination of bilirubin	Failure to eliminate bilirubin causes elevation in serum bilirubin and jaundice
Metabolism of steroid hormones	
Estrogens and progesterone	Altered liver function may cause disturbances in gonadal function
Testosterone	
Glucocorticoids	Altered excretion of glucocorticoids may cause Cushing's syndrome
Aldosterone	Sodium retention and edema; hypokalemia
Metabolism of drugs	Alterations in liver function may alter plasma binding of drugs owing to a decrease in albumin production
	Decreased removal of drugs that are metabolized by the liver
Carbohydrate metabolism	Hypoglycemia may develop when glycogenolysis and gluconeogenesis are impaired
Stores glycogen	
Synthesizes glucose from	
Amino acids	There may be abnormal glucose tolerance curve due to impaired uptake and release of glucose by the liver
Lactic acid	
Glycerol	
Fat metabolism	
Formation of lipoproteins	Impaired synthesis of lipoproteins
Conversion of carbohydrates and proteins to fat	
Synthesis of cholesterol	
Formation of ketones from fatty acids	
Protein metabolism	
Deamination of proteins	
Formation of urea from ammonia	Elevated blood ammonia levels
Synthesis of plasma proteins	Decreased levels of plasma proteins, particularly albumin, which contributes to edema formation
Synthesis of clotting factors	Bleeding tendency
Fibrinogen	
Prothrombin	
Factors V, VII, IX, X	
Storage of minerals and vitamins	Signs of deficiency of fat-soluble and other vitamins that are stored in the liver

(NAD), that are needed for other metabolic processes, such as gluconeogenesis. At blood levels commonly obtained by drinking, the generation of hydrogen ions by the liver often exceeds hydrogen ion disposition.[3]

The rate of alcohol metabolism is about the same for all persons, except the practicing alcoholic. The rate-limiting step in the process is the availability of the enzyme alcohol dehydrogenase, which is located in the cytosol of the liver cells (Fig. 38-4). The average person can metabolize about 18 gm of alcohol per hour (it takes about 2 hours to metabolize one mixed drink). With prolonged and excessive ingestion of alcohol, the liver seems to develop a supplemental system for metabolizing alcohol, and is able to almost double the rate at which it is metabolized. With

Figure 38–4.   The process of alcohol metabolism.

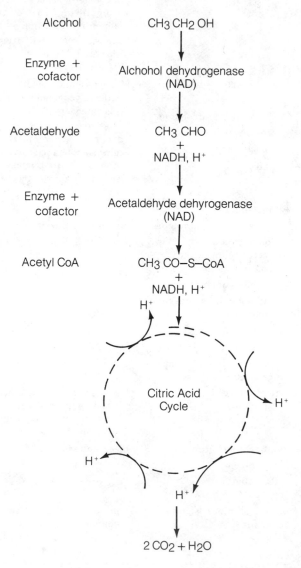

cessation of drinking, the rate of alcohol metabolism rapidly returns to normal.

One of the main effects of alcohol is the accumulation of fat within the liver. When alcohol is present, it becomes the preferred fuel for the liver, displacing substrates such as fatty acids, which are normally used for this purpose. Triglycerides accumulate in the liver, probably as a result of increased production and because of increased trapping of fatty acids within the liver cells.

Since alcohol competes for utilization of cofactors normally needed by the liver for other metabolic processes, it tends to disrupt the other functions of the liver. An altered redox state (reduction and oxidation, with accumulation of hydrogen ions) and the preferential utilization of NAD for alcohol metabolism can result in increased production and accumulation of lactic acid in the blood. The increased lactate levels tend to impair uric-acid excretion by the kidney, which probably explains why excessive alcohol consumption frequently aggravates or precipitates gout. By decreasing the availability of the cofactor NAD, alcohol impairs the liver's ability to form glucose from amino acids and other glucose precursors. Thus, alcohol-induced hypoglycemia and alcoholic ketoacidosis can develop when excess alcohol ingestion occurs during periods of depleted liver glycogen stores. This may become a particular problem for the alcoholic who has been vomiting and has not eaten for several days. Alcohol also increases the body's requirements for the B vitamins and increases urinary losses of magnesium, potassium, and zinc.

There has been considerable controversy over the interaction of diet as it relates to liver changes observed with chronic alcoholism. In fact, one of the arguments that heavy drinkers often use to justify their habit is that with proper attention to diet, they can avoid the undesirable effects that alcohol produces on the liver. In the past, it has been difficult to study and document the influence of nutrition on liver changes that arise with chronic alcohol abuse. However, very recent animal research has demonstrated that full-blown cirrhosis of the liver can develop even when the diet is adequate.[4] This suggests that the alcohol itself plays an important role in liver injury. Studies using alcohol-fed baboons had led to the discovery of alcohol-related changes in one of the enzymes of protein metabolism, gamma-glutamyl transpeptidase transferase (Table 38-2). Serum levels of this enzyme became elevated with prolonged heavy drinking, and this enzyme test has been used in rehabilitative and industrial settings to indicate active alcoholism.[4]

Production of bile

The liver produces about 600 ml to 800 ml of yellow–green bile daily. Bile contains water, bile salts, bilirubin, cholesterol, and various inorganic acids. Of these, only bile salts are important in digestion.

Bile salts. The liver forms about 0.5 gm of bile salts daily. Bile salts are formed from cholesterol, which is either supplied by the diet or is synthesized by the liver. Bile salts serve an important function in digestion: they aid in *emulsifying dietary fats* and they are necessary for *formation of the micelles* that transport fatty acids and fat-soluble vitamins to the surface of the intestinal mucosa for absorption. About 94% of bile salts that enter the intestine are reabsorbed into the portal circulation by an active transport process that takes place in the distal ileum. From here, the bile salts pass into the liver where they are recycled. Normally, bile salts travel this entire circuit about 18 times before being expelled in the feces.[5] This system for recirculation of bile is called the *enterohepatic circulation*.

Removal of bile

Bilirubin. Bilirubin is the substance that gives bile its color. It is formed from senescent red blood cells. In the process of degradation, the hemoglobin from the red blood cell is broken down to form biliverdin, which is rapidly converted to *free bilirubin* (Fig. 38-5). The free bilirubin, which is insoluble in plasma, is transported in the blood attached to plasma albumin. As blood passes through the liver,

Figure 38–5.   The process of bilirubin formation, circulation, and elimination.

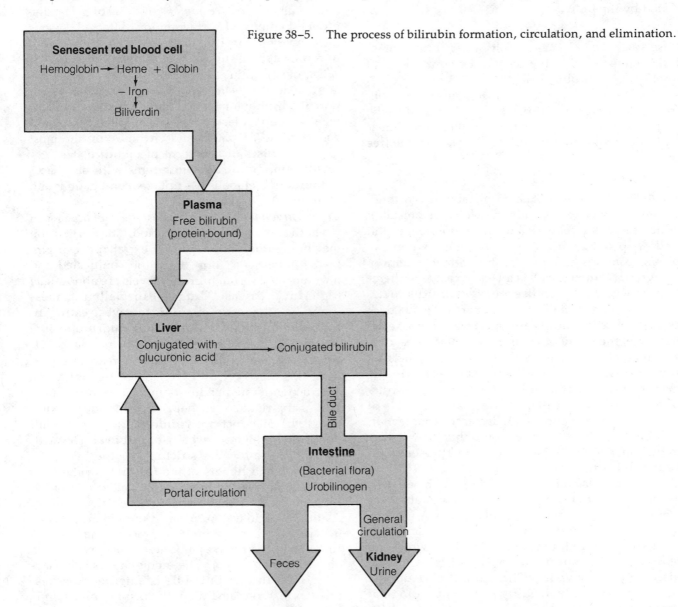

the free bilirubin is absorbed by the hepatocytes and is released from the albumin-carrier molecule. Once inside the hepatocyte, the bilirubin is conjugated with either glucuronic acid or glucuronic sulfate, a process that enables the bilirubin to become soluble in bile. The conjugated bilirubin is then secreted into the canaliculi of the liver as a constituent of bile, and in this form it passes through the bile ducts into the small intestine. The bacterial flora in the intestine converts bilirubin to urobilinogen, which is highly soluble. Urobilinogen is either reabsorbed into the portal circulation or is excreted in the feces. Most of the urobilinogen that is reabsorbed is returned to the liver to be re-excreted into the bile. A small amount of urobilinogen, about 5%, is reabsorbed into the general circulation and is then excreted by the kidneys.

Plasma bilirubin. Usually, only a small amount of bilirubin is found in the serum, the normal level of total serum bilirubin being 0.3 to 1.3 mg per dl. A simple test, the *van den Bergh test*, measures both free and conjugated bilirubin that is present in the total bilirubin. The *direct* van den Bergh test measures the conjugated bilirubin; the *indirect*, the free bilirubin.

Jaundice. Jaundice is due to an abnormally high accumulation of bilirubin in the blood, as a result of which there is a yellowish discoloration to the skin and deep tissues. Jaundice develops when the plasma contains about twice the normal amount of bilirubin. Normal skin has a yellow cast, and therefore early signs of jaundice are often difficult to detect. This is especially true in persons with dark skin. Because bilirubin has a special affinity for elastic tissue, the sclera of the eye, which contains considerable elastic fibers, is usually one of the first structures wherein jaundice can be detected. The four chief causes of jaundice are (1) excess destruction of red blood cells, (2) decreased uptake of bilirubin by the liver cells, (3) decreased conjugation of bilirubin, and (4) obstruction of bile flow, either in the canaliculi of the liver or in the intra- or extrahepatic bile ducts.

Hemolytic jaundice occurs when red blood cells are destroyed at a rate in excess of the liver's ability to remove the bilirubin from the blood. It may follow a hemolytic blood transfusion reaction, occur in diseases such as hereditary spherocytosis, in which the red cell membranes are defective, or in hemolytic disease of the newborn (Chap. 20). *Kernicterus* is a condition characterized by severe neurological symptoms which are due to high blood levels of

unconjugated bilirubin; because the unconjugated bilirubin is lipid-soluble, it is able to enter nerve cells and cause brain damage. A physiological jaundice may be seen in infants during the first week of extrauterine life, and is related to the immaturity of the infant's liver and its inability to remove and conjugate sufficient amounts of bilirubin. In recent years it has become evident that sunlight breaks down bilirubin into products that can be excreted in stool and urine; this knowledge formed the basis of *phototherapy* for these juandiced newborns. Phototherapy can be used to treat babies with physiological jaundice or hemolytic jaundice caused by the Rh factor. This simple and easily accomplished treatment is successful in many cases.

Gilbert's disease is inherited as a dominant trait and results in a *reduced uptake* of bilirubin. The disorder is benign and fairly common. Affected persons have no symptoms other than a slightly elevated unconjugated bilirubin, and hence jaundice. *Conjugation* of bilirubin is impaired whenever liver cells are damaged (*hepatocellular jaundice*), when transport of bilirubin into liver cells becomes deficient, or when there is a lack of enzymes needed to conjugate the bile. Hepatitis and cirrhosis are the most frequent causes of this form of jaundice. Hepatocellular jaundice usually interferes with all phases of bilirubin metabolism—uptake, conjugation, and excretion.

Obstructive jaundice or *cholestatic jaundice* is seen when the flow of bile is obstructed. The obstruction may be of either intrahepatic or extrahepatic origin. In the *intrahepatic* form, both the conjugated and unconjugated serum bilirubin levels are abnormally high. Liver disease, drugs—especially the anesthetic halothane—oral contraceptives, estrogen, anabolic steroids, isoniazid, and chlorpromazine are all possible causative factors. *Extrahepatic cholestatic jaundice* is due to obstruction to bile flow between the liver and the intestine, with the obstruction located at any point between the junction of the right or left hepatic duct and the point where the bile duct opens into the intestine. With this form, conjugated levels of bilirubin are elevated. Among the causes are strictures of the bile duct, gallstones, and tumors of the bile duct or the pancreas. Blood levels of bile acids are elevated in both intrahepatic and extrahepatic cholestatic jaundice. As the bile acids accumulate in the blood, pruritus develops. A history of pruritus preceding jaundice is common in obstructive jaundice of *either intrahepatic* or *extrahepatic* origin. The stools are usually clay-colored because so little bile is entering the intestine, and, at the same time, the urinary bilirubin is increased. Also common to both intra- and extra-

Table 38–2   Tests of Liver Function

Type of Test	Tests	Significance
Enzyme	Serum glutamic-oxaloacetic transaminase (SGOT)	Released into the serum when there is liver damage Elevated in hepatitis, cirrhosis, liver necrosis May also be elevated in myocardial infarction, skeletal muscle disease, and hematopoietic disorders
	Serum glutamic-pyruvic transaminase (SGPT)	Elevation indicates death of liver cells Elevated in hepatocellular disease, infectious hepatitis, liver injury, and liver congestion
	Alkaline phosphatase	Rises when excretion of the enzyme is impaired due to biliary obstruction Useful in differentiating hepatocellular and obstructive jaundice
	Lactic acid dehydrogenase (LDH)	The isoenzymes LDH_1 and LDH_2 are found primarily in liver, skeletal muscle, and lung; test is sensitive enough to detect increased fraction in infectious hepatitis before jaundice appears
	Y-glutamyl transpeptidase transerase (YGT)	The liver is the main source of this enzyme; it facilitates the transport of amino acids across the cell membrane; used to detect alcoholic liver disease and alcohol consumption
Bilirubin	Total	Measures total serum bilirubin
	Direct	Measures conjugated bilirubin (an increase usually associated with liver disease or obstruction of bile duct)
	Indirect	Measures free bilirubin (an increase usually associated with increased destruction of red blood cells)
	Icterus index	Measures the degree of jaundice by comparing yellowness of the serum with that of a standard-yellow-color compound
	Tests for bilirubin in urine	Usually, there is no bilirubin in urine; when present it represents conjugated bilirubin since free bilirubin that is attached cannot be filtered in the glomerulus; presence suggests liver disease or obstructive jaundice
	Urinary and fecal urobilinogen	Absence of fecal urobilinogen indicates obstruction of biliary tract An increase in fecal urobilinogen indicates excessive bilirubin production An increase in urinary urobilinogen in absence of an increased fecal urobilinogen indicates liver disease
Blood Ammonia		The liver normally removes ammonia from the blood and converts it to urea; blood ammonia levels are often elevated in severe liver disease
Blood Coagulation	Prothrombin time	Liver disease causes impaired synthesis of clotting factors V, VII, IX, X, prothrombin (II), and fibrinogen; prothrombin time is affected by most of these factors; the test is used to assess risk of bleeding
Dye Clearance	Sodium sulfobromophthalein (Bromsulphalein, BSP)	Liver function test, which is based on the liver's ability to remove dye from the blood
	Indocyanine green (IGG)	Also measures ability of liver to remove dye from blood (used less frequently than BSP)
Plasma Proteins	Total plasma proteins Albumin	Measures total plasma proteins, including albumin, globulins, and fibrinogen Plasma proteins are synthesized by the liver Albumin is decreased in cirrhosis
	Globulins	Alpha and beta globulins are increased in infectious or obstructive jaundice and decreased in liver failure, which interferes with their synthesis
Liver Scan	Blood vessel structural scan	Measures the size, shape, and filling defects of the liver after intravenous injection of a radioactive substance; a radioactive detector (or scanner) outlines the liver and spleen
	Rose bengal liver function scan (I–131–rose bengal excretion test)	Rose bengal is a radioactive dye which is cleared from the blood by the liver; the size, shape, and filling of the liver, gall bladder, and small intestine are determined by scanning following intravenous injection of the dye

hepatic jaundice is an abnormally high level of serum alkaline phosphatase. Alkaline phosphatase is produced by the liver and excreted with the bile, thus when there is obstruction to bile flow, the blood alkaline phosphatase becomes elevated.

Tests of liver function

The history and physical examination will, in most instances, provide clues about liver function. Diagnostic tests help to assess liver function and the extent of liver disease. A liver biopsy affords a means of examining liver tissue without necessitating surgery. Table 38-2 describes the common tests of liver function and their significance.

Alterations in liver function

Although the liver is among the organs most frequently damaged, only about 10% of hepatic tissue is required for the liver to remain functional.[1] Of the numerous pathologic processes to which the liver may be subject—including vascular disorders, inflammation, metabolic disorders, toxic injury, and neoplasms—three diseases have been selected for inclusion in this section: acute hepatitis, cirrhosis, and cancer.

Hepatitis

Viral hepatitis is an acute inflammatory disease usually caused by hepatitis virus A (HVA), hepatitis virus B (HVB), or other nonA–nonB virus(es) which have not yet been elucidated. Viruses, such as cytomegalovirus, herpes simplex, and rubella virus, may be rarely implicated. Table 38-3 describes the salient features of both hepatitis A and B.

Hepatitis A

Hepatitis A has a brief incubation period. It is usually spread by the fecal-oral route. Drinking contaminated milk or water and eating shellfish from infected waters are fairly frequent causes. Institutions housing large numbers of people (usually children) are sometimes striken by an epidemic of HVA. At special risk are persons traveling abroad who have never previously been exposed to the virus.

Hepatitis B

Hepatitis B represents a more serious problem than HVA; it has a longer incubation period and is more likely to cause serious illness, and to become chronic. The sources of HVB are chronic carriers and persons with active hepatitis B. Moreover, infected blood is also a source. Hence, persons who habitually abuse certain drugs by injecting them directly into the blood stream are at special risk, because they frequently use needles contaminated by the blood of fellow addicts without first sterilizing the needles. It can also be transmitted by contaminated medical equipment. This is one reason why disposable needles and syringes are preferable. Persons on hemodialysis are also at high risk, in part because they often require blood transfusions and in part because their immune system is deficient. HVB has also been found in the saliva, urine, semen, menstrual blood, and other secretions of persons with

the disease. Mother-to-infant transmission occurs, but whether transmission occurs in utero or during the birth process is not known.

Acute hepatitis

The injurious effects of both type A and type B hepatitis viruses are believed to arise because of an immune reaction in which the hepatitis virus in some way alters the antigenic properties of the hepatocytes. The extent of inflammation and necrosis, therefore, varies depending upon the individual immune response.

The clinical manifestations of both hepatitis A and B have been divided into four phases: (1) the incubation period, (2) the preicterus period, (3) the icterus period, and (4) the convalescent period. Table 38-3 summarizes each of these phases.

Treatment

The treatment of hepatitis is largely symptomatic. Bedrest, which at one time was a mainstay in treatment, has now largely been replaced with a more liberal program, which permits patients to pace their own activity. Most patients will elect to limit activity because of fatigue. Dietary restrictions are usually minimal. If oral intake becomes inadequate, glucose solutions may be administered intravenously. Patients are instructed to avoid strenuous exercise, and alcohol and other hepatotoxic agents.

Prevention

The most effective way to prevent hepatitis is to prevent opportunities for transmission of the virus. Because *contamination* (of blood, needles, other equipment) affords the virus ready access to the body, as previously described, the health-care worker should follow proper procedures when handling syringes and needles that have been used for drawing blood or injecting medications. Gloves should be worn when handling blood samples. Routine screening of blood donors has reduced the incidence of post-transfusion hepatitis B. There is increasing evidence, however, that other nonA–nonB virus(es) may be responsible for the transfusion-induced hepatitis.

Gamma globulin is usually administered to close personal contacts of persons with hepatitis A. It may be advisable for persons traveling to countries where hepatitis A is endemic to receive a protective dose of gamma globulin within 2 weeks of arrival in that country, and to receive booster doses if their stay is an extended one. The standard gamma globulin does not appear to afford protection against

Table 38–3 Manifestations of Viral Hepatitis A and B

Features	Hepatitis A	Hepatitis B	Common Manifestations
Mode of transmission	Excreted in the stool 2 weeks prior to and for 1 week after onset of clinical disease; transmitted by fecal-oral route, contaminated water, milk, shellfish	Present in the serum; transmitted by blood transfusion and blood products, needles, and other inoculation equipment; can also be transmitted by intimate sexual partners or family members; mother-to-infant transmission	
Persons at risk	Young children and persons in institutions	Parenteral drug abusers; persons on hemodialysis; health-care workers	
Carrier state	Not known to occur	Develops in about 5% to 10% of persons who have the disease	
Incubation period*	15 to 40 days (average, 30–38 days)	43 to 160 days (average, 90 days)	Headache Nausea Vomiting

Preicterus period		Manifestations more severe, including
		  skin rash
		  arthralgia
		Test for HVB positive
			3 to 12 days
			Fever
			Headache
			Epigastric distress
			Anorexia, nausea, vomiting
			Intolerance to fatty foods
			Diminished sense of smell
			Loss of taste for cigarettes
			Elevation of SGOT, SGPT, LDH$_1$ and LDH$_2$

Icterus period			2 to 6 weeks Jaundice Dark urine Clay-colored stool Elevated total bilirubin
Convalescent period			Abdominal pain and tenderness
Other		May progress to carrier state and chronicity Risk of later development of hepatocarcinoma in persons who develop chronic hepatitis	

*Richman A: Infectious hepatitis. Hospital Medicine 14, No. 3:72, 1978

hepatitis B. However, hepatitis B immune globulin, which is not widely available, is effective if administered in a large dose within 10 days of exposure.

Cirrhosis

The World Health Organization defines cirrhosis as "a diffuse process characterized by fibrosis and conversion of normal liver architecture into structurally abnormal nodules."[6] Although cirrhosis is usually associated with alcoholism, it can develop in the course of other disorders, including viral hepatitis, toxic reactions to drugs and chemicals, biliary obstruction, and cardiac disease. Cirrhosis also accompanies metabolic disorders that cause deposition of minerals in the liver; two of these disorders are hemochromatosis (iron deposition) and Wilson's disease (copper deposition).

There are three types of cirrhosis: postnecrotic, biliary, and portal. Each of these has a different etiology, but in the end, each causes liver failure and the ultimate outcome is much the same. Following a brief discussion of postnecrotic and biliary cirrhosis, we shall take portal (alcoholic) cirrhosis as our prototype.

Postnecrotic cirrhosis

This form of cirrhosis is characterized by replacement of liver tissue with small to large nodules of fibrous tissue, with a resultant markedly deformed and nodular liver. Postnecrotic cirrhosis accounts for some 10% to 30% of cases of cirrhosis. It may follow viral hepatitis (type B or nonA–nonB type) or an autoimmune disease, or may be a toxic response to drugs and other chemicals. It is a predisposing factor in hepatic cancer, when it is caused by hepatitis type B.

Biliary cirrhosis

Biliary cirrhosis has its start in the bile ducts, occurring as a primary or a secondary disorder and accounting for about 10% to 20% of cases of cirrhosis. *Primary biliary cirrhosis* is seen most commonly in women 40 to 60 years of age. The cause is unknown. It is characterized by inflammation and scarring of the septal and intralobular bile ducts. The liver becomes enlarged and takes on a green hue. The earliest symptoms are pruritus, followed by a dark urine and pale stools. Once symptoms become clinically evident, life expectancy is about 5 years.[7] So far as is known, in some persons the existence of the disease is detectable only through laboratory studies, since there are no symptoms. *Secondary biliary cirrhosis* develops as the result of prolonged obstruction of bile flow either within the liver or in

the extrahepatic ducts. It is most commonly due to gallstones, stricture of the bile ducts, or neoplasms that obstruct bile flow. A secondary infection may develop and ascend causing further liver damage.

Portal or alcoholic cirrhosis

Cirrhosis is the fourth leading cause of death among adult Americans and the third leading cause of death among men 35 to 55 years of age. The most common cause of cirrhosis is excessive alcohol consumption. At least 75% of deaths attributable to alcoholism are caused by cirrhosis.[8] It is estimated that there are 10 million alcoholics in the United States. Interestingly, not all alcoholics develop cirrhosis, suggesting that other conditions such as genetic and environmental factors contribute to its occurrence. In fact, one-third of alcoholics never develop cirrhosis; in another one-third, there are fatty liver changes but not cirrhosis; and the remaining one-third are those who have cirrhosis.[9] Most deaths from alcoholic cirrhosis are attributable to liver failure, bleeding esophageal varices, or kidney failure.

Alcoholic cirrhosis is sometimes referred to as *Laennec's cirrhosis*. Although the mechanism whereby alcohol exerts its toxic effects on liver structures in somewhat unclear, the changes that develop can be divided into three stages: (1) fatty changes, (2) alcoholic hepatitis, and (3) cirrhosis.

Stage of fatty changes. During this stage, there is enlargement of the liver due to excessive accumulation of fat within the liver cells. Alcohol replaces fat as a fuel for liver metabolism and impairs mitochondrial ability to oxidize fat. There is evidence that high ingestion of alcohol can cause fatty liver changes even in the presence of an adequate diet. For example, young nonalcoholic volunteers had fatty liver changes after 2 days of consuming 18 to 24 oz of alcohol, even though adequate carbohydrates, fats, and proteins were included in the diet.[10] The fatty changes that occur with ingestion of alcohol do not usually produce symptoms and are reversible once the alcohol intake has been discontinued.

Stage of alcoholic hepatitis. Alcoholic hepatitis is the intermediate stage between fatty changes and cirrhosis. It is characterized by inflammation and necrosis of liver cells, and thus is always serious and sometimes fatal. The necrotic lesions are generally patchy, but may involve an entire lobe. The cause is unknown. It is often seen after an abrupt increase in alcohol intake, and is common in "spree" drinkers. "Ballooning" of hepatocytes, and the toxic effects of the intermediates of alcohol metabolism, such as acetaldehyde, are believed to be contributory factors. This stage is usually characterized by hepatic tenderness, pain, anorexia, nausea, fever, jaundice, ascites, and liver failure; but some patients may be asymptomatic. There is a marked increase in the serum glutamic oxaloacetic transaminase. Within 1 to 20 years, 80% of persons with alcoholic hepatitis who continue to drink will have liver changes consistent with cirrhosis.[9]

Stage of cirrhosis. Cirrhosis is the direct result of liver injury due to the fatty changes and alcoholic hepatitis. The liver becomes yellow–orange, fatty, and diffusely scarred. Its normal structure is distorted by bands of fibrous tissue, which separate areas of regenerated cells. As the disease progresses, the liver shrinks. As normal tissue is replaced by scar tissue, there is obstruction to blood flow through the liver and formation of extrahepatic shunts, which serve as alternative routes for return of portal blood to the heart.

Clinical manifestations

There may be no symptoms for long periods of time, and when symptoms do appear, they are vague at first, with complaints of fatigability and weight loss. At this point, the liver is often palpable and hard. Diarrhea is frequently present, although some persons may complain of constipation. There may be abdominal pain due to liver enlargement or stretching of Glisson's capsule. This pain is located in the epigastric area or in the upper right quadrant and is described as being dull and aching, and causing a sensation of fullness. The late manifestations of cirrhosis are related to portal hypertension and liver cell failure. Portal hypertension causes complications such as esophageal varices and ascites; in hepatocellular failure, there is decreased production of bile, plasma proteins, and blood-clotting factors, and interference with removal of bilirubin, ammonia, and other substances. The manifestations of cirrhosis are discussed in the section that follows and are summarized in Table 38-4.

Portal hypertension. Portal hypertension describes a condition in which there is an increase (10 mm Hg to 12 mm Hg across the liver) in portal-vein pressure.[7] The presence of bands of fibrous tissue and fibrous nodules within the liver induces a gradual increase in portal-vein pressure with development of (1) collateral channels between the portal and systemic veins, (2) ascites, and (3) splenomegaly.

Development of collateral channels. With gradual obstruction of blood flow in the liver, the pressure in the portal vein becomes increased and large collateral channels develop between the portal veins and the systemic veins in the esophagus and lower rectum, and in the umbilical veins of the falciform ligament that attaches to the anterior abdominal wall. There is splenomegaly due to congestion of the splenic vein. The esophageal veins, being thin-walled, are vulnerable to formation of varicosities (see Chap 9). These *esophageal varices* are subject to rupture, with massive and sometimes fatal hemorrhage. This acute bleeding is the most significant complication of portal hypertension. The presence of the collaterals between the inferior and internal iliac veins may give rise to *hemorrhoids*. In some persons, the fetal umbilical vein is not totally obliterated; it forms a channel portal vein and the vein on the anterior abdominal wall (Fig. 38-6). These dilated veins around the umbilicus are called *caput medusae*. Finally, portopulmonary shunts may arise, causing blood to bypass the pulmonary capillaries, thereby interfering with blood oxygenation and producing cyanosis.

Surgical treatment of portal hypertension consists of creating a portal–systemic shunt (an opening between the portal and a systemic vein). While this procedure does not improve liver function, it does decrease the pressure within the esophageal veins and thus prevents esophageal hemorrhage. The two procedures that are done most frequently are portacaval shunt and splenorenal shunt. In a *portacaval* shunt, an opening is created between the portal vein and the vena cava. A *splenorenal* shunt involves removal of the spleen and anastomosis of the splenic vein to the left renal vein. It is often done when there is enlargement of the spleen, and prevents further thrombocytopenia and leukopenia. One of the untoward sequelae that develop in some 10% of persons with a portal-systemic shunt is hepatic-systemic encephalopathy. As will be discussed, the neurological manifestations of this disorder are believed to result from absorption of ammonia and other neurotoxic substances from the gut directly into the systemic circulation without going through the liver.

Splenomegaly. The splenomegaly observed in cirrhosis results from the shunting of blood into the splenic vein, which gives rise to such hematological disorders as anemia, thrombocytopenia, and leukopenia.

Ascites and peripheral edema. Ascites is an accumulation of fluid within the peritoneal cavity. This fluid is a transudate of plasma, constantly being exchanged with fluid from the vascular compartment, and com-

Table 38–4 Manifestations of Portal Cirrhosis

Primary Alteration in Function	Manifestation
Portal hypertension	
Development of collateral vessels	Esophageal varices
	Hemorrhoids
	Caput medusae (dilated cutaneous veins around the umbilicus)
Increased pressure in the portal vein and decreased levels of serum albumin	Ascites
	Peripheral edema
Splenomegaly	Anemia
	Leukopenia
	Thrombocytopenia
Hepatorenal syndrome	Elevated serum creatinine
	Azotemia
	Oliguria
Portal-systemic shunting of blood	Hepatic-systemic encephalopathy
Hepatocellular dysfunction	
Impaired metabolism of sex hormones	Female: menstrual disorders
	Male: testicular atrophy, gynecomastia, decrease in secondary sex characteristics
	Skin disorders: vascular spiders and palmar erythema
Impaired synthesis of plasma proteins	Decreased levels of serum albumin with development of edema and ascites
	Decreased synthesis of carrier proteins for hormones and drugs
Decreased synthesis of blood-clotting factors	Bleeding tendencies
Failure to remove and conjugate bilirubin from the blood	Jaundice
Impaired bile synthesis	Malabsorption of fats and fat-soluble vitamins
Impaired metabolism of drugs cleared by the liver	Risk of drug reactions and toxicities
Impaired gluconeogenesis	Abnormal glucose tolerance
Decreased ability to convert ammonia to urea	Elevated blood ammonia levels

posed of electrolytes and albumin similar in composition to plasma. In cirrhosis, the two major factors contributing to ascites are (1) impaired synthesis of albumin by the liver such that the plasma colloidal osmotic pressure falls, and (2) obstruction of venous flow through the liver. This obstruction causes an increased production of lymph, with oozing of serous fluid from the liver surface. The decreased colloidal osmotic pressure causes fluid to leak out of the capillaries in the splanchnic (visceral) circulation. Added to these is a rise in aldosterone, which augments kidney retention of sodium and water. Among causes postulated to be responsible for the increased aldosterone levels are an impairment of aldosterone inactivation by the liver, and production by the liver of a humoral substance that stimulates aldosterone secretion. The increased aldosterone leads to a potassium deficiency. Because

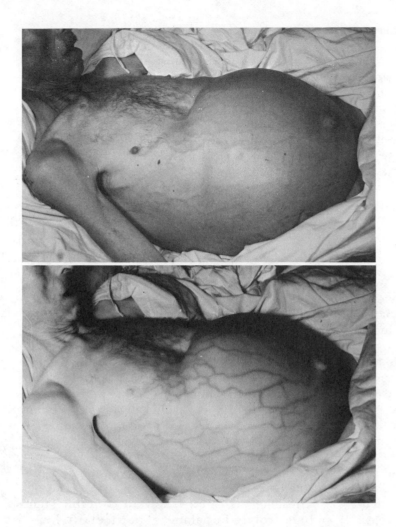

Figure 38–6. Collateral abdominal veins on the anterior abdominal wall in a patient with alcoholic liver disease as recorded by black and white photography (*top*) and infrared photography (*bottom*). (Schiff L: Diseases of the Liver, 4th ed, p 345. Philadelphia, JB Lippincott, 1975)

of the fall in serum albumin and the retention of sodium and water, peripheral edema develops, particularly in the dependent parts of the body, such as the feet.

Treatment of ascites usually focuses on dietary restriction of sodium and administration of diuretics. Water intake may also need to be restricted. To counteract the rise in aldosterone, an aldosterone-blocking diuretic along with one of the thiazide diuretics is usually prescribed. Oral potassium supplements are often given to prevent hypokalemia, since the potassium level probably has fallen before diuretic therapy is begun. Paracentesis may be done for diagnostic purposes, but is seldom done to treat the ascites, since it may cause a shift in fluid from the vascular compartment to the peritoneal cavity, along with complications such as infection and hemorrhage.

Hepatorenal syndrome. The hepatorenal syndrome refers to a functional state of renal failure that is sometimes seen during the terminal stages of cirrhosis and ascites. It is characterized by progressive azotemia, increased serum creatinine levels, and oliguria. Although the basic cause is not known, a decrease in renal blood flow is believed to play a part. Ultimately, when renal failure is superimposed on liver failure, there is impaired elimination of bilirubin along with azotemia and elevated levels of blood ammonia; this often precipitates hepatic coma.

A surgical procedure called the *LaVeen* continuous peritoneal-jugular shunt has recently been devised, in which the peritoneal fluid is shunted from the abdominal cavity through a one-way pressure-sensitive valve into a silicone tube that empties into the superior vena cava. The procedure is reported to relieve refractory ascites in persons with cirrhosis and to reverse the pathophysiological manifestations of the hepatorenal syndrome.[11]

Endocrine disorders. Endocrine disorders are frequent accompaniments of cirrhosis, particularly disturbances in gonadal function. In women there may be menstrual irregularities (usually amenorrhea), loss of libido, and sterility. In men, the testosterone level usually falls, the testes atrophy, and there is loss of libido, impotence, and gynecomastia.

Skin disorders.   Liver failure brings on numerous skin disorders. These lesions, called variously *vascular spiders*, *telangiectasia*, *spider angiomas*, and *spider nevi*, most often are seen in the upper half of the body. These lesions consist of a central pulsating arteriole from which smaller vessels radiate. (It should be kept in mind that spider angiomas may be seen in pregnancy even when liver function is normal.) *Palmar erythema* is redness of the palms, probably due to an increased blood flow resulting from higher cardiac output. *Clubbing* of the fingers may be seen in persons with cirrhosis. *Jaundice* is usually a late manifestation of liver failure.

Hematological disorders.   Anemia, thrombocytopenia, coagulation defects, and leukopenia may arise in the presence of cirrhosis. *Anemia* may be due to blood loss, excessive red blood cell destruction, and impaired formation of red blood cells. A folic-acid deficiency may lead to severe megaloblastic anemia. Changes in the lipid composition of the red cell membrane increase hemolysis. Since factors V, VII, IX, X, prothrombin, and fibrinogen are synthesized by the liver, their decrease in liver disease contributes to bleeding disorders. Malabsorption of the fat-soluble vitamin K contributes further to the impaired synthesis of these clotting factors. Often there is also a *thrombocytopenia* that occurs as the result of splenomegaly. Thus, the cirrhotic patient is subject to purpura, easy bruising, hematuria, and abnormal menstrual bleeding (women), and is vulnerable to bleeding from the esophagus and other segments of the gastrointestinal tract.

Fetor hepaticus refers to a characteristic musty, sweetish odor of the breath in the patient in advanced liver failure, due to breakdown products of metabolism manufactured by intestinal bacteria.

Hepatic-systemic encephalopathy.   Hepatic-systemic encephalopathy refers to the totality of central nervous system manifestations of cirrhosis. It is characterized by neural disturbances ranging from a lack of mental alertness to confusion, coma, and convulsions. A very early sign of hepatic encephalopathy is asterixis. There may be a loss of memory of varying degrees coupled with personality changes, such as euphoria, irritability, anxiety, and lack of concern about personal appearance and self. There may also be impairment of speech and inability to perform certain purposeful movements. The encephalopathy may progress to decerebrate rigidity and finally to a terminal deep coma.

The essential cause of hepatic encephalopathy is not yet known. The presence of neurotoxins, which appear in the blood because the liver has lost its detoxifying capacity, is believed to be a related factor. As has been stated, hepatic encephalopathy develops in about 10% of persons having a portal-systemic shunt.

One of these neurotoxins is ammonia. We may trace its development as follows: One function of the liver is to convert ammonia, a byproduct of protein metabolism, to urea. Ammonia is produced in the intestine and kidneys. In the intestine, the bacterial flora converts proteins to ammonia, which normally diffuses back into the portal blood and thence to the liver, where it is converted to urea before entering the general circulation. This is the normal situation. However, should a pathologic process develop wherein blood from the intestine bypasses the liver, or the liver is no longer able to convert the ammonia to urea, the ammonia is able to reach the brain through the general circulation and there to exert its toxic effects. This is why hepatic encephalopathy is aggravated by a large protein meal, by bleeding from the gastrointestinal tract, and during periods of dehydration. When hypokalemic alkalosis is present, it causes increased renal production of ammonia. Narcotics and tranquilizers are poorly metabolized by the liver, and administration of these drugs may cause central nervous system depression and precipitate hepatic encephalopathy.

Treatment is directed toward correcting fluid and electrolyte imbalances, particularly hypokalemia, and limiting ammonia production in the gastrointestinal tract by limiting protein intake. A nonabsorbable antibiotic, such as neomycin, may be given to eradicate bacteria from the bowel and thus prevent this cause of ammonia production. Another drug that may be given is lactulose. It is not absorbed from the small intestine, but moves directly to the large intestine where it is catabolized by the colon bacteria to small organic acids which cause production of large, loose stools with a low pH. The low pH is believed to convert ammonia to ammonium ion, which is not absorbed by the blood.[12]

Cancer of the Liver

Primary cancer of the liver, which accounts for 2% of all cancers, is relatively rare in the United States. There are two primary types of cancer of the liver—hepatocarcinoma, which arises from the liver cells; and cholangiocarcinoma, which is a primary cancer of the bile duct cells. Sometimes cellular components of both types are present. Hepatocarcinoma is strongly associated with postnecrotic cirrhosis due to hepatitis B and with hemochromatosis. A small number of cases have been reported to occur in women taking oral contraceptives. By far, the most common basis of liver cancer is metastases, usually from the lung or the breast.

The initial symptoms are weakness; anorexia; fatigue; bloating; a sensation of abdominal fullness; and a dull, aching abdominal pain. Usually, the liver is enlarged at the time these symptoms appear, and there is a low fever without apparent cause. A serum protein is present in fetal life, called serum-alpha fetoprotein, and normally it is barely detectable in the serum after the age of 2 years; but it is present in some 70% of cases of hepatocarcinoma.[1]

Primary cancers of the liver are usually far advanced at the time of diagnosis; the 5-year survival rate is about 1%, with most patients dying within 6 months. The treatment of choice is subtotal hepatectomy of 85% to 90% of the liver, if conditions permit.[13] The cancer is not radiosensitive. Chemotherapeutic drugs, among them methotrexate and 5-fluorouracil (5-FU) may be administered by cannula placed in the hepatic artery.

In summary, the liver is the largest and, in function, one of the most versatile organs in the body. It secretes bile and synthesizes fats, plasma proteins, and glucose. It metabolizes drugs, and removes, conjugates, and secretes bilirubin into the bile. The liver is subject to most of the disease processes that affect other body structures, such as vascular disorders, inflammation, metabolic diseases, toxic injury, and neoplasms. Two of the most common liver diseases are hepatitis and cirrhosis. Acute viral hepatitis is caused by hepatitis A and hepatitis B viruses. Spread of hepatitis A occurs by oral-fecal transmission; it has a short incubation period and is usually followed by complete recovery. Hepatitis B has a longer incubation period and is spread through contact with contaminated blood, serum, instruments, and body secretions. Its symptoms are more severe and it may progress to the carrier or chronic state. Cirrhosis caused by hepatitis B is associated with increased risk of hepatocarcinoma. Cirrhosis is the fourth leading cause of death in the United States. It is characterized by fibrosis and conversion of the normal hepatic architecture into structurally abnormal nodules. There are three types of cirrhosis—postnecrotic, biliary, and portal or alcoholic cirrhosis, of which the most common is alcoholic cirrhosis. Regardless of cause, the manifestations of end-stage cirrhosis are similar and result from portal hypertension and liver cell failure.

Gall Bladder and Biliary System

The secretion of bile is essential for digestion of dietary fats and absorption of fats and fat-soluble vitamins from the intestine. Bile produced by the

Figure 38–7.   The liver and biliary system including the gall bladder and bile ducts. (Chaffee EE, Lytle IM: Basic Physiology and Anatomy, 4th ed. Philadelphia, JB Lippincott, 1980)

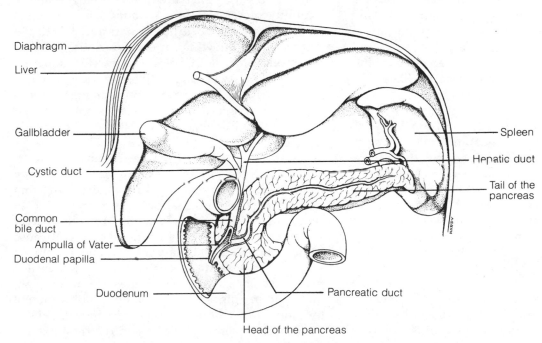

Diaphragm

Liver

Gallbladder

Cystic duct

Common bile duct

Ampulla of Vater

Duodenal papilla

Duodenum

Head of the pancreas

Spleen

Hepatic duct

Tail of the pancreas

Pancreatic duct

hepatocytes flows into the canaliculi, then to the periphery of the lobules, which drain into larger ducts, until it reaches the right and left hepatic ducts. These ducts unite to form the common duct (Fig. 38-7). The common duct, which is about 10 cm to 15 cm in length, descends and passes behind the pancreas and enters the descending duodenum. The pancreatic duct joins the common duct in the ampulla of Vater, which empties into the duodenum through the duodenal papilla. Muscle tissue at the junction of the papilla, called the sphincter of Oddi, regulates the flow of bile into the duodenum. A second sphincter (sphincter of Boyden), which is just above the point where the pancreatic duct fuses with the common duct, controls the flow of bile into this area of the common duct. When this sphincter is closed, bile moves back into the gall bladder.

The gall bladder is part of the biliary system. It is a distensible, pear-shaped muscular sac located on the ventral surface of the liver. It has a smooth muscle wall and is lined with a thin layer of absorptive cells. The cystic duct joins the gall bladder to the common duct. The function of the gall bladder is to store and concentrate bile. When full, it can hold 20 ml to 50 ml of bile. Entrance of food into the intestine causes contraction of the gall bladder and relaxation of the sphincter of Oddi. The stimulus for gall bladder contraction is primarily hormonal. Products of food digestion, particulary lipids, stimulate cholecystokinin release from the mucosa of the duodenum. The role of other gastrointestinal hormones in bile release is less clearly understood. Passage of bile into the intestine is largely regulated by the pressure within the common duct. Normally, the gall bladder serves to regulate this pressure: it collects and stores bile as the pressure increases and it causes an increase in pressure when it contracts. Following gall bladder surgery, the pressure in the common duct changes, causing the common duct to dilate. The flow of bile is then regulated by the sphincters in the common duct.

Two very common disorders of the biliary system are *cholelithiasis* (gallstones) and *cholecystitis* (inflammation of the gall bladder). Together, these diseases affect about 16 million persons living in the United States and account for some 16% to 18% of admissions to short-stay hospitals for treatment of digestive diseases.[8] Close to 400,000 cholecystectomies are performed in this country each year.[14]

Composition of Bile and Formation of Gallstones

Gallstones are due to precipitation of substances contained in bile, mainly cholesterol and bilirubin. Bile contains bile salts, cholesterol, bilirubin, lecithin, fatty acids, water, as well as electrolytes, normally found in the plasma. The cholesterol found in bile has no known function; it is assumed to be a byproduct of bile salt formation and its presence is linked to the excretory function of bile. Normally insoluble in water, cholesterol is rendered soluble by the action of bile salts and lecithin, which combines with it to form micelles. In the gall bladder, water and electrolytes are absorbed from the liver bile, causing the bile to become more concentrated. Because neither lecithin nor bile salts are absorbed in the gall bladder, their concentration becomes increased along with that of cholesterol, and in this way, the solubility of cholesterol is maintained.

The bile of which gallstones are formed is usually supersaturated with either cholesterol or bilirubinate. The majority of gallstones, about 75%, are composed primarily of cholesterol, and the other 25% are pigment, or calcium bilirubinate, stones. Many stones have a mixed composition. Three factors contribute to the formation of gallstones: (1) abnormalities in the composition of bile, (2) stasis of bile, and (3) inflammation of the gall bladder. Formation of cholesterol stones is associated with obesity and is seen more frequently in women, especially women who have had multiple pregnancies or who are taking oral contraceptives. All of these situations cause the liver to excrete more cholesterol into the bile. Drugs such as clofibrate, which lower serum cholesterol levels, also cause increased cholesterol excretion into the bile. Malabsorption disorders stemming from ileal disease or intestinal bypass surgery, for example, tend to interfere with absorption of bile salts, which are needed to maintain the solubility of cholesterol. Inflammation of the gall bladder alters the absorptive characteristics of the mucosal layer, allowing for excessive absorption of water and bile salts. Cholesterol gallstones are extremely common among native Americans, which suggests that a genetic component may have a role in gallstone formation. Pigment stones are seen in persons with hemolytic disease and hepatic cirrhosis.

Many persons with gallstones have no symptoms. Gallstones cause symptoms when they obstruct bile flow. Small stones not more than 8 mm in diameter pass into the common duct, producing symptoms of indigestion and biliary colic. Larger stones are more likely to obstruct flow and cause jaundice. The pain of biliary colic is generally abrupt in onset, increasing steadily in intensity until it reaches a climax in 30 to 60 minutes. The upper right quadrant, or epigastric area, is the usual location of the pain, often with referred pain to the back, above the waist, the right shoulder, and the right scapula or midscapular region. A few persons will experience pain on the left side. The pain usually persists for 2 to 8 hours, to be followed by upper right quadrant soreness.

Cholecystitis

Cholecystitis is inflammation of the gall bladder. It may be either acute or chronic, and both types are associated with formation of gallstones. Acute cholecystitis may be superimposed on chronic cholecystitis.

Acute cholecystitis is almost always associated with complete or partial obstruction of bile flow. It is believed that the inflammation is caused by chemical irritation from the concentrated bile, along with mucosal swelling and ischemia due to venous congestion and lymphatic stasis. The gall bladder is usually markedly distended. Bacterial infections may arise secondarily to the ischemia and chemical irritation. The bacteria reach the injured gall bladder through the blood, lymphatics, or bile ducts, or from adjacent organs. Among the common pathogens are staphylococci and enterococci. The wall of the gall bladder is most vulnerable to the effects of ischemia, as a result of which there is mucosal necrosis and sloughing. The process may lead to gangrenous changes and perforation of the gall bladder.

The *symptoms of acute cholecystitis* vary with the severity of obstruction and inflammation. It is often precipitated by a fatty meal and may be initiated with complaints of indigestion. Pain, initially similar to that of biliary colic, is characteristic of acute cholecystitis. It does not, however, subside spontaneously, and it responds poorly or only temporarily to potent analgesics. When the inflammation progresses to involve the peritoneum, the pain becomes more pronounced in the right upper quadrant. The right subcostal region is tender, and there is spasm of the muscles that surround the area. *Vomiting* occurs in about 75% of patients and jaundice in some 25%. *Fever* and an abnormally high *white blood cell* count attest to the presence of inflammation. Total serum bilirubin, serum transaminase, and alkaline phosphatase are usually elevated.

The manifestations of *chronic cholecystitis* are more vague than those of *acute cholecystitis*. There may be intolerance to fatty foods, belching, and other indications of discomfort. Often there are episodes of colicky pain with obstruction of biliary flow due to gallstones. The gall bladder, which in chronic cholecystitis usually contains stones, may be enlarged, shrunken, or of normal size. The passage of a stone into the common duct causes obstruction of bile flow and may contribute to carcinoma of the gall bladder.

Diagnosis and treatment

Radiologic techniques provide a means for visualizing the outline of the biliary tract. Ten to 15 percent of gallstones contain sufficient calcium to be visible on plain x-ray films. *Oral cholecystography* is effective when there are no symptoms of active gall bladder disease. The evening before the films are to be taken, tablets containing a contrast dye are administered orally. The dye is absorbed in the gut, excreted in the bile, and concentrated in the gall bladder. If stones are present, they will be outlined on the x-ray film. The gall bladder will not be outlined if the dye is not absorbed, if the common duct is obstructed, or if the gall bladder cannot concentrate the dye. *Intravenous cholangiography* involves the intravenous injection of a contrast dye, which is excreted by the liver. X-ray films are taken immediately following the injection, and during a period of up to 4 hours, to afford sufficient time for the gall bladder to concentrate the dye. *Operative cholangiograms* are done at the time of gall bladder surgery to afford immediate visualization of the ductal system and detection of filling defects and the presence of stones in the hepatic and common duct. *T-tube cholangiography* can be done after gall bladder surgery when the T-tube is in place, in which case the dye is injected into the T-tube. *Transhepatic cholangiography* involves the insertion of a needle through the eighth or ninth rib space into a bile duct in the center of the liver. A dye is injected into the duct for the purpose of visualizing the ductal structures and diagnosing strictures or neoplastic obstruction of the bile ducts. *Ultrasound* may be employed to demonstrate gallstones and biliary tract dilatation.

The usual treatment of choice for symptomatic cholelithiasis and cholecystitis is surgical removal of the gall bladder—*cholecystectomy*. If the inflammation is acute, the surgery is delayed, unless complications demand immediate surgery. This allows time for the inflammatory process to subside. Recently, there has been interest in administering *chenodeoxycholic acid* to dissolve radiolucent cholesterol stones. This drug causes bile to become unsaturated by decreasing cholesterol production while increasing bile salt excretion. It dissolves most stones within a year or two. However, it is not being administered to women of childbearing years because of fears that it may adversely affect the fetal liver.

In summary, the biliary tract serves as a passageway for delivery of bile from the liver to the intestine. This tract consists of the bile ducts and gall bladder. The most common causes of biliary tract disease are cholelithiasis and cholecystitis. Three factors contribute to the development of gallstones: (1) abnormalities in the com-

position of bile, (2) stasis of bile, and (3) inflammation of the gall bladder. Cholelithiasis predisposes to obstruction of bile flow, causing biliary colic and acute or chronic cholecystitis. Cholecystectomy is usually the treatment of choice for symptomatic cholelithiasis in persons who are good surgical risks. Chenodeoxycholic acid has recently become available for use in dissolving cholesterol gallstones. Its effect on the liver of the fetus has not been established, therefore, it is not being prescribed for women of childbearing years.

:The Pancreas

The pancreas lies transversely in the posterior part of the upper abdomen. The head of the pancreas is at the right of the abdomen; it rests against the curve of the duodenum in the area of the ampulla of Vater and its entrance into the duodenum. The body of the pancreas lies beneath the stomach. The tail touches the spleen. The pancreas is virtually hidden because of its posterior position. Unlike many other organs, it cannot be palpated. Because of the position of the pancreas and its large functional reserve, symptoms of disease do not usually appear until the disorder is far advanced. This is pariculary true of cancer of the pancreas.

The pancreas is both an endocrine and an exocrine organ. Its function as an endocrine organ was discussed in Chapter 35. The exocrine pancreas is made up of lobules, which consist of acinar cells. These cells secrete digestive enzymes into a system of microscopic ducts. These ducts are terminal branches of larger ducts that drain into the main pancreatic duct which extends from left to right through the substance of the pancreas (Fig. 38-7). In most people, the main pancreatic duct empties into the ampulla of Vater, although in some persons it empties directly into the duodenum. The pancreatic ducts are lined with epithelial cells that secrete water and bicarbonate and thereby modify the fluid and electrolyte composition of the pancreatic secretions. The pancreatic secretions contain proteolytic enzymes that break down dietary proteins, including trypsin, chymotrypsin, carboxypolypeptidase, ribonuclease, and deoxyribonuclease. The pancreas also secretes pancreatic amylase, which breaks down starch, and lipase, which hydrolyzes neutral fats into glycerol and fatty acids. The pancreatic enzymes are secreted in the inactive form and become activated once in the intestine. This is important, since the enzymes would digest the tissue of the pancreas itself were they to be secreted in the active form. The acinar cells secrete a trypsin inhibitor, which prevents trypsin activation. Since trypsin activates other proteolytic enzymes, the trypsin inhibitor prevents subsequent activation of those other enzymes. Two types of pancreatic disease are discussed in this chapter: acute and chronic pancreatitis and cancer of the pancreas.

Acute Hemorrhagic Pancreatitis

Acute pancreatitis is a severe and life-threatening disorder which is associated with escape of activated pancreatic enzymes into the pancreas and surrounding tissues. These enzymes cause fat necrosis, or autodigestion, of the pancreas and produce fatty depots in the abdominal cavity with hemorrhage from the necrotic vessels. Although there are a number of factors associated with the development of acute pancreatitis, the two most important are biliary tract disease with reflux of bile into the pancreas, and alcoholism. Biliary reflux is believed to activate the pancreatic enzymes within the ductile system of the pancreas. Gallstones that obstruct the common duct account for 40% to 60% of cases of acute pancreatitis.[1] The precise mechanisms whereby alcohol exerts its action are largely unknown. Alcohol is known to be a potent stimulator of pancreatic secretions, and at the same time it often causes partial obstruction of the sphincter of Oddi. Acute pancreatitis is also associated with hyperlipidemia, hyperparathyroidism, infections (particularly viral), abdominal and surgical trauma, and drugs such as steroids and the thiazide diuretics.

An important disturbance related to acute pancreatitis is the loss of a large volume of fluid into the retroperitoneal, peripancreatic spaces, and the abdominal cavity. The onset is usually abrupt and dramatic, and it may follow a heavy meal or an alcoholic binge. There is severe epigastric and abdominal pain often radiating to the back. The pain is aggravated when the person is lying supine; it is less severe when sitting and leaning forward. Abdominal distention accompanied by hypoactive bowel sounds is common. Tachycardia; hypotension; cool, clammy skin; and fever are often evident. Signs of hypocalcemia may develop, probably as a result of the precipitation of serum calcium in the areas of fat necrosis. Mild jaundice may appear after the first 24 hours owing to biliary obstruction. The serum amylase becomes elevated within the first 24 hours, and serum lipase within 72 to 94 hours. Both enzymes remain elevated during the destructive stage of the disease and return to normal within 2 to 5 days following the acute attack. Urinary clearance of amylase is increased. Since the serum amylase may be elevated due to the presence of other serious illnesses, the urinary amylase may be measured. Hyperglycemia and an elevated serum bilirubin may be present. About 5% of persons with acute pancreatitis die of the acute effects of peripheral vascular collapse. Serious complications include acute respiratory distress syndrome and acute tubular necrosis.

Treatment consists of measures directed at pain relief and restoration of lost plasma volume. Meperidine (Demerol), rather than morphine, is usually given for pain relief because it causes fewer spasms of the sphincter of Oddi. Papaverine, nitroglycerin, barbiturates, or anticholinergic drugs may be given as supplements to provide smooth muscle relaxation. Oral foods and fluids are withheld and gastric suction is instituted to treat distention of the bowel and prevent further stimulation of secretion of pancreatic enzymes. Intravenous fluids and electrolytes are administered to replace those that have been lost from the circulation and to combat the hypotension and shock. Intravenous colloid solutions are given to replace the fluid that has become sequestered in the abdomen and retroperitoneal space. Percutaneous peritoneal lavage has been tried as an early treatment of acute pancreatitis with encouraging results. Should a pancreatic abscess develop, it must be drained, usually through the flank. Pseudocysts that develop and persist must be treated surgically.

A *pseudocyst* is a collection of pancreatic fluid in the peritoneal cavity, enclosed in a layer of inflammatory tissue. Autodigestion or liquefaction of pancreatic tissue may be the cause. The pseudocyst most often is connected to a pancreatic duct so that it continues to increase in mass. The symptoms depend on its location. For example, jaundice may occur when a cyst develops near the head of the pancreas in close approximation to the common duct. Pseudocysts may resolve or may require surgical intervention.

Chronic Pancreatitis

Chronic pancreatitis is characterized by progressive destruction of the pancreas. It can be divided into two types: chronic calcifying pancreatitis and chronic obstructive pancreatitis. In *chronic calcifying pancreatitis*, calcified protein plugs (calculi) form in the pancreatic ducts. This form is seen most often in alcoholics. *Chronic obstructive pancreatitis* is associated with stenosis of the sphincter of Oddi. The lesions are prominent in the head of the pancreas. It is usually due to cholelithiasis and is sometimes relieved by removal of the sphincter of Oddi.

Chronic pancreatitis is manifested in episodes that are similar, albeit of lesser severity, to those of acute pancreatitis. There are persistent, recurring episodes of epigastric and upper left quadrant pain. Anorexia, nausea, vomiting, constipation, and flatulence are common. The attacks are often precipitated by alcohol abuse or overeating. Eventually, the disease progresses to the extent that both endocrine and exocrine pancreatic functions become deficient. At this point, signs of diabetes mellitus and the malabsorption syndrome become apparent. Pancreatic enzymes are given to treat the malabsorption, and the diabetes is treated with insulin. Narcotic addiction is a potential problem in persons with chronic pancreatitis.

Cancer of the Pancreas

There has been a marked increase in cancer of the pancreas during the past 30 years. Statistics from the American Cancer Society indicate that mortality has increased 27% in men and 19% in women compared to the figures of 30 years ago.[16] Presently, it is the fourth leading cause of cancer death in the United States. Cancer of the pancreas is usually far advanced when diagnosed, and the 5-year survival rate is less than 2%. The cause of pancreatic cancer is unknown. Recently, an association between coffee and cancer of the pancreas has been made. The relative risk associated with drinking two cups of coffee per day was 1.8 times normal; with three or more cups, it was reported to be 2.7 times normal.[17]

Cancer of the pancreas usually has an insidious onset, with anorexia, weight loss, flatulence, and nausea as symptoms. A dull, aching epigastric pain is present in about 70% to 80% of cases.[18] Overt diabetes mellitus is found in one-fifth of persons with pancreatic cancer, and almost all persons with the disease have an abnormal glucose tolerance.[18]

Because of the proximity of the pancreas to the common duct and the ampulla of Vater, cancer of the head of the pancreas tends to obstruct bile flow; this causes distention of the gall bladder and jaundice. The jaundice is frequently the presenting symptom in cancer of the head of the pancreas, and it is usually accompanied by complaints of pain and by pruritus. Cancer of the body of the pancreas generally impinges on the celiac ganglion, causing pain. The pain usually worsens with ingestion of food or with assumption of the supine position. Cancer of the tail of the pancreas has usually metastasized before causing symptoms.

Most cancers of the pancreas have metastasized by the time of diagnosis. Therefore, treatment is usually palliative and consists of high-voltage irradiation and chemotherapy. Surgical resection of the tumor is done when the tumor is localized.

In summary, the pancreas is both an endocrine and an exocrine organ. Diabetes mellitus is the most common disorder of the endocrine pancreas, and it occurs independently of disease of the exocrine pancreas. The exocrine pancreas produces digestive enzymes that are secreted in an inactive form and transported to the small intestine through the main pancreatic duct, which usually empties into the ampulla of Vater, and then into the duodenum through the sphincter of Oddi. The most common diseases of the exocrine pancreas are acute and chronic pancreatitis, and cancer. Both acute and chronic pancreatitis are associated with biliary reflux and chronic alcoholism. Acute pancreatitis is a dramatic and life-threatening disorder in which there is autodigestion of pancreatic tissue. Chronic pancreatitis causes progressive destruction of both the endocrine and exocrine pancreas. It is characterized by episodes of pain and epigastric distress that are similar to but less severe than that which occurs with acute pancreatitis. Cancer of the pancreas has shown a marked increase in incidence during the past 30 years. It is usually far advanced at the time of diagnosis and, as a result, the 5-year survival rate is less than 2%.

:Study Guide

After you have studied this chapter, you should be able to meet the following objectives:

: : Describe the anatomy of the liver.

: : Describe the function of the liver as it relates to alcohol metabolism.

: : Describe the enterohepatic circulation.

: : Explain the formation and degradation of bilirubin.

: : Compare hemolytic jaundice and obstructive jaundice with reference to their clinical manifestations.

: : Summarize the salient features of hepatitis A and hepatitis B with which the health professional should be acquainted.

: : Characterize postnecrotic cirrhosis and biliary cirrhosis.

: : Summarize the three stages of alcoholic cirrhosis.

: : Describe the clinical manifestations of alcoholic cirrhosis with reference to development of collateral channels.

: : Explain the development of ascites in alcoholic cirrhosis.

: : State a clinical definition of the hepatorenal syndrome.

: : Explain the basis of bleeding disorders in alcoholic cirrhosis.

: : Characterize hepatic-systemic encephalopathy.

: : Explain the significance of the presence of serum-alpha fetoprotein in an adult.

: : Explain the physiology of the gall bladder.

: : Describe the formation of gallstones.

: : Compare the symptoms of acute cholecystitis with those of chronic cholecystitis.

: : Describe the exocrine function of the pancreas.

: : Describe the clinical manifestations of acute pancreatitis.

: : Compare chronic calcifying pancreatitis and chronic obstructive pancreatitis.

: : State a significant statistic relating to pancreatic cancer.

:References

1. Robbins SL, Cotran RS: Pathologic Basis of Disease, ed 2, pp 1011, 1014, 1065–1066, 1097, 1101. Philadelphia, WB Saunders, 1979
2. Iber F: In alcoholism, the liver sets the pace. Nutrition Today 6, No. 1:2, 1971
3. Lieber CS: Alcohol, protein metabolism, and liver injury. Gastroenterology 79, No. 2:373, 1980
4. Lieber CS: Pathogenesis and early diagnosis of alcoholic liver injury. N Engl J Med 298, No. 16:888, 889, 1978
5. Guyton AC: Textbook of Medical Physiology, ed 5, p 872. Philadelphia, WB Saunders, 1981
6. Anthony PP, et al: The morphology of cirrhosis: Definition, nomenclature, and classification. Bull WHO 55, No. 4:522, 1977
7. Jeffries GH: Diseases of the liver. In Beeson PB, McDermott W, Wyngaarden JB (eds): Cecil Textbook of Medicine, ed 15, pp 1639, 1670. Philadelphia, WB Saunders, 1979
8. Report to the Congress of the United States of the National Commission on Digestive Diseases, vol 2 (A), p 305, and vol 4 (2A), p 395. National Institute of Health, Public Health Service. DHEW Publication No. (NIH) 79–1884
9. Leevy CM, Kangasundororm N: Alcoholic hepatitis. Hosp Pract 13, No. 10:115, 117, 1978
10. Rubin E, Lieber CS: Alcohol-induced hepatic injury in nonalcoholic volunteers. N Engl J Med 278:869, 1968

11. Wapnick S, Grosberg S, Kinney M, LaVeen HH: LaVeen continuous peritoneal-jugular shunt. JAMA 237, No. 2:131, 1977

12. Hardison GM: Cirrhosis—treating the ascites and encephalopathy. Med Times 107, No. 5:23, 1979

13. Adams JT: Cancer of the digestive glands. In Rubin P (ed): Clinical Oncology, ed 5, p 103. New York, American Cancer Society, 1978

14. Motson RW, Way LW: Differential diagnosis of gall bladder disease. Hospital Medicine 13, No. 3:26, 1977

15. Iber FL: Axioms on biliary tract disease. Hospital Medicine 15, No. 6:52, 1979

16. Bowden L: Cancer of the Pancreas. New York, American Cancer Society, 1972

17. MacMahon B, et al: Coffee and cancer of the pancreas. N Engl J Med 304, No. 11:630, 1981

18. Douglas HO, Karakousis C, Nava H: Guide to diagnosis of pancreatic cancer (part 2). Hospital Medicine 14, No. 1:40, 1978

Klingenstein J, Dienstag JL: Viral hepatitis: The meaning of serologic markers. Consultant 20, No. 10:53, 1980

McBride CM: Cancer of the liver. Hospital Medicine 13, No. 11:32, 1977

McElroy DB: Nursing care of patients with viral hepatitis. Nurs Clin North Am 12, No. 2:305, 1977

Pierce L: Anatomy and physiology of the liver. Nurs Clin North Am 12, No. 2:259, 1977

Regan PT, DiMagno EP: Acute pancreatitis: Diagnosis and treatment 15, No. 8:30, 1979

Schiff ER, Chiprut R: Chronic hepatitis: Guidelines for diagnosis and management. Hospital Medicine 14, No. 9:59, 1978

Shahinpour N: The adult patient with bleeding esophageal varices. Nurs Clin North Am 12, No. 2:331, 1977

Willson RA: Acute fulminant liver failure. Hospital Medicine 13, No. 10:8, 1977

:Suggested Readings

Altshuler A, Hilden D: The patient with portal hypertension. Nurs Clin North Am 12, No. 12:317, 1977

Banks PA: Answers to questions on pancreatitis. Hospital Medicine 14, No. 5:8, 1978

Bennison LJ, Grundy MD: Risk factors for the development of cholelithiasis in man. Part I. N Engl J Med 299, No. 21:1161, 1977

Bennison LJ, Grundy MD: Risk factors for the development of cholelithiasis in man. Part II. N Engl J Med 299, No. 22:1221, 1977

Boyer CA, Oehlberg SM: Interpretation and clinical relevance of liver function tests. Nurs Clin North Am 12, No. 2:275, 1977

Daniel E: Chronic problems in rehabilitation of patients with Laennec's cirrhosis. Nurs Clin North Am 12, No. 2:345, 1977

Dolan P: Conquering cirrhosis of the liver. Nursing '76 11:44, 1976

Douglass HO, Karakousis CP, Nava H: Guide to diagnosis of pancreatic cancer. Part 1. Hospital Medicine 13, No. 12:8, 1977

Douglass HO, Karakousis CP, Nava H: Guide to diagnosis of pancreatic cancer. Part 2. Hospital Medicine 14, No. 1:40, 1978

Gelfand MD: Gallbladder disease; Diagnostic guide. Hospital Medicine 15, No. 1:8, 1979

Hardison GM: Cirrhosis: Treating the ascites and encephalopathy. Med Times 107, No. 5:23, 1979

Hunter GR, Gaisford WD: Guide to the diagnosis and management of obstructive jaundice. Hospital Medicine 13, No. 6:82, 1977

Kaplowitz N: Cholestatic liver disease. Hosp Pract 13, No. 8:83, 1978

Katz J: How to manage the complications of chronic pancreatitis. Consultant 20, No. 5:141, 1980

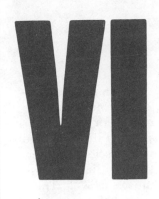

VI

Alterations in Neuromuscular Function

The nervous system in coordination with the endocrine system provides the means for all of the integrative aspects of life. It controls not only skeletal muscle movement, but the activity of cardiac and visceral smooth muscle as well. The nervous system makes possible the reception, integration, and perception of sensory information; it provides for memory and problem-solving; and it facilitates the adjustment to an ever-changing external environment. No part of the nervous system functions separately from other parts, and in the human, who is a thinking and feeling creature, the effects of emotion can exert a strong influence on both neural and hormonal control of body function. On the other hand, alterations in both neural and endocrine function (particularly at the biochemical level) can exert a strong influence on psychological behavior. Since the nervous system is subject to many different disorders, which are too numerous to be covered in this text, the content of the unit has been carefully selected to cover the following topics: 1) properties of nervous tissue, 2) structure and organization of the nervous system, 3) mechanisms of pain, 4) disorders of cerebral function, 5) alterations in motor function, and 6) chronic organic brain syndrome. Alterations in muscular function, while not presented separately, have been integrated throughout the chapters in this unit.

39

Robin L. Curtis

Properties of Nervous Tissue

To understand the brain and nervous system, we must understand how neurons are constructed, how they work, and how they communicate with one another. The human brain consists of several trillion cells, each of which must communicate with several thousand others. The average nerve cell ranges in size from 2/100 mm to 4/100 mm, and a synapse measures no more than 1/1000 mm.[1]

This chapter is divided into two parts: the first describes the cells of the nervous system and their

response to injury, and the second describes the generation and transmission of nerve impulses.

Neurons have branching cytoplasmic-filled processes, the dendrites and the axons, which project from the cell body and which are unique to the nervous system. The axonal processes are particularly designed for rapid communication between other neurons and the many body structures that are innervated by the nervous system. *Afferent*, or *sensory*, neurons carry information to the CNS (Fig. 39-1). *Efferent*, or *motor*, neurons carry information away from the CNS (Fig. 39-2). Interspersed between the afferent and efferent neurons is a network of *interconnecting neurons*, which serve to modulate and control the body's response to changes in the

Figure 39–1. Diagram of a typical afferent neuron that carries information from surface receptors (in this case the skin) to the CNS. The cell body and axons are in the PNS, while the central axon penetrates into the CNS wherein myelin is provided by oligodendroglial cells. (From Chaffee EE, Lytle IM: Basic Physiology and Anatomy, 4th ed. Philadelphia, JB Lippincott, 1980)

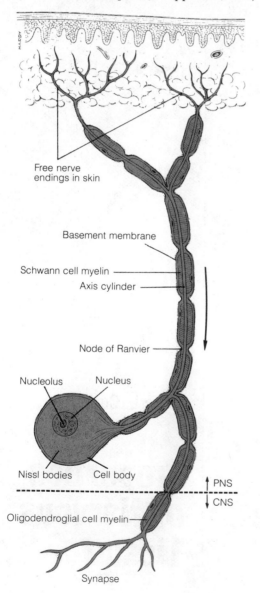

Figure 39–2. Myelinated efferent neuron, with axon entering the PNS to innervate skeletal muscle cells. (From Chaffee EE, Lytle IM: Basic Physiology and Anatomy, 4th ed. Philadelphia, JB Lippincott, 1980)

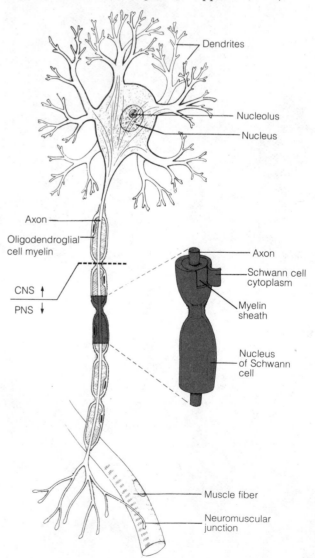

internal and external environments. In the human, who is a thinking and feeling creature, these interconnecting networks facilitate the establishment of response patterns and allow for the storage of information upon which learning and memory are based. Learning permits the modification of response patterns and allows for adaptation to an ever-changing environment. Complex neural networks provide the means for subjective experiences, such as perception and emotion. These also provide for intelligence, judgment, and anticipation of events.

:Nervous Tissue Cells

Nervous tissue contains two types of cells—neurons and supporting cells. The neurons are the functional cells of the nervous system. Neurons exhibit membrane excitability and conductivity, and secrete neuromediators and hormones, such as epinephrine and antidiuretic hormone. The *supporting cells*, such as the Schwann cells in the PNS and the glial cells in the CNS, function to *protect* the nervous system and *supply nourishment* for the neurons.

Neurons

Neurons have three distinct parts—the cell body and its cytoplasmic-filled processes, the dendrites and the axons. These processes form the functional connections, or synapses, with other nerve cells, with receptor cells, or with effector cells.

The *cell body*, or *soma*, contains a large, vesicular nucleus and one or more distinct nucleoli, a well-developed endoplasmic reticulum with ribosomes. The nucleus has the same DNA code content that is present in other cells of the body. The nucleoli, which are composed of both DNA and RNA, are associated with protein synthesis. There are large masses of ribosomes, which are prominent in many neurons. These acidic RNA masses, which are involved in protein synthesis, stain as dark *Nissl* bodies with basic histological stains (see Fig. 39-2).

The *dendrites* (treelike) are multiple, branched extensions of the nerve body; they are afferent in nature and conduct information *toward* the cell body. The dendrites and cell body are studded with *synaptic terminals* from axons and dendrites of other neurons (Fig. 39-3).

The *axon* is a long efferent process that projects from the cell body and that carries impulses away from the cell. There is usually only one axon to a nerve cell. Most axons undergo multiple branching, resulting in many axonal terminals. The cytoplasm of the cell body extends to fill both the dendrites and the axon (see Fig. 39-1 and 39-2). The reader will note that there are no Nissl bodies in the *axon hillock*, which is the point where the axon joins the cell body. The proteins and other materials that are used by the axon are synthesized in the cell body and then flow down the axon through its cytoplasm.

The cell body of the neuron is equipped for a high level of metabolic activity. This is necessary since the cell body must synthesize the cytoplasmic

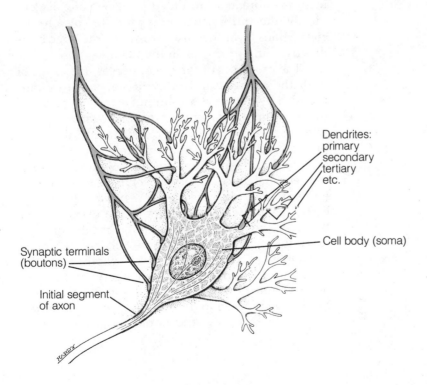

Figure 39–3.   Synaptic terminals in contact with the dendrites and cell body of an efferent neuron. (From Chaffee EE, Lytle IM: Basic Physiology and Anatomy, 4th ed. Philadelphia, JB Lippincott, 1980)

Dendrites:
primary
secondary
tertiary
etc.

Cell body (soma)

Synaptic terminals
(boutons)

Initial segment
of axon

and membrane constituents that are required for maintaining the function of the axon and its terminals. Some of these axons extend for a distance of 1 m to 1.5 m and have a volume that is sometimes 200 to 500 times greater than the cell body itself. An active process, called axonal flow, serves as a transport and communication system between the various parts of the axon and cell body. It moves amino acids, polypeptides, and other substances through the axon. A reverse axonal flow also exists and serves to transport materials from the axonal terminals back to the cell body. It is believed that the process of axonal flow not only facilitates the movement of metabolites between the cell body and the axonal terminals, but also serves as an internal communication system between the two parts of the neuron. In secretory neurons, such as those in the hypothalamic pituitary stalk, axonal flow carries antidiuretic hormone or oxytocin from the cell body to terminals in the posterior pituitary, where these hormones are released.

Figure 39–4.   The Schwann cell migrates down a larger axon to a bare region, settles down and encloses the axon in a fold of its plasma membrane. It then rotates around and around, wrapping the axon in many layers of plasma membrane, with most of the Schwann cell cytoplasm squeezed out. The resultant thick, multiple layered coating around the axon is called myelin.

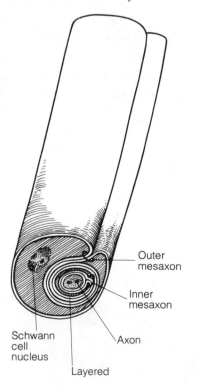

Outer mesaxon

Inner mesaxon

Schwann cell nucleus

Axon

Layered

Supporting Cells

Supporting cells of the nervous system, the Schwann cells of the PNS, and the several types of glial cells of the CNS, provide the neurons with protection and nourishment. The supporting cells segregate the neurons into isolated metabolic compartments, which are required for normal neural function. Together with the tightly joined endothelial cells of the capillaries in the CNS, these supporting cells may contribute to what is called the blood brain barrier. This term is used to emphasize the impermeability of the nervous system to large and potentially harmful molecules. In addition, the many-layered myelin wrappings of the Schwann cells of the PNS and the oligodendroglia of the CNS provide the myelin sheath segments that serve to increase the velocity of nerve impulse conduction in the axons having larger diameters.

Normally, the nerve cell bodies in the peripheral nervous system are collected into *ganglia*, such as the dorsal root and autonomic ganglia. Each of the cell bodies and processes of the peripheral nerves is surrounded or enclosed in cellular sheaths of supporting cells. The cells that surround the ganglion cells are called *satellite cells*. The satellite cells secrete a basement membrane that apparently protects the cell body from diffusion of large molecules. Collagen, secreted by fibroblasts, protects the nerve from mechanical forces. Thus, in the PNS, all parts of a neuron and its supporting cells are surrounded by an *endoneural sheath* made up of continuous basement membrane surrounded by layers of collagen. Finally, the entire ganglion is protected by a heavy collagenous layer that also surrounds the large bundles of neural processes in the PNS.

The processes of the larger nerves, the axons of both the afferent and efferent neurons, are surrounded by the plasma membrane and cytoplasm of the Schwann cells, which are close relatives of the satellite cells. The Schwann cell surrounds the nerve process and then twists many times in "jelly-roll" fashion (Fig. 39-4). The Schwann cells line up along the neuronal process, and each of these cells, in turn, forms its own discrete *myelin segment*. The end of each myelin segment attaches to the plasma membrane of the neuronal process by means of tight junctions. Successive Schwann cells are separated by short gaps, the *nodes of Ranvier*, where the myelin is missing. The nodes of Ranvier serve to increase nerve conduction by allowing the impulse to jump from node to node in a process called *saltatory conduction*. In this way, the impulse can travel more rapidly through the extracellular fluid than it could if it were required to move systematically along the entire nerve process. This increased conduction velocity greatly reduces reaction time, or time between the application of a stimulus and the subsequent motor response. The short reaction time that occurs when there is a rapid conduction velocity is of particular importance in peripheral nerves with long distances (sometimes 1 m to 2 m) for conduction between the CNS and distal effector organs (Fig. 39-5).

In addition to its role in increasing conduction velocity, the myelin sheath aids in nourishing the neuronal process. Since there are essentially no glycogen stores within the cytoplasm of the neuron, the major source of energy for the membrane of the neuronal process must be supplied by the supporting cells, in this case the myelin sheath, or from the vascular system at the nodes of Ranvier. In some pathologic conditions, the myelin may degenerate or be destroyed, leaving a section of "bare" axonal process that eventually dies unless remyelination takes place. Thus, the metabolic intervention of the supporting cells is essential for the long-term survival of the neuron and its processes.

Each of the end-to-end series of Schwann cells is enclosed within a continuous tube of basement membrane, which is surrounded by a multiple-layered collagen-rich *endoneurial tube* (Fig. 39-6). These endoneurial tubes are bundled together with blood vessels and lymphatics into nerve *fascicles*, which are surrounded by a collagenous *perineural sheath*. Usually, several fascicles are further surrounded by the heavy, protective *epineural sheath* of the peripheral nerve. The protective layers that surround the peripheral nerve processes are continuous

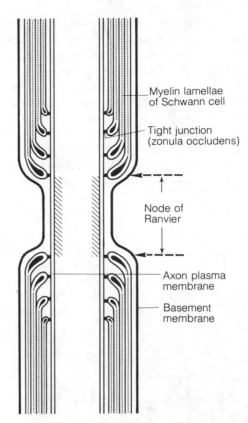

Figure 39-5. Schematic drawing of a longitudinal section through a node of a myelinated axon of the PNS. Tight junctions between myelin lamellae of the Schwann cell and the axon plasma membrane seal in the intracellular fluids within the internodal region. Extracellular fluids of the PNS communicate directly with the bare axon at the node. In the CNS, no basement membrane is present surrounding the internode and nodal regions.

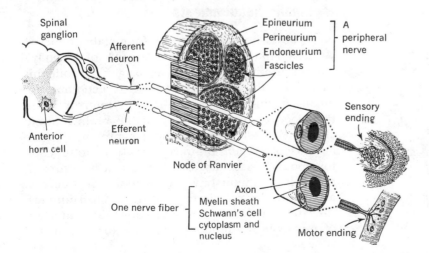

Figure 39-6. Peripheral nerve sheaths. The heavy connective tissue epineurium sheathes the whole nerve trunk. The perineurium sheathes bundles of axons or fasciculi. A large fasciculus is enlarged and cut away to illustrate its internal structure and two smaller fasciculi at the bottom of the diagram. The innermost connective tissue layer, the endoneurium, is made up of several layers of connective tissue fibers and fibrocytes that surround each individual "fiber" or myelinated axon. Unmyelinated fibers are not visible at this magnification. (From Chaffee EE, Lytle IM: Basic Physiology and Anatomy, 4th ed. Philadelphia, JB Lippincott, 1980)

with the connective tissue capsule of the sensory endings and the connective tissue that surrounds the effector structures, such as the skeletal muscle cell. Centrally, the connective tissue layers continue along the dorsal and ventral roots of the nerve and fuse with the meninges that surround the spinal cord and brain. The endoneurial tube does not penetrate the CNS. Absence of these tubular collagenous structures is thought to be a major factor in the less-effective axonal regeneration that occurs within the CNS as compared with the PNS.

Figure 39–7.   Diagram showing the supporting cells of the nervous system: a row of oligodendroglial cells is seen on the left, and a fibrous astrocyte on the right. (Modified from Penfield W: Brain 47:430, 1924. From Ham A, Cormack DH: Histology, 8th ed. Philadelphia, JB Lippincott, 1979)

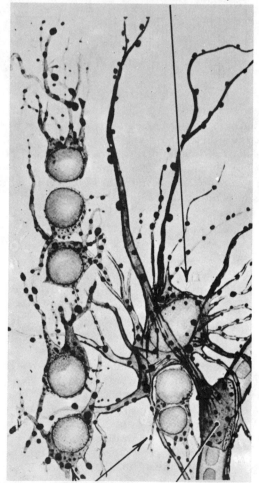

Fibrous astrocyte

Oligodendroglial cells

Perivascular foot on blood vessel

The supporting cells of the CNS consist of the neuroglial cells—oligodendroglia, astroglia, and microglia—and the ependymal cells.

The *oligodendroglial cells* form the myelin for the CNS. Instead of forming a single myelin segment for each neuron, these cells reach out with several processes, each wrapping around a different axon, and form a multilayered myelin segment around each axon (Fig. 39-7). The coverings of the nerve processes in the CNS also function in speeding the velocity of nerve conduction in a manner similar to that of the peripheral myelinated fibers. *Myelin* has a high lipid content, which gives it a *whitish* color, and thus the name *white matter* is given to the masses of myelinated fibers of the spinal cord and brain.

A second type of glial cell, the *astroglia*, is particularly prominent in the *gray matter*, or more central portion of the brain. These large cells have many processes, some reaching to the surface of the capillaries, others reaching to the surface of the nerve cells, and still others filling most of the intercellular space of the CNS (see Fig. 39-7). The astrocytic linkage between the blood vessels and the neurons may provide a transport mechanism for the exchange of oxygen, carbon dioxide, metabolites, and so on. The astrocytes are capable of filling their cytoplasm with microfibrils, and masses of these cells form the special type of scar tissue that develops in the CNS when brain tissue is destroyed.

A third type of glial cell, the *microglia*, is really a *phagocytic cell* (histiocyte) that migrates into the CNS and is available for cleaning up debris following cellular damage and death.

The ependymal cells line the ventricular system and the choroid plexus. These cells are involved in the production of *cerebral spinal fluid*.

Metabolic Requirements

Nervous tissue has a high need for metabolic energy. Although the brain comprises only 2% of the body's weight, it consumes 20% of its oxygen. Despite this high need, the brain cannot store oxygen nor can it engage in anaerobic metabolism. An interruption in the blood or oxygen supply to the brain leads to clinically observable signs and symptoms. In the absence of oxygen, brain cells continue to function for about 10 seconds. Unconsciousness occurs almost simultaneously when cardiac arrest occurs, and death of brain cells begins within 4 to 6 minutes. Interruption of blood flow also leads to accumulation of metabolic by-products that are toxic to neural tissue.

Glucose is the major fuel source for the nervous system, yet the nervous system has no provisions for storing glucose. Unlike muscle cells, it has no glycogen stores and must rely on glucose from the blood or glycogen stores of supporting cells. Persons receiving insulin for diabetes may experience signs of neural dysfunction and unconsciousness (insulin reaction or shock) when blood glucose drops due to an insulin excess.

Nerve Injury and Regeneration

Neurons exemplify the general principle that the more specialized the function of a cell type, the less able it is to regenerate. In neurons, cell division ceases by the time of birth and from then on the cell body of a neuron is unable to divide and replace itself. Although the entire neuron cannot be replaced, it is often possible for the axon of peripheral nerves to regenerate as long as the cell body remains viable.

When a peripheral nerve is destroyed by a crushing force or by a cut that penetrates the nerve, the portion of the nerve fiber that is separated from the cell body rapidly undergoes degenerative changes at the same time that the central stump and cell body of the nerve are able to survive (Fig. 39-8). Since the cell body synthesizes the material required for nourishing and maintaining the axon, it is likely that the loss of these materials results in the degeneration of the separated portion of the nerve fiber.

Following injury, the Schwann cells that are distal to the site of damage are also able to survive, but their myelin degenerates in a process called *wallerian degeneration*. The Schwann cells assist other phagocytic cells in the area in the clean-up of the debris caused by the degenerating axon and myelin. As they remove the debris, the Schwann cells multiply and fill the "empty" endoneurial tube. At this point, nothing further happens, unless a regenerating nerve fiber penetrates into the endoneurial tube, in which case, the Schwann cells reform the myelin segments around the fiber.

Meanwhile, the cell body of the neuron responds to the loss of part of its nerve fiber by shifting into a phase of greatly increased protein and lipid synthesis. It does this by dispersing the masses of ribosomes, which stain as Nissl granules. They cease to be stainable and disappear in a process called *chromatolysis*. In the process, the nucleus moves away from the axonal side of the cell body, as though displaced by the active synthetic apparatus of the cell. These changes reach their height within

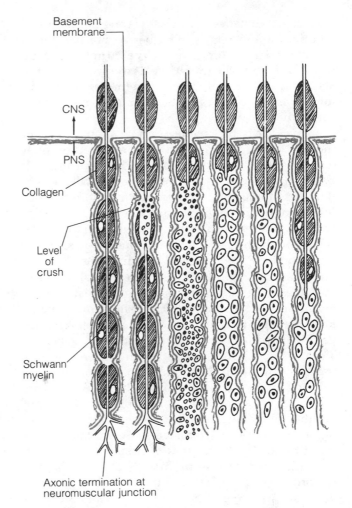

Figure 39–8. Diagram showing the changes that occur in a nerve fiber that has been severed and then regenerates.

about 10 days of injury and continue until regrowth of the nerve fiber ceases.

In the process of regeneration, the injured nerve fiber develops one or more new branches, which grow into the developing scar tissue. If a crushing injury has occurred and the endoneurial tube is intact through the trauma area, the outgrowing fiber will grow back down this tube to the structure that was originally innervated by the neuron. If, however, the injury involves the severing of a nerve, then the outgrowing branch must come in contact with its original endoneurial tube if it is to be reunited with its original receptor sites. The rate of outgrowth of regenerating nerve fibers is about 1 mm to 2 mm per day so that the recovery of conduction to a target structure depends not only on regrowth into the proper endoneurial tube, but also on the distance involved. It can take weeks or months for the regrowing fiber to reach the end organ and for communicative function to be re-established. Further time is required for the Schwann cells to form new myelin segments and for the axon to recover its original diameter and conduction velocity.

The successful regeneration of a nerve fiber in the PNS depends upon many factors. If a nerve fiber is destroyed relatively close to the neuronal cell body, the chances are that the nerve cell will die, and if it does, it will not be replaced. If a crushing type of injury has occurred, partial and often full recovery of function occurs. A cutting type of trauma to a nerve is an entirely different matter. Connective tissue scar forms rapidly at the wound site and when it does, only the most rapidly regenerating axonal branches are able to get through to the intact distal endoneurial tubes. A number of scar-inhibiting agents have been used in an effort to reduce this hazard but have met with only moderate success. In another attempt to improve nerve regeneration, various types of tubular implants have been placed to fill longer gaps in the endoneurial tube. The most successful of these has been a transplanted section of another peripheral nerve or a section of cadaver nerve. The latter is irradiated to destroy all cells in order to reduce the sources of tissue rejection. Perhaps the most difficult problem is the alignment of the proximal and distal endoneurial tubes such that a regenerating fiber can return down its former tube and innervate its former organ. This problem is similar to realigning a large telephone cable that has been cut, in such fashion that all of the wires are reconnected exactly as before the separation. An efferent nerve fiber that formerly innervated a skeletal muscle, which regrows down an endoneurial tube formerly occupied by an afferent fiber, will stop growing, and eventually its cell body will die. Likewise, a sensory fiber that ends up growing down an endoneurial tube that connects with a skeletal muscle fiber will undergo the same fate. If, however, these fibers grow down endoneurial tubes that innervate the appropriate type of target organ, reinnervation and function may return, even though the fibers have "changed places." Under the best of conditions, a 10% regeneration to the appropriate organ is considered a success once a peripheral nerve has been severed. Even so, considerable function will return with this amount of reinnervation.

In summary, nervous tissue is composed of two types of cells, neurons and supporting cells. Neurons are composed of three parts: a cell body which controls cell activity, the dendrites which conduct information to- *ward the cell body, and the axon which carries impulses from the cell body. The supporting cells consist of the Schwann cells of the PNS and the glial cells of the CNS. The supporting cells protect and nourish the neurons and aid in segregating them into isolated compartments, which is necessary for normal neuronal function. The function of the nervous system demands a high amount of metabolic energy. Glucose is the major fuel for the nervous system, and although the brain comprises only 2% of body weight, it consumes 20% of its oxygen supply. In general, neurons exemplify the principle that the more specialized the function of a cell type, the less its ability to regenerate. Although the entire neuron is unable to undergo mitosis and regenerate when injury occurs, it is often possible for the axons of the peripheral nervous system to regenerate provided the cell body remains viable. Axonal regeneration and reinnervation of target structures is much more likely to be successful in the PNS where connective tissue of the endoneurial tube provides a conduit to the target structures. Absence of connective tissue in the CNS decreases the likelihood of successful regeneration. Scar tissue, whether glial (CNS) or connective tissue (PNS), is a major deterrent to successful regeneration to the former target structures.*

:The Excitable Properties of Nervous Tissue

Neurons are classified as excitable tissue. This means that they are able to initiate and conduct electrical impulses. Basic to an understanding of nerve function is an appreciation of the events that occur during excitation and initiation of an action potential in a nerve or muscle cell. The discussion in this chapter focuses on action potentials that occur in nerves; the reader is asked to remember that many of the same type of phenomena occur in other types of excitable tissue, such as muscle.

An impulse, or action potential, represents the lateral, or lengthwise, movement of electrical charge along the plasma membrane. This phenomenon is based on the rapid flow, sometimes called *conductance*, of charged ions through the membrane in a progressive manner along the length of the neuron's axon. In excitable tissue, ions such as sodium, potassium, chloride, and calcium carry the electrical charges that are involved in the initiation and transmission of such impulses.

Membrane Potentials

There is a *potential* or difference in *electrical charge* that exists across the cell or plasma membrane in most, if not all, cells of the body. This difference is called the *membrane potential* and is measured in *millivolts* (mV). One mV is equal to one thousandth of a volt. Because the cell membrane is very thin, the charges that are of *opposite polarity (+ and −)* tend to become aligned on either side of the membrane (Fig. 39-9). By convention, the resting membrane potential is written with a minus (−) sign, indicating that the inside of the membrane is negative, or has less charge than the outside of the membrane. The membrane potential is analogous to the voltage difference (in this case, 6 or 12 volts) that is present across the + and − terminals of a car battery. The ability of excitable tissue to exhibit rapid changes, within milliseconds (mSec), or thousandths of a second, in the membrane potential allows for the initiation and transmission of action potential.

The membrane potential is determined by three factors: the polarity of the ions on either side of the membrane, the concentration of charge across the membrane, and the permeability of the membrane for the flow of the current-carrying ions, such as sodium and potassium. It is thought that there are *pores or channels* in the cell membrane through which the *current-carrying ions flow* and that the sodium and potassium ions use different channels as they move through the membrane. It is also thought that these channels are guarded by *electrically charged "gates"* that open or close with changes in the membrane potential (Fig. 39-10). In the resting, or unexcited, state the membrane is more permeable to the flow of the intracellular potassium ions than it is to that of the extracellular sodium ions. This leads to a continual movement of positively charged ions to the outside of the membrane. As a result, there is a minute excess of positive charge that accumulates along the outside of the membrane.

The *ATP driven sodium−potassium membrane pump removes sodium from the inside of the cell, returns potassium to the inside of the cell,* and is essential for generating the resting membrane potential. This pump actively removes sodium that has entered the cell during the resting state; it aids in the re-establishment of the resting membrane potential following an action potential or any change of these ions between the inside and outside of the membrane.

Excitability

When charges of opposite polarity (+ and −) are aligned across the membrane, it is said to be *polarized*. The changes that occur in the membrane of excitable tissue during an action potential can be divided into three phases—the resting or polarized state, depolarization, and repolarization (Fig. 39-11).

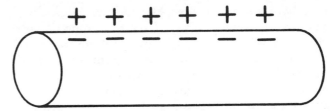

Figure 39–9.   Alignment of charge along the cell membrane.

The *resting membrane potential* is characterized by the relatively low permeability of the membrane to the rapid flow of charged ions. During this phase, there is about 70 mV less charge on the inside of the membrane (−70 mV) as compared to the outside. This difference in concentration of charge is necessary for the establishment of current flow once the membrane becomes permeable to the flow of charged ions.

The *threshold potential* (about −60 mV) represents the membrane potential at which the neuron is stimulated to fire. Stimuli that excite a neuron produce marked increases in membrane permeability and an increased flow of sodium through the membrane, causing it to become less negative and moving it toward the threshold potential. When the

Figure 39–10.   A hypothetical model of a sodium channel through the plasma membrane of an axon. A narrow pore (0.3 × 0.5 nm) with negatively charged wall provides selectivity to hydrated sodium ions. When the gate is opened during the initial stage of depolarization, the flow of sodium is greatly increased.

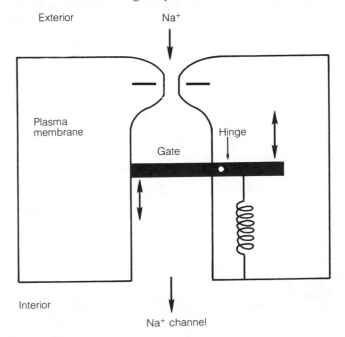

threshold level is reached, the sodium gates swing open and there is a rapid inflow of positively charged sodium ions through the membrane and into the cell. In neurons, the sodium ion gate remains open for only about a quarter of a millisecond, then closes quickly. During this period, the membrane potential rapidly shifts toward zero and beyond so that the membrane is positively charged. At the same time, a slower operating increase in outflow of potassium ions moves the potential back toward zero. Once a neuron reaches the minimal threshold for excitation, it is committed to fire and its response will be maximal. This is called the *all or none law*.

Depolarization represents the phase of the action potential during which the membrane is highly permeable to the sodium ions. During this phase, there is reversal of the membrane potential and the inside of the membrane becomes positive (about +20 mV).

Figure 39–11. Diagram of the time course of the action potential recorded at one point of an axon with one electrode inside and one on the outside of the plasma membrane. The rising part of the action potential is called the spike. The rising phase plus approximately the first half of the repolarization phase is equal to the absolute refractory period. The remaining portion of the repolarization phase to the resting membrane potential is equal to the negative after potential. Hyperpolarization is equal to the positive after potential.

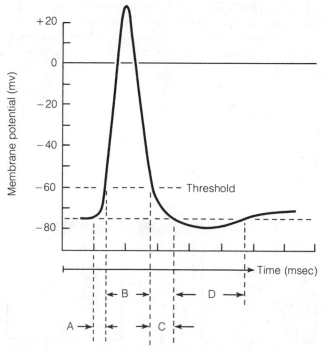

A = Generator potential that exceeds threshold
B = Absolute refractory period (active potential and partial recovery)
C = Negative-relation refractory period
D = Positive-relation refractory period

The third phase of the action potential is called *repolarization*. During this phase, the polarity of the resting membrane potential is re-established. This is accomplished as sodium permeability quickly returns to normal, while potassium permeability increases. The outflowing positively charged potassium ions return the membrane potential toward negativity. The sodium gates close. The sodium–potassium pump gradually re-establishes the resting ionic concentrations on each side of the membrane.

The membrane of excitable tissue must be sufficiently repolarized before it can be re-excited. In the process of repolarization, the membrane remains refractory (will not fire) until the repolarization is about one-third complete. This period of approximately one-half millisecond is called the *absolute refractory period*. There is an additional period of time during the recovery period in which the membrane can be excited, but only by a stronger-than-normal stimulus. This period is called the *relative refractory period*.

The excitability of a neuron or muscle fiber depends on the amount of change that must occur in the membrane potential to reach the threshold level needed for initiation of an action potential. When the resting membrane potential becomes extremely negative, the membrane is said to be hyperpolarized (Fig. 39-11). When this happens, re-excitation becomes more difficult or does not occur. *Hypopolarization*, on the other hand, represents the situation in which the resting membrane potential *becomes less negative*. When it approaches the threshold potential, the membrane becomes extremely excitable and may undergo spontaneous depolarization.

Alterations in membrane excitability. There are a number of factors that alter membrane excitability. Among these are (1) changes in the resting membrane potential and (2) change in the permeability of the membrane.

Serum levels of potassium exert a strong influence on repolarization (and the resting membrane potential) of excitable tissue. In situations in which there is a decrease in serum levels of potassium, the resting membrane potential becomes more negative, and nerve and muscle fibers become hyperpolarized, sometimes to the extent that they cannot be re-excited. *Familial periodic paralysis* is a hereditary condition in which extracellular potassium levels periodically fall to low levels, causing muscle paralysis (Chap. 22). An increase in potassium, on the other hand, interferes with the repolarization of the membrane; it causes hypopolarization, and the resting membrane potential moves closer to threshold levels and then to zero. When this happens, the strength of the action potential is decreased. This is because there is a decrease in the concentration of charge between the two sides of the membrane, and consequently less charge is available to move through the membrane during each action potential. Should the resting potential be reduced so that it approaches zero, the membrane will remain depolarized. This situation is similar to what happens when the car battery goes "dead" and needs to be recharged. Elevations in serum potassium exert their greatest effect on the conduction system of the heart. The force of cardiac contractions becomes weaker until eventually repolarization is inadequate to maintain excitability, and the heart stops in diastole.

Neural excitability is markedly altered by changes in membrane permeability. Calcium ions decrease membrane permeability to sodium ions. If there are not sufficient calcium ions available, the permeability of the membrane becomes increased and, as a result, membrane excitability increases—sometimes to the extent that spontaneous muscle movements (tetany) occur. *Local anesthetic agents* (such as procaine or cocaine) act directly on the membrane to decrease its permeability to sodium.

Impulse conduction

During the depolarization process, the rapid flow of sodium ions induces local currents which travel through the adjacent cell membrane and this, in turn, causes the sodium channels in this part of the membrane to open, and depolarization occurs. Thus, the impulse moves progressively along the nerve, depolarizing the membrane ahead of the action potential. The impulse is conducted longitudinally along the membrane from one part of the axon to other parts. In unmyelinated fibers, this sequence of events moves the impulse progressively along the axon. Conduction in myelinated fibers follows a similar pattern, but because of the high resistance in the myelinated segments, the current flow jumps from node to node (saltatory conduction) as was described earlier. This is a more rapid process, and myelinated axons conduct up to 50 times faster than unmyelinated fibers.

Neurotransmitters

Neurotransmitters, or neuromediators, are chemical messengers of the nervous system. These transmitters are synthesized in the cell body of the neuron and released from terminals of the axon upon arrival of an action potential. They exert their effect as they attach to *transmitter-specific membrane receptors* on other cells, particularly those of other neurons.

The distinction betweeen the neurons and endocrine cells is somewhat blurred. Many neurons, such as those of the adrenal medulla, secrete neuromediators into the blood stream just as endocrine cells do.

The neurotransmitters are rapidly removed from the synaptic cleft following their release (Fig. 39-12). Some transmitters, such as acetylcholine, are hydrolyzed by enzymes, in this case, acetylcholinesterase. Other mediators, such as epinephrine, are largely taken up into the presynaptic nerve terminals and are reused or diffuse away.

Neuromediators exert their action through membrane receptors that are similar to those discussed for hormones in Chapter 32. The action of a neurotransmitter is determined by the receptor site. For example, the neuromediator acetylcholine is excitatory when it is released at a myoneural junction and it is inhibitory when it is released into the sinoatrial node of the heart. Some neuromediators act as modulators rather than initiators (or inhibitors) of a neural action.

Recently, it has been found that neurons possess receptor sites for many *hormones*. Receptors, for example, which mediate indirect steroid effects have been characterized in brain and pituitary tissue for four out of the five classes of steroid hormones: estrogens, androgens, progestin, and glucocorticoids.[1] These receptors are similar to those that have been identified on nonneuronal cells.

Although neurons respond to circulating neuromediators, communication between neurons has particular advantages over communication with the endocrine system. This is because neurons have axonal processes that extend and secrete neurotransmitters directly on the surface of a target cell. In this way, selected neurons are stimulated and others with the same type of receptor sites remain unstimulated. This discreteness in location of neural secretion is quite different from the diffuse action of the endocrine hormones, which are released into the blood stream and which have contact with *all* cells of the body with the appropriate receptors that are perfused with blood containing the hormone; it allows for much more complex circuitry to be established in the nervous system than could occur without this specificity.

Sensory Receptors

Information from the internal and external environment reaches the nervous system through a variety of sensory receptors. Receptors from the *special senses* provide the body with vision, hearing, smell, and taste. Other types of receptors provide input needed for maintaining normal levels of blood gases, blood pressure, position sense, muscle tone, and others.

These receptors receive and transform energy from the environment into an action potential in an afferent neuron, which carries the impulse to the CNS. There are two types of impulses that contribute to sensory input to the CNS. One is the *local potential* of the receptor and the other is the *propagated afferent nerve impulse*.

In order for an impulse to be generated in a receptor, the stimulus must be appropriate: the adequate stimulus is the form of energy which, at the lowest intensity, will result in an action potential (*e.g.*, light for photoreceptors and sound for audioreceptors) and in adequate intensity to trigger propagated action potentials carried to the CNS by the afferent neuron. Sensory receptors may be the terminal part of the neuron (naked nerve endings of pain fibers), or they may be associated with non-neural tissue, such as the connective tissue matrix of the pacinian corpuscle that surrounds the neuron, or they may be separate sensory cells which are innervated by the afferent neurons (glomus chemoreceptors of the carotid body, hair cells of the auditory apparatus, and so on). The sensory cells are very sensitive to a particular type of energy (adequate stimulus). For example, thermoreceptors respond to temperature changes; photoreceptors in the retina of the eye respond to light waves; mechanoreceptors, such as those in the skin and subcutaneous tissue, sense changes in pressure and touch; and chemoreceptors in the taste buds respond to changes in the chemical composition of food. The sensory input to the brain is influenced not only by the selective nature of the various receptors, but by the number, frequency, and pattern of impulses. The intensity and pattern of stimulation provide a coding system whereby information about the internal and external environment is transmitted to the central nervous system. At high energy levels almost all receptors will respond to other forms of stimuli. Pressure on the eyeball, for example, is experienced as light.

Some receptors discharge continuously as long as the stimulus is applied; these are the *slowly adapting receptors*. Other receptors discharge only at the time the stimulus is initially applied and then cease to discharge even though the stimulus continues; these are the *rapidly adapting receptors*. Slowly adapting receptors provide information about steady-state conditions, whereas rapidly adapting receptors are designed for sensing changing conditions in the environment.

Synapse

A chemical synapse serves as a *one-way* communication link between neurons. The *synapse* consists of *presynaptic* and *postsynaptic* terminals. The synaptic cleft separates the pre- and post-synaptic membranes. The presynaptic terminal secretes neurotransmitters into the synaptic cleft. Diffused transmitters unite with receptors on the postsynaptic membrane, and this causes either excitation or inhibition of the postsynaptic neuron by producing hypopolarization or hyperpolarization, respectively (Fig. 39-12).

A neuron's cell body and dendrites are covered by thousands of synapses, any or many of which can be active at any moment in time. Because of this rich synaptic capability, each neuron resembles a little computer in which there are many circuits of neurons, which interact with each other. It is the complexity of these interactions that gives the system its "intelligence" in terms of the subtle integrations that are involved in producing behavioral responses, and it is the complexity of these interactions that makes the prediction of stimulus-response relationships somewhat hazardous in the absence of a millisecond-to-millisecond knowledge of the excitatory and inhibitory activity that takes place on the surfaces of each neuron in a functional circuit. It is amazing, with billions of these little computers capable of becoming involved in such a response, that

Figure 39–12.   Diagram of synapse, showing the pre- and postsynaptic neuron. (From Chaffee EE, Lytle IM: Basic Physiology and Anatomy. 4th ed. Philadelphia, JB Lippincott, 1980)

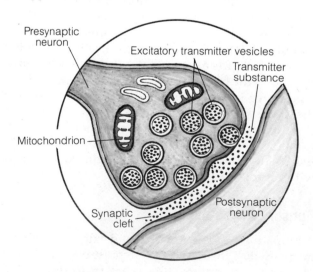

Presynaptic neuron

Excitatory transmitter vesicles

Transmitter substance

Mitochondrion

Synaptic cleft

Postsynaptic neuron

predictions are possible at all. It is even more astounding that the basic microcircuitry involved in the nervous system is reliably reproduced during the development of each new organism. To put it more dramatically, humans produce human babies that behave like human babies—not like baby rabbits or baby eagles.

There are several types of synapses. Axonic terminals of an afferent neuron can develop in close apposition to the dendrites (*axodendritic synapse*), to the cell body (*axosomatic synapse*), or the axon (*axo-axonic synapse*) of a CNS neuron. The mechanism of communication between the *presynaptic* axonic terminal and the *postsynaptic* neuron is similar in all three types of synapses. In all three, the action potential sweeps into the axonic terminals of the afferent neuron and triggers rapid secretion of neurotransmitter molecules from the axonic, or presynaptic, surface. Conversion of action potentials into secretion is called coupling and although it is not completely understood, it is believed that the release of calcium ions is involved.

The neuromediators are synthesized in the cytoplasm of the axonic terminal and are stored in small membrane-bound vesicles, the *synaptic vesicles*. Usually, the same transmitter compound is secreted from all axonic terminals of the same neuron. All afferent neurons do not, however, secrete the same neurotransmitter. Some neuromediators are rapidly inactivated by enzymes on the synaptic membranes. In synapses where inactivating enzymes are not present, the messenger molecules diffuse away from synaptic terminals, and then portions of these transmitter molecules may re-enter the presynaptic terminal to be reincorporated into a new transmitter.

During secretion, these vesicles of the presynaptic terminal move toward and fuse with the synaptic membrane and release their transmitter contents into the narrow *synaptic cleft*. The transmitter molecule diffuses through the intercellular fluid to the membrane of the postsynaptic neuron and unites with receptor sites that are specific for that particular transmitter. The combination of the neurotransmitter with the receptor sites causes partial depolarization of the postsynaptic membrane. This is called an *excitatory postsynaptic potential*, or *EPSP*. All afferent transmitters are excitatory to the CNS neurons with which they synapse.

The postsynaptic membrane region of any single dendrite-cell body synapse is not capable of inciting an action potential by itself. The inward depolarizing sodium ion current of the EPSP results in action currents back out the plasma membrane,

and the density of this outward current decreases with distance from the synapse. The outward current is especially strong in the *initial segment* of the neuron's axon, an area devoid of synaptic endings. It is at this initial segment that the action potential can be initiated (see Figs. 39-2 and 39-3). The currents resulting from any one EPSP (sometimes called a generator potential) are usually insufficient to pass threshold and thus cause depolarization to occur in the axon's initial segment. However, if several EPSPs occur simultaneously, the area of depolarization can become large enough and the currents at the initial segment can become strong enough to exceed the threshold potential and initiate a conducted action potential. This summation of depolarized areas is called *spatial summation*. The EPSPs can also summate and cause an action potential if they come in close temporal relation to each other. This temporal aspect of the occurrence of two or more EPSPs is called *temporal summation*.

Many CNS neurons possess hundreds or thousands of synapses on their dendritic and soma surfaces. Some of these synapses are *inhibitory* in the sense that the combination of their transmitter with receptor sites causes the local membrane to become hyperpolarized and decreases the probability of an action potential by the postsynaptic neuron. This is called an *inhibitory postsynaptic potential*, or *IPSP*. The IPSPs can also undergo spatial and temporal summation with each other and with EPSPs, reducing the effectiveness of the latter by a roughly algebraic summation. If the sum of EPSPs and IPSPs keeps the depolarization at the initial segment below threshold levels, the generation of an action potential does not occur.

The *spatial* and *temporal* summation required in the distribution and timing of synaptic activity serves as a sensitive and very complicated switch, requiring just the right combination of incoming activity before it releases its own message in the form of the action potential. The frequency of action potentials in the axon, on the other hand, is an all-or-none language (digital language), which can vary only as to presence or absence of such impulses and their frequency.

In summary, nervous tissue is able to initiate and conduct impulses, and is classified as excitable tissue. The excitable properties of nervous tissue rely on membrane properties which provide for separation of charges with opposite polarity on either side of the cell membrane, positive on the outside and negative on the inside. In the resting, or unexcited state, the nerve cell membrane is relatively impermeable to the flow of electrical charge.

The resting membrane potential is about −70 mV. The threshold potential represents a change in the membrane potential (usually to a −60 mV) which is sufficient to cause the nerve to fire. During the depolarization phase of the action potential, the membrane becomes highly permeable to the inward flow of sodium ions, causing the polarity across the membrane to become reversed, so that it is positive on the inside and negative on the outside. Repolarization represents the phase of the action potential during which the resting membrane polarity is re-established. During this phase potassium ions flow out of the cell and the sodium-potassium pump accelerates the extrusion of sodium ions from the cell. Receptors are special neuronal structures designed for providing the body with sensory input from the internal and external environments. Sensory receptors provide the body with hearing, vision, smell, and taste. Other receptors monitor blood gases, blood pressure, position sense, muscle tone, and other information. Neuromediators are chemical messengers which serve to control neuronal function; they selectively cause either excitation or inhibition of action potential generation. A synapse is a one-way communication link between neurons; it has both presynaptic and postsynaptic terminals. Neuromediators released from the presynaptic terminal of one neuron diffuse across the synaptic cleft and unite with receptor sites of the postsynaptic terminal of another neuron as a means of communicating information between the two neurons. Thus the neuron integrates the ongoing synaptic activity on its dendritic and soma surface, resulting in the production or nonproduction of an action potential. The latter travels rapidly along the cell's axon to trigger the release of transmitter substance on the postsynaptic surface of the next neuron in a circuit. This combination of integration of synaptic activity and rapid communication to discretely positioned sensory terminals permits the complex circuitry as well as rapid communication characteristic of neural tissue function.

Lastly, at present we have only scratched the surface as compared to what we may ultimately learn about the details of neuronal circuitry: how it is formed and how it is modified by internal and external environmental factors during development and maturation. The alterations that must occur in neuronal circuitry during learning and forgetting also are not yet understood.

:Study Guide

After you have studied this chapter, you should be able to meet the following objectives:

: : Name and describe the anatomy of the three parts of a neuron.

: : State the function of the supporting cells of the nervous system.

: : Describe the function of the Schwann cells with reference to the nodes of Ranvier.

: : State the purpose of saltatory conduction.

: : Describe the function of the myelin sheath.

: : Describe the consequences of an interruption to the brain's blood supply.

: : State a general principle related to cell regeneration.

: : Explain the sequence of events in chromatolysis.

: : Explain the rationale underlying the use of scar-inhibiting agents and tubular implants in regeneration of nerve fibers.

: : Define *conductance*.

: : State the determinants of the membrane potential.

: : Explain the *all or none law*.

: : Compare depolarization and repolarization.

: : Define *adequate stimulus*.

: : Describe the interaction of the presynaptic and the postsynaptic terminals.

: : Explain the occurrence of both spatial and temporal summation.

:Reference

1. Report on Convulsive and Neuromuscular Disorders to the National Advisory Neurological and Communicative Disorders and Stroke Council, p 103. National Institute of Health, National Institute on Communicative Disorders and Stroke, U.S. Department of Health, Education, and Welfare, Public Health Service, NIH Publication No. 79–1913

:Suggested Readings

Ganong WF: The nervous system. Los Altos, CA, Lange Medical Publications, 1977

Kandel ER, Schwartz JH: Principles of neural science. New York, Elsevier North-Holland, 1981

Schmidt RF (ed): Fundamentals of neurophysiology, ed. 2. New York, Springer-Verlag, 1978

Shephard GM: The synaptic organization of the brain, ed. 2. New York, Oxford University Press, 1979

40

Robin L. Curtis

Structure and Organization of the Nervous System

The nervous system is the most highly organized system in the body, regulating and controlling most of the other systems. Its functions are concerned with the reception of information from the internal and external environments, the transmission of information, and the integration of sensation and of effector responses. No computer of human design is able to process such an immense amount and variety of information with the same degree of precision, flexibility, and creativity as that found in the nervous system. Hundreds of billions of neurons are involved in these processes with all but a few million of them packed into the cavities of the cranium and spinal column.

This chapter is divided into three parts: (1) the development and structural organization of the nervous system, (2) the basic organization of the CNS, using somatic and autonomic systems as examples, and (3) brief consideration of the complex, higher-order, functional organization of the brain.

:Development and Structural Organization of the Nervous System

The nervous system can be divided into two parts—*the central nervous system* (CNS) and *the peripheral nervous system* (PNS). The CNS consists of the brain and spinal cord, which are located within the protected environment of the axial skeleton (cranium and spinal column). The PNS contains neurons and neuronal processes that are located outside the axial skeleton in the body wall (soma) and viscera. The basic design of the nervous system is for the concentration of computational and control functions within the CNS. In this design, the PNS functions as an input–output system for relaying input to the CNS and for transmitting output messages which control effector organs, such as muscles and glands, in the periphery. There are both somatic and visceral nerves. The *somatic nerves* innervate the skeletal muscle, and smooth muscle and glands of the skin and body wall. The *visceral nerves* supply the visceral organs of the body, transmitting information through the autonomic nerves in the PNS to control the smooth and cardiac muscle as well as the glands of the visceral organs. This visceral system is largely of reflex or "involuntary" function.

Hierarchy of Control

The development of the nervous system can be traced far back into evolutionary history, during which newer functional features were superimposed on more primitive ones. Greater complexity resulted from modification and enlargement of older organization and structures. In a moving organism, rapid reaction to environmental danger, to potential food sources, or to a sexual partner was required for survival of the species. Thus, the front, or rostral, end of the CNS became specialized as a means of sensing the external environment and controlling reactions to it. In time, the ancient organization, which is largely retained in the spinal cord segments, was expanded in the forward segments of the nervous system. Of these, the most forward have undergone the most radical modification and have developed into the forebrain: the diencephalon and the cerebral hemispheres. The dominance of the front end of the CNS is reflected in a hierarchy of control levels—brain stem over spinal cord, forebrain over brain stem. Because the newer functions were added on the outside of older functional systems and because the newer functions became concentrated at the rostral end of the nervous system, they are much more vulnerable to injury. These three principles—(1) no part of the nervous system functions independently of the other parts, (2) newer systems control older systems, and (3) the newer systems are more vulnerable to injury—form a basis for understanding many of the manifestations that occur when there is injury to or disease of the nervous system.

Development of the Nervous System

The central nervous system develops as a hollow tube, the cephalic portion of which becomes the brain and the more caudal part the spinal cord. In the process of development, the basic organizational pattern of the body is that of a longitudinal series of segments, each repeating the same fundamental organizational pattern: a body wall or *soma* containing the axial skeleton and neural tube, separated by a body cavity from the *viscera*, made up of the gut and its associated organs. Although the early muscular, skeletal, vascular, and excretory systems and the nerves that supply these parts have this segmental pattern (Fig. 40-1), it is the nervous system that most clearly retains this organization in the adult. The central nervous system and its associated peripheral nerves are thus made up of 43 or so segments, 33 of which form the spinal cord and spinal nerves, and 10 the brain and its cranial nerves.

On cross-section, the hollow embryonic neural tube can be divided into a central canal or ventricle that contains the cerebrospinal fluid and the wall of the tube. The latter develops into the gray or cellular portion and the white matter, the tract systems of the CNS (Fig. 40-2). The dorsal half of the gray matter is called the *dorsal horn*; it receives afferent nerve terminals and distributes and processes this incoming information. The ventral portion, or *ventral horn*, contains efferent neurons and is largely concerned with outward communication to the body segment and its effector organs, the muscles and glands of the body segment reached by the axons of ventral horn neurons. Many of the CNS neurons develop axons which grow longitudinally as the developing tract systems that intercommunicate between neighboring and distal segments of the neural tube. As this occurs, the neural tube becomes segmented with a repeating pattern of entering *afferent neuron axons*, forming the *dorsal roots* of each succeeding segmental nerve, and exiting *efferent neuron axons*, forming the *ventral roots* of each succeeding segmental nerve. The nerve cells in the gray matter are arranged longitudinally in *cell columns*, with nerve cells having similar functions being grouped together. The axons of the cell column neurons can project out into the white matter of the CNS, forming the longitudinal tract systems. Both the cell columns and the longitudinal tracts extend along the entire length of the nervous system (Fig. 40-2).

Structural Organization of the Nervous System

Association neurons of the dorsal horn.
The effectiveness of a CNS-mediated response to changed environmental conditions depends upon the functional integrity of the neurons and effector cells in

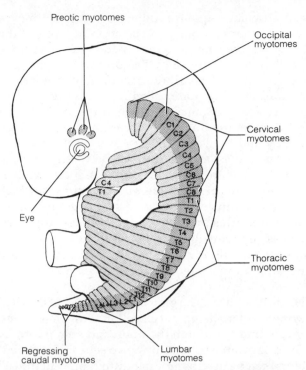

Figure 40–1. The developing muscular system in a 6-week-old embryo. The segmental muscle masses or myotomes, which give rise to most skeletal muscles, reflect the basic segmental organization of the body and head. Efferent cranial nerves innervating the myotomes of the head are as follows: preotic myotomes (nerves III, IV, and VI), and the occipital myotomes (XII). (After Moore K: The Developing Human. Philadelphia, WB Saunders, 1977)

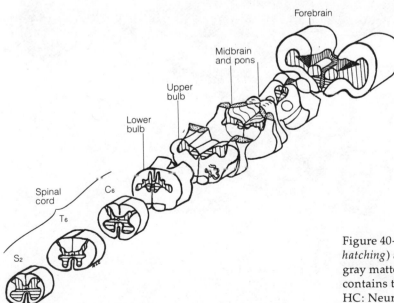

Figure 40–2. The adult human CNS. The dorsal (*vertical hatching*) and ventral (*horizontal hatching*) horns of the gray matter are surrounded by the white matter that contains the longitudinal tracts. (Adapted from Elliott HC: Neuroanatomy. Philadelphia, JB Lippincott, 1969)

the particular sequence, called a *reflex*, that moves from afferent neurons to association neurons of the dorsal and ventral gray matter to effector neurons and then to effector cells. The dorsal horn neurons that receive and distribute the afferent message in the cord and brain are called *input association neurons*. A group of small neurons in the ventral horn that provide the linkage between the CNS network activity and the lower motor neuron activation are called *output association neurons*. Between the input association neurons and the output association neurons are chains of small internuncial neurons, which are arranged in complex circuits. It is the internuncial neurons that provide the discreteness, appropriateness, and intelligence of responses to stimuli. Most of the billions of CNS cells in the spinal cord and brain gray matter are internuncial neurons.

The cell columns. The gray matter of each of the CNS segments is made up of cell columns, which extend longitudinally through the brain and spinal cord. A box of 24 colored soda straws (two sets of 12 different colors) can be used as an analogy to represent the cell columns. Using this analogy, each lateral half of the nervous system (right and left sides) is represented in mirror fashion by one set of the 12 colored straws. If these straws were cut crosswise (equivalent to a transverse section through the nervous system) at several places along their length, the spacial relationship between these straws would be repeated in each section.

The cell columns can be further grouped according to their location in the dorsal (posterior) and ventral (anterior) portions of the nervous system (Fig. 40-3). In the brain, the position of those cell columns is somewhat distorted by the developmental changes that occur. The columns in the dorsal horn of the CNS contain *input association neurons* for *afferent fibers entering* the central nervous system. The *ventral horn* contains cell columns of *output association cells and efferent neurons* concerned with control of the activity in fibers leaving the central nervous system. Our interest lies in two sets of association neurons, the *general somatic input association* (GSIA) neurons and the *general visceral input association* (GVIA) neurons. The GSIA neurons are con-

Figure 40–3. Cell columns of the central nervous system. The columns in the dorsal horn contain input association neurons: special sensory (SSIA), general sensory (GSIA), special visceral (SVIA), and general visceral (GVIA). The ventral horn contains the efferent neurons: the general visceral efferent (GVE), special visceral efferent (SVE), and general somite efferent (GSE).

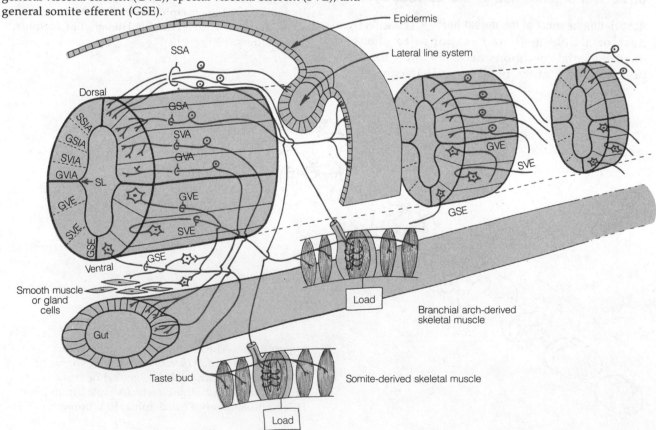

Table 40-1   The Segmental Nerves and Their Components

Segment	Segmental Nerve	GSA	GVA	GVE	GSE	Other	Innervation	Function
1	*Forebrain* I. Olfactory					SVA	Olfactory mucosa	Smell
2								
3	*Midbrain* V. Trigeminal—ophthalmic division					SSA	Extrinsic eye muscles; upper muscles of facial expression	Sensory input for eye movement control
		X					Skin on forehead, upper face, and conjunctiva	Reflexes and somesthesia
	III. Oculomotor			X			Sphincter of iris; ciliary muscle	Pupillary constriction, accommodation
					X		Extrinsic eye muscles	Motor innervation of eye muscles and lid
4	*Pons* V. Trigeminal—maxillary division					SSA	Muscles of facial expression	Sensory input for control of facial expression
		X					Skin, nose, upper jaw, nasal cavity	Somatic reflexes; somesthesia
	—mandibular					SSA	Muscles of mastication	Sensory input for control of mastication
		X					Skin of lower jaw, inside mouth, anterior ⅔ of tongue	Somatic reflexes; somesthesia
						SVE	Muscles of mastication, tensor, tympani	Mastication; protection of auditory apparatus
	IV. Trochlear				X		Extrinsic eye muscles	Control of superior oblique
5	*Caudal pons* VIII. Vestibular, cochlear					SSA	Vestibular end organs; organ of Corti	Vestibular reflexes and sensation; auditory reflexes and hearing
	—int. intermedius	X						Somesthesia
						SVA	Taste buds; anterior ⅔ tongue; palate	Gustation
			X				Nasopharynx	Sneeze reflex; sensation
				X			Nasopharynx; lacrimal gland	Lacrimation
	VII. Facial			X			Muscles of facial expression; stapedius	Facial expression; protective reflex for auditory apparatus
	VI. Abducens				X		Extrinsic eye muscle	Control lateral eye movement
6	*Middle medulla* IX. Glossopharyngeal					SSA	Pharyngeal muscle	Sensory input for movement control
		X					External ear; external acoustic meatus	Somesthesia
						SVA	Taste buds; posterior ⅓ tongue; oral pharynx	Gustation, particularly bitter
			X				Oral pharynx	Gag reflex; sensation
				X			Parotid salivary gland; pharyngeal mucosa	Salivation
						SVE	Pharyngeal muscle (stylopharyngeus)	Swallowing

(continued)

Table 40–1 The Segmental Nerves and Their Components (continued)

Segment	Segmental Nerve	GSA	GVA	GVE	GSE	Other	Innervation	Function
7,8,9,10	*Caudal medulla* X. Vagus					SSA	Pharyngeal, laryngeal muscles	Sensory input for movement control
		X					External ear; external acoustic meatus	Reflexes; somesthesia
						SVA	Taste buds: laryngeal pharynx, larynx	Gustation
			X				Laryngeal pharynx, larynx, trachea, bronchi, lung, esophagus, stomach, small intestine, ascending colon; ½ transverse colon	Input for reflexes; movement control of swallowing, phonation other
				X			Heart, gall bladder, liver, pancreas, spleen, kidney	Autonomic parasympathetic control of smooth muscle, cardiac muscle, and glands
						SVE	Pharyngeal, laryngeal muscles	Control of swallowing, phonation, other
	XII. Hypoglossal				X		Extrinsic, intrinsic muscles of tongue	Tongue reflexes and movements
Spinal Segmental								
C₁–C₄	*Upper cervical* C₁–C₄					SSA	Neck muscles	Sensory input for movement control
		X					Neck and back of head	Reflexes, somesthesia
	IX. Spinal accessory					SVE	Sternocleidomastoid; trapezius	Control of head, shoulder movement
	C₁–C₄				X		Neck muscles	Control of head; shoulder movement
C₅–C₈	*Lower cervical* C₅–C₈					SSA	Muscles of upper limb; pectoral muscles	Sensory input for movement control
		X					Upper limb	Reflexes; somesthesia
					X		Muscles of upper limb	Control of movement
T₁–L₂	*Thoracic, upper lumbar*					SSA	Muscles of thorax, abdomen, back	Sensory input for movement control
		X					Thorax, abdomen, back	Reflexes; somesthesia
			X				All of viscera	Input for visceral reflexes; sensation from stomach through transverse colon
				X			All of viscera; all of soma of body and head	Visceral reflexes; control of vasomotor, sweating, piloerection; all of body
					X		Muscles of thorax and back	Control of posture, movement
L₃–S₁	*Lower lumbar* S₁					SSA	Muscles of lower back and abdomen, lower limb	Sensory input for movement control
		X					Lower back, abdomen, lower limb	Reflexes; somesthesia

(continued)

Table 40–1   The Segmental Nerves and Their Components (continued)

Segment	Segmental Nerve	GSA	GVA	GVE	GSE	Other	Innervation	Function
					X		Muscles of lower back and lower limb	Control of posture and movement
S$_2$–S$_4$	*Sacral 2–4*					SSA	Muscles: perineum, genitalia, pelvic diaphragm	Sensory input for movement control
		X					Perineum, genitalia, pelvic diaphragm	Reflexes; somesthesia
			X				Distal half transverse colon; descending colon; rectum; pelvic viscera, including bladder, uterus, prostate	Visceral reflexes; visceral sensation; autonomic control of lower visceral organs
					X		Skeletal muscles; perineum; genitalia; pelvic diaphragm	Reflex and movement control
S$_5$, Co$_1$, Co$_2$	*Lower sacral, coccygeal*					SSA	Muscles of sacrum	Sensory input for movement control
		X					Lower sacrum; anus	Reflexes; somesthesia
					X		Skeletal muscles; lower sacrum	Postural and movement control

GSA: General Soma Afferent
SSA: Special Soma Afferent
GVA: General Visceral Afferent
SVA: Special Visceral Afferent
GVE: General Visceral Efferent (Autonomic)
SVE: Special Visceral Efferent (Branchial)
GSE: General Somatic Efferent

cerned with sensory input from the body wall and the GVIA neurons, with sensory input from the viscera. The efferent cell columns can also be subdivided into those containing efferent cells innervating skeletal muscle of the body wall—*general somite efferent* (GSE)—and those providing the first link in communication with smooth or cardiac muscle and glands—*general visceral efferent* (GVE), otherwise known as the *autonomic nervous system*. Other cell columns, such as those handling special somatic afferent activities, such as audition, or specialized visceral afferent information, such as taste (gustation), are not discussed in this text. Table 40-1 describes the segmental nerves and their components.

Longitudinal tracts.   The gray matter of the cell columns in the CNS is surrounded by bundles of myelinated and unmyelinated axons (white matter) that travel longitudinally along the length of the neural axis. This white matter can be divided into three layers—an inner, a middle layer, and an outer layer (Fig. 40-4). The inner, or *archi*, layer contains short fibers that project for a maximum of about five segments before re-entering the gray matter. The mid-

dle, or *paleo*, layer projects six or more segments. Both the archi and the paleo layer fibers have many branches, or *collaterals*, which enter the gray matter of intervening segments. The outer, or *neo*, layer contains large-diameter axons that can travel the entire length of the nervous system (Table 40-2).

The longitudinal layers are arranged in bundles. A fiber tract contains axons that have the same destination, origin, and function. These longitudinal tracts are named systematically to reflect their origin and destination, with the site of origin being named first and the site of destination second. For example, the spinothalamic tract originates in the spinal cord and terminates in the thalamus. The corticospinal tract originates in the cerebral cortex and ends in the spinal cord.

The inner layer.   The inner layer of white matter contains the axons of neurons of the gray matter that interconnect with neighboring segments of the nervous system. The axons of this layer permit the pool of motor neurons of several segments to work together as a functional unit. They also permit the afferent neurons of one segment to trigger reflexes

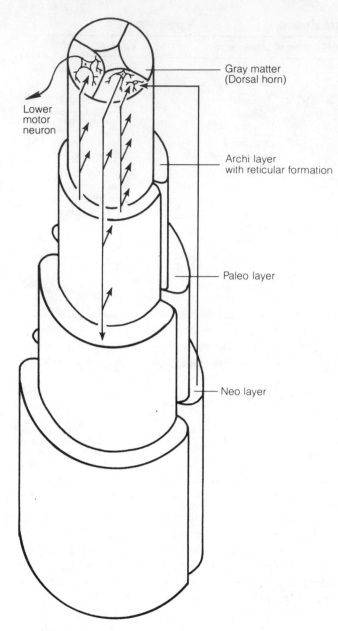

Lower motor neuron

Gray matter (Dorsal horn)

Archi layer with reticular formation

Paleo layer

Neo layer

Figure 40–4. The three concentric subdivisions of the tract systems of the white matter. Migration of neurons into the archi layer converts it into the reticular formation of the white matter.

which activate motor units in neighboring as well as the same segments. With reference to evolution, this is the oldest of the three layers, and thus, it is sometimes referred to as the archi-level layer. It is the first of the longitudinal layers to become functional and it appears to be limited to reflex types of movements. Reflex movements of the fetus (quickening) that begin during the fifth month of intrauterine life involve the inner archi-level layer.

The inner layer of the white matter differs from the other two layers in one important aspect. Many of the neurons in the embryonic gray matter migrate out into this layer, resulting in a rich mixture of gray and white fibers called the *reticular formation*. The circuitry of most reflexes is contained in the reticular formation. In the brain stem, the reticular formation becomes quite large and contains major portions of vital reflexes, such as those controlling respiration, cardiovascular function, swallowing, and vomiting, to mention a few.

A functional system called the *reticular activating system* (RAS) operates in the lateral portions of the reticular formation of the medulla, pons, and especially the midbrain. Convergence of information from all sensory modalities, including those of the somesthetic, auditory, visual, and visceral afferent nerves, bombards neurons of this system. The RAS has both descending and ascending portions. The descending portion communicates with all spinal segmental levels through higher-level reticulospinal tracts and serves to facilitate many of the cord-level reflexes. For example, it speeds up reaction time and stabilizes postural reflexes. The ascending portion, sometimes called the *centroencephalic system*, accelerates brain and particularly thalamic and cortical activity. This is reflected by the appearance of "awake" brain-wave patterns. Thus, sudden stimuli not only result in protective and "attentive" postures, but also increase awareness.

The middle layer. The middle layer of the white matter contains most of the major fiber tract systems required for sensation and movement. It contains the spinoreticular and spinothalamic tracts. This system consists of larger-diameter and longer suprasegmental fibers, which ascend to the brain stem and which are largely functional at birth. In terms of evolutionary development, these tracts are quite old, and therefore this layer is sometimes called the paleo layer. It facilitates many of the primitive functions, such as the "auditory startle reflex," which occurs in response to a loud noise. This reflex consists of turning the head and body toward the sound, dilating the pupils of the eyes, "catching of the breath," and "quickening of the pulse."

The outer layer. The outer layer of the tract systems is the newest of the three layers in terms of evolutionary development, and hence is sometimes called the neo layer. It becomes functional at about the second year of life and it contains the pathways that are needed for bladder training. Myelination of the neo layer suprasegmental tracts, which include many of those required for the most delicate coordination

Table 40–2   **Characteristics of the Concentric Subdivisions of the Longitudinal Tract System in White Matter of the Nervous System**

Characteristics	Archi-level Tracts	Paleo-level Tracts	Neo-level Tracts
Segmental span	Intersegmental (less than five segments)	Suprasegmental (five or more segments)	Suprasegmental
Number of synapses	Multisynaptic	Multisynaptic but fewer than archi-level tracts	Monosynaptic with target structures
Conduction velocity	Very slow	Fast	Fastest
Examples of functional systems	Flexor withdrawal reflex circuitry	Spinothalamic tracts	Corticospinal tracts

and skill, is not complete until sometime around the tenth to the twelfth year of life. This includes the development of tracts needed for fine manipulative skills, such as the finger–thumb coordination required for the use of many tools and the toe movements needed for acrobatics. Being the newest to evolve and being outside the brain and spinal cord, these tracts are the most vulnerable to injury. When these outer tracts are damaged, the paleo and archi tracts often remain functional, and rehabilitation methods can result in quite effective use of the older systems. Delicacy and refinement may be gone but basic function remains. For example, a very important outer system, or neosystem, the corticospinal system, permits the fine manipulative control required for writing. If this is lost, paleo-level systems remaining intact permit grasping and holding of objects. Thus, the hand can still be used to perform its basic functions.

Collateral communication between tracts.   Axons in the archi and paleo layers characteristically possess many collateral branches, which move into the gray cell columns or synapse with the reticular formation as the axon passes each succeeding CNS segment. Should a major axon be destroyed at some point along its course, these collaterals provide multisynaptic, alternative pathways that bypass the local damage. Neo-level tracts do not possess these collaterals, but are instead highly discrete as to the target neurons with which they communicate. Because of their discreteness, damage to the neo tracts causes permanent loss of function. Damage to the archi or paleo systems, on the other hand, is usually followed by slow return of function presumably through the use of these collateral connections. For example, the surgical section of pathways carrying pain impulses

(spinothalamic paleo-level tracts) can be used for temporary relief of intractable pain. The pain experience usually returns after some weeks or months. When it does return, it is often poorly localized and sometimes more unpleasant than it had been initially. Consequently, this surgical procedure, which is called a tractotomy, is usually reserved for persons who are not expected to survive for longer than a few months.

:Basic Organization of the Central Nervous System

Both the fragile and vital brain and spinal cord are enclosed within the protective confines of rigid bony structures of the skull and vertebral column. Although these structures afford protection for the tissues of the CNS, they also afford the potential for development of ischemic and traumatic nerve damage. This is because these structures cannot expand to accommodate the increase in volume that occurs when there is swelling within the nervous system or the expanded volume that occurs when there is bleeding within the confines of these structures. The bony structures themselves can also cause injury to the nervous system. Fractures of the skull and vertebral column can compress sections of the nervous system, or they can splinter and cause penetrating injuries. Surgical removal of the protective cover of the skull is called *craniotomy*, and that of the arches of bone of each vertebra (neural laminae) covering the spinal cord is called *laminectomy*. This is done to relieve pressure on the CNS or to remove tumors, blood clots, or foreign objects around or within the CNS.

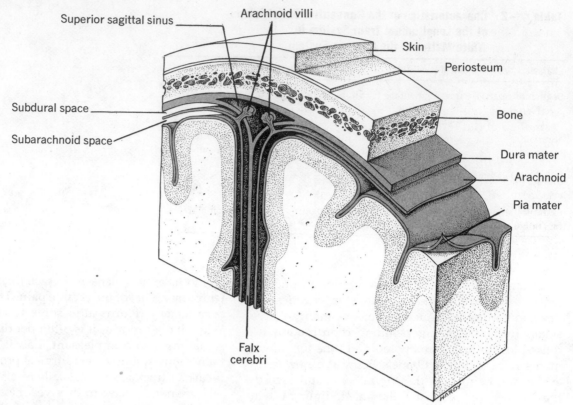

Figure 40–5. The cranial meninges. Arachnoid villi shown within the superior sagittal sinus are one site of cerebrospinal fluid absorption into the blood. (Chaffee EE, Lytle IM: Basic Physiology and Anatomy, 4th ed. Philadelphia, JB Lippincott, 1980)

The Meninges

Inside the skull and vertebral column, the brain and spinal cord are loosely suspended and further protected by several connective tissue sheaths called the meninges (Fig. 40-5). The surfaces of the spinal cord, brain, and segmental nerves are covered by a delicate, connective-tissue layer called the *pia mater* (delicate mother). The surface blood vessels and those that penetrate the brain and spinal cord are also encased in this protective tissue layer. A second very delicate, nonvascular, and waterproof layer, called the *arachnoid* because of its spider-web appearance, encloses the entire CNS. The cerebrospinal fluid (CSF) is contained within the subarachnoid space. Immediately outside the arachnoid is a continuous sheath of strong connective tissue, the *dura mater* (tough mother), which provides the major protection for the brain and spinal cord.

The Cerebrospinal Fluid

The brain and spinal cord float in a clear and colorless fluid, the cerebrospinal fluid, which fills the subarachnoid space. The cerebrospinal fluid is similar in many respects to the extracellular fluid (Table 40-3). The CSF serves to cushion and protect the brain and spinal cord. It may also be involved in a number of other control mechanisms. For example, blood glucose levels are reflected in the CSF, and hypothalamic centers have been shown to respond to these glucose levels, possibly contributing to hunger and eating behaviors.

Table 40-3 Composition of Cerebrospinal Fluid Compared to Plasma

Substance	Plasma	Cerebrospinal Fluid
Protein mg/dl	7500.00	20.00
Na^+ mEq/l	145.00	141.00
Cl^- mEq/l	101.00	124.00
K^+ mEq/l	4.50	2.90
HCO^- mEq/l	25.00	24.00
pH	7.4	7.32
Glucose mg/dl	92.00	61.00

The CSF is secreted by ependymal cells in the choroid plexus, which is located in the ventricles of the brain. The waterproof arachnoid has protuberances, called the arachnoid villi, that penetrate the inner dura and the venous walls of the superior sagittal sinus; it is here that most of the CSF is reabsorbed into the vascular system (see Fig. 40-5). Although about 500 ml of CSF is secreted each day, the total volume in the spinal canal and ventricular system is only about 150 ml, so that the CSF is completely replaced about three times a day.

The Spinal Cord and Spinal Nerves

In the adult, the spinal cord is located in the upper two-thirds of the vertebral canal of the body's vertebal column (Fig. 40-6). It extends from the foramen magnum at the base of the skull to a cone-shaped termination, the conus medullaris, which is usually located at the level of the first or second lumbar vertebra in the adult. The filum terminale, which is composed of nonneural tissues and pia mater, continues caudally and attaches to the second sacral vertebra.

Development of the spinal cord

The early embryo has three basic tissue layers: an outer ectoderm, a middle mesoderm, and an inner endoderm. The nervous system forms along the longitudinal axis of the early-developing embryo as a thickening of the ectoderm, or outer cell layer; this layer of thickened epithelium has a midline groove with ridges on each side. The edges of these ridges fuse over the top, turning the groove into a tube, called *the neural tube*. The neural tube extends the length of the embryo, with the rostral portion becoming the brain, and the caudal end, the spinal cord. As the nervous system develops, the neural tube sinks below the surface and becomes surrounded by bony elements of the axial skeleton, and is then covered with skin. The fusion process that forms the neural tube begins at what becomes the high thoracic and cervical levels, and proceeds like a zipper downward toward the sacral areas, while simultaneously "zippering" rostrally toward the brain end (Fig. 40-7). Eventually, the open ends of the tube close at the front end of the brain and at the caudal end of the spinal cord. The hollow cavity of the tube becomes the central canal in the spinal cord segments and the primitive ventricular system in the brain.

Closure defects.

Various abnormalities of the fusion process can occur. They include (1) failure of the skeletal elements to close, called a *spina bifida* or split

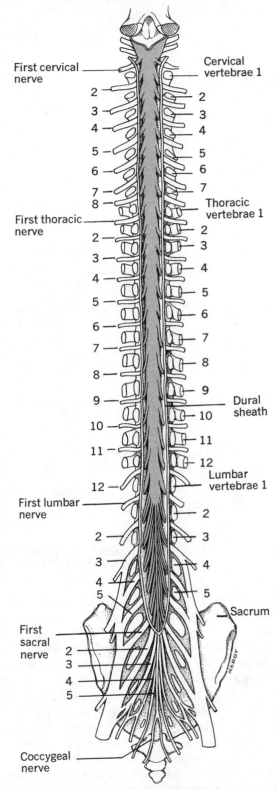

Figure 40–6.   The spinal cord lying within the vertebral canal. The spinal processes and meninges have been opened. The spinal nerves are numbered on the left and the vertebrae on the right. (Chaffee EE, Lytle IM: Basic Physiology and Anatomy, 4th ed. Philadelphia, JB Lippincott, 1980)

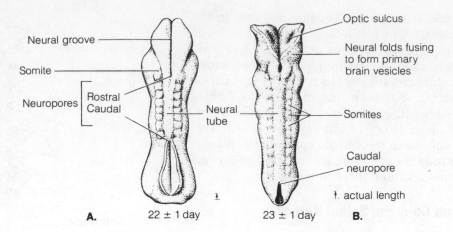

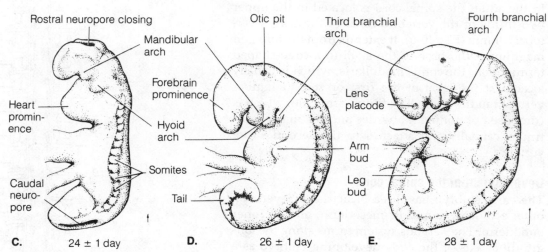

Figure 40–7. Drawings of a 4-week-old embryo. *A* and *B* dorsal views during stage 10 of development (22 to 23 days), showing 8 to 12 somites, respectively, *C*, *D*, and *E*, lateral views during stages 11, 12, and 13 (24 to 28 days), showing 16, 27, and 33 somites, respectively. (Moore KL: The Developing Human: Clinically Oriented Embryology, 2nd ed, p 317. Philadelphia, WB Saunders, 1977)

spine, (2) formation of a CSF-filled sac covered by meninges (spina bifida with meningocele), and (3) complete nondevelopment of the neural tube and associated structures (spina bifida with myeloschisis or split marrow). If only a closure defect of the bony neural lamina occurs, called spina bifida occulta, the spinal cord develops normally, but the CNS is more vulnerable to trauma at that point. This defect often does not become apparent until an accident occurs with possible sensory or paralytic effects. The more severe defects must be repaired surgically shortly after birth in order to reduce the problems of repeated infection and damage to the CNS. If the neural tube does not close, the internal structures do not mature properly and, even following successful surgical repair, permanent flaccid paralysis results, and often nontransmission of sensory information occurs through the defect with a resul-

tant anesthesia of the affected parts. Table 40-4 describes the various types of closure defects at spinal and cranial levels.

Structure of the spinal cord

The spinal cord is oval or rounded in shape, and on transverse section is noted to have a gray interior portion which is shaped like a butterfly or letter H (Fig. 40-8). Some of the neurons that make up the gray matter of the cord have processes that leave the cord, enter the peripheral nerves, and supply tissues, such as autonomic ganglia. Other neurons in the gray portion of the cord are concerned with input or reflex mechanisms. The white matter of the cord contains fiber tracts, which transmit information between segments of the cord or to higher levels of the central nervous system, such as the brain stem or cerebrum.

Table 40-4 Closure Defects at Spinal and Cranial Levels

Level	Neural Tube Closure	Meninges Closure Cyst	Skeletal Elements Closure vs Dysraphia	Skin Closure	Clinical
Spinal	Closed	Closed—none	Closed	Closed	Normal
	Closed	Closed—none	Open (rachischisis or spina bifida)	Closed	Spina bifida occulta
	If extends the entire length of the spinal column: Total rachischisis				
	Closed	Closed—cyst (meningocele)	Open	Closed	Spina bifida cystica with meningocele
	Closed but incorporated into cyst (myelocele)	Closed—cyst (meningocele)	Open	Closed	Spina bifida with meningo-myelocele
	Open (myeloschisis) (if not formed: amyelia)	Open	Open	Open	Spina bifida with myeloschisis
	If extends the entire length of the spinal cord: Total myeloschisis				
Cranial	Closed	Closed—none	Closed	Closed	Normal
	Closed	Closed—none	Open (cranioschisis)	Closed	Craniobifida
	Closed	Closed—cyst (cephalocele)	Open	Closed	Craniobifida with cephalocele
	Closed; incorporated into cyst (encephalocele)	Closed—cyst	Open	Closed	Craniobifida with encephalocele
	Closed—no cerebral hemispheres; enlarged single ventricle (holocephaly)				Holocephaly
	Open—overgrowth of alar lamina extraversion of cerebral hemispheres (pseudoencephaly)				Pseudoencephaly
	Open—no medullary plate (anencephaly)				Anencephaly
	If extends the entire length of the neural tube: Craniorachischisis with myeloschisis				

Source: Willis RA: The Borderland Between Embryology and Pathology, ed 2. Washington, D.C., Butterworths, 1962.

The horns of the cord that extend posteriorly are called the *dorsal* horns and those that extend anteriorly, the *ventral* horns. The dorsal horns contain input association neurons that receive afferent nerve terminals through the dorsal roots and other interconnecting neurons. The dorsal horns contain the GSIA and GVIA neurons that were described earlier. The ventral horns contain output association neurons of the GSOA and GVOA type. A central portion of the cord, which connects the dorsal and ventral horns and which surrounds the central canal, is called the *intermediate gray*. In the thoracic area, the small, slender projections that emerge from the intermediate gray are called the *intermediolateral columns* or *horns*. These columns contain the efferent neurons (GVE) of the sympathetic nervous system.

The amount of gray matter that is present in the cord is largely determined by the amount of tissue that is innervated by a given segment of the cord. There are increased amounts of gray matter in the lower lumbar and upper sacral segments which supply the lower extremities, and in cervical segment five to thoracic segment one, where the innervation of the upper limbs is located.

The volume of white matter in the spinal cord also increases progressively as it moves toward the brain because of the addition of more and more ascending axons and because the mass of descending axons, which terminate in the segments, becomes greater.

During the developmental process, the spinal cord stops growing in length before growth of the

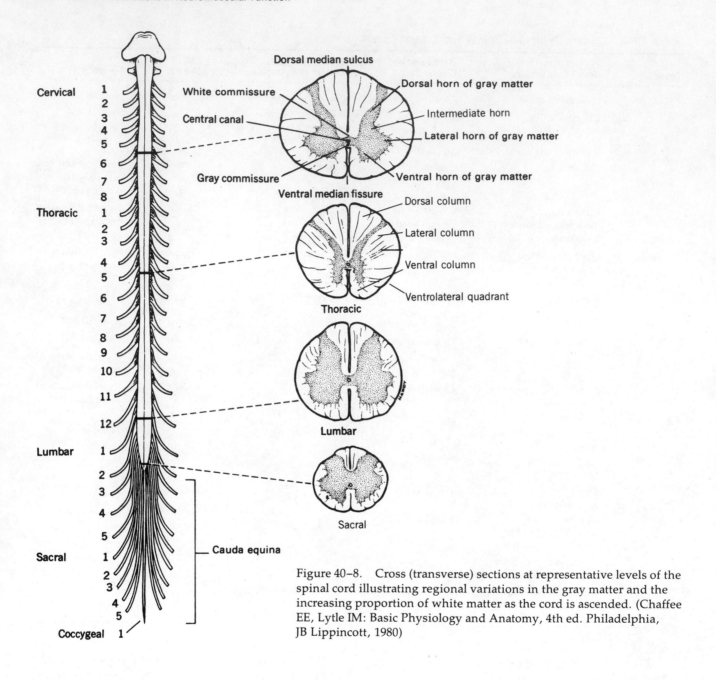

Cervical
1
2
3
4
5
6
7
8

Thoracic
1
2
3
4
5
6
7
8
9
10
11
12

Lumbar
1
2
3
4
5

Sacral
1
2
3
4
5

Coccygeal 1

Dorsal median sulcus
White commissure
Central canal
Gray commissure
Ventral median fissure

Dorsal horn of gray matter
Intermediate horn
Lateral horn of gray matter
Ventral horn of gray matter

Dorsal column
Lateral column
Ventral column
Ventrolateral quadrant

Thoracic

Lumbar

Sacral

Cauda equina

Figure 40–8. Cross (transverse) sections at representative levels of the spinal cord illustrating regional variations in the gray matter and the increasing proportion of white matter as the cord is ascended. (Chaffee EE, Lytle IM: Basic Physiology and Anatomy, 4th ed. Philadelphia, JB Lippincott, 1980)

spinal axial skeleton reaches its adult dimensions. This results in a disparity between the positions of each succeeding cord segment and the exit of its dorsal and ventral roots through the corresponding intervertebral foramen. This disparity becomes progressively more pronounced at the more caudal levels. In the adult, the spinal cord usually ends at the level of the first or second lumbar segment. From this point, the dorsal and ventral roots angle downward

from the cord, forming what is called the *cauda equina*, or horse's tail. The pia mater that covers the caudal end of the spinal cord continues as the filum terminale through the spinal canal, and attaches to the coccygeal vertebrae. However, the arachnoid and its enclosed subarachnoid space, which is filled with CSF, do not close down on the filum terminale until they reach the second sacral vertebra. This results in formation of a pocket of cerebral spinal fluid, the dural *cisterna spinalis*, which extends from about the second lumbar to the second sacral vertebra.

Because of the abundant supply of spinal fluid and the fact that the spinal cord does not extend this far, this area is often used for sampling the cerebral spinal fluid. A procedure called a *spinal tap*, or *puncture*, can be done by inserting a special type of needle into the dural sac at the level of L$_3$ and L$_4$. The spinal roots, which are covered with pia mater, are in relatively little danger of trauma from the needle used for this purpose.

Protective structures. The spinal cord and the dorsal and ventral roots are covered with connective tissue sheath, the pia mater, which also carries the vascular supply to the white and gray matter of the cord. On the lateral sides of the spinal cord, extensions of the pia mater, the *dentate ligaments*, attach the sides of the spinal cord to the bony wall of the spinal canal (Fig. 40-11). Thus, the cord is suspended by both the dentate ligaments and the segmental nerves. A fat- and vessel-filled epidural space intervenes between the spinal dura mater and the inner wall of the spinal canal. Each vertebral body has two *pedicles* which extend laterally and support the transverse processes of the neural laminae, which arch medially and fuse together to continue as the spinal process. The gaps between each of the vertebra and its body parts are

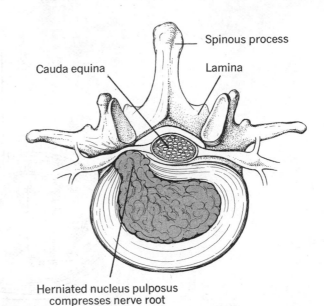

Figure 40–10.   A ruptured intervertebral disc. The soft central portion of the disc is protruding into the vertebral canal, where it exerts pressure on a spinal nerve root. (Chaffee EE, Lytle IM: Basic Physiology and Anatomy, 4th ed, p 103. Philadelphia, JB Lippincott, 1980)

filled with tough ligaments. Thus, the spinal cord lives within the protective confines of this series of concentric flexible tissue and bony sheaths. A gap, the interverbral foramen, occurs between each two succeeding pedicles, allowing for exit of the segmental nerves and veins and entrance of arteries.

The bony structure of the closely approximated vertebrae provides good protection for the spinal cord, nerve roots, and posterior root ganglia. Major weight bearing is accomplished through the column of vertebral bodies, and flexibility of the vertebral column is provided by fibrocartilaginous *intervertebral discs*, which lie between each two succeeding centra (see Fig. 40-6). A firm, gelatinous structure called the nucleus pulposis gives substance to the disc; it is held in place by a strong ventral, longitudinal ligament and a weaker dorsal, longitudinal ligament which acts to interconnect neighboring verte bral bodies.

Herniation of the nucleus pulposus.   If the dorsal ligament, which supports the vertebral column, becomes weakened, the nucleus pulposus can be squeezed out of place, a condition often referred to as a "slipped disc" (Fig. 40-10). When this happens, the nucleus pulposus usually moves laterally and dorsally, causing irritation or crushing of a segmental nerve root. This irritation causes spontaneous firing

Figure 40–9.   Spinal cord and meninges. (Chaffee EE, Lytle IM: Basic Physiology and Anatomy, 4th ed, p 234. Philadelphia, JB Lippincott, 1980)

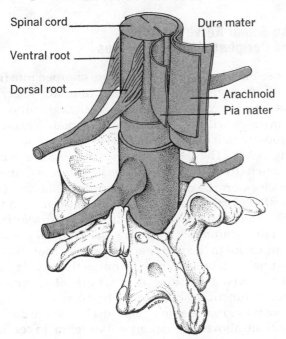

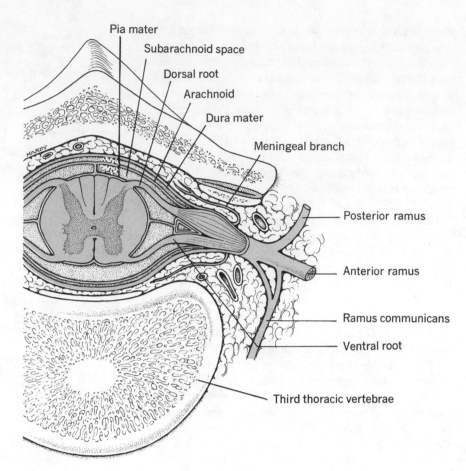

Figure 40–11. Cross section of vertebral column at the level of the third thoracic vertebra, showing the meninges, the spinal cord, and the origin of a spinal nerve and its branches or rami. (Chaffee EE, Lytle IM: Basic Physiology and Anatomy, 4th ed, p 235. Philadelphia, JB Lippincott, 1980)

(Figure labels: Pia mater, Subarachnoid space, Dorsal root, Arachnoid, Dura mater, Meningeal branch, Posterior ramus, Anterior ramus, Ramus communicans, Ventral root, Third thoracic vertebrae)*

of the afferent axons and severe pain along the length of the nerve. Crushing damage to the dorsal roots results in reduction or loss of sensation, and crushing of the ventral roots produces weakness. The signs and symptoms associated with a "slipped disc" are localized to the body segment that is innervated by the nerve roots. If the "slipped disc" moves straight back and compresses or destroys a part of the spinal cord, longitudinal communication along the ventral white matter of the cord is most likely to be blocked.

The level at which a "slipped disc" occurs is important. Usually, it occurs at the lower levels of the lumbar spine where both the mass being supported and the bending of the vertebral column are greatest. When the injury occurs in this area, only the cauda equina will be irritated or crushed. Since these elongated dorsal and ventral roots contain endoneurial tubes of connective tissue, regeneration of the nerve fibers is likely, although the distance to the innervated muscle or skin of the lower limbs requires several weeks or months for full recovery to occur. A "slipped disc" into the spinal canal at higher levels can destroy the ventral white matter or can

completely sever the cord. Here, regeneration is insignificant, and paralysis and anesthesia of the more caudal body regions may be permanent.

The Spinal Nerve Roots and Peripheral (Spinal) Nerves

The segments of the spinal cord are grouped into five parts: 8 cervical, 12 thoracic, 5 lumbar, 5 sacral, and 2 to 3 coccygeal segments. Each segment communicates with its corresponding body segment through a pair of segmental nerves, one on each side (Fig. 40-9). The spinal nerve in the intervertebral foramen divides into two branches, or roots, one of which enters the dorsolateral surface of the cord (*the dorsal root*), carrying afferent neuron axons into the CNS. The other leaves the ventrolateral surface of the cord (*the ventral root*), carrying the axons of efferent neurons out to the periphery. These two roots fuse at the intervertebral foramen, forming the *mixed spinal nerve*—mixed because it has both afferent and efferent functions. Because the first cervical (C_1) spinal nerve exits the spinal canal just below the base of the skull, above the first cervical vertebra, in cervical segments the nerve is given the number of the bony vertebra just below it. Numbering was changed for all lower levels, however. Thus, an *extra* cervical nerve, the C_8 nerve, exists above the T_1 vertebra, and all subsequent nerves are numbered for the vertebra just above its point of exit.

A general organization plan is retained in all the segments. Using a thoracic-level segment as an example, the dorsal and ventral roots forming a peripheral nerve fuse at the *dorsal root ganglion* in a mixed spinal root, which contains both *afferent* and *efferent* neuronal processes (Fig. 40-12). Just outside the exit from the spinal cord, the spinal nerve divides into a *small dorsal primary ramus*, which carries efferent and afferent neuronal processes into the dorsal musculature and skin of the body, and a *larger ventral primary ramus*, which innervates the lateral and ventral parts of the body. Cutaneous branches of these rami innervate the skin and cutaneous fascia of the associated blood vessels and connective tissues. Other branches innervate the joints, the marrow cavities of the bones, and the meninges of the spinal canal. Branches from the anterior primary ramus interconnect with the peripheral nervous system innervating the great vessels, genitourinary organs, and the gut and its derivatives.

Spinal cord reflexes

Between 30 and 50 thousand sensory or afferent neuron cell bodies live in each of the pair of connective tissue-enclosed colonies, or *dorsal root ganglia*, that are located on each side of the spinal cord in the opening (intervertebral foramina) between adjacent

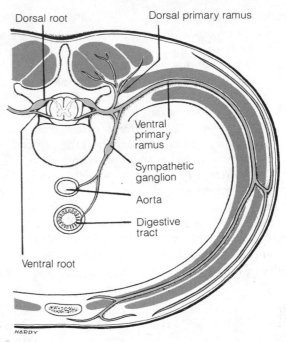

Figure 40–12.   Schematic cross section through the vertebral column and the left side of the trunk, showing anterior and posterior rami of one spinal nerve. Also shown are fibers leading to a sympathetic ganglion and to internal organs. (Chaffee EE, Lytle IM: Basic Physiology and Anatomy, 4th ed, p 235. Philadelphia, JB Lippincott, 1980)

Figure 40–13.   Diagram of a flexor-withdrawal reflex. (Chaffee EE, Lytle IM: Basic Physiology and Anatomy, 4th ed, p 240. Philadelphia, JB Lippincott, 1980)

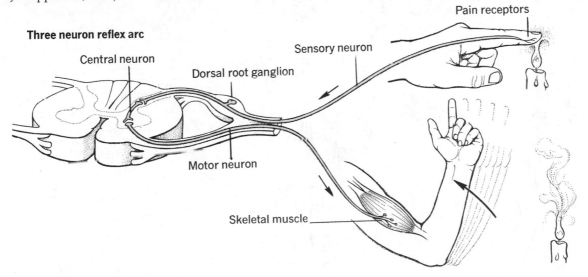

vertebrae. Each afferent neuron sends protoplasmic peripheral processes to receptors in the associated side of the body segment. If a skin receptor, such as that which responds to increased temperature, is stimulated by skin contact with a hot object, a series of events takes place in the nervous system (Fig. 40-13). First, a local change occurs in the receptor, which is converted to action potentials, transmitted through the peripheral nerve toward the cell body in the dorsal root ganglia and then through its axon into the spinal cord segment. At this point, internuncial or interconnecting neurons can trigger an action potential in a lower motor or efferent neuron that passes through a ventral root to a mixed (afferent and efferent) segmental nerve. Contraction of the muscles innervated by branches of this nerve results in movement of the skin surface away from

the stimulus. This protective reflex is called the *flexor-withdrawal reflex*. This is an example of the many spinal cord reflexes that make standing, stepping, scratching, and walking possible.

Ascending (sensory) pathways

General soma afferent (GSA) neurons. Each segment of the body, with few exceptions, contains a pair of dorsal root ganglia within which live the GSA (general soma afferent) neurons, innervating the body wall, or soma, of that segment. As a result, these stripes of segmental nerve-innervated regions, or *dermatomes*, occur in regular sequence from coccygeal 2, upward through the upper cervical segments. In the adult, these stripes overlap each other somewhat and also become distorted by the outgrowth of the limbs (Fig. 40-14). Yet these der-

Figure 40–14.   Cutaneous distribution of spinal nerves (dermatomes). (Barr M: The Human Nervous System, p 253. New York, Harper & Row, 1979)

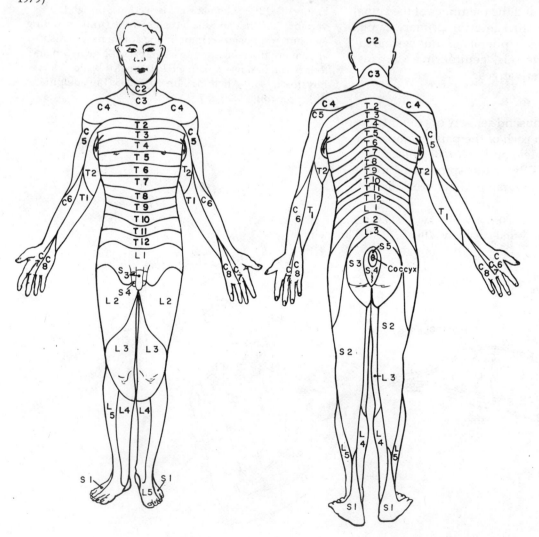

matomes reflect the basic segmental organization of the body and of the nervous system. Clinical neurological examination of the patient uses this segmental sequence of afferent innervated zones to quickly test the integrity of the entire series of spinal nerves. A pin point pressed against the skin of the sole which results in a flexor-withdrawal reflex and a complaint of pain confirms the functional integrity of the sacral dorsal root ganglion cell afferent terminals in the skin of the foot, the entire pathway of the afferent nerve neuron's peripheral axon to the S_1 dorsal root ganglion, and beyond the central axon through the S_1 dorsal root and into the spinal cord. It also means that the GSIA cells receiving this information are functioning and the reflex circuitry of the cord segments (L_5–S_2) involved is functioning. Further, the lower motor neurons (GSE) of the L_4–S_1 ventral horn are operational, and their axons conduct through the ventral roots, the mixed spinal nerve, and the muscle nerve to the muscles effecting the withdrawal response. The communication between the lower motor neuron and the muscle cells is functional also. All of this information is obtained in a fraction of a second by pressing the pin point and observing the quick reflex response. If this is done at each segmental level, or dermatome, moving upward along the body and neck, and the reflexes are all in the normal range, the functional integrity of all of these spinal nerves, their roots, and the spinal gray matter of that side must be within normal limits—from coccygeal 2 through the high cervical levels. Similar dermatomes cover the face and scalp, and these, although innervated by cranial segmental nerves, are tested in the same manner.

Central mechanisms of general somatic afferent (GSA) neurons.   Primary afferent signals from receptors in the body wall are distributed to one or more dorsal horn association neuron cell columns. Each of these columns has characteristic patterns of central projections. The general somatic input association column (GSIA) relays afferent signals (1) to local reflex circuits, providing rapid, lower motor neuron responses, (2) to more rostral parts of the reflex hierarchy, permitting more complex, organized response patterns, (3) to the reticular activating system, contributing to general alerting of forebrain systems, and (4) to the thalamus, where sensation and perceptive functions begin. A specialized association column provides a fifth projection to basic coordination systems.

The skin, fascial sheets, muscles, tendons, joint capsules, periosteum, marrow cavities, and parietal lining of the body cavities receive GSA neuron ter-

minals. The peripheral axon of a GSA neuron branches many times before innervating a circumscribed arc, of skin, for instance. Action potentials originating from receptors in any of these branches are conducted through the dorsal root into the spinal cord. This neuron, in a sense, cannot discriminate from which peripheral branch the impulse originated. Thus, it functions as a unit—*the sensory unit*. It is easy to fool such a mechanism. When the "funny bone" (ulnar nerve on the medial side of the elbow) is traumatized, the person experiences pain at the elbow but also "tingling" radiating from the palm and fingers. The CNS has interpreted the burst of impulses as coming from the GSA terminals in the hand. This *"referral" to the innervated periphery* explains why a pinched sacral nerve at the sacrum results in shooting pain down the back of the leg and foot, a condition called sciatica. Irritation of the stump of a nerve following limb amputation is interpreted as an annoying sensation in the nonexistent *phantom limb*.

Discrimination of location of a stimulus is based on the sensory field innervated by an afferent neuron. Intensity discrimination is based on the rate of impulses in the afferent neuron and this is related to the intensity of the stimulus applied. Some afferent neurons maintain a more or less steady rate of firing to an uninterrupted stimulus. These *slow-adapting* afferent neurons are in contrast to *rapid-adapting* afferent neurons, which signal only the onset and conclusion of a stimulus. Slow-adapting afferent neurons are required to maintain stable posture, for instance, while rapid-adapting afferent neurons are required to signal moving, brief, or vibrating stimuli.

The qualitative aspects of different types of stimuli are based on differential sensitivity of the terminals of different afferent neurons. This is called the stimulus *modality*. Some afferent neurons are particularly sensitive to increased skin temperature, and these signals are interpreted as "warm" or hot. Others are particularly sensitive to slight indentations of the skin and their signals are interpreted as "touch." Cool–cold, sharp or bright pain, burning–aching pain, delicate touch, deep pressure, joint movement, joint position, muscle stretch, and tendon stretch sensations are based on the specific sensitivities of different GSA neurons. Each of these sensations is based on a different population of afferent neurons or on central integration of several modalities occurring at the same time.

The input association column neurons of the dorsal horn (GSIA) distribute the afferent signals to differing reflex circuits—pain to the flexor-withdrawal circuit, deep pressure to a stepping reflex circuit, and so on. All GSA input signals are projected by other central neurons to higher levels of the nervous system as necessary input to more complex reflex patterns. This spinoreticular projection, for instance, permits a fallen animal to regain its footing and depends on midbrain-level circuits. Stepping on a tack not only results in quick flexion of the injured limb but also extension of the opposite limb, taking over body weight support. The same information is projected by spinoreticular fibers to brainstem levels, where the circuitry for "catching" the breath, sudden rise in blood pressure, and phonation (crying out) occur. This illustrates the concept of the *hierarchy of reflexes* in which the same afferent information contributes to more and more complex reaction patterns, each at a more rostral location and controlling various components organized at lower levels.

Protopathic pathway.   The GSIA cell column is the indirect source of spinoreticular projections to the reticular activating system referred to above. In addition, it relays the afferent information to the forebrain, where *sensation* and *perception* occur. Two parallel pathways reach the thalamic level and sensation, each taking a different route. The *protopathic pathway*[1] is a multisynaptic pathway, for the most part, by which local spinal afferent signals are relayed up the ventrolateral paleo-level tract systems to both the *lateral* and the *intermediate* nuclei of the thalamus. For the sensation of pain, the axons travel almost exclusively up the opposite side of the nervous system. For the more crude aspects of touch, both sides of this protopathic system are used. This is a slow-conducting pathway with many collateral branches feeding information into the reticular formation of segments along the way. Few fibers travel all the way to the thalamus. Most synapse on reticular formation neurons which send their axons on toward the thalamus. The lateral nuclei of the thalamus receiving this information are capable of contributing a crude, poorly localized sensation ("something touched my hand") (opposite side to the thalamic nuclei). These same nuclei are in intimate communication with areas of the parietal cerebral cortex, and these are necessary for the sensation to be clear, well localizable, and graded in intensity. The spinothalamic tract system, or protopathic pathway, also projects into the intermediate nuclei of the thalamus, which have close connections with the limbic cortical systems. It is this circuitry which gives sensation its affective or emotional aspects (*e.g.*, the "hurtfulness" of pain, the particular unpleasantness of itch or heavy pressure, and the pecu-

liar pleasantness of tickle). For most sensations, the protopathic pathway is multisynaptic and, therefore, slow and crudely graded. This is called the *paleospinothalamic* fiber system. A recently evolved, more rapid and discrete *neospinothalamic* system of fibers in this pathway provides sharp, highly localizable pain sensation.

Apparently most of the *perceptive* aspects of body sensation, or *somesthesia*, require the function of "associational" cortex as well as other thalamic nuclei. The perceptive aspect or meaningfulness of a stimulus pattern involves integration of present sensation with past learning. Your past learning plus present tactile sensation gives you the perception that you are sitting on a soft chair seat and not on a bicycle seat, for instance.

Epicritic pathway.   A more rapid pathway to the thalamus, which involves afferent axons travelling up the dorsal columns of white matter and synapsing in the GSIA nuclei in the medulla with further large-diameter projection through the brain stem without collateral branches, is called the *epicritic pathway*. Sensory information arriving at the thalamus by this route is much more discretely localizable, and more delicately analyzable in terms of intensity grades. This pathway has little projection into the intermediate thalamic nuclei, with a high dependency on parietal cortical function. This is the only pathway taken by sensations of joint movement (kinesthesis); of body position (proprioception); of vibration; and of delicate, discriminative touch, such as is required to correctly differentiate between the touching of the skin at two neighboring points vs only one point (two-point discrimination). Many lesions in the CNS differentially damage these two pathways, protopathic vs epicritic, and since the routes are different, this helps in the localization of the pathological process. The epicritic pathway is a neo-level system and is much more vulnerable to injury.

Abnormal somesthetic sensation.   Abnormalities of somesthetic sensation can involve (1) reduced sensitivity (hypesthesia), (2) increased sensitivity beyond normal (hyperesthesia) or disordered (dysesthesia), often very unpleasant sensitivity (paresthesia). These conditions can result from congenital, pharmacological, traumatic, or metabolic modifications of peripheral nerve transmission and excitability, or of the function of the CNS ascending systems. Congenital absence of pain (congenital analgesia) is a rare but dangerous disorder, because an affected person is often unaware of minor infections or trauma, with resulting serious damage to body

Table 40-5   Terminology of Abnormalities of Sensation

	Word or Root	Diminished Sensation	Excessive Sensation	Disordered or Unpleasant Sensation	Loss of Sensation
General somatic afferent (GSA)					
Tactile (touch)	-esthesia	hypesthesia	hyperesthesia	dysesthesia or paresthesia	anesthesia
Position	proprioception stereognosis	—	—	phantom limb dysstereognosis	—
Sense of movement	kinesthesis	—	—	—	—
Vibration	—	—	—	—	—
Temperature	-thermia	hypothermia	hyperthermia	—	athermia
General somatic or visceral afferents (GSA, GVA)					
Pain	-algesia	hypalgesia	hyperalgesia	dysalgesia neuralgia causalgia	analgesia
Special visceral afferents (GVA)					
Taste	-geusia	hypogeusia	hypergeusia	—	ageusia
Olfaction	-nosmia	hyponosmia	hypernosmia	—	anosmia
Special sensory afferents (SSA)					
Audition	-acusis	hypacusis	hyperacusis	tinnitus	anacusis (deafness)
Vestibulation	—	—	—	vertigo (dizziness)	—
Vision	-opsia	hypopsia	hyperopsia	phosphenes (seeing stars or lights when subjected to cranial percussion	anopsia hemianopsia, scotoma

parts through lack of attention and care. The nomenclature for reduced acuity in the various subdivisions of somesthetic sensation is presented in Table 40-5. For some categories of sensation, no special term exists; this is true of the sensation of vibration, for example. Some forms of somesthetic sensation are dependent upon input from multiple receptors. The sense of the "shape" and "size" of an object in the absence of visualization, called *stereognosis*, is based on afferent information from muscle, tendon, and joint receptors. A screwdriver has a different shape from a knife, not only in the texture of its parts (tactile sensibility), but also in its shape. This complex, interpretive perception requires not only proprioceptive input but also prior experience.

In the clinical setting, additional terms may be used to describe some alterations in sensory modalities. High-pitch deafness is a condition often encountered in the aged in which there is a differential loss of acoustic sensitivity at the higher frequencies. Exposure to intense sound at certain frequencies can lead to permanent reduction in auditory acuity at those frequencies ("boilermaker's deaf-ness"), a condition which often occurs in industrial workers or musicians who do not wear adequate ear protectors. The distinction between hypacusis or deafness due to pathology of the middle ear sonic transmission system as contrasted to degeneration of the acoustic end organ or neural pathway is implied by the terms *transmission deafness* vs *nerve deafness*. A blind spot not normally present in the visual field is called a *scotoma*. If an entire half of the visual field of one eye is missing, the term *hemianopsia* is used; this defect is usually due to pathology of the central visual pathways in the brain.

Abnormally high excitability, either centrally or peripherally, can result in the sensation without obvious peripheral stimulation. The sensation of ringing in the ears (*tinnitus*) or of sudden sharp and often painful somesthetic sensations during local ischemia or during peripheral nerve regeneration (paresthesias) is fairly common. Direct trauma or irritation of the central nervous system portions of an ascending system can also result in sensations which are usually unpleasant and without any meaning or perception attached. Irritation of associational parts of the cerebrum can result in perceptual hallucinations. These hallucinations may indicate the presence and sometimes the location of irritative lesions. For example, repeated sensations of strong and extremely unpleasant odors not sensed by others in the room may be an early symptom of irritation of the olfactory association cortex by a meningeal tumor.

Special soma afferents (SSA). Sensory neurons that send branches of their central axon into the special soma input association (SSIA) cell column of the dorsal horn are called special soma afferent neurons (SSA). These include the afferent neurons from the vestibular and auditory end organs of the inner ear and also the primary afferent neurons innervating specialized muscle stretch receptors, called *muscle spindles*. These have in common the SSIA neuron projection of information to the cerebellum. The cerebellum is largely responsible for coordinating the timing of movement of various groups of muscles. The functions of the cerebellum are not subject to voluntary control. Temporal smoothness in changing motor unit firing and, therefore, the shifting of strength of muscle contraction in various muscles involved in a movement is an essential part of coordinated movement. The major function of this part of the CNS is the precise control of sequential timing of motor unit firing during movement patterns.

With reference to an ongoing movement, muscles are classified into *agonists*, which promote the movement; *antagonists* which resist it; and *synergists*, which assist the agonistic muscles by stabilizing a joint or by contributing minor force to the movement. Keeping track of all of this during complex movements and smoothing the ongoing sequence of motor unit firing is the responsibility of the cerebellar circuits. This is called the *synergistic aspect of coordination*.

There are a number of sensory pathways that project input to the cerebellum and that are integrated into body movement. The vestibular nuclei, which receive information from the labyrinth system of the inner ear, are intimately concerned with cerebellar function, providing input that makes possible adjustive changes in ongoing movements during alterations in head position. The auditory system, a specialized derivative of the vestibular system for sonic stimulus analysis, has a reduced projection to the cerebellum. Directional information about the location of sound is used during response patterns related to turning toward or away from the stimulus.

A necessary and major input to cerebellar function is required from muscle, tendon, and joint re-

ceptors. This feedback system provides the informational background for cerebellar control of ongoing movement. It is not surprising, therefore, to find that the SSIA column is present at all cord and brainstem levels with muscle, tendon, and joint afferent neurons.

The stretch reflex. The stretch reflex is considered essential for maintenance of normal muscle tone and posture. Most skeletal muscles contain large numbers of specialized stretch receptors scattered throughout the muscle substance, called *muscle spindles*. These encapsulated receptor organs contain miniature skeletal muscle fibers which are surrounded at their middle by helical receptive terminals (annulospiral endings) of very-large-diameter afferent neurons (Group Ia). The muscle spindles are attached to the connective tissue within the skeletal muscle so that stretching a muscle stretches its muscle spindles, resulting in an increased impulse rate in the Ia afferent fibers. All of the miniature muscle fibers of one spindle are innervated by the same Ia afferent, and each Ia afferent innervates only one spindle. These afferent neurons enter the spinal cord through the dorsal root and have several branches, one of which reaches the SSIA cell column for communication with the cerebellum. At the segment of entry, other large collateral branches make monosynaptic contact with each of the lower motor neurons which have motor units in the muscle containing the spindle source of input. Strong facilitory drive by the stretch afferent neurons on these lower motor neurons increases motor unit firing, opposing the stretch of the muscle. Axons from the spindle fibers also travel up the dorsal cell columns to the medulla, and as they travel many collaterals are dropped into the dorsal horn of the succeeding segment, influencing reflex function at each level.

The stretch reflex is useful in that it stabilizes joint position. A joint rotation will stretch one or more flexor, extensor, or rotator muscles and this is immediately opposed by contraction of the stretched muscle. The greater the stretch, the greater the strength of motor unit response. This reflex is continuously available to all muscles in the body, neck, and head. It stabilizes assumed posture against gravitational pull or against any other force that tends to move bones around joints.

Clinically, the *status of the stretch reflex* is evaluated by asking a person to relax while supporting the limb except at the joint being investigated. The distal part of the extremity is then moved passively around the joint. Normally, it is possible for the examiner to feel mild opposition to this movement. This is called *muscle tone* and can be less than normal

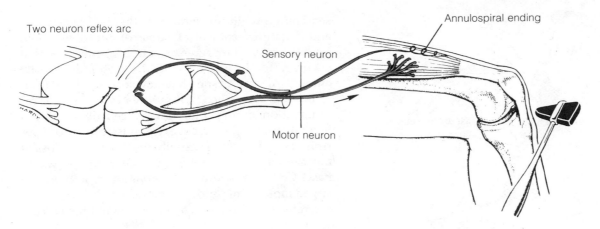

Figure 40–15.   Testing the stretch reflex with a reflex hammer.
(Chaffee EE, Lytle IM: Basic Physiology and Anatomy, 4th ed, p 240.
Philadelphia, JB Lippincott, 1980)

(*hypotonia*) or absent (*flaccidity*). It can also be excessive (*hypertonia*) or extreme (*rigidity, spasticity*, or *tetany*). The latter three terms include extremes of hypertonia plus other distinguishing characteristics.

A second method for assessing stretch reflex excitability is to tap briskly with a reflex hammer on the tendon of a muscle, which is almost immediately followed by a sudden contraction or "muscle jerk" (Fig. 40-15). Here the stretch reflex has been "tricked" by the sudden tug on the tendon. A synchronous burst of Ia activity from spindles in the muscle results in essentially simultaneous firing of a large number of motor units. The stretch reflex was "tricked" into responding, as though the joint had been suddenly rotated. The classic "knee jerk" is just one example of many places where tendons can be reached and tested with a reflex hammer. These muscle jerk reflexes are called *deep tendon reflexes* (DTRs) and provide a useful means for observing stretch reflex excitability.

The deep tendon reflexes can provide an amazing amount of information in a brief period of time. If a DTR is within normal range, you know that (1) the stretch afferent peripheral process in the peripheral, including the muscle, nerves, is normal; (2) the dorsal root ganglion function is normal; (3) the dorsal root function is normal; and (4) the dorsal, intermediate, and ventral horns are functioning appropriately, as are the ventral root and lower motor neuron cell body and axon. It also means that the neuromuscular synapse is functioning normally and that the muscle fibers are capable of normal contraction. It is possible to test the function of all the spinal nerves and spinal cord segments and most of the cranial nerves and brain stem segments in a short

time, using this method of assessment. If abnormality of excitability is detected, further tests are required to determine the nature and location of the pathological process.

Descending (motor) pathways

The *general somatic efferent (GSE) neurons* are found in the *ventral horns* of the gray matter of the spinal cord and brain stem. These neurons are called *lower motor neurons* (LMN). Their axons pass through the segmental nerves to enter and innervate the skeletal muscle cells, including the limbs, back, abdominal muscles, and intercostals. Each LMN undergoes multiple branching before innervating single skeletal muscle cells (Fig. 40-16). Thus, each LMN can innervate and control from 10 to 2,000 individual muscle cells. In general, large muscles, those containing hundreds and thousands of muscle cells and providing gross motor movements, have large motor units. This is in sharp contrast to smaller muscles, such as those in the hand and the tongue and muscles that move the eye, in which the motor units are small and permit very discrete control. An LMN and the muscle fibers it innervates is called a *motor unit*.

The LMNs are surrounded by small CNS neurons, called *internuncial neurons*, which synapse with the cell body or dendrites of the efferent cells. Action potentials in the axons of these internuncial neurons exert either excitatory or inhibitory effects on the LMN. Although some CNS systems communicate directly with the LMN, almost all LMN activity is controlled by systems communicating through excitatory or inhibitory internuncial neurons. These internuncial general somatic output association (GSOA) neurons represent the final stage of communication between elaborate CNS neuronal

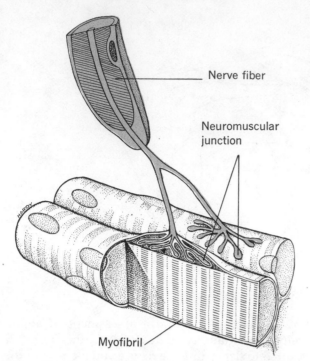

Figure 40–16. Diagram of a neuromuscular junction (motor end plate) in striated muscle. Each lower motor neuron undergoes multiple branching before innervating single muscle cells, and each can control 10 to 2000 individual muscle cells. (Chaffee EE, Lytle IM: Basic Physiology and Anatomy, 4th ed, p 130. Philadelphia, JB Lippincott, 1980)

circuits and the transmission of information to the skeletal muscle cells of the motor unit.

During early embryological development, outgrowing GSE axons innervate partially mature muscle cells, which if not innervated, will not mature and will eventually die. Randomly contracting muscle cells become "enslaved" by the innervating neurons and from then on, the muscle cell will contract only when stimulated by that particular neuron. If the LMN dies or its axon is destroyed, the skeletal muscle cell is again free of neural domination. When this happens, it begins to have spontaneous contractions on its own. It also begins to lose its contractile proteins and after several months, degenerates. This is called *denervation atrophy*. If a peripheral nerve or muscle nerve is crushed and the endoneurial tubes remain intact, the outgrowing axonic branches may reinnervate the muscle cell. If the nerve is cut, however, the likelihood of axonic reinnervation by the original axon is slight, and muscle cell loss is likely to occur. If some intact LMN axons remain within the muscle, nearby denervated muscle cells apparently emit what is called a *trophic signal*, probably some form of chemical, which signals the intact axon to

send outgrowing collaterals into the denervated area and "capture" control of some of the denervated muscle fibers. The degree of axonic regeneration that occurs after injury to an LMN depends on the amount of scar tissue that develops at the site of injury and how quickly reinnervation occurs. If reinnervation occurs after muscle cell degeneration had taken place, no recovery is possible. Thus, peripheral nerve section usually results in some loss of muscle cell function, which is experienced as weakness. Collateral sprout reinnervation results in enlarged motor units and, therefore, a reduction in the discreteness of muscle control following recovery.

Trophic effects. If a normally innervated muscle is not used for long periods of time, muscle cell diameter becomes reduced (*disuse atrophy*) and although the muscle cells do not die, they become weakened. With appropriate exercise, muscle strength will return. Exercise beyond the normal results in enlargement of the muscle-fiber diameter with the addition of contractile substance, and muscle strength increases. There are limits, however, and when muscle *hypertrophy* becomes excessive, the largest of the muscle cells can undergo degeneration.

Hyperexcitability due to injury or infection. Infection or irritation of the cell body of the LMN or its axon can lead to hyperexcitability, which causes rapid contractions of the muscle units to occur. These are often seen through the skin as twitching and squirming on the muscle surface. They are called *fasciculations*. Toxic agents, such as the tetanus toxin (*Clostridium tetani*), produce extreme hyperexcitability of the LMN, which results in firing at maximum rate. The resultant extreme contraction of the muscles is called *tetany*. Tetany of muscles on both sides of a joint produces immobility or tetanic paralysis. The poliomyelitis virus, when it attacks an LMN, first irritates the LMN, causing fasciculations to occur. These fasciculations are often followed by neuronal death. Weakness results. If muscles are totally denervated, total weakness, called *flaccid paralysis*, occurs.

Myasthenia gravis. Myasthenia gravis is a disease process that affects the communication between the terminal and innervated muscle cell. The disease is thought to be due to a deficiency in the acetylcholine (ACh) receptor sites on the muscle side of the neuromuscular junction. In the normal person, each neuromuscular junction contains about 38 million receptor sites. In myasthenia gravis this number may be reduced to levels as low as 20% of normal.[2] This decrease in receptor sites is believed to be caused by an autoimmune mechanism. This immune response has two effects: it blocks the receptor site, and it causes destruction of the receptor site.

The incidence of myasthenia gravis is about 1 in 10,000 and it is seen most frequently in young adults. The disability persists throughout life, although there may be periods of improvement followed by periods of worsening. This disease causes weakness of the muscles. There are no sensory changes or hyperactive reflexes. The most common manifestations are weakness of the eye muscles, with ptosis (dropping of the eyelids) and diplopia caused by weakness of the extraocular muscles. Chewing and swallowing may be difficult. Weakness in limb movement is usually more proximal than distal so that there is difficulty in climbing stairs, lifting objects, and so on. As the disease progresses, the muscles of the lower face may be affected, causing speech impairment. When this happens, the person often supports the chin with one hand to assist in speaking.

There are two treatment methods for myasthenia gravis. One involves the administration of drugs that prevent the normally rapid breakdown of ACh (*i.e.*, neostigmine and pyridostigmine). The other form of treatment is designed to halt the immune response and induce a remission in the disease; it includes adrenocorticosteroid and immunosuppressive drugs as part of the regimen. Surgical removal of the thyroid gland also may be done. Significant improvement has been noted in two-thirds of myasthenic persons who were so treated.[3]

Persons with myasthenia gravis may develop sudden respiratory difficulty, called myasthenic crisis, which is severe enough to require mechanical ventilation. This usually occurs during a period of stress, such as infection or following surgery. The crisis is usually a transient one and subsides if adequate ventilatory support can be maintained.

The Brain

The brain is divided into three parts: the forebrain, which forms the two cerebral hemispheres, thalamus and hypothalamus; the midbrain; and the hindbrain, which is divided into the pons and the medulla. The structure and organization of the brain become clearer when considered in the context of embryonic development.

The important concept to be kept in mind is that the more rostral, recently elaborated parts of the neural tube gain *domination*, or *control*, over regions and functions at lower levels. They *do not replace* the more ancient circuitry, but merely dominate it. Thus, following damage to the more vulnerable

parts of the forebrain, as occurs in "brain death," a brain stem organism remains capable of respiration and survival if environmental temperature is regulated and if nutrition and other aspects of care are provided. All aspects of intellectual function, including experience, perception, and memory, are usually permanently lost, however.

In the process of development, the most rostral part of the embryonic neural tube—in humans approximately ten segments—undergoes extensive modification and enlargement to form the brain. The brain stem is a modification of the neural tube segments. In the early embryo, three swellings, or primary vesicles, develop, subdividing these ten segments into the prosencephalon (forebrain), which contains the first two segments; the metencephalon, or midbrain, which develops from segment 3; and the rhombencephalon, or hindbrain, which develops from segments 4 to 10.

The central canal of the prosencephalon develops two pairs of lateral outpouchings, which carry the neural tube with them: the optic cup, which becomes the optic nerve and retina, and the telencephalic vesicles, which become the cerebral hemispheres with their enlarged CSF-filled cavities, the first, second, or lateral vesicles. The remaining neural tube of these three segments is called the diencephalon ("between brain"), and it becomes the adult thalamus and hypothalamus. The neurohypophysis (posterior pituitary) grows as a midline ventral outgrowth at the junctions of segments 1 and 2. A dorsal outgrowth, the pineal body, develops between segments 2 and 3, at the diencephalic–mesencephalic junction.

The third neural tube segment, which forms the midbrain, retains its basic spinal segment-like organization. Segment 4, the rhombencephalon, becomes much enlarged and flattened laterally, giving the fourth ventricle its rhomboid shape. This segment, called the metencephalon, or pons, also grows up and over the fourth ventricle and is a major contributor to the adult cerebellum.

The remaining segments, 5 through 10, become the adult medulla oblongata, with the widened fourth ventricle narrowing down to form a central canal, which continues through the spinal cord segments. The most rostral segment (number 5) of the medulla fuses with the pons and is often called the caudal pons. It also contributes to the caudal part of the cerebellum. The junction of segment 10 of the brain stem with the cervical spinal segments occurs at the foramen magnum, the large opening in the skull through which the neural tube passes (Fig. 40-17).

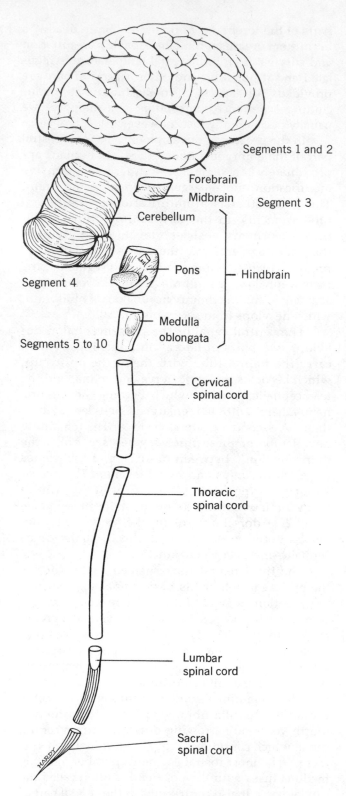

Figure 40–17. The central nervous system. The parts of the brain and the spinal cord have been separated. (Chaffee EE, Lytle IM: Basic Physiology and Anatomy, 4th ed, p 203. Philadelphia, JB Lippincott, 1980)

Each of these brain-stem segments, except for segment 2, retains at least some portion of the basic segmental nerve organization. Our ancient ancestry is reflected in the cranial nerve and upper cervical segmental nerves, because the original pattern was for many branches to occur directly from the neural tube, with each containing a particular component, or functional grouping, of axons. Thus, one segment would have paired branches to somite muscles, another a set to gill arch muscles, and yet another a set to visceral structures, and so on. The classic pattern of the spinal nerve organization, which consists of a pair of dorsal and a pair of ventral roots, is a more recent evolutionary development that has not occurred in the cranial nerves. Consequently, the arbitrarily numbered 1 through 12 cranial nerves retain the ancient pattern, and more than one cranial nerve can branch from a single segment. The truly segmental nerve pattern of the cranial nerves is further clouded by the loss of all branches from segment 2 and most of the branches from segment 1. In segments 6 through 10, longitudinal fusions between segments and loss of components at some segments reflect the specialization of the head end of the organism through nearly a billion years of evolutionary history. It should also be noted that the classic second cranial nerve, the optic nerve, is not really a segmental nerve branch at all, but is a brain tract connecting the retina (modified) brain with the first forebrain segment from which it developed.

The ventral half of the neural tube gray matter, the basal lamina, which becomes the ventral horn, remains relatively unchanged through the brain segments. Most of the brain, as seen grossly, represents tremendous enlargements, outpouchings, outgrowths, and cortex formation derived from the dorsal horns.

Both the central and peripheral nervous systems differentiate very early in embryonic life and hold a critical position in providing a necessary stimulus for differentiation of many other body tissues, particularly the skeletal muscles. By the end of the third month of gestation, the gross structure of the brain and spinal cord is established. The remaining period of intrauterine growth involves increases in cell numbers of both neurons and glial cells to a final neural to glial ratio of 1:20, as well as the development of the basic circuitry and myelination of the major tract systems of the spinal cord and brain stem. A phenomenal increase in brain weight occurs during the 3- to 5-month period of intrauterine life. At birth, the average brain weighs about 300 gm, approximately 12.5% of total body weight. During postuterine life, growth continues but at a decreasing rate, while body growth continues. As a result, the adult human brain weight (1450 gm to 1500 gm in the male, and 1200 gm to 1300 gm in the female) is only about five times that at birth and yet is only about 2.4% of total body weight. Maximum brain weight is reached between ages 20 and 29 and is then followed by a gradual decrease in weight with advancing years.

During the later two-thirds of intrauterine life, the cerebral cortex increases its volume relative to that of deeper structures; this is achieved by a greatly increased surface area, which occurs with increasing development of the number and depth of infoldings. The ridge between these infoldings, or grooves, is called a gyrus; a groove is called a sulcus. The adult cerebral cortex, with its many gyri and sulci, is equivalent to an area of about 160,000 mm² and contains approximately 16.5 billion neurons.[4] The most recently enlarged parts of the neocortex develop later in postnatal life, particularly the portions of the frontal, parietal, and temporal cortex that grow out and cover the insula. The cerebellar cortex also undergoes a tremendous increase in area during the latter part of embryonic life and infancy, achieving an area of 84,000 mm², again with the development of many deep sulci and narrow gyri. The cerebellar cortex of the adult contains approximately 100 billion neurons.

The brain stem

The adult brain stem is a distorted, enlarged, and elaborated version of the spinal cord. It contains the neuronal circuits required for the basic breathing, eating, and locomotive functions required for survival. It also is surrounded on the outside by the long tract systems that interconnect the forebrain with lower parts of the CNS (Fig. 40-18).

The medulla

The medulla oblongata represents the caudal 5 segments of the brain part of the neural tube, and thus the cranial nerve branches entering and leaving it have similar functions, as do the spinal nerve segmental nerves. General somite innervating lower motor neurons (GSE) from the lower segments of the medulla innervate the skeletal muscles of the tongue via the *twelfth cranial nerve*. In the most rostral segment of the medulla, lower motor neurons reach forward through the sixth cranial nerve to the skeletal muscle, which moves the eye outward or laterally. Afferent and efferent neurons (GVA; GVE) innervating the gastrointestinal tract enter and leave the medulla via the *tenth* or *vagus cranial nerve*. Neurons in the medulla also provide innervation for the heart and lungs. Slightly more rostral, the *ninth cranial nerve* has similar function for the oral pharynx and caudal third of the tongue mucosa, including the taste buds. This nerve innervates the parotid gland,

Figure 40–18. Midsagittal section of the brain. (Chaffee EE, Lytle IM: Basic Phsiology and Anatomy, 4th ed, p 214. Philadelphia, JB Lippincott, 1980)

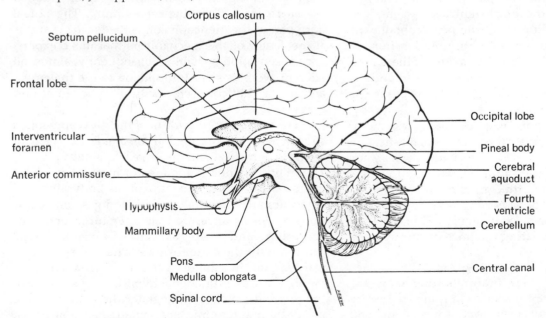

which provides the major supply of saliva. At the rostral end of the medulla, the *intermedius nerve* again has a similar pattern of innervating the nasopharynx and the taste buds of the palate and forward two-thirds of the tongue. It also innervates the lacrimal gland and the salivary glands under the tongue. A large *facial nerve* innervates the muscles of facial expression over all of the head. It can be thought of as the sphincter nerve for the head, controlling the muscles of the eye in opening and closing, the nose, the lips, and the external ear (minor function).

Although the ventral horn area in the medulla is relatively small, the dorsal horn area is enlarged because of the great amount of information pouring in through these cranial nerves. Outside of the central gray matter, the archi, or inner, layer of longitudinal tracts, which forms the reticular formation of the medulla, is greatly enlarged. This contains the circuitry for most of the basic life-support reflexes—respiration, heart rate, gagging, swallowing, coughing, hiccuping, vomiting, salivating. Two longitudinal ridges along the medial part of the undersurface of the medulla, called the *pyramids*, represent the pathways of the neo system, which bring the cerebral cortical control to these cranial nerves and spinal lower motor neurons. The tracts within the pyramids are the corticobulbar and corticospinal.

The pons

The pons, or bridge, developed from the fourth neural tube segment. The central canal of the spinal cord, which is greatly enlarged in the pons and rostral medulla, forms the fourth ventricle. An enlarged area on the ventral surface of the pons contains the pontine nuclei, which receive information from all parts of the cerebral cortex. The axons of these neurons form a massive bundle that swings around the lateral side of the fourth ventricle to enter the cerebellum.

Internally, the pons contains the lower motor neurons, which innervate the muscles of mastication via the *fifth cranial nerve*. The major somesthetic innervation of the forehead, face, and mouth enters the pons through the fifth cranial nerve. The reticular formation of the pons is very large and contains the circuitry necessary for incising and masticating food and for manipulating the jaws during speech.

The cerebellum

The cerebellum, or "little brain," sitting above the 4th ventricle, is a complicated computer necessary for interrelating visual, auditory, somesthetic, and vestibular information with ongoing motor activity such that highly skilled movement is smoothly performed.

The midbrain

The midbrain developed from the third segment of the neural tube and is not very differently organized from a spinal cord segment. The central canal is reestablished as the cerebral aqueduct, interconnecting the fourth ventricle with the third ventricle, just rostral. The central gray matter contains the lower motor neurons that innervate most of the skeletal muscles that move the optic globe about and raise the eyelids. These axons leave the midbrain through the *third cranial nerve*, and this also contains autonomic axons controlling pupillary constriction and ciliary-muscle focusing of the lens. Massive fiber bundles of the cerebral peduncles pass from the forebrain to the pons along the ventral surface of the midbrain. On the dorsal surface, four "little hills," the superior and inferior colliculi, are areas of cortex formation. The inferior colliculus is involved in directional turning and, to some extent, the experiencing of the direction of sound sources. The superior colliculus is an essential part of the reflex mechanisms that control eye movements when the visual environment is being surveyed.

The forebrain

The two forward-most brain stem segments form an enlarged dorsal horn–ventral horn structure with a narrow, deep, enlarged central canal, the third ventricle separating the two sides. This region is called the *diencephalon*, or "between brain." The dorsal horn part of the diencephalon is the *thalamus* and is at the center of the mechanisms that make experience or sensation possible. Consequently, almost all afferent systems send information to the thalamus, and it is richly connected with all other forebrain areas.

The ventral horn portion of the diencephalon is subdivided into the medial *hypothalamus*, next to the third ventricle, and the more lateral *subthalamus*. The hypothalamus is the area of master-level integration of homeostatic control of the body's internal environment. Maintenance of blood gas concentrations, water balance, body temperature, food consumption, and major aspects of hormone level control, with the close tolerances necessary for normal function in a highly variable external environment, requires a functional hypothalamus. Many of the efferent functions integrated here involve the use of both autonomic and somatic motor systems.

The subthalamic area is a part of movement control systems related to the basal ganglia discussed below.

The two *cerebral hemispheres* are lateral outgrowths of the diencephalon that become so massive as to dominate the appearance of the forebrain. These hemispheres are hollow, containing the *lateral ventricles* (ventricles I and II), which are interconnected with the third ventricle of the diencephalon by a small opening, the interventricular foramen (of Munro).

The hemispheres are separated by the heavy longitudinal fold of the dura mater, called the *falx cerebri*. The falx cerebri carries the inferior sagittal venous sinus in its lower edge and the superior sagittal sinus at its junction with the outer dural lining of the cranial cavity. The corpus callosum is a massive commissure, or bridge, of myelinated axons interconnecting the cerebral cortex of the two sides of the brain. Two smaller commissures, the anterior and posterior commissures, connect the two sides of

the more specialized regions of the cerebrum and diencephalon (Fig. 40-19).

A section through the cerebral hemisphere will reveal a surface of *cerebral cortex*, a subcortical layer of *white matter* made up of masses of myelinated axons, and deep masses of gray matter, the *basal ganglia* (caudate, putamen, globus pallidus), which border on the internal, lateral ventricle.

The cerebral cortex exposed to view from the side is a recently evolved layered neocortex. It is arbitrarily divided into lobes named for the bones of the skull that cover them. The frontal lobe lies in front of the central sulcus and can be subdivided into the frontal pole, rostrally; and the *superior*, *middle*, and *inferior frontal gyri* laterally; which continue on the undersurface over the eyes as the orbital cortex.

The *precentral gyrus*, immediately bordering the central sulcus, is the *primary motor cortex* from which axons of large cortical neurons leave the cerebrum to reach the intermediate and ventral horns of all brain

Figure 40–19.   Oblique coronal section through the cerebrum and brain stem. Commissural and projection fibers are shown in color. (Chaffee EE, Lytle IM: Basic Physiology and Anatomy, 4th ed, p 204. Philadelphia, JB Lippincott, 1980)

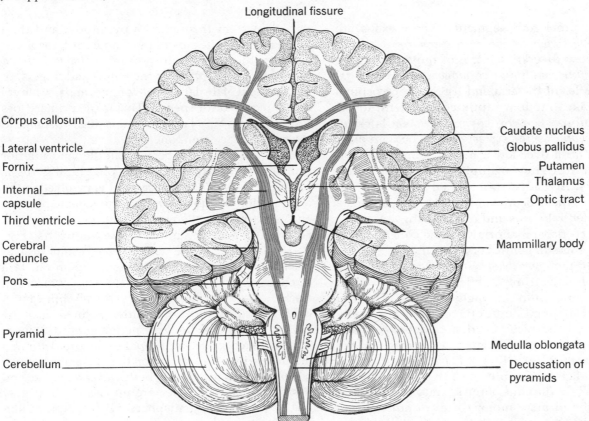

Longitudinal fissure

Corpus callosum

Lateral ventricle

Fornix

Internal capsule

Third ventricle

Cerebral peduncle

Pons

Pyramid

Cerebellum

Caudate nucleus

Globus pallidus

Putamen

Thalamus

Optic tract

Mammillary body

Medulla oblongata

Decussation of pyramids

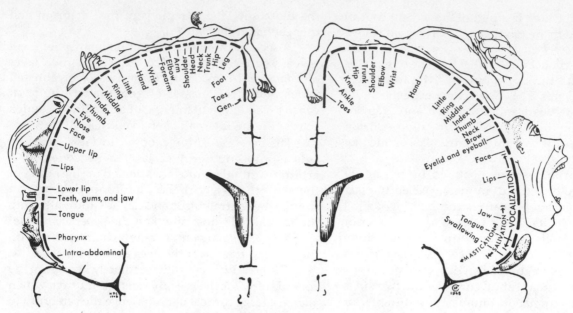

Figure 40–20.   Sensory (*left*) and motor (*right*) representations as determined by stimulation studies on the human cortex at surgery. Compare the sensory homunculus (*left*) to the motor homunculus (*right*). Note the relatively large area devoted to the lips, thumb, and fingers. (Penfield E, Rasmussen T: The Cerebral Cortex of Man. New York, Macmillan, 1955, Copyright © by Macmillan Publishing Co., Inc., renewed 1978 by Theodore Rasmussen)

stem and spinal cord segments. These axons are known collectively as the *corticospinal system* and provide very discrete control of movement, particularly, *fine manipulative movement*. For distal flexor muscles of the arm and leg, the corticospinal system makes monosynaptic contact with lower motor neurons. The corticospinal system is called the *upper motor neuron system* (UMN) because of its discrete control over lower motor neuron function during the initiation of highly skilled voluntary movements. Actually, corticospinal axons originate in all parts of the neocortex, but nearly 60% originate in the precentral gyrus and neighboring areas. The pattern of corticospinal origin in the cortex reflects the discreteness of control of lower motor neurons, innervating the *opposite side of the body*. Relatively less control of the trunk is reflected in a small trunk area of the cortex, and extremely high level of control of the tongue, thumb, index finger, and large toe by larger areas. The resultant distorted body "map" represented in the primary motor cortex is called the *motor homunculus* (Fig. 40-20). The lower limb of the opposite side is represented near the vertex, and the face, laterally at the edge of the lateral sulcus. Loss of a part of the primary motor cortex or of the large-diameter myelinated axons that pass through the cerebral white matter, down the ventral surface of

the brain stem through the pyramids, and then down the opposite side of the spinal cord, results in a loss of the capacity to perform *delicate, refined movements*, particularly of the hands and fingers, of the toes, and of the laryngeal, tongue, and jaw movements required for speech. This is the primary loss resulting from UMN lesions and is due to damage to the motor cortex component.

The area of the superior, middle, and inferior frontal gyri just in front of the precentral gyrus is called the *premotor area* because it is involved in the organization of more complex movement patterns and is an important source of control for patterned activity of primary motor cortex neurons (Fig. 40-21). Damage to premotor cortex results in *dyspraxia* or *apraxia*. Such patients can manipulate a screwdriver, for instance, but cannot *use it* to loosen a screw. They can handle a pencil well, but cannot use it to write with. Higher-order motor skills of the opposite side of the body are permanently damaged.

The major sources of input to the premotor and motor cortices are nuclei of the thalamus, which receive information from both the cerebellum and basal ganglia. The latter are masses of deep gray matter within the hemisphere, with complex interconnections with motor and premotor cortices, the thalamus, and the reticular formation of the brain

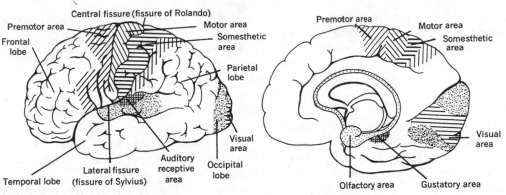

Figure 40–21.   Diagram of the localization of function in the cerebral hemisphere. Various functional areas are shown in relation to the lobes and fissures. (*Left*) lateral view; (*right*), medial view. (From Chaffee EE, Greisheimer EM: Basic Physiology and Anatomy, 3rd ed, p 199. Philadelphia, JB Lippincott, 1974)

stem. At present, their function is believed to be the organization of movement patterns characteristic of the species: the swinging of the arms during walking, the follow-through of the arms and body during the throwing of a ball, or the swinging of a club.

The *parietal lobe* of the cerebrum lies behind the central sulcus and above the lateral sulcus. The strip of cortex bordering the central sulcus is called the *primary sensory cortex* because this receives very discrete projections from the lateral nuclei of the thalamus of somesthetic information. Again, the density of this input reflects the density of somesthetic receptors on the body surface and in the body wall. The tongue, the lips, and the palmar surface of the thumb, index finger, and large toe have the largest receptive areas. The *sensory homunculus* is organized with the leg at the vertex and the face laterally, next to the lateral sulcus (see Fig. 40-20). This cortical area must be functional for discrete, highly discriminative sensation to occur, originating from the opposite side of the body and face. If the area is damaged, sensation still occurs, probably at the thalamic level, but the delicacy of discrimination of location, intensity, and subtle aspects of the given situation are lost. Such a patient cannot tell the differences in texture between sandpaper and velvet, or localize delicate touch other than to a vague, general area of the body. The sense of vibration is lost because this is really a delicate, temporal discrimination. The sense of the position or movement of body parts is also lost. This information is derived from joint, muscle, and tendon receptors and involves subtle discriminations as to joint movement and muscle tension.

A small cortical area just above the lateral sulcus and posterior to the primary somesthetic area seems to be involved in discrimination of the intensity and fine localization of *painful stimuli*. Electrical stimulation of this parietal cortex results only in a sharp, localized sensation but not of the "painfulness" or "hurtfulness" of a nociceptive stimulus. The latter aspects of experience involve the limbic areas of the cerebrum and thalamus.

Just behind the primary somesthetic cortex is a region of "association" cortex, which is interconnected with thalamic nuclei and the primary sensory area. This region is necessary for *perception* or meaningfulness to be appreciated. Lesions in this area lead to *somesthetic agnosia* (gnosis, perception). With this area damaged, a patient can describe the size, shape, or texture of a screwdriver without seeing it but is unable to explain its use—the perception of the word "screwdriver" is lost. However, if the patient can see the tool, he then can explain its function. So it is not the loss of meaning per se but of somesthetically derived meaning that is damaged.

The *temporal lobe* lies below the lateral sulcus and merges with the parietal and occipital lobes. It has a polar region and three primary gyri: superior, middle, and inferior. It is separated from limbic areas on the ventral surface by the collateral or rhinal sulcus. The *primary auditory cortex* involves the part of the superior temporal gyrus that extends into the lateral sulcus. This is particularly important for fine discrimination of sound frequency. Octaves are represented at equal intervals along this cortex, and damage results in deficient but not lost pitch discrimination from sound entering the opposite ear. The more exposed part of the superior temporal gyrus involves the *auditory "association,"* or perceptive, area. The gnostic aspects of hearing (*e.g.*, the meaningfulness of a certain sound pattern, as that of a steam train or a dropped fork) require function of this area. The remaining portion of the temporal cortex has a more vague function, apparently important in long-term memory recall. Irritation or stimulation can result in vivid hallucinations of long-past events.

The *occipital lobe* is posterior to the temporal and parietal lobes and is only arbitrarily separated from them. The medial surface contains a deep sulcus extending from the limbic cortex to the occipital pole, the *calcarine sulcus*, which houses the *primary visual cortex*. Stimulation of this cortex causes the experiencing of bright lights in the visual field. Destruction results in "cortical blindness" in which the patient "sees nothing" yet has normal visual reflexes to bright light or moving objects. Just above and below and extending onto the lateral side of the occipital pole is the *"association" cortex for vision*. This area is closely connected with the primary visual cortex and with complex nuclei of the thalamus. Its integrity is required for the gnosic visual function—the meaningfulness of visual sensation (*e.g.*, is the streaking object "a bird, a plane, or a . . .?").

The neocortical areas of the parietal lobe, between the somesthetic and the visual cortices, have a function in interrelating the texture or "feel" of an object with its visual image. Between the auditory and visual association areas, the parieto-occipital region is necessary for interrelating the sound and the image of an object or person.

It should be noted that the cortices of the frontal, parietal, and temporal lobes surrounding the older cortex of the *insula*, deep in the lateral fissure, represent the most recently evolved parts of the cerebral cortex. These areas contain primary and associative functions for motor control and somesthesias for the lips and tongue, and for audition; thus, they are particularly involved in *speech mechanisms*, discussed later.

The medial aspect of the cerebrum is organized as three concentric bands of cortex, the limbic lobe, surrounding the interconnection between the lateral and third ventricles (the interventricular foramen). The innermost band just above and below the cut surface of the corpus callosum is folded out of sight but is an ancient, three-layered cortex. Just outside that is a band of transitional cortex, which includes the cingulate and parahippocampal cortices. The neocortex, responsible for limbic function, includes the orbital cortex on the underside of the frontal lobe. Outside this is the neocortex of the hemisphere merging into the more specific areas briefly described above. This limbic lobe has intimate connections with the intermedial nuclei of the thalamus, called the intralaminar nuclei, with deep nuclei of the cerebrum (amygdaloid nuclei, septal nuclei),

Figure 40–22. Cranial dura mater. Skull is open to show the falx cerebri and the right and left portions of the tentorium cerebelli, as well as some of the cranial venous sinuses. (Chaffee EE, Lytle IM: Basic Physiology and Anatomy, 4th ed, p 219. Philadelphia, JB Lippincott, 1980)

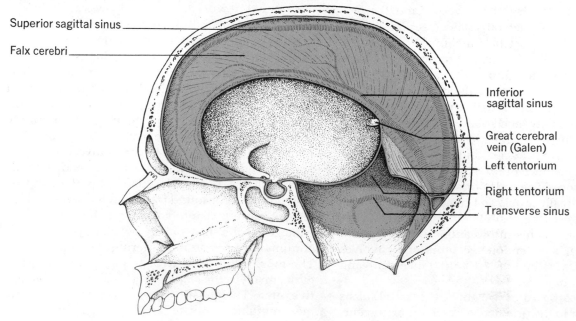

Superior sagittal sinus

Falx cerebri

Inferior sagittal sinus

Great cerebral vein (Galen)

Left tentorium

Right tentorium

Transverse sinus

and with the hypothalamus. In general, this region of the brain is involved in *emotional experience* and in the control of emotion-related behavior. Stimulation of specific areas in this system can lead to feelings of dread, high anxiety, or exquisite pleasure.

The only cortical regions not discussed, the region of the *frontal pole* and that in front of the associative motor cortex, are called the *premotor* frontal cortices. These areas are associated with particular thalamic nuclei, which also are related to the limbic system. In general terms, the prefrontal cortex appears to be involved in anticipation and prediction of the consequences of behavior. This "future-oriented" region is particularly depressed by many drugs, including a goodly dose of ethyl alcohol. Removal of the cortex leads to a less "worrying" personality, preoccupied with the present and giving little thought to the future.

The meninges

Within the skull the dura of the cranial cavity is continuous with the spinal dura. In this area, the arachnoid is closely adherent to the inner surface of the dura, including its various folds. The cranial dura often splits into two layers, and the outer layer serves as the periosteum of the inner surface of the skull (Fig. 40-22).

The inner layer of the dura forms two folds. The first, a longitudinal fold, the *falx cerebri*, intervenes between the cerebral hemispheres and fuses with a second transverse fold, called the *tentorium cerebelli*. The latter acts as a hammock, supporting the occipital lobes above the cerebellum. The tentorium forms a tough septum, which divides the cranial cavity into the anterior and middle fossa, or hollow, which lies above the tentorium, and a posterior fossa, which lies below. The tentorium attaches to the petrous portion of the temporal bone and the dorsum sellae of the cranial floor, with formation of a semicircular gap, or incisura, at the midline to permit the midbrain to pass forward from the posterior fossa. The resultant compartmentalization of the cranial cavity is the basis for the commonly used terms *supratentorial*—above the tentorium—and *infratentorial*—below the tentorium. The cerebral hemispheres and the diencephalon are supratentorial structures, and the pons, cerebellum, and medulla are infratentorial. The strong folds of the inner dura, the tentorium and falx cerebri, support and protect the brain, which is floating in cerebrospinal fluid within the enclosed space. During extreme trauma, however, the sharp edges of these folds can damage the brain as it floats inside the cranium. Space-occupying lesions such as enlarging tumors or he-

matomas can squeeze the brain against these edges or through the small opening of the tentorium, the incisura. As a result, brain tissue can be compressed, contused, or destroyed, often with permanent deficits.

The Ventricular System and Cerebrospinal Fluid

The lining of the embryonic neural tube undergoes multiple foldings in several areas to develop into structures called the choroid plexuses, which are present in the ventricular system and which secrete the cerebrospinal fluid (Fig. 40-23).

The CSF produced in the ventricles must flow through the interventricular foramen, the third ventricle, the cerebral aqueduct, and the midbrain and fourth ventricle to escape from the neural tube. Openings, or foramina, are present: two at the lateral corners of the fourth ventricle, the two lateral foramina of Luschka, and the medial foramen of Magendie in the midline at the caudal end of the fourth ventricle. These openings allow the CSF to flow into the subarachnoid space. About 20% of the CSF passes down into the subarachnoid space that surrounds the spinal cord, mainly on its dorsal surface, and then moves back up to the brain along its ventral surface.

Reabsorption of the CSF into the vascular system occurs largely along the sides of the superior sagittal sinus in the anterior-middle fossa. To reach this area, the CSF must pass along the sides of the medulla and pons, and then pass through the tentorial incisura that surrounds the midbrain. The major part of the flow continues along the sides of the hypothalamus to the region of the optic chiasma and then laterally and dorsally along the lateral fissure and over the parietal cortex to the superior sagittal sinus region. Here the waterproof arachnoid has protuberances, the *arachnoid villi*, which penetrate the inner dura and venous walls of the superior sagittal sinus.

The reabsorption of CSF into the vascular system occurs along a pressure gradient. The normal CSF pressure is about 150 mm H_2O throughout the system, while the venous pressure in the superior sagittal sinus is about 90 mm H_2O. The microstructures of the arachnoid villi are such that if the CSF pressure falls below approximately 50 mm H_2O, the passageways collapse and reverse flow is blocked. The villi, therefore, function as one-way valves, permitting CSF outflow into the blood, but not allowing blood to pass into the subarachnoid spaces.

The brain literally floats in CSF, and the CSF

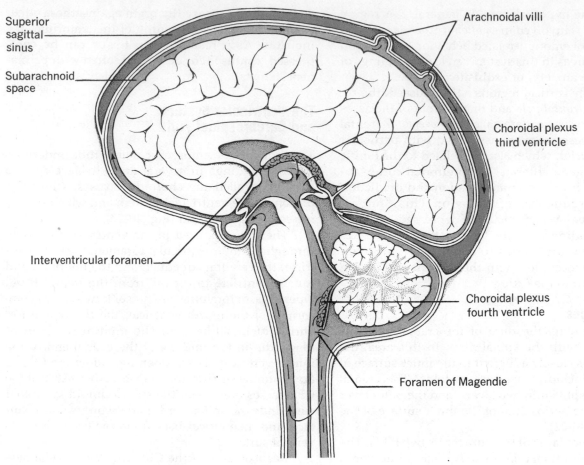

Superior sagittal sinus

Subarachnoid space

Interventricular foramen

Arachnoidal villi

Choroidal plexus third ventricle

Choroidal plexus fourth ventricle

Foramen of Magendie

Figure 40–23.   Diagram of the flow of cerebrospinal fluid from the time of its formation from blood in the choroid plexuses until its return to the blood in the superior sagittal sinus. (Note: Plexuses in the lateral ventricles are not illustrated.) (Chaffee EE, Lytle IM: Basic Physiology and Anatomy, 4th ed, p 221. Philadelphia, JB Lippincott, 1980)

provides support for the ventricular system. When the CSF is removed from the ventricles or the subarachnoid spaces, as during a spinal puncture, the partially collapsed brain tugs on the meninges, stretching the free nerve endings in the inner dura, especially along its major vessels, and giving rise to a rather severe headache. Refilling of the CSF is fairly rapid, and the headache rarely lasts more than a day or so.

Hydrocephalus

An abnormal increase in CSF volume within any part or all of the ventricular system is called *hydrocephalus*. Hydrocephalus is not a disease, but the result of a pathologic process that causes production of CSF at a rate greater than its rate of removal. The two causes of hydrocephalus are overproduction of CSF and obstruction to its flow through the ventricular system, around the brain in the subarachnoid space or through the arachnoid villi.

There are two types of hydrocephalus: communicating and noncommunicating. *Communicating hydrocephalus* occurs when there is obstruction to flow within the subarachnoid space. The obstruction can be caused by congenital malformation, infection, or tumors encroaching upon the ventricular system. *Noncommunicating hydrocephalus* occurs when the CSF is not reabsorbed into the arachnoid villi. This can occur if too few villi are formed, if postinfective (meningitis) scarring occludes them, or because the villi become obstructed by fragments of blood or infectious debris. The signs depend on the type of hydrocephalus, the age of onset, and the extent of increase in CSF pressure. The usual treatment is a shunting procedure, which provides an alternate route for CSF back into the circulation.

The Autonomic Nervous System

Control of the visceral functions of the body is largely vested in the autonomic nervous system, of which there are two divisions, the sympathetic and the parasympathetic nervous systems. Their functions differ. Generally, the functions of the sympathetic nervous system are designed to enable the body to deal with emergency or stress situations. The parasympathetic nervous system, on the other hand, is more concerned with the restorative functions of the body. While it is the sympathetic system that increases the heart rate and blood pressure needed for the "fight or flight" response, it is the parasympathetic system that controls the gut and replenishing of the body's energy stores. The control of visceral function, like that of skeletal muscle contraction, requires both afferent (general visceral afferent, or GVA) and efferent (general visceral efferent, or GVE) endings.

The innervation of visceral organs and the great vessels involves visceral afferent dorsal root ganglion cells and a special type of efferent system, the general visceral efferent (GVE) component of the autonomic nervous system. The role of the CNS in modulating the function of these organs and systems is different from the absolute control that the lower motor neuron exerts on skeletal muscle contraction. Therefore, the autonomic nervous system and its reflexes are considered separately. We will find that the distinction between autonomic and somatic function becomes blurred when the higher levels of integrated response mechanisms are considered. Indeed, almost all somatic reflexes have a visceral component and vice versa.

General visceral afferent (GVA) neurons

There is a rich innervation of the visceral organs and great vessels by dorsal root ganglion cells. Many of these visceral afferent neurons terminate in specialized chemoreceptive organs, such as the carotid body and aortic bodies or in pressure-sensitive endings in the carotid and aortic baroreceptors. Visceral afferent terminals are also present in the mucosal smooth muscle and connective tissue layers of the gastrointestinal tract. In the respiratory system, the trachea, bronchi, and lungs are richly innervated by afferent endings.

Visceral afferent neurons are located in the ganglia of the intermedius, the ninth and tenth cranial nerves, the thoracic and upper lumbar dorsal root ganglia, and the dorsal root ganglia of sacral levels 2, 3, and 4. Essentially, all visceral organs receive dual afferent innervation which travels with both sympathetic and parasympathetic portions of the autonomic nervous system.

The central axons of these GVA cells enter the dorsal horn gray matter or its equivalent in the medulla and synapse in the visceral association cell column (GVIA) of the same or neighboring segments to those of entry. The association cells, utilizing multisynaptic pathways: (1) project into local reflex circuits, (2) project into spinoreticular projections to higher levels of the brain stem, and contribute to hierarchical control mechanisms of visceral reflexes (the spinoreticular projection has a mild contribution to facilitating the ascending reticular system); and (3) project to the thalamus by way of the *protopathic pathway*, the spinothalamic system of both sides of the cord and brain stem.

The contribution of visceral afferent endings to sensation is disproportionately small, considering the richness of afferent input from these regions. It reaches a sensation level in the thalamus which has a projection to a small parietal cortical area near the insula. Visceral sensation has a very strong emotional component, and the intermediate thalamic nuclei receive visceral signals and communicate with the limbic system. Sensations of fullness, pressure, and pain, and those associated with deep structure stimulation during evacuation and during sexual activity can have intensely unpleasant or pleasant aspects and can precipitate short-term as well as long-term behavioral consequences.

Despite complete dual GVA innervation of the entire length of the gut, sensation from the viscera is separated into three parts: (1) input to the cranial nerves from the pharynx, larynx, and esophagus; (2) input to the thoracic-lumbar segments from the stomach, small intestine, and ascending and mid-transverse colon; and (3) input to sacral segments 2 through 4 from the descending colon and rectum, bladder, and uterus. Although there is no explanation available for this separation of GVA-derived sensation, it is useful to understanding. For example, pain and discomfort arising from the uterus and associated organs is experienced only from the afferent neurons entering at sacral levels. Therefore, pharmacological blockade of these roots or the spinal cord at low lumbar levels prevents pain information from being relayed through the protopathic pathways from these levels so that the pain associated with childbirth can be avoided. Because of the various levels of input, GVA information from these same organs continues to enter the cord at the lower thoracic and high lumbar levels, probably contributing to normal vasomotor reflex control, which is maintained in these organs during blockade of visceral pain sensation.

General visceral efferent (GVE) neurons

General visceral efferent neurons of the ventral horn are also called *preganglionic* neurons. These preganglionic neurons send their axons into the PNS to innervate a second postganglionic neuron in autonomic ganglia. The axons of these postganglionic neurons innervate viscera, blood vessels, heart, smooth muscles, and glands.

The efferent neurons of the parasympathetic nervous system originate in cranial and sacral segments of the cell columns, whereas the sympathetic neurons have origin in thoracic-lumbar segments. Axons of the preganglionic sympathetic neurons leave the segmental nerve to reach a chain of ganglia containing postganglionic sympathetic neurons, called the *sympathetic* or *paravertebral chain*. Because of the myelinated axons, this connection is called a *white ramus* (branch) (Fig. 40-24). The axons of the postganglionic sympathetic neurons proceed toward the visceral organs through a *visceral ramus*. Some of the postganglionic neurons have migrated closer to the gut to form sympathetic ganglia, which are scattered along the dorsal aorta and its branches (celiac, superior mesenteric, aorticorenal, and inferior mesenteric ganglia, others). Sympathetic postganglionic axons leave these ganglia to innervate the smooth muscle and gland cells of visceral organs supplied by these vessels. The adrenal medulla contains postganglionic sympathetic neurons. These sympathetic postganglionic neurons secrete their transmitters, norepinephrine (NE) and epinephrine (E), directly into the blood stream. The characteristics of the GVE sympathetic and parasympathetic nervous systems are summarized in Table 40-6.

Functions of the sympathetic nervous system

In general, increased activity in the sympathetic nervous system shifts blood from the visceral organs into organs closely involved in meeting a challenge to survival (such as the skeletal muscles and the

Figure 40–24.   Autonomic elements of the spinal nerves. In the thoracolumbar region, each ventral nerve root carries a contingent of efferent sympathetic fibers. These pass to the neighboring sympathetic trunk as a white ramus. Some of the fibers synapse in ganglia of corresponding levels, but others emerge from the trunk without synapsing. Fibers emerge from the ganglia to pass to plexuses, or to rejoin the nerves as gray rami passing to peripheral or meningeal structures. In the cervical and sacral regions the ventral roots give off no white ramus. But fibers from other levels synapse in the ganglia and secondary fibers pass off as gray rami to join the nerve trunks. (Elliott HC: Neuroanatomy. Philadelphia, JB Lippincott, 1969)

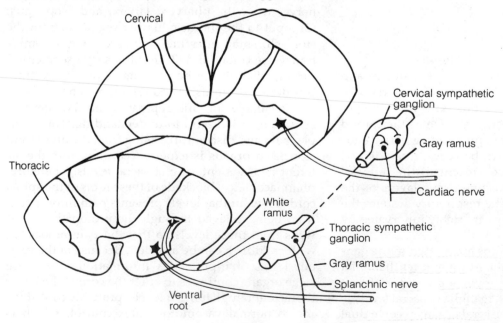

Table 40-6   General Characteristics of GVE Sympathetic and Parasympathetic Nervous Systems

Characteristic	Sympathetic Outflow	Parasympathetic Outflow
Location of preganglionic cell body in GVE column	Thoracic 1–12, lumbar 1 & 2	Cranial nerves: III, intermedius, IX and X, sacral segments 2, 3, 4
Relative length of preganglionic axon	Short; to sympathetic (paravertebral) chain of ganglia or to aortic (prevertebral) chain of ganglia	Long; to ganglion cells in ganglia near or in organ innervated
Transmitter between preganglionic terminals and postganglionic neuron	Acetylcholine (ACh)	Acetylcholine (ACh)
Transmitter of postganglionic neuron	ACh (sweat glands); NE (most synapses); NE and E (secreted by adrenal medulla)	ACh
General function	Mobilization of resources in anticipation of challenge to survival (preparation for "fight-or-flight") (catabolic)	Conservation of resources, renewal and recovery from mobilization (anabolic)
Specific examples:		
Iris	Dilation (radial muscle)	Constriction (sphincter muscle)
Salivation	Slight, viscid secretion	Fluid secretion
Gut	Reduced peristaltic activity and glandular secretion	Increased peristaltic activity, secretory activity
Sphincters of gut	Constriction	Relaxation
Heart rate	Increased rate	Decrease
Blood pressure	Increase	Decrease
Bronchi	Dilation of bronchial muscle	Constriction
Blood vessels:		
Skin	Constriction	None
Skeletal muscle	Dilation	None
Viscera	Constriction	None
Effect on adrenal medullary secretion	Secrete NE and E	None
Piloerector muscles	Erection of hair	None

central nervous system). Thus, the sphincters of the stomach, intestine, anus, and bladder become constricted, and the rate of secretion of glands involved in digestion diminishes. One of the major functions of sympathetic innervation to these visceral organs is in the control of vasoconstriction and, therefore, of blood flow. Sympathetic innervation of the SA and particularly of the AV nodes of the heart provides strong acceleratory stimulation to heart rate.

This survival function of high sympathetic nervous system activity requires that postganglionic axons must also dilate the bronchial airway and increase the secretion of the adrenal medulla, the cells of which are, in reality, postganglionic sympathetic neurons.

Emergency situations require the shunting of blood flow away from the skin and into the muscles and brain. This reduces the rate of bleeding should a wound occur, and increases those particular resources required for either fighting or fleeing a threat to survival. Postganglionic sympathetic neu-

rons of the sympathetic (paravertebral) ganglionic chain must therefore reach the body wall, or soma, and its organs; they do so by re-entering the segmental nerve via the gray ramus to be distributed with the peripheral nerves to the blood vessels of the skin, muscles, and CNS (dilatory in skeletal muscles; constrictive in vessels of the skin). They also innervate the piloerector muscles which, when contracted, cause the hair to fluff—characteristic of an angry, challenging animal or of a cold animal—enhancing insulation by trapping air in the fur. Remnants of these functions in the human include "creeping" of hair, especially on the back of the neck during moments of fear or anger, and raising of "goose bumps" (short, thin hair shafts) when cold. Postganglionic axons of the autonomic system are unmyelinated and therefore have a gray cast; hence the appellation of gray ramus to the interconnecting link between the sympathetic chain ganglia and the segmental nerves traversed by these axons (Fig. 40-25).

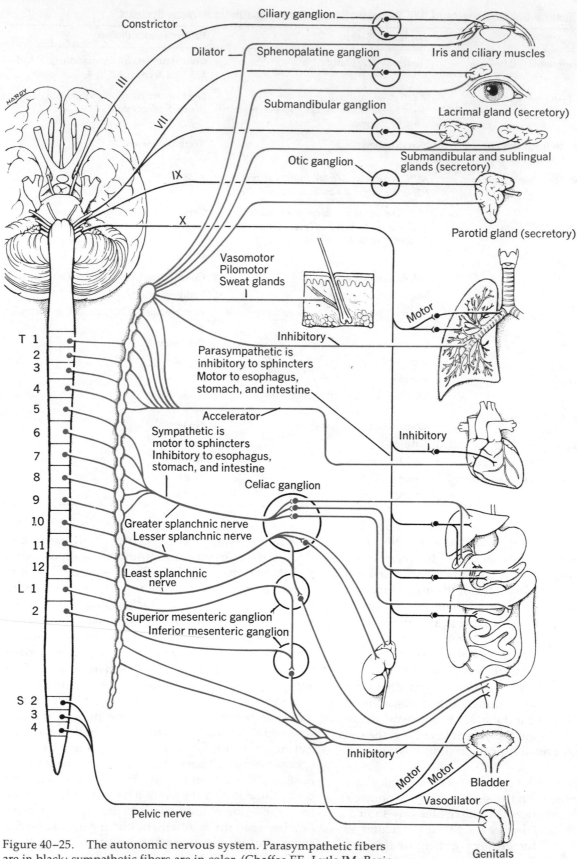

Figure 40–25. The autonomic nervous system. Parasympathetic fibers are in black; sympathetic fibers are in color. (Chaffee EE, Lytle IM: Basic Physiology and Anatomy, 4th ed, p 252. Philadelphia, JB Lippincott, 1980)

The sympathetic outflow from the GVE cell column occurs only from the first thoracic to the second lumbar segments, yet the sympathetic innervation involves all regions of the viscera and soma. This innervation is accomplished by longitudinal spread of preganglionic axons along the sympathetic chain of ganglia into cervical and sacral segments. Postganglionic sympathetic axons of the cervical and lower lumbar–sacral chain ganglia spread further through nerve plexuses along continuations of the great arteries. Thus, cranial structures, particularly blood vessels, are innervated by the spread of postganglionic axons along the internal and external carotid arteries into the face and into the cranial cavity.

Functions of the parasympathetic nervous system

The parasympathetic portions of the GVE cell column are at the forward and caudal ends. Thus, parasympathetic preganglionic neurons of cranial nerve and sacral nerve distribution are located within the brain stem and sacral segments 2, 3, and 4 of the cord. Preganglionic neurons of these cells distribute with the third, intermedius portion of the facial nerve complex, ninth, and tenth cranial nerves to the viscera of the head (salivary glands, lacrimal glands, mucosal glands, and smooth muscle of the nasal, oral, and laryngeal pharynx) and to the visceral organs of the thoracic and abdominal cavities (trachea and lungs; esophagus; heart; stomach; small intestine; the ascending and transverse portions of the large bowel).

These preganglionic axons innervate postganglionic parasympathetic neurons, which lie in a series of autonomic ganglia of the head (ciliary, submandibular, pterygopalatine, and otic ganglia) or in the tissues of the thoracic and abdominal organs. Parasympathetic vagus (tenth cranial nerve) preganglionic axons innervate postganglionic parasympathetic neurons imbedded in the wall of the heart near the AV and SA nodes, for example. The latter innervate the nearby nodal tissue and slow the heart rate. For most of these visceral organs, increased parasympathetic activity results in increased glandular secretion necessary for efficient digestive function or other anabolic and restorative activity, such as constriction of the pupil, constriction of the bronchi, increased salivary secretion, and opening the sphincters of the gut. The preganglionic sacral axons of this system leave the sacral segmental nerves by gathering into the pelvic nerves, which lead to the autonomic plexuses along the great vessels. They spread to the hindgut and its derivatives, the pelvic viscera (bladder, uterus, urethra, prostate, distal portion of the transverse colon, descending colon,

and rectum). In the walls of these organs, postganglionic parasympathetic neurons send their axons to the smooth muscle and gland cells facilitating digestive functions, and urinary and fecal release.

Thus the autonomic system dually innervates the visceral organs: the sympathetic system by spreading from the middle region of the neural tube (T_1–L_2 spinal segments), longitudinally to all parts of the foregut and middle and hindgut and associated organs. The parasympathetic system originates at the two ends (cranial nerves, sacral nerves) and spreads toward the middle. Both innervate the entire viscera but with somewhat opposing function: the parasympathetic system tends to facilitate anabolic recovery and regenerative functions of the unthreatened organism, and the sympathetic system facilitates preparation for encounters with survival-threatening challenges.

Recently, increased attention to the microcircuitry of the autonomic ganglia has revealed a much higher level of complexity than the above account might suggest. It has been demonstrated that within the sympathetic ganglia and within the parasympathetic ganglionic plexuses in the wall of the gut, the enteric plexuses, inhibitory and feedback circuits, and local afferent neurons continue to function as sources of local reflexes when isolated from the CNS. The peripheral autonomic system thus appears to have considerable computing capacity and autonomous function, with the CNS input via preganglionic axons as a modulating rather than a total controlling influence on local function.

The hierarchy of visceral reflexes

Reflex control of the bladder after recovery from spinal cord transection will serve as an example of local spinal-level visceral reflexes. The visceral afferent neurons and parasympathetic efferent neurons of the second through fourth sacral segments are involved, and the reflex circuitry is contained in these cord segments. As the bladder is filling, constriction of the internal sphincter is maintained and the general state of smooth muscle tone in the bladder is reflexly and gradually relaxed. Stretch receptors in the bladder wall increase their activity as filling continues, and a threshold for the *emptying reflex* usually occurs with a retained urine volume of 250 cc. The emptying reflex involves relaxation of the internal sphincter of the urethra and contraction of the bladder wall. Voiding is incomplete, however, and the retention of a small volume of urine increases the probability of chronic infection. When the bladder is filling, the internal sphincter is not able to completely prevent urine outflow, so that some dribbling occurs. If descending control from brain stem levels is intact, the internal sphincter is more effective and, in addition, forebrain control of the somite efferent lower motor neurons can reinforce this effect by contraction of the striated muscles of the external sphincter.

Medullary-level organization of evacuative functions brings the local emptying reflex under rostral control. Spinoreticular projection brings in a continuous flow of bladder wall stretch information; reticulospinal, paleo-level tracts reaching to sacral levels can inhibit or stimulate the reflex as a part of a more general voiding response, which includes placing the body in an appropriate posture. Hypothalamic control dominates the voiding behavior pattern, blocking it in times of emergency and facilitating it at other times. Limbic and other forebrain systems provide an even higher level of control, inhibiting the reflex in spite of dangerous overfilling under strong social pressure about the "appropriateness" of the situation, for example. Other somatic efferent components also can be brought in to modify the process. Increased intra-abdominal pressure can be exerted by the muscles of the abdominal wall, thoracic cage, and diaphragm to cause emptying.

Organization of many life-support reflexes occurs in the reticular formation of the medulla and pons. These areas of reflex circuitry, often called "centers," produce the complex combinations of autonomic and somatic efferent functions required for respiration, gag, cough, sneeze, swallow, and vomit reflexes as well as the more purely autonomic control of the cardiovascular system. At the hypothalamic level these reflexes are integrated into more general response patterns of rage, defense, eating, drinking, voiding, and sexual mounting and copulation, and so on. Forebrain and especially limbic system control of these behaviors involves learning to inhibit or facilitate release of the behavior patterns according to social pressures or general emotion-provoking situations.

The basic hierarchical control of autonomic function is based on local circuits interrelating visceral afferent and autonomic efferent activity. Progressively greater complexity in the responses and greater precision in their control occurs at higher and higher levels of the brain stem. For much autonomic-mediated visceral function, the hypothalamus stands as the region of master control. Yet it is under forebrain domination involving still more complex stimuli as well as the full effects of past learning. It should also be emphasized that most "visceral" reflexes also contain contributions from the striated muscle innervating lower motor neurons as part of the response pattern. In other words, the distinction

between visceral and somatic reflex hierarchies becomes less and less meaningful at the higher levels of hierarchical control and behavioral integration.

:Higher Order Functions and Their Relationships to the Structure of the Nervous System

The relationship between nervous system structure and specificity of function is the theme of this chapter. Yet, as more complex functions are considered, the reader should have noted that reference to areas or circuits became progressively more vague. This may be due to our current lack of knowledge or to the nonspecificity of function of many forebrain regions. Attempts to interrelate neural structure and function, particularly in the forebrain, often fall into two "schools": the "lumper" school tends to deny anything other than the most vague relationship. Emphasis here is on the vast redundancy of neuronal circuits and on the lack of highly specific functional loss with highly localized lesions, particularly of the associational cortex and basal ganglia. Theoretical frameworks here emphasize "field effects" and information storage or analysis based on interacting patterns of mass neuronal activity. The other school, perhaps equally extreme, can be called the "splitters." They tend to seek minute correlations between structure and function, often beyond the scientific data base. The "truth" may eventually be found to lie somewhere between these extremes.

One of the greatest dangers in making assumptions about the nervous system is to underestimate the complexity of neuronal circuits and networks. There are many examples of microcircuits between small populations of neurons that are now becoming evident.[5] Macrocircuits involving dispersed groups or regions are also known for some neural systems. As an analogy, a radio set works. You remove the transistor and it does not function. Does the function of the set therefore reside in that transistor? Replace the transistor and remove another part, a condensor for instance. Again the set doesn't work. Now, is the function of the system residing in that condensor? The answer is that the different subcircuits of the set accomplish different aspects of the function of the set: there are feedback control systems to maintain the current flow in one part of the set, or the overall voltage control regardless of temperature changes or, in better sets, in spite of aging of certain components. In the nervous system, the crispness and delicacy of function is the net result of many circuits, each containing redundant circuits for safety against local damage. Just as the function of the radio set cannot be adequately assessed with a hammer, neither can much of the neural circuitry of the brain be assessed with our present rather crude experimental methods. On the other hand, methods of assessing changes in function of an area of the nervous system as a result of a localized cerebral vascular accident or tumor growth provide information about important components of the functional systems, but do not tell us what all of the components of the system actually do.

In spite of these limitations, some evidence of localization of complex functions of the forebrain, for example, has accumulated. Lateral dominance, or the tendency to use one hand, eye, or foot over its contralateral competitor, is evidenced in humans, monkeys, and even mice. Studies of identical twins raised apart and of persons who have had major side-by-side bridging of the neocortex or had the corpus callosum removed for therapeutic purposes, generally confirm the biological anatomical basis for side preference. In general, the left cerebral hemisphere tends to be dominant for speech and symbolic logic functions in the vast majority of persons.[6] In fact, the actual size of the two hemispheres differs, with the speech dominant hemisphere possessing more mass of brain substance in the parieto-occipito-temporal region on the side of auditory speech analysis. This holds true for all but left-handed persons. The right hemisphere, on the other hand, seems in most persons to be involved in spacial integration and in the less logical and more intuitive aspects of intellectual function. Examples occur rather frequently in which large destruction in the association cortex on the nondominant side results in an agnosia for the entire left side of the body. In these persons, the left hand when it comes into visual view is treated as "a hand," but not "my hand." Because of this lack of recognition, there is often neglect in shaving, washing, and dressing that side of the body. On the motor side of function, the assembly of words required for meaningful speech, called the *praxia of speech (phasia)*, appears to require the services of the opercular part of the premotor cortex, which is sometimes called Broca's area, usually located on the left side of the brain.

In spite of what is known about dominance, speech, and other areas of motor and sensory function, most important higher order functions such as memory and personality remain mysterious as to their anatomical-functional relationships. For exam-

ple, certain circuits in the limbic system are essential for the recall of recently acquired information. Although the circuits are fairly well known, how they function and how the basic information storage occurs is not known. Thus the significant others of most brain-damaged patients judged to be "normal" following recovery from trauma or surgery to the nervous system will report that their "loved one" has changed, indicating that subtle alterations have occurred in function, some of which may have been due to the damage involved. For example, personality changes following major or multiple minor damage are common. Explaining the mechanisms responsible for these changes remains a challenge for future research.

In summary, the CNS develops from the ectoderm of the early embryo by the formation of a hollow neural tube which closes and sinks below the surface of its longitudinal axis. The side walls of the neural tube develop to form the neural circuitry of the brain stem and spinal cord; it is subdivided into the dorsal horn which receives and processes incoming or afferent information and the ventral horn which handles the final stages of output processing and contains the LMN which innervate the effector muscles and glands. The cavity of neural tube layer of CSF secreting ependymal cells develops to form the ventricles of the brain and the spinal canal.

The rostral 10 segments of the neural tube become the brain by enlargement of the dorsal horn portion into elaborate outgrowths and outpouchings. The cerebellum forms by enlargement over the roof of the fourth ventricle, fusion at the midline, and then the migration of neurons to the surface forming the highly folded cerebellar cortex. This structure provides important control of the sequencing and timing of motor unit activity required for coordinated motor skills. A paired outgrowth of the dorsal horn in the forward-most neural tube segment forms the optic cup from which the retina, iris, and optic nerve are derived. A second pair of lateral outpouchings from the dorsal horn develop into the cerebral hemispheres. The dorsal horn portion becomes the basal ganglia, the outer tract systems become the cerebral white matter, and neurons migrate through the latter to form the highly differentiated cerebral cortex which lies just under the pia mater. The medial portion of the cerebral cortex retains its close relationship with the olfactory input and becomes the limbic lobe. The lateral portion of the cerebral cortex becomes the six-layered neocortex. The cortex and the dorsal horn portion of the neural tube or brain stem are intimately connected in the structure called the thalamus. The thalamocortical circuits of the neocortex of the frontal lobe are involved in the initiation of movement and anticipation of behavior and its consequences. Thalamocortical circuits of the parietal lobe are essential to the delicate analysis of somesthetic and proprioceptive sensation and perception. The occipital lobe interacts with thalamic nuclei to provide sensation and perception of visual stimuli. The temporal lobe–thalamic interaction provides discriminative analysis of auditory sensation and perception as well as long-term memory functions. Cortical regions among the parietal, occipital, and temporal lobes interrelate these sensory domains and, on the dominant (usually left) side of the brain, verbal function. On the nondominant side, the corresponding areas are essential for spatial and perhaps imaginative function.

The PNS is derived from neural crest ectodermal cells which migrate into the soma and viscera during embryonic development to contribute to many structures and become the afferent neurons of the dorsal root ganglia and postganglionic efferent neurons of the autonomic ganglia. Each of the 43 or more body segments is interconnected to corresponding CNS or neural tube segments by segmental afferent and efferent nerves. The segmental nerves of the foremost 10 segments form the cranial nerves. Afferent neurons of the dorsal root ganglia are of four types: general soma afferents (GSA), which are the input source of somatic reflexes of somesthetic sensation; special soma afferents (SSA), which send information to the cerebellum and motor control systems; general visceral afferents (GVA), which provide an input source for the autonomic and visceral afferents; and special visceral afferents (SVA), which initiate their own reflexes, salivation for example, and which are sources of taste and olfactory sensation. These four classes of afferents deliver their signals to four groups of neurons in the dorsal horn which occur in a regular positional pattern of cell columns extending through the dorsal horn along the length of the CNS. The input association cells of these columns distribute the afferent signals into reflex circuits, as well as to various control systems and the thalamus of the forebrain where basic sensation occurs. Efferent neurons of the ventral horn send their axons back into body segments, to effector cells of the soma or viscera. The LMN that are located in the ventral horn innervate skeletal muscles, and supply the preganglionic sympathetic and parasympathetic neurons which innervate the smooth muscle, cardiac muscle, and gland cells of the viscera and body wall.

Longitudinal communication between CNS segments is provided by neurons which send the axons into nearby segments via the innermost layer of the white matter, the ancient archi-level system of fibers; these cells provide for coordination between neighboring segments. Neurons have invaded this layer and the mix of these cells and axons, called the reticular formation, is the location of much of the important reflex circuitry of the spinal cord and the brain stem. Paleo-level tracts,

which are located outside this layer, provide the longitudinal communication between more distant segments of the nervous system; this layer includes most of the important ascending and descending tracts. The recently evolved neo-level systems, which become functional during infancy and childhood, travel on the outside of the white matter and provide the means for very delicate and discriminative function. The outside position of the neo-tracts, as well as their lack of collateral and redundant pathways, makes them the most vulnerable to injury.

The autonomic nervous system, which is subdivided into the parasympathetic and sympathetic nervous systems, provides for the control of visceral function, including the activity of the gut and its secretory glands, the heart, blood vessels, and smooth muscle of the body wall. The sympathetic nervous system provides for the "fight or flight response" and the parasympathetic for the restorative functions of the body. Both systems utilize a second neuron (postganglionic cell). These are the paravertebral sympathetic chain which lies at the side of the axial skeleton and the prevertebral sympathetic ganglia which are located near major vessels and somewhat distant from the effector organs, and the parasympathetic ganglia which are located near or in the visceral organs. The two systems work in either a complementary or opposing manner to provide balanced control of visceral, vascular, and secretory functions. The coordination of autonomic reflexes is based on a rich afferent visceral system and a hierarchy of reflex control regions culminating in the hypothalamus of the forebrain. This region is, in turn, under the control of cerebral circuits, particularly those of the limbic system.

:Study Guide

After you have studied this chapter, you should be able to meet the following objectives:

: : Compare the functions of the CNS with those of the PNS.

: : Explain the hierarchy of control levels of the CNS.

: : State the purpose of a reflex.

: : State the function of GSIA and GVIA neurons.

: : Name the layers of the white matter.

: : Name the layer of white matter that is involved in fine manipulative skills.

: : Explain why a tractotomy may sometimes relieve intractable pain.

: : Name the procedure that may be done to remove the arch of bone of each vertebra.

: : Describe the protection of the brain afforded by the meninges.

: : Trace the development of the spinal cord in the embryo.

: : Describe the closure defect called spina bifida.

: : Trace the steps involved in the development of the spinal cord.

: : Explain how the spinal cord is protected.

: : Describe the condition often called slipped disc.

: : Describe the organization of the spinal segments.

: : Name the reflex that causes the skin surface to move away from a stimulus.

: : State the significance of the dermatomes in neurological examination.

: : State the functions of the GSIA.

: : Explain the use of the phrase *hierarchy of reflexes*.

: : Compare the epicritic pathway with the protopathic pathway.

: : Explain the use of the phrase *synergistic aspect of coordination*.

: : By citing a clinical example, demonstrate why it is important for the health professional to understand the physiology of the stretch reflex.

: : Explain the sequence of events involved in denervation atrophy.

: : Describe the clinical condition called *tetany*, with reference to the underlying cause.

: : Explain the pathology involved in myasthenia gravis.

: : Describe the organization of the brain on the basis of embryonic development.

: : Describe the anatomy of the forebrain, the midbrain, and the hindbrain.

: : Explain the concept of motor homunculus and sensory homunculus.

: : Name the layers of the meninges.

: : Trace the circulation of the CSF.

: : Explain the pathology involved in hydrocephalus.

: : Compare the functions of the sympathetic and the parasympathetic divisions of the ANS.

: : Describe the function of the GVA and the GVE neurons.

: : Explain the survival function of the sympathetic nervous system.

: : Describe the innervation due to the autonomic nervous system.

: : Explain the hierarchy of visceral reflexes by use of an example.

:References

1. Head H, Holmes G: Sensory disturbances from cerebral lesions. Brain 34:1–51, 1911
2. Report on Convulsive and Neuromuscular Disorders to the National Advisory Neurological and Communicative Disorders and Stroke Council, p 53. National Institute of Health, National Institute on Communicative Disorders and Stroke, U.S. Department of Health, Education, and Welfare, Public Health Service, NIH Publication No. 79–1913
3. Rowland LP: Diseases of the muscle and neuromuscular junction. In Beeson PB, McDermott W, Wyngaarden JB (eds): Cecil Textbook of Medicine, p 928. Philadelphia, WB Saunders, 1979
4. Blinkov SM, Glezer II: The Human Brain in Figures and Tables, p 201. New York, Basic Books, 1968
5. Shepherd GM: The Synaptic Organization of the Brain. New York, Oxford University Press, 1979
6. Whitaker HA, Selnes OA: Anatomical variations in the cortex: Individual differences and the problem of localization of language function. Ann NY Acad Sci 280:844-854, 1976

:Suggested Readings

Bannister R: Brain's Clinical Neurology, ed 5. New York, Oxford University Press, 1978

Blackwood W, Corsellis JAN (eds): Greenfield's Neuropathology, ed 3. Chicago, Year Book Medical Publishers, 1976

Blinkov SM, Glezer II: The Human Brain in Figures and Tables. New York, Basic Books, 1968

Carpenter MB: Human Neuroanatomy, ed 7. Baltimore, Williams & Wilkins, 1976

Eliasson SG, Prensky AL, Hardin WB, Jr.: Neurological Pathophysiology. New York, Oxford University Press, 1974

Eyzaguirre C, Finone SJ, ed 2. Physiology of the Nervous System. Chicago, Year Book Medical Publishers, 1975

Garoute P: Survey of Functional Neuroanatomy. Greenbrae, Jones Medical Publishers, 1981

Lewis AJ: Mechanisms of Neurological Disease. Boston, Little, Brown, 1976

Menkes JH: Textbook of Child Neurology, ed 2. Philadelphia, Lea and Febiger, 1980

Moore KL: The Developing Human, ed 2. Philadelphia, WB Saunders, 1977

Mountcastle VB (ed): Medical Physiology, ed 14. St. Louis, CV Mosby, 1980

Sarnat NB, Netsky MG: Evolution of the Nervous System, ed 2. New York, Oxford University Press, 1981

Schmidt RF (ed): Fundamentals of Neurophysiology. New York, Springer-Verlag, 1978

Thompson JS: Core Textbook of Anatomy. Philadelphia, JB Lippincott, 1977

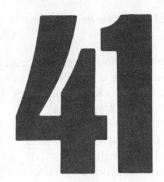

Sheila M. Curtis

Mechanisms
of Pain

Pain is elusive and complex. Physically, pain can be a burn, a toothache, a migraine headache. Psychologically, it can be the loss of a parent, loss of a child, witnessing another's suffering.

About 75 million Americans suffer from pain of some kind; their pain disabilities cause the loss of approximately 700 million work days each year. The cost of pain in lost production and charges for medications (prescription and over-the-counter), physicians and other care providers, and hospitals totals about 57 million dollars every year. Pain is a symptom common to most ailments: about 23 million Americans have backaches; 28 million, arthritis; and 24 million, severe headaches. In the United States close to 400,000 persons die of cancer every year, and most will experience intense pain in the course of the disease or before they die. Despite the magnitude and prevalence of chronic pain and disability, the National Institute of Health has allocated only about 0.02% of its annual budget to studies of the basic mechanisms of pain.[1]

Because pain is common to so many diseases, a full chapter is devoted to it in this text, centering on its mechanisms, theories about it, its manifestations, and its forms.

:What Is Pain?

Historically, pain has often been looked upon as a punishment or a means of atonement. The term itself—Greek, poinē; Latin, poena; French, peine—means punishment. Some western cultures have viewed pain as something to be avoided at all costs.

Aristotle regarded pain as the antithesis of pleasure, while Freud discussed the pleasure principle in relation to the avoidance of pain. Numerous clinicians have noted a link between emotion and pain, in which the pain sensation itself is only a part, and perhaps not even the main one, of the total pain experience. Some have observed that responses to pain were learned or patterned according to the norms of the person's cultural group. Zborowski, in his studies of Italian and Jewish women, found that both groups had low levels of pain tolerance and complained loudly when in pain. Interestingly, this behavior occurred for different reasons. The Italian women were relatively satisfied once their pain was relieved, while the Jewish women pursued the matter further, demanding to know its meaning.[2]

Pain is a personal, subjective, and unpleasant experience evoking unpleasant sensory, emotional, and motor responses. It involves not only anatomic structures and physiologic behaviors, but psycho-logical, social, cultural, and cognitive factors as well. And it has been repeatedly demonstrated that learning is a very important factor in a person's response to painful stimuli.

Pain can be a prepotent, overwhelming experience, often disruptive to customary behavior. When severe, pain demands and directs all of one's attention to it.

Definitions of Pain

What is pain? What is its purpose? Is it of any use? Does it help or harm? Scientific disciplines have attempted to answer these and other questions about pain. The many definitions of pain flowing from these efforts serve to highlight its complex nature. Yet, in the face of intense interest in and research on pain, we still have much to learn about this very human, very common experience. The puzzle of pain persists.

Pain has been studied from neurophysiological, psychological, sociological, anthropological, and historical perspectives, yet one simple and satisfactory definition has eluded all efforts. From the practical clinical point of view, health professionals must appreciate the findings of other disciplines in order to approach their clients in an integrated, holistic manner. Emphasizing one aspect of the person's pain experience while ignoring others is not likely to meet with success. For this reason, efforts continue to be made to develop unified theories of pain and behavior related to it.

Given the complex nature of the phenomenon called pain, it should not be surprising that a single or simple definition does not describe it. Sharp, burning, pricking, stabbing, piercing, pounding, throbbing—these are but a few of the adjectives that describe the physical aspects of pain, while suffering, agonizing, debilitating, demoralizing, unbearable, and terrifying connote something of the mental and psychological sides of pain.

What can the health professional do to make sense out of all of this? Is there a functional, workable definition which can adequately serve the health disciplines, as well as the suffering person?

Sternbach has given us an academic definition in which pain is described as follows: "An abstract concept which refers to (1) a personal, private sensation of hurt; (2) a harmful stimulus which signals current and impending tissue damage; (3) a pattern of responses which operate to protect the organism from harm."[3] Useful as this definition is, it fails to describe all facets of the experience called pain.

Margo McCaffery, a nurse in private practice

with more than 20 years of experience in the management of pain, has provided one of the most clinically useful definitions to date. She states, "Pain is whatever the experiencing person says it is, existing whenever he says it does."[4] Clinically, there are advantages to this definition. It is broad enough to cover the client's expression of pain, verbal or nonverbal; but perhaps more important, it indicates that the client is believed, which is critical to developing the trust relationship so important in managing pain. Merskey[5] believes that if pain is accepted as a psychological phenomenon with physiological correlates, rather than vice versa, some clinical problems can be prevented (*i.e.*, the patient will not be considered a malingerer or a liar if no objective cause for the pain can be found).

Purpose of Pain

In spite of its unpleasantness, pain can serve a useful purpose, for it warns of impending tissue injury and causes the individual to seek relief. An inflamed appendix, for example, would progress in severity, could rupture, and eventually might cause death were it not for the warning afforded by the pain.

Pain is probably the most common symptom that motivates an individual to seek professional help; its location, radiation, duration, and severity give important clues about its etiology. Indeed, it probably sends sufferers to the physician's office more often and with greater speed than any other symptom.

Theories About Pain

One difficulty in arriving at a workable definition of pain is that research findings have not been available to support clinical observations. The available theories have not adequately explained the pain experience as observed by health professionals.

Specificity Theory (Descartes, 1644; Van Fry, 1894) and Pattern Theories (Goldscheider, 1896; Noordenhoos, 1959; Livingston, 1943; others) explained some of the observed phenomena, primarily on a neurophysiological basis, but no unifying theory existed which could clarify all or most of the phenomena experienced, or observed to be experienced, by persons in pain.

In 1965, Melzack and Wall developed a theory to which they gave the name Gate Control Theory, and for the first time a theory became available to address the many remaining questions.[6] Gate Control Theory accounted for many neurophysiological, cognitive, and affective components of pain and so was greeted with enthusiasm. The theory proposes that there are neural mechanisms that can modulate input to the central nervous system. Stimuli such as vibration and massage are transmitted by large-diameter afferent axons, while pain information is carried by small-diameter myelinated and unmyelinated afferent axons. The spinal relay of pain information is said to be modulated or blocked by proportionately greater activity in the large-diameter afferent fibers. Influences descending from the forebrain are also postulated to be capable of blocking or modulating the relay of painful information. Recent findings have disclosed certain conflicting pieces of evidence related to Gate Control Theory. Nevertheless, Melzack believes that the concept of input modulation or gating holds, although revision of some of its physiological details may be needed.[7]

:Basic Pain Mechanisms and Responses

The mechanisms of pain are many and complex. There are the receptors that monitor the stimuli for pain, the pathways that carry pain impulses, the integration of the pain experience in the brain, and, finally the personal reaction to pain.

Pain Receptors

The receptors for pain are said to be *nociceptive*. They are widely distributed in the skin, some internal organs, the periosteum, and the meninges. The nociceptors are nerve endings of A delta and C fibers which *transduce* (convert) information about cell damage into a stimulus, and the person responds to the stimulus with the *flexor withdrawal reflex*. The *adequate stimulus* for this withdrawal reflex is threatened cell damage. It is a protective mechanism designed to remove the endangered tissue from the damaging stimulus. *Other stimuli*, such as temperature and pressure, also give rise to nociceptive reflexes when overstimulated to the point of tissue damage. For example, skin temperature of 45°C or greater usually evokes the flexor withdrawal reflex response. Nociceptive information transmitted to the thalamus or forebrain is usually experienced as pain. It should be noted that the mechanism(s) involved in the initial excitation of peripheral receptors, and the transmission of noxious stimuli to the central nervous system by the primary afferent fibers require further clarification.

Transmission of Pain Signals

When, for example, one's finger gets caught in a car door, the first component of the pain experience is a sharp, bright, localized, and unpleasant sensation known as *first or fast* pain. This is followed by a dull, aching, diffuse, and particularly unpleasant sensation known as *second or dull* pain. The presence of two pain pathways seems to explain these two components of pain. The more distal the stimulus from the brain, the more temporally separated are the fast and slow components. It is generally accepted that first or fast pain is primarily carried by the A-delta pain fibers, which are 2 to 5 μm in diameter and which transmit at a rate of 12 to 30 meters per second. The second or slow pain is thought to be primarily transmitted by the small C fibers, which are 0.4 to 1.2 μm in diameter and which transmit at a rate of 0.5 to 2 meters per second.

The A-delta pain fibers feed into pathways mainly associated with the spatial and temporal aspects of pain. The C fibers tend to feed into multisynaptic pathways to the thalamus, the limbic system, and the hypothalamus; these pathways have more to do with the emotional and autonomic aspects of the pain experience.

Although the *pain pathways* to the brain are *diffuse*, the main pathways are the neospinothalamic, the paleospinothalamic, and the spinoreticular systems. The neospinothalamic system is primarily concerned with the temporal, spatial, and intensity discrimination of the pain experience. After several synapses at the segmental level, projection neurons send their axons into the *spinothalamic tracts* of the opposite side of the spinal cord. This tract travels to the *lateral thalamus*, where the basic sensation of pain occurs. Interconnections between the lateral thalamus and an area in the *parietal cortex* are necessary to add precision and discrimination to the pain sensation. Association parts of the parietal cortex are essential to the perception or meaningfulness of the experience. For example, if a mosquito bites a person's index finger on the left hand and only the thalamus is functional, the person will complain of pain somewhere on the hand. With the primary sensory cortex functional, the person can localize it to the precise area on the index finger. The association cortex, on the other hand, is necessary for the person to interpret the sensation and "buzzing" that preceded the pain as being related to a mosquito bite. See Figure 41-1.

The *paleospinothalamic system* is more concerned with the emotional and autonomic aspects of the pain experience. It projects multisynaptically to the intermediate part of the thalamus, a region rich in connections with the limbic and hypothalamic areas. This adds the "hurtfulness" aspect to the pain.

The *reticulospinal system* projects bilaterally to the reticular formation of the brain stem. This system, in conjunction with the collaterals of the paleospinothalamic system, facilitates avoidance reflexes at all levels. It also contributes to an increase in the electroencephalographic activity associated with alertness.

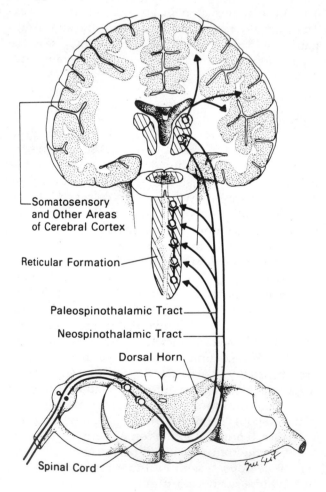

Figure 41-1. The spinothalamic system, one of the several ascending systems that carry pain impulses. One spinothalamic tract runs to the thalamic nuclei and has fibers that project to the somatosensory cortex. Another tract sends collateral fibers to the reticular formation and other structures, from which further fibers project to the thalamus. These fibers finally influence the hypothalamus and limbic system, as well as the cerebral cortex. (Rodman MJ, Smith DW: Pharmacology and Drug Therapy in Nursing, 2nd ed, p 263. Philadelphia, JB Lippincott, 1979)

Somatosensory and Other Areas of Cerebral Cortex

Reticular Formation

Paleospinothalamic Tract

Neospinothalamic Tract

Dorsal Horn

Spinal Cord

Sources of Pain

Characteristics of pain are related to its source. The sources of pain are commonly divided into three general categories: cutaneous, deep somatic, and visceral pain.

Cutaneous pain arises from superficial structures, such as the skin and subcutaneous tissues. It can be accurately localized and may have either an abrupt or a slow onset. It tends to be a sharp, bright pain with a burning quality. It may be distributed along the dermatomes, the areas of the skin supplied by a single segment or spinal root. Boundaries of pain may not be as clear-cut as the dermatomal diagrams would seem to indicate since there is an overlap of nerve fiber distribution between the dermatomes. A paper cut on the finger is an example of easily localized superficial or cutaneous pain.

A second source of pain is the deep *somatic* structures, such as periosteum, muscles, tendons, joints, and blood vessels. Deep somatic pain tends to be more diffuse than cutaneous pain. Examples of stimuli that produce deep somatic pain are strong pressure exerted on bones or ischemia to a muscle. This is the type of pain one experiences from a sprained ankle. Radiation of pain from the original site of nociceptive stimulation can occur. For example, damage to a nerve root can cause the person to experience pain radiating along its fiber distribution.

The third type of pain, called *visceral*, or splanchnic, pain, originates in the viscera. We are most accustomed to thinking of visceral pain as emanating from the abdominal cavity. However, visceral pain tends to be diffuse, especially in early stages. Unlike cutaneous pain, it is often accompanied by autonomic responses, such as nausea, vomiting, sweating, pallor, possibly shock. Small, unmyelinated pain fibers subserve visceral pain and travel along with the nerves of the autonomic system. Pain from the lower end of the esophagus and pain below the midtransverse colon tends to travel the course of cranial nerves IX and X and parasympathetic nerves entering the sacral region of the spinal cord. Pain fibers entering the thoracolumbar region of the spinal cord travel the course of the sympathetic nerves. Common examples of visceral pain are renal colic, pain due to cholecystitis, pain associated with acute appendicitis, and ulcer pain. The viscera are diffusely and richly innervated, but cutting or burning of viscera is unlikely to cause pain, as occurs when similar noxious stimuli are applied to cutaneous or superficial structures. However, strong abnormal contractions of the GI system or ischemia affecting the walls of the viscera can induce severe pain. Anyone who has suffered from either severe GI distress or ureteral colic can readily attest to the misery involved.

Reactions to Pain

Pain threshold and *pain tolerance* are not the same thing, although the terms are often used interchangeably. *Pain threshold* is usually defined as the least-intense stimulus that will cause pain. Although pain threshold is still controversial, it is generally accepted that the threshold is similar in most normal persons, particularly under controlled experimental situations. For example, upon exposure to heat of increasing intensity, most people state that the sensation of heat converts to sensation of pain at approximately 45°C.

Pain tolerance is usually defined as the maximum intensity or duration of pain that the subject is willing to endure—the point beyond which the person wants something done about the pain. Tolerance is not necessarily indicative of the severity of the pain. Psychological, familial, cultural, and environmental factors significantly influence the intensity of pain an individual is willing to tolerate.

Physical reactions to pain may be manifested in biting of lips, clenching of teeth, and facial expressions, such as frowning or wrinkling the brows. Protective body movements can be both involuntary and voluntary. The flexor withdrawal reaction, as discussed in Chapter 40, moves the part away from the pain source; it is involuntary. Voluntary movements are those such as changes in posture and relaxation exercises, which often relieve discomfort.

Physiological responses to pain involve activation of the *sympathetic* nervous system which evokes the "fight or flight" response, with catecholamine release from the adrenal medulla. What happens is this: as blood is shifted from nonvital to vital parts of the body, the vessels of the skin and the abdominal viscera (spleen, kidney, intestine) constrict, while those of the heart, skeletal muscles, lungs, and brain dilate. The face is pallid, the pupils dilated. Respiration, heart rate, and strength of contraction increase. Muscle tension rises and energy stores are mobilized to supply blood glucose. A relative decrease in parasympathetic activity may result in a loss of appetite, nausea, and vomiting. Gastrointestinal motility and digestive gland secretion also diminish. After a period of time, there occurs a *parasympathetic* or rebound response, in which respiration, pulse rate, and blood pressure may fall below the "prepain" level. This is likely when pain is of short duration but intense.

Pain that persists or is repetitive calls up *adaptation of response*, with observable decreases in sympathetic signs and symptoms. On the other hand, the pain *receptors* show little if any adaptation. Reactions to long-term pain tend to be hormonal rather than neural in nature. With time, physiological and psychological coping mechanisms evolve, but these behavioral responses *do not* indicate pain relief. The person may merely be too fatigued to respond.

Figure 41–2. Areas of referred pain. *Top*, anterior view; *bottom*, posterior view. (Chaffee EE, Lytle IM: Basic Anatomy and Physiology, 4th ed, p 266. Philadelphia, JB Lippincott, 1980)

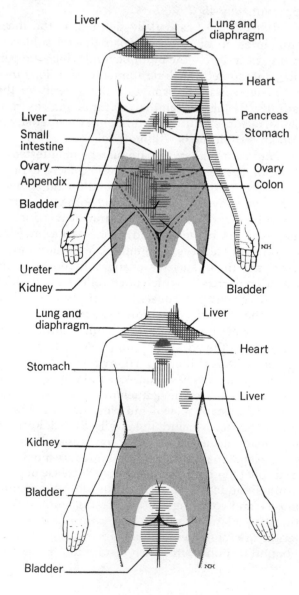

Occasionally, pain is associated with *neurogenic shock* due to inhibition of the medullary vasomotor center with decreased vasomotor tone. This mechanism is not well understood; it is believed that it might cause circulatory collapse, despite the presence of sympathetic activity.

During rapid eye movement (REM) or dream sleep, the electroencephalograph (EEG) records very active brain activity. Certain disorders in which pain predominates—such as angina and ulcer—appear to be *exacerbated* during this phase of *paradoxical sleep*.

Psychosocial reactions to pain are deeply influenced by a person's familial, religious, and cultural background, as well as by past experiences with pain. A verbal person may be able to accurately describe the location, duration, and intensity of the pain, as well as the ability or willingness to tolerate it. A change in the tone of voice may be as revealing as the words spoken. A person whose immediate family and forebears have been free of cancer will attach less significance to pain than one whose family is riddled with cancer.

Pain that necessitates absence from work will probably be of greater importance to one who is paid an hourly wage than to one who has ample health insurance and sick time available.

Vocalizations comprise a group of responses, such as crying, groaning, grunting, and gasping. Their frequency, loudness, and duration can assume importance in situations where the person is either too young or too confused to be verbally competent.

Referred Pain

Referred pain is that pain perceived at a site on the skin surface distant from the area from which it originated but innervated by the same spinal segment. Pain originating in the abdominal or thoracic viscera tends to be diffuse and poorly localized, and is often perceived at a site far removed from the affected area. For example, the pain associated with myocardial infarction is often referred to the left arm.

Referred pain may arise *alone or concurrent with* pain located at the origin of the noxious stimuli. Although the term *referred* is usually applied to pain originating in the viscera, it may also be applied to pain arising from the deep somatic structures. An example is referred pain for which the stimulus arises in muscles, joints, or periosteum.

An understanding of pain reference is of great value in diagnosing illness, because afferent neurons from visceral or deep somatic tissue enter the spinal cord at the same level as those from the cutaneous areas to which the pain is referred.

This relationship can be demonstrated by tracing the development of organ systems in the embryo (Fig. 41-2). Let us say that the client has peritonitis, but complains of pain in the shoulder. Internally, there is irritation or inflammation of the diaphragm. In the embryo, the diaphragm originates in the neck, and its central portion is innervated by the phrenic nerve, which enters the cord at the level of the fifth to seventh cervical segment (C 5–7). As the fetus develops, the diaphragm descends to its adult position between the thoracic and abdominal cavities, innervated by the phrenic nerve. Therefore, fibers entering the spinal cord at the C 5–7 level carry information from the neck area, as well as from the diaphragm. Although *visceral* pleura, pericardium, and peritoneum are said to be relatively free of pain fibers, *parietal* pleura, pericardium, and peritoneum *do react* to nociceptive stimuli. Visceral inflammation can involve parietal or somatic stuctures, and this may in turn give rise to diffuse local or referred pain. For example, irritation of the parietal peritoneum owing to appendicitis often gives rise to pain directly over the inflamed area in the right lower quadrant. Also, such stimuli can evoke pain *referred* to the umbilical area.

Another type of pain is *muscular spasm*, or guarding, when somatic structures are involved. *Guarding* is a protective-reflex rigidity and its purpose is to protect the affected body part (*e.g.*, an abscessed appendix or a sprained muscle). This protective guarding may give rise to the pain of muscle *ischemia*.

Pain from the viscera may be localized only with difficulty. There are several explanations for this. First, innervation of visceral organs is very poorly represented at forebrain (sensation) levels. A second explanation, held by some researchers, is that the brain does not easily "learn" to precisely localize sensations originating from organs that at best are only imprecisely visualized. For example, a cut on the third finger of the right hand can be readily seen, identified, and localized, whereas an inflamed internal organ can be localized only vaguely. A third explanation is that sensory information from thoracic and abdominal viscera can travel by two pathways to the central nervous system. The first route is called the *visceral* or *true visceral pathway*. According to this hypothesis, the "pain information" travels with the fibers of the autonomic nervous system, and the pain is felt at a site on the surface of the body distant to the pain locus. Pain felt along the

inner left arm following a myocardial infarction is an example.

The second route, the parietal pathway, which is somatic, is not usually considered to be a pathway for visceral pain, but may be the pain route in inflammation of *parietal* pleura, pericardium, or peritoneum. Sensations traveling along this pathway can be localized directly over the affected part, a common example being pain in the right lower quadrant or in the umbilical area associated with an inflamed appendix.

It is always possible that referred pain can be one of the consequences of an anatomical anomaly; therefore, the reader should guard against jumping to conclusions. Needless to say, although pain may be the prepotent stimulus that prompts the person to seek professional help, a careful history and examination are needed to correctly assess the problem.

:Alterations in Pain Mechanisms and Response

Organic or Somatogenic Pain versus Functional or Psychogenic Pain

Organic or *somatogenic* pain is that which originates in the body or the soma. *Functional* or *psychogenic* pain is that which is attributed to the psyche or emotions. In both situations, the physical sensation of pain is the same. The individual may be unaware that the origin of the pain is emotional, and may experience it as if the pain were truly originating from an organic disorder. Many persons who suffer from pain of psychogenic origin have had developmental difficulties during adolescence. It is of importance to note that persons in pain usually experience both its physical and its emotional aspects. It is difficult to conceive of pain as being either purely organic or purely functional. McCaffery's statement that "pain is whatever the experiencing person says it is and exists whenever he says it does" is particularly applicable here.[4]

"Positive placebo reactors" may be found among those suffering from either organic or functional pain. Research has demonstrated the importance of higher central nervous system control over sensory input. Whereas in the past there was no adequate explanation for the behavior of positive placebo reactors, and in fact such persons sometimes were regarded as malingerers, the discovery of endogenous modulators of pain, such as endorphins and enkephalins, suggests that placebos may trigger the release of pain-modulating substances, which cause the pain to diminish. (See "Placebo Response" later in this chapter.

Alterations in Pain Sensitivity

Sensitivity to pain varies among people, as well as in the same person, under different circumstances and in different parts of the body. *Analgesia* is a lack of pain without loss of consciousness. *Hyperalgesia* is an increased sensitivity to pain, which may be one of two types, primary or secondary. Tenderness in an area of infection and inflammation is an example of primary hyperalgesia; an abnormality of the central nervous system, of secondary hyperalgesia. *Hypoalgesia* is a decreased sensitivity to pain.

Inherited insensitivity to pain may take the form of congenital indifference to pain or congenital insensitivity to it. In the former, transmission of nerve impulses appears normal but appreciation of painful stimuli at higher levels appears absent. In the latter, there appears to be a peripheral nerve defect such that transmission of painful nerve impulses does not result in perception of pain. Whatever the cause, in either case there may be severe and extensive tissue damage without the person's being aware of it. Obviously, pain is not serving its protective function in these circumstances.

Alterations in Pain Perception or Response

Pain may occur with or without an apparently *adequate stimulus*; on the other hand, even in the presence of an *adequate* noxious stimulus, pain may be absent. Most familiar to us is pain following adequate noxious stimulation. For example, a hand touched by a flame will be quickly withdrawn. The interesting feature of this reaction is that the hand is moved away from the painful stimulus in whichever direction is appropriate—up, down, or to either side, as demanded by the situation.

Pain without an apparently adequate stimulus is puzzling. It may be that in an area hypersensitive due to inflammation or another cause, a normally subthreshold stimulus is sufficient to trigger the sensation of pain. This response is thought to be chemically mediated, possibly the result of tissue damage in the surrounding area.

As stated above, persons who lack the ability to perceive pain are at constant risk. Trauma, infection, even loss of a body part or parts may be the eventual outcome of this lack.

Persons with diabetes mellitus may develop neurological deficits, most commonly in the nerves that supply the feet. As a consequence, the diabetic may have no sensation in the feet—which explains why diabetics are constantly cautioned about the necessity of meticulous foot care to prevent trauma. In other disease processes, pain pathways may be accidentally or deliberately destroyed to prevent noxious stimuli from relaying messages to the forebrain.

Cultural and environmental factors may play a role in pain perception, too. For example, a native American who values stoicism is unlikely to cry out in public when subjected to a painful stimulus, whereas this may be an acceptable response in an Italian–American.

Pain can provide reassurance. In one study, the members of a group of men, matched as to injuries, gave very different responses depending upon the circumstances of their wounding.[8] Trauma inflicted on the battlefield evoked denial of pain and refusal of medications; the same types of injuries inflicted in civilians evoked complaints of pain and requests for pain relief. These striking differences have been attributed to the high emotional state at the time of injury as well as to the significance each person attached to the injuries. For the soldier, being wounded afforded a face-saving escape from unpleasant, life-threatening situations. It meant being transported to a relatively safe environment, perhaps even home. But a civilian with the same type of injury felt that life-style, as well as income, was under threat.

:Headache

Headache is discussed here because it is a type of pain that is recognized almost universally. Although headache is so common, its cause is not really known. There are many types of headache, of which the more common appears to be muscle contraction or tension headache and migraine headache. It is estimated that 50% to 90% of adult Americans experience headache at some time, at a cost of millions of workdays lost and billions of dollars spent on headache relief.[1]

Tension or muscle contraction headaches

Tension headaches commonly result from sustained contractions of the skeletal muscles of the scalp and neck. The usual source of this tensing of muscles is an unconscious reaction to stress. However, any activity that requires the head to be held in one position such as typing, repairing jewelry, or using a microscope, can cause a muscle contraction headache.

Migraine headaches

There is more than one type of migraine headache, but for the purpose of this text they are discussed in general. Women are affected more frequently than men, in a ratio of 10:1, and a family history of migraine headaches, photophobia, anorexia, and pallor is not uncommon. These headaches cause a throbbing pain; nausea and vomiting are frequent accompaniments. Neurological deficits may be noted.

There may be two phases to the migraine experience. During the prodromal phase or stage there can be vascular spasm, decreased cerebral blood flow, and sensory or motor alterations. During the headache phase, there is vasodilatation and increased cerebral blood flow.

Most such headaches are thought to be due to changes in blood flow and, therefore, changes in oxygen availability. The pain receptors are sensitive to this diminution of oxygen. The blood vessels become restricted, serotonin is released, and finally there is vasodilatation. If serotonin is blocked, the headache may be prevented.

Migraine headache sufferers are advised to avoid tyramine-containing foods, such as red wine, certain cheeses, smoked herring, and foods seasoned with monosodium glutamate, and to stay away from smoke-filled rooms and other stimuli known to trigger migraines. Practicing biofeedback and changing one's life-style may help to decrease the frequency of the headaches. Drugs may be useful but are usually more effective before the headache is full-blown.

:Acute Versus Chronic Pain

The pain research of the past 25 years has emphasized the importance of differentiating acute pain from chronic pain and of dealing with them separately. This is because they differ from each other in etiology, mechanisms, pathophysiology, and function, and because the diagnosis of and therapy for each is distinctive (Table 41-1).

Acute pain is ordinarily defined as pain of less than six months' duration. It consists of unpleasant sensory, perceptual, and emotional components, with associated somatic, autonomic, psychological, and behavioral responses.

Acute pain is caused by noxious or tissue-damaging stimuli, and its purpose is to serve as a protective or warning system. Besides alerting the

Table 41-1 Characteristics of Acute and Chronic Pain

Characteristic	Acute Pain	Chronic Pain
Onset	Recent	Continuous or intermittent
Duration	Short duration	Six months or more
Autonomic responses	Consistent with sympathetic fight or flight response* Increased heart rate Increased stroke volume Increased blood pressure Increased pupillary dilation Increased muscle tension Decreased gut motility Decreased salivary flow (dry mouth)	Habituation of autonomic responses
Psychological component	Associated anxiety	Increased irritability Associated depression Somatic preoccupation Withdrawal from outside interests Decreased strength of relationships
Other types of response		Decreased sleep Decreased libido Appetite changes

*Responses are approximately proportional to intensity of the stimulus.

individual to the existence of actual or impending tissue damage, it prompts seeking of professional help. The pain's location, intensity, duration, and radiation, as well as those factors that aggravate or relieve it, are essential diagnostic clues. Unlike chronic pain, it is extremely rare for acute pain to be due to psychological factors alone. Acute pain is often accompanied by *anxiety*, which usually disappears when the pain is relieved.

Chronic pain is defined as pain of six months' duration or longer. The pain may be continuous (*e.g.*, due to arthritis) or intermittent (*e.g.*, due to periodic sternal puncture). Unlike acute pain, persistent pain usually serves no useful function. To the contrary, it imposes severe physiological, psychological, familial, and economic stresses on the person, and may exhaust his resources. Unlike acute pain, psychological and environmental influences often play a significant role in chronic pain and in the development of behaviors associated with it. Chronic pain is associated with *depression* and despair more than with anxiety. Amazingly, this depression often can be lifted almost spontaneously if the pain is removed.

It is extremely important to appreciate that persons suffering chronic pain may not exhibit the somatic, autonomic, or affective behaviors one associates with acute pain. One reason for this is that the stress response cannot be maintained for long periods of time. As was described earlier, either parasympathetic rebound or adaptation occurs.

Then too, certain behaviors, viewed as acceptable in patients with severe but short-lived pain, would not be expected or considered appropriate in the chronic situation. The patient's own description of the pain experience should be heeded, since the expected psychophysiological responses may or may not be present.

One proposed classification of chronic pain divides the affected persons into two broad groups according to life expectancy (brief versus normal). This may be significant and will be discussed under Treatment.

:Treatment of Pain

It is often not possible to eliminate the cause of pain, and efforts to relieve it may take any of several forms—physical, psychological, pharmacological, surgical, stimulation-induced analgesia, and a multidisciplinary approach. The decision about which approach should be tried is based on the duration, characteristics, cause, and mechanisms of the pain,

if known; the age and social responsibilities of the individual; the prognosis; any previous therapy; and psychological considerations.

Ideally, removal of the sources of noxious stimuli, including anything that causes exacerbation, would be effective. When this is not possible, attempts are made to moderate the reaction to pain.

It may be necessary to interrupt pain pathways by such methods as spinal blocks, use of local anesthetics, and surgical intervention. Drug treatment can include the use of narcotics and of nonnarcotic analgesics, anti-inflammatory and vasoconstrictive agents, antidepressant and antianxiety drugs, and sometimes anticonvulsant drugs.

Surgical Intervention

Surgery to remove the cause or block the transmission of pain is fairly frequent. Surgery for severe intractable pain of either peripheral or central origin has met with some success. Persons with phantom-limb pain, severe neuralgia, or causalgia sometimes suffer so intensively that they consider suicide as their only means of escape. In these extreme cases, surgery may be the only remaining treatment that seems to offer relief from their agony. Nevertheless, surgical methods to relieve pain are usually considered a last resort because damage to nerve cell bodies is irreversible. Although severed axons may regenerate, full recovery is highly unlikely, and after a few weeks or months the pain often returns and may be more disturbing than the condition for which the surgery was done, as has been described. However, pain is often completely relieved, as occurs with removal of a tumor pressing on nerve fibers or removal of an inflamed appendix, for example.

Surgery to block transmission of pain signals along peripheral or central pathways may be successful. Peripherally, nerve section (*neurotomy*) or section of a dorsal root ganglion (*rhizotomy*) is not uncommon, and some success has been reported for this type of surgery in tic douloureux, herpes zoster, and neuralgia.

At the spinal cord level, *cordotomy* and *tractotomy* may require very deep incisions into the cord to give adequate relief. With such deep surgery, bladder function may be affected. The success of these types of surgery depends on the source of the pain and the cord level involved. Electrical stimulation and/or pharmacologic agents are often used either to determine the appropriate surgical site or to eliminate the need for surgery.

Hypophysectomy, the removal of the pituitary, has an interesting history. It was done originally in efforts to prevent metastasis in certain hormone-dependent malignancies, including some breast cancers. It was found, rather unexpectedly, that the pain was often immediately and totally relieved. Hypophysectomy, now employed to relieve intractable pain from other sources, has had some success. The mechanism of pain relief is not yet understood.

Treatment with Drugs

Use of drugs to control pain is only one aspect of the overall program for pain relief. These agents have been used for many years to relieve pain of short duration, enabling the person to achieve mobility, as, for example, after surgery, when exercises such as coughing and deep breathing may be required.

An analgesic is defined as a drug that acts upon the nervous system to decrease or eliminate pain without inducing loss of consciousness. In general, analgesics have no powerful curative effects.

Analgesics are categorized as narcotic or non-narcotic, addictive or nonaddictive, prescription or over-the-counter, strong or weak, and peripherally or centrally acting.

The ideal analgesic would be potent yet non-addicting, and would have few side effects. It would be effective yet would not alter the state of awareness. Tolerance would not occur. Finally, it would not be expensive.

Aspirin (acetylsalicylic acid, ASA) is an example of a non-narcotic, nonaddictive, over-the-counter medication that is effective both peripherally and centrally. ASA also has antipyretic and anti-inflammatory properties.

Morphine (morphine sulfate) is an example of a narcotic that is addictive and can be obtained only by prescription. Morphine acts centrally, decreasing concern about pain experience more than it diminishes the pain itself.

There is much evidence that for effective relief of severe pain, narcotics given routinely before the pain becomes extreme are far more effective than when given in a sporadic fashion; patients seem to require fewer doses and are better able to resume regular activities earlier.

Other Types of Treatment

Exercise, postural changes, heat, cold, massage, traction, and braces and splints are *physical* measures to control or relieve pain.

Psychological treatment involves individual and group therapy, biofeedback, hypnosis, operant conditioning, and relaxation exercises.

Endorphins and Enkephalins

The endorphins ("morphine-like") and enkephalins ("in the head") are a group of endogenous peptides that have opiate-like activity. The globus pallidus seems to contain the most enkephalins, while the endorphins are more heavily concentrated in the hypothalamus. The presence of these morphine-like substances tends to mimic the peripheral and central effects of morphine and other opiate drugs. Opiate receptors have been identified in nervous tissue of various parts of the CNS, and in the plexuses of the gastrointestinal tract. Their presence tends to have a depressant effect.

Placebo response

An interesting phenomenon that deserves comment is the placebo response (placebo = I will please). A placebo is an inert substance. At one time "placebo reactors" were thought to be malingerers or to have psychogenic or functional pain which was more imaginary than real—hence their "pain" was relieved by a placebo. Newer research indicates that all of us are, to a greater or lesser degree, placebo reactors.

Placebos should not be given to determine whether pain is imaginary or real, mild or severe, nor to assess a patient's personality or possible psychopathology. They may induce physiological and psychological reactions, such as changes in blood pressure, respiration, heart rate, gastrointestinal activity, and temperature as well as pain relief.

Stimulation-induced analgesia

The early 1970s have been called the "stimulation-induced analgesia (SIA) period of investigation" by Chapman.[9] Electrical acupuncture and transcutaneous electrical stimulation (TES) are included under this term.

Acupuncture. Electrical stimulation may gradually increase the pain threshold to almost double.[9] This stimulation-induced analgesia is one of the oldest known pain relief methods. It consists of brief, intense stimulation of trigger points by injection of normal saline, dry needling, or intense cold, which in many cases brings prolonged relief. The Chinese have practiced acupuncture—insertion of needles into certain body areas followed by manual manipulation—for centuries. In the mid-1970s, interest in this modality peaked on the basis of reports of complete surgical analgesia by use of acupuncture alone. However, later findings indicate that complete analgesia is unlikely. The Chinese are now practicing electroacupuncture, in which electrical impulses are passed through the needles. Acupressure over the same sites has also been done. Analgesic effects are greater over specifically designated sites than over alternative sites.

Transcutaneous electrical nerve stimulation.
Transcutaneous electrical nerve stimulation units (TENS) have been developed, which are convenient and relatively economical to use. These units, the size of a small transistor radio or a cigarette package, deliver a measurable amount of current to a target, and can be transported and operated easily.

The system usually consists of three parts, *electrodes* connected by *lead wires* to a *stimulator*. The electric current delivered by the generator can be varied in *frequency* and *intensity*. It increases the activity in the large-diameter afferent fibers, which have a lower stimulation threshold and hence relay information more quickly than the small-diameter nociceptive afferent fibers.

As you will recall, pain information is transmitted by small-diameter A-delta and C fibers. The large-diameter afferent A fibers carry information mediating touch, pressure, and kinesthesis. Transcutaneous electrical nerve stimulators function on the basis of preferentially firing off impulses in the larger fibers carrying nonpainful information. According to the Gate Control Theory, increased activity in these large fibers is expected to "close the gate"—to block or modulate transmission of painful information to the forebrain. Although this theory provides one possible explanation for the phenomenon, it is still controversial, and alternative mechanisms for the success of the method have been proposed. It is suggested that the peripheral nerve fibers fatigue or that there is increased production of endogenous substances such as endorphins.

TENS has the advantage that it is noninvasive, is easily regulated by the individual or the health professional, and is quite effective in some forms of acute and chronic pain. Its use can be taught preoperatively, affording a reduction in both hospital days and postoperative analgesic medication.

Life Expectancy as a Basis of Treatment for Pain

Surgery for relief of pain. According to this classification, those with chronic pain but a normal life expectancy probably should not have treatment involving central nervous system damage or destruction. The aftermath of this type of surgery may be more distressing than the pain for which it was done. (Of course, persons suffering from chronic pain may not easily believe that this is so.) Those whose life expectancy is brief may benefit from surgery. Regenerating nerve fibers may give rise to extremely uncomfortable sensations (dysesthesias), but when the period of survival is short, surgery may be warranted.

Drug therapy for relief of pain. Life expectancy is again an important factor. Because there is undue concern about the possibility of addiction, many chronic pain sufferers with a short life expectancy receive inadequate pain relief. Though social factors rather than medical treatment are the primary cause of drug addiction, many patients do not get enough medication, of the proper strength, to meet their needs. Lipton,[10] McCaffery,[4] and others have shown that it is quite appropriate to provide as much narcotic as is necessary to patients with severe, intractable pain whose life expectancy is very limited.

One views the chronic pain patient with a normal life expectancy somewhat differently. For example, if the person suffers from low back pain, sciatica, or some other condition that is not life threatening, ordinarily it would not be appropriate to prescribe narcotics. Such a person is more likely to feel a need to gradually increase the amount and frequency of medication, so the possibility exists that addiction may occur.

In severe pain associated with a short-term condition, narcotics may be given when necessary, and withdrawn as the pain decreases. Narcotic addiction is unlikely in such a case.

Multidisciplinary approach
Over 30 years ago, the notion of a *multidisciplinary approach* to complex chronic pain problems was first put into practice. Today a number of pain clinics have been established. This team approach utilizes the knowledge and expertise of many health professionals to diagnose and manage complex types of pain. Besides being useful clinically, the team approach is effective both in teaching and in collaborative research. The acute pain model assumes an objective cause that can be treated and diminished or eliminated within a short time, but, unfortunately, the most perplexing difficulties are those related to chronic pain. Nevertheless, the multidisciplinary approach has had a measure of success in treatment of chronic pain.

In summary, pain is an elusive and complex phenomenon; it is a symptom common to many illnesses.

Pain is a highly individualized experience, shaped by a person's culture and previous life experiences and as such is very difficult to measure. Pain can be either acute or chronic, and the latter is particularly difficult to manage. Controversy continues as to whether chronic pain should be viewed as a physiological phenomenon with psychological correlates, or as a psychological phenomenon with physiological correlates. There is a growing body of data which suggests that the latter definition may eliminate many of the chronic pain management problems.

Current treatment modalities include physical, psychological, pharmacological, neurosurgical, and stimulation-induced analgesic methods singly or in combination. Currently, the greatest success in the management of problems related to pain is achieved with the use of multidisciplinary teams.

:Study Guide

After you have studied this chapter, you should be able to meet the following objectives:

: :   Explain Gate Control Theory.

: :   Describe the action of nociceptors in response to "pain information."

: :   Trace the transmission of pain signals, with reference to the neospinothalamic, paleospinothalamic, and reticulospinal pathways.

: :   State examples of visceral, cutaneous, and somatic pain.

: :   Compare pain threshold and pain tolerance.

: :   Explain the cultural factors that may influence a person's response to pain.

: :   Explain the occurrence of referred pain.

: :   State examples of alterations in sensitivity to pain or its perception that may place the affected person at risk.

: :   Describe the reaction of the sympathetic nervous system to a painful stimulus.

: :   State possible causes of migraine headache.

: :   Differentiate *chronic* pain from *acute* pain.

: :   Name two or more surgical procedures that may block transmission of painful stimuli.

: :   Describe the phenomenon called stimulation-induced analgesia.

: :   Explain the rationale underlying the use of TENS.

:References

1. The Interagency Committee on New Therapies for Pain and Discomfort: Report to the White House. National Institute of Health, Public Health Service, U.S. Department of Health, Education, and Welfare, May 1979, IV–38
2. Zborowski M: Cultural components in response to pain. J Social Issues 8:16, 1952
3. Sternbach R (ed): The Psychology of Pain. New York, Raven Press, 1978
4. McCaffery M: Nursing Management of the Patient with Pain, ed 2. Philadelphia, JB Lippincott, 1979
5. Merskey H: Pain and personality, pp 123–124. In Sternbach RA: The Psychology of Pain. New York, Raven Press, 1978
6. Melzack R, Wall PD: Science 150:971–979, 1965
7. Melzack R, Dennis SG: Neurophysiological foundations of pain. In Sternbach RA (ed): The Psychology of Pain. New York, Raven Press, 1978
8. Beecher HK: JAMA 161:1609–1613, 1956
9. Chapman CR: Contribution of research on acupunctural and transcutaneous electrical stimulation to the understanding of pain mechanisms and pain relief. In Roland F, Beers J, Bassett EG: Mechanisms of Pain and Analgesic Compounds, pp 7–183. New York, Raven Press, 1979
10. Lipton S: The Control of Chronic Pain, p 83. Chicago, Year Book Medical Publishers, 1979

:Suggested Readings

Bonica JJ: Current status of pain therapy. In The Interagency Committee on New Therapies for Pain and Discomfort. Report to the White House, May, 1979

Bonica JJ: Important clinical aspects of acute and chronic pain. In Beers RF and Bassett EG (eds): Mechanisms of Pain and Analgesic Compounds. New York, Raven Press, 1979

Boyd DB, Merskey H, Nielson JS: The pain clinic: an approach to the problem of chronic pain. In Smith WL, Merskey H, Gross SC (eds): Pain: Meaning and Management. New York, SP Medical and Scientific Books, 1980

Carruthers SG: Clinical pharmacology of pain. In Smith WL, Merskey H, Gross SC (eds): Pain: Meaning and Management. New York, SP Medical and Scientific Books, 1980

Chapman DR: Pain: the perception of noxious events. In Sternbach RA (ed): The Psychology of Pain. New York, Raven Press, 1978

Cohen FL: Postsurgical pain relief: patients' status and nurses' medication choices. Pain 9:2:265–274, 1980

Ferreira SH: Site of analgesic action of aspirin-like drugs and opioids. In Beers RF, Bassett EG (eds): Mechanisms of Pain and Analgesic Compounds. New York, Raven Press, 1979

Gardner GG, Gross SC: Child pain: treatment approaches. In Smith WL, Merskey H, Gross SC (eds): Pain: Meaning and Management. New York, SP Medical and Scientific Books, 1980

Hart LK, Reese JL, Fearing MO: Concepts Common to Acute Illness: Identification and Management. St. Louis, CV Mosby, 1981

Herz A, Schulz R, Blasig J: Changes in neuronal sensitivity in opiate tolerance/dependence. In Beers RF, Bassett EG (eds): Mechanisms of Pain and Analgesic Compounds. New York, Raven Press, 1979

Hunt GE: Pain and the aged patient. In Smith WL, Merskey H, Gross SC (eds): Pain: Meaning and Management. New York, SP Medical and Scientific Books, 1980

Ignelzi RJ, Atkinson JH: Pain and its modulation. Part 1. Afferent mechanisms. Neurosurgery 6:5:577–583, 1980

Ignelzi RJ, Atkinson JH: Pain and its modulation. Part 2. Efferent mechanisms. Neurosurgery 6:5:584–590, 1980

Jacox AK: The assessment of pain. In Smith WL, Merskey H, Gross SC (eds): Pain: Meaning and Management. New York, SP Medical and Scientific Books, 1980

Janko M, Trontelj JV: Transcutaneous electrical nerve stimulation: A microneurographic and perceptual study. Pain 9:2:219–230, 1980

Jasinski DR: Morphine and nonaddicting analgesics: a current prospective. In Beers RF, Bassett EG (eds): Mechanisms of Pain and Analgesic Compounds. New York, Raven Press, 1979

Kim S: Pain: theory, research and nursing practice. Advanc Nurs Sci 2:2:43–59, 1980

Knox VJ, Handfield-Jones CE, Shum K: Subject expectancy and the reduction of cold pressor pain with acupuncture and placebo acupuncture. Psychosom Med 41:477–485, October 1979

Lewis AJ: Mechanisms of Neurological Disease. Boston, Little, Brown, 1976

McCaffery M: Nursing Management of the Patient with Pain. Philadelphia, JB Lippincott, 1972

McCaffery M: Nursing Management of the Patient with Pain, ed 2. Philadelphia, JB Lippincott, 1979

Melzack R: The Puzzle of Pain. New York, Basic Books, 1973

Melzack R, Dennis SG: Neurophysiological foundations of pain. In Sternbach RA (ed): The Psychology of Pain. New York, Raven Press, 1978

Melzack R, Wall PD: Pain mechanisms: A new theory. Science 150:971–979, 1965

Merskey H: The nature of pain. In Smith WL, Merskey H, Gross SC (eds): Pain: Meaning and Management. New York, SP Medical and Scientific Books, 1980

Merskey H: Psychological and psychiatric aspects of pain control. In Smith WL, Merskey H, Gross SC (eds): Pain: Meaning and Management. New York, SP Medical and Scientific Books, 1980

Olson GA, Olson RD, Kastin AJ, Coy DH: The opioid neuropeptides enkephalin and endorphin and their hypothesized relation to pain. In Smith WL, Merskey H, and Gross SC (eds): Pain: Meaning and Management. New York, SP Medical and Scientific Books, 1980

Pilowsky I: Psychodynamic aspects of the pain experience. In Sternbach RA (ed): The Psychology of Pain. New York, Raven Press, 1978

Rodman MJ, Smith DW: Pharmacology and Drug Therapy in Nursing, ed 2. Philadelphia, JB Lippincott, 1979

Sanders SH, Webster JS, Framer E: Analysis of nurses' knowledge of behavioral methods applied to chronic and acute pain patients. J Nurs Educ 19:4:46–50, 1980

Sicuteri F: The nature of pain in headache and central panalgesia. In Beers RF, Bassett EC (eds): Mechanisms of Pain and Analgesic Compounds. New York, Raven Press, 1979

Smith WL, Duerksen DL: Personality and the relief of chronic pain: predicting surgical outcome. In Smith WL, Merskey H, Gross SC (eds): Pain: Meaning and Management. New York, SP Medical and Scientific Books, 1980

U.S. Government Printing Office. The Interagency Committee on New Therapies for Pain and Discomfort. Report to the White House. May, 1979

Wolf ZR (ed): Pain management. Topics Chron Nurs 2:1:1–95, 1980

Wallenstein SL, Heidrich GD, Kaiko R, Haude RW: Clinical evaluation of mild analgesics: The measurement of clinical pain. Brit J Clin Pharmacol 10:Suppl 2:319S–327S, 1980

42

Mary Wierenga

Disorders of Cerebral Function

Normally, neurons respond appropriately to changes in stimuli from the internal and external environment. Periods of wakefulness and sleep are regulated by need, and even during sleep, a person can be aroused with relative ease. The threshold of excitation of neurons is such that responses can be controlled. The extremes of normal responses are coma or unconsciousness, which can be considered an inappropriate extension of sleep, and epilepsy, in which neurons become paroxysmally hyperexcitable. Among the causes of coma and epilepsy are injuries and infections of the nervous system. This chapter discusses head injury, brain infections, epilepsy, and coma.

:Head Injury

The more critical an organ or system is to the body as a whole, the more provisions nature makes to protect its structures. The brain is protected by the skull, meninges, and cerebrospinal fluid (CSF). When the integrity of this protective system is broken, usually as the result of trauma, brain damage may occur; the ultimate results may range from a minor psychomotor deficit to total dependency.[1] Hemiparesis (weakness of one side of the body); aphasia; hemianopia (blindness or defective vision in half of the visual field); unconsciousness, either immediate or delayed; post-traumatic epilepsy; and postconcussion syndrome are frequent sequelae of head injury.

Although the skull and the CSF provide protection for the brain, they can also contribute to trauma in some injuries, known as *contrecoup injuries*. In this type of injury the side of the brain opposite the side of the head that was struck is injured. This occurs because the brain floats freely in the CSF, while the brain stem is stable. Thus, the skull, being lighter in mass than the brain, is hit first, causing the brain to be thrown against the opposite side of the skull and then to rebound. As the brain strikes the rough surface of the cranial vault, brain tissue, blood vessels, nerve tracts, and other structures become bruised and torn.

Head injury may be due to either penetration (open head injury) or impact (closed head injury), and each affects the brain, meninges, CSF, and skull in different ways.

For descriptive purposes, head injuries are divided into primary, or *direct*, injuries in which damage is due to impact, and *secondary injuries*, in which damage results from the subsequent brain swelling (cerebral edema), intracranial hematomas (blood clots), infection, cerebral hypoxia, and ischemia.[2] Because secondary injuries follow rapidly, usually within hours of the direct injury, it is often difficult to distinguish the damage done by each. The distinction between direct and secondary injuries is crucial, however, since the main objective of treatment is to prevent or minimize secondary brain injury.

Direct Injuries

One of the most serious types of direct injury is skull fracture. In one neurosurgical unit, 80% of fatal injuries were associated with fractures of the skull.[3] Skull fractures can be divided into three groups: simple linear, compound, and comminuted. A *simple linear skull fracture* is a break in the continuity of the bone. Multiple linear fractures, which cause splintering or crushing of bone, are classified as *comminuted fractures*. When bone fragments are depressed into the brain tissue, the fracture is said to be *depressed*. When an opening is present through the skull or mucous membrane of the sinuses, the fracture is termed a *compound fracture*. A compound fracture may be linear or comminuted.

Usually, radiological examination is needed to confirm the presence and extent of a skull fracture. This is of importance because of the possible damage to the underlying tissues. A frequent complication of fractures is the leakage of CSF from the nose (rhinorrhea) or ear (otorrhea) with resultant infection. One of the ways to differentiate between CSF and mucus drainage from the nose is to collect a specimen and test it for glucose. Glucose is normally present in the CSF, but is absent in mucus. There may be lacerations to vessels in the dura, most often to the middle meninges, with resulting intracranial bleeding. Damage to cranial nerves may also result from skull fractures.

Concussion–contusion

Even if there is no break in the skull, a blow to the head can cause severe and diffuse brain damage. Such closed injury can be classified as (1) mild, moderate, or severe; or (2) concussion or contusion. There is some overlap in these classifications. For example, the terms mild head injury and concussion may be used interchangeably.

In *mild head injury*, there may be momentary loss of consciousness without demonstrable neurological symptoms or residual damage, except for possible residual amnesia. Microscopic changes can usually be detected in the neurons and glia within hours of injury. Although recovery usually takes place within 24 hours, mild symptoms, such as headache, irritability, and insomnia, may persist for months.

Moderate head injury is characterized by a longer period of unconsciousness and may be associated with neurological manifestations, such as hemiplegia. In this type of injury, there are many small hemorrhages and some swelling of brain tissue (cerebral edema).

In *severe head injury*, there is cerebral contusion (bruising of the brain), and tearing and shearing of brain structures. It is often accompanied by symptoms such as hemiplegia. These injuries frequently occur with other types of trauma—to the extremities, the chest, and the abdomen, for example. Extravasation of blood may occur; if the contusion is severe, the blood may coalesce, similar to intracerebral hemorrhage.[3] Similarly, when there is laceration of the brain directly under the area of injury, especially if the skull is fractured, hemorrhage may be so extensive as to merit the designation of *hematoma*. The contusion is often distributed along the rough, irregular inner surface of the brain, so is more likely to occur in the occipital area than in the frontal lobes.[3] Contusions are usually multiple and may be bilateral.

Frequently there is ischemic necrosis in the center of a contused area, with eventual scar-tissue formation. These scars are predisposing factors in post-traumatic epilepsy.

Secondary Injuries

The significance of contusion depends on the extent of secondary injury due to edema, hemorrhage, and infection. Two types of hematomas may result from hemorrhage—epidural and subdural.

Epidural hematoma (extradural hematoma)

Epidural hematomas are usually caused by a severe head injury in which the skull is fractured. An *epidural* (extradural) hematoma is one that develops between the skull and the dura, outside the dura (Fig. 42-1). It is usually due to a tear in the middle meningeal artery and, since the bleeding is of arterial origin, there is rapid compression of the brain. Epidural hematomas are more common in young persons because in them the dura is not as firmly attached to the skull surface as it is in older persons, and, as a consequence, the dura can be easily stripped away from the inner surface of the skull, allowing the hematoma to form.[2]

Typically, a person with an epidural hematoma presents the following picture: a history of head injury, a brief period of unconsciousness followed

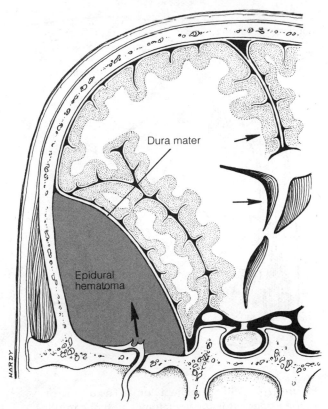

Figure 42–1.   Epidural hematoma. The dark area in the lower left is the hematoma. Note the broken blood vessel and the shift in the midline structures of the brain. (Cosgriff JH, Anderson DL: The Practice of Emergency Nursing. Philadelphia, JB Lippincott, 1975)

by a lucid period where consciousness is regained, after which there is a rapid progression to unconsciousness. The lucid interval is not always present but when it is, it is of great diagnostic value. With rapidly developing unconsciousness there are focal symptoms related to the area of the brain involved. These symptoms can include ipsilateral (same side) pupil dilatation and contralateral (opposite side) hemiparesis. If the hematoma is not removed the condition progresses, with increased intracranial pressure and tentorial herniation, and finally, death.

Subdural hematoma

The area between the dura and the arachnoid is the subdural space. A subdural hematoma is the result of a tear in the arachnoid which allows blood from the small bridging veins between the dura and the pia to collect in the subdural space (Fig. 42-2). It is slower to develop than an epidural hematoma because the tear is in the venous system, whereas epidural hematomas are arterial. Subdural hematomas are classified as acute, subacute, or chronic. Symp-

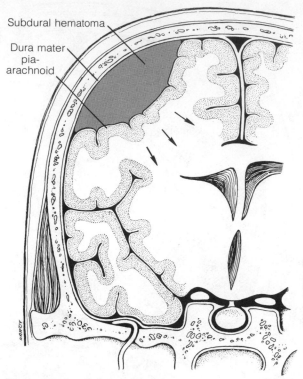

Subdural hematoma

Dura mater
pia-
arachnoid

Figure 42–2. Subdural hematoma. The dark area in the upper left is the hematoma. Note the midline shift of brain structures. (Cosgriff JH, Anderson DL: The Practice of Emergency Nursing. Philadelpha, JB Lippincott, 1975)

toms of acute subdural hematoma are seen within 24 hours of the injury, while subacute hematoma does not produce symptoms until 2 to 10 days following injury. These types of hematoma are frequently discussed together. Symptoms of chronic subdural hematoma may not arise until several weeks after the injury. These classifications are based partially on temporal and partially on pathological considerations.

Acute subdural hematomas have a rapid progression and carry a high mortality because of the severe secondary injuries associated with edema and increased intracranial pressure. The clinical picture is similar to that of epidural hematoma except that there is usually not a lucid interval. In *subacute* hematoma, there may be a period of improvement in the level of consciousness and neurological symptoms, only to be followed by deterioration if the hematoma is not removed.

Symptoms of *chronic subdural hematoma* develop weeks after a head injury, so much later, in fact, that the person may not remember having had a head injury. This is especially true of older persons with brittle vessels. Seepage of blood into the subdural

space occurs very slowly. Since the blood in the subdural space is not absorbed, fibroblastic activity begins and the hematoma becomes encapsulated. Within this encapsulated area, the cells are slowly lysed and a fluid with a high osmotic pressure is formed. This creates an osmotic gradient, with fluid from the surrounding subarachnoid space being pulled into the area; in turn, the mass increases in size, exerting pressure on the cranial contents.

In some instances, the clinical picture is less defined, with the most prominent symptom being a decreasing level of consciousness indicated by drowsiness, confusion, and apathy. Headache may also be present.

Postconcussion Syndrome

Following a head injury, complaints of headache, dizziness, poor concentration and memory, fatigue, and irritability are usual, although their extent and duration have considerable variation. Because these complaints are vague and subjective, they have sometimes been regarded as being of psychological origin. Recent findings, however, support the belief that there is an organic basis for the postconcussion symptoms.[3] Sequelae that have a definite physical basis include hemiparesis, dysphasia, hemianopia, cranial nerve palsy, and epilepsy.

Increased Intracranial Pressure

The rigid structure of the skull prevents its expansion when the intracranial pressure increases. The intracranial pressure can increase due to impaired production, circulation, or absorption of the CSF or result from edema caused by brain tumor, stroke, or injury. When the edema is due to a brain tumor, it tends to be localized in the immediate area, while that due to head injury usually increases rapidly and is generalized in one hemisphere. Localized edema due to brain tumors often responds to corticosteroids, whereas these drugs have little effect on generalized edema.

A progression or worsening of increased intracranial pressure can be detected by changes in (1) the level of consciousness, (2) the pupils, (3) the vital signs, and (4) motor function. The level of consciousness may deteriorate from alertness through confusion, lethargy, obtundation, stupor, and coma. The *pupillary change* of greatest importance is unilateral dilatation. (The third cranial nerve [oculomotor], which controls pupillary constriction, runs along the tentorial ridge. In increased intracranial pressure, there may be downward displacement of the cerebral cortex, which exerts pressure on this nerve, causing unilateral pupil dilatation.) This is a primary sign of impending herniation. The motor signs include changes in strength and coordination of voluntary movements.

Blood pressure and heart rate should be monitored frequently when there is a possibility of increased intracranial pressure, as these vital signs reflect the body's attempt to compensate for the increased pressure. The effect on the vital signs can be explained in terms of the three fluid compartments within the brain: interstitial, vascular, and cerebrospinal fluid. Because of the rigid nature of the skull, the total quantity of fluid must remain relatively constant, although there may be a compensatory shift in fluid volumes between the compartments. An increase in interstitial fluid, for example, is accompanied by a decrease in vascular volume and CSF. Compensation fails when the volume of CSF has been lowered as much as possible and vascular volume has been reduced to a point where it causes ischemia of brain structures.

One of the late reflexes seen with marked increases in intracranial pressure is the *CNS ischemic response*, which is triggered by ischemia of the vasomotor center. The neurons in the vasomotor center respond directly to ischemia by producing a marked increase in mean arterial blood pressure, sometimes to levels as high as 270 mm Hg. The Cushing reaction is a type of CNS ischemic response. It results from a severely increased intracranial pressure that compresses blood flow to the brain. If the increase in blood pressure initiated by the CNS ischemic reflex is greater than the pressure surrounding the compressed vessels, blood flow will be re-established. The CNS ischemic response is a "last ditch" effort by the nervous system to maintain cerebral circulation. It is accompanied by a widening of the pulse pressure and a reflex bradycardia.

This *widening of the pulse pressure* and the *decrease in heart rate* are important but late indicators of increased intracranial pressure. There may also be respiratory changes, and temperature may or may not rise.[4]

In summary, head injury may be classified as direct, *due to the immediate effects of the injury, skull fracture, concussion, or contusion; or as* secondary, *due to edema, hemorrhage, and infection.*

:Infections

Infections of the CNS may be classified according to the structure involved: the meninges—meningitis; the brain parenchyma—encephalitis; the spinal cord—myelitis; both brain and spinal cord—encephalomyelitis. They may also be classified by the type of invading organism, whether bacteria, viral, or other. In general, the pathogens enter the CNS via the blood stream by crossing the blood-brain barrier in a systemic disease, or by direct invasion through skull fracture, bullet hole, or, more rarely, through contamination during surgery or lumbar puncture. This section focuses on meningitis and encephalitis.

Meningitis

Meningitis, also called leptomeningitis, is an infection of the pia mater, the arachnoid, and the subarachnoid space. The meningococcus is the most frequent causative pathogen in adolescents and adults; in infants and the elderly, it is the pneumococcus; and in young children, it is the hemophilus, specifically *Hemophilus influenzae*. Staphylococci and streptococci are less common causes.

In an adult, the symptoms are those of meningeal irritation: fever, headache, lethargy, stiff neck (nuchal rigidity), and vomiting. The headache is frequently described as "the worst ever." Children may have less specific symptoms, with fever the most common and vomiting the second most frequent. Infants have few specific symptoms. The health professional should consider meningitis whenever these symptoms are present. An analysis of CSF will confirm or rule out meningitis and will identify the organism. Other observations should include (1) the presence of infection, (2) alterations in behavior or level of consciousness, and (3) neurological symptoms.

As the disease progresses, there may be nausea and vomiting, photophobia, convulsions, petechiae, and arthritis. Kernig's sign and Brudzinski's sign will determine whether or not there is meningeal irritation. *Kernig's sign* is elicited when the leg cannot be extended while the patient is lying with the hip flexed at a right angle. A positive *Brudzinski's sign* is seen when forcible flexion of the neck results in flexion of the hip and knee.

As the pathogens enter the subarachnoid space, they cause inflammation, characterized by a cloudy, purulent exudate. Thrombophlebitis of the bridging veins and dural sinuses may develop, followed by congestion and infarction in the surrounding tissues. Ultimately, the meninges thicken and adhesions form. These adhesions may impinge on the cranial nerves, giving rise to cranial nerve palsies, or may impair the outflow of CSF, giving rise to hydrocephalus.

Encephalitis

Generalized infection of the parenchyma of the brain or spinal cord is almost always caused by a virus. The infection takes one of these forms: (1) inflammation due to direct invasion, as in encephalitis; (2) a postinfectious noninflammatory process, as in Reye's syndrome; (3) a postinfectious inflammatory process, as in encephalomyelitis; and (4) a slow-growing infection with a prolonged incubation period and running a chronic course.[5]

The pathologic picture includes local necrotizing hemorrhage, which ultimately becomes generalized, with prominent edema. There is progressive degeneration of nerve cell bodies. The histologic picture, though rather general, demonstrates some specific characteristics; for example, the poliovirus selectively destroys the cells of the anterior horn of the spinal cord.[6]

Encephalitis, like meningitis, is characterized by fever, headache, and nuchal rigidity. In addition, there is a wide range of neurological disturbances, such as lethargy, disorientation, seizures, dysphasias, focal paralysis, delirium, and coma. The nervous system is subject to invasion by many viruses, such as arbovirus, poliovirus, and rabies virus. The mode of transmission varies: it may be the bite of a mosquito, tick, or rabid animal; it may be enteral, as in poliomyelitis. A very common cause of encephalitis in the United States is herpes simplex virus.

In summary, infection may be classified according to the structure involved (meningitis, encephalitis) or the type of invading organism. The damage caused by infection may predispose to hydrocephalus, seizures, or other neurological defects.

:Seizures

A seizure may be defined as the spontaneous, uncontrolled, paroxysmal, transitory discharge from the cortical centers in the brain. This uncontrolled activity causes symptoms based on the location of the involved area—there may be bizarre muscle movements, strange sensations and perception, and loss of consciousness.

A seizure is not a disease, but a symptom of an underlying disorder. Although seizures are commonly associated with epilepsy, the two are not necessarily the same. For example, metabolic abnormalities are a major cause of a pathological condition that gives rise to seizures and that is reversible.

Examples include electrolyte imbalance, hypoglycemia, hypoxia, hypocalcemia, and acidosis. Toxemia of pregnancy, water intoxication, uremia, and CNS infections (meningitis, for example) may also precipitate a seizure. The rapid withdrawal of sedative–hypnotic drugs, such as alcohol or barbiturates, is another cause.[7] In children, a high fever (temperature over 104°F) may precipitate a seizure.

Seizure activity may be initiated by abnormal cells within the brain called *epileptogenic foci*. This abnormal activity is believed to be caused by alterations in membrane permeability or in distribution of ions across the cell membrane.

There are four patterns of abnormal activity. In one, the abnormal discharge may arise from the central areas of the brain, with *immediate alterations in the level of consciousness*. A second pattern may be localized in a specific part of the brain and produce a focal seizure.[8] The third type of abnormal discharge begins as a localized seizure and extends to a generalized seizure. Finally, if the site of the discharge is the reticular formation, there will be a *generalized* seizure with diffuse and nonspecific disturbances of cerebral function. Regardless of the type of seizure, the basic cause is always excessive electrical discharges from the brain.

Epilepsy

Recurrence of seizures without evidence of reversible metabolic activity is called *epilepsy*. These seizures are caused by paroxysmal and transitory disturbance of brain function which develops suddenly and disappears spontaneously. Unlike other types of seizure, epilepsy exhibits a definite tendency to recur and is not usually associated with systemic disease. The two chief types of epilepsy are *structurally induced* seizures and *idiopathic* seizures.

A structurally induced seizure results from cerebral scarring owing to head injury, cerebral vascular accident, infection, degenerative CNS disease, or recurrent childhood febrile seizures. This type of seizure is also called *secondary epilepsy*. The likelihood that epilepsy will develop owing to cerebral trauma depends on the severity of the underlying injury or disease, whether or not there was unconsciousness, and whether the dura was penetrated. Genetic influences play a role, too.

The age of onset can be a clue to the type or cause of the seizure. Seizures occurring between birth and 6 months of age are probably due to *congenital defects* or birth injury. Seizures between the ages of 2 and 20 years may be the result of *genetic* and other unidentified causes and are called *idiopathic*. *Primary* epilepsy is the term that describes such recurrent seizures, and 80% of all cases of epilepsy are thought to be idiopathic—apparently there is a "low threshold" for epilepsy, as indicated by genetic studies. After the age of 20, seizures are usually due to structural damage or trauma, tumor, or stroke.

Classification

The classification of seizures established by the International League Against Epilepsy combines clinical and electroencephalographic (EEG) manifestations. The two chief categories—generalized and focal/partial epilepsy—are based on the site of origin in the brain (Table 42-1).

Focal/partial epilepsy.

Focal/partial seizures have a local origin resulting from a specific lesion or focus in the brain. There is usually a warning aura preceding the seizure proper. The aura helps to localize the area of the brain where the focus is located. The symptomatology of focal/partial seizures is known as either elementary or complex.

Elementary symptomatology seizures have their foci located in the motor or sensory portions of the cerebral cortex, resulting in focal sensory or motor symptoms. If the focus is in the motor strip portion, the earliest symptom is motor movement corresponding to the location of the focus on the contralateral side. If the focus is in the sensory portion of the brain, there may be no apparent clinical manifestations. Sensory symptoms correlating with the focus area on the contralateral side of the brain may be described. Partial seizures with elementary symptomatology may remain localized or focal in nature, or may spread throughout the brain. If the latter occurs, there may be a postictal (postseizure) period of drowsiness, fatigue, confusion, semipurposeful activity, and transient paresis—symptoms related to the suppression of brain activity in the area of the seizure origin.

Complex symptomatology seizures usually have their focus in the temporal lobe, giving rise to a wide variety of unusual behaviors, hallucinations, sensations, and automatism. The behavior of a person during a seizure with complex symptomatology is not purposeful—such as playing with clothing. It sometimes happens that a person with complex symptomatology is misunderstood, and is believed to require psychiatric hospitalization.

Generalized epilepsy.

The seizures of generalized epilepsy occur without a focal origin. They are bilaterally symmetrical, without gradual buildup. These seizures range from *minor motor seizures*, such as

Table 42-1 International Classification of Epileptic Seizures

I. Partial seizures (seizures beginning locally)
  A. Partial seizures with elementary symptomatology*
    1. With motor symptoms
    2. With sensory symptoms
    3. With autonomic symptoms
    4. Compound forms
  B. Partial seizures with complex symptomatology (temporal lobe or psychomotor seizures)**
    1. With impairment of consciousness only
    2. With cognitive symptomatology
    3. With affective symptomatology
    4. With "psychosensory" symptomatology
    5. With "psychomotor" symptomatology
    6. Compound forms
  C. Partial seizures, secondarily generalized
II. Generalized seizures (bilaterally symmetrical; without local onset)
    1. Absence (petit mal) seizures
    2. Myoclonic seizures
    3. Infantile spasms
    4. Clonic seizures
    5. Tonic seizures
    6. Tonic-clonic (grand mal) seizures
    7. Atonic seizures
    8. Akinetic seizures
III. Unilateral seizures (those involving one hemisphere)
IV. Unclassified epileptic seizures (due to incomplete data)

*Generally without impairment of consciousness.
**Generally with impairment of consciousness.
Adapted with permission from Gastaut H: Clinical and electroencephalographical classification of epileptic seizures. Epilepsia 11:102, 1970.
Norman SE, Browne TR: Seizure disorders. Am J Nurs 81, No. 5:986, 1981

absence (petit mal seizure), *myoclonic*, and *akinetic seizure*, to *major motor* or *clonic-tonic seizure* (grand mal seizure).

In a *minor motor* seizure, there is abnormal discharge activity throughout the brain, but the manifestations are so subtle that it may pass unnoticed. There is often a brief loss of contact with the environment, but no loss of consciousness. The seizure usually lasts only a few seconds and then the person is able to resume normal activity. The *absence seizure*, which is characterized by a brief loss of contact with the environment, typically occurs only in children, and either is outgrown or evolves into generalized major motor seizures. In a *myoclonic seizure*, there is bilateral rapid jerking of the extremities, but no loss of consciousness. If the seizure persists and gains strength, it may progress to a clonic-tonic seizure. In *akinetic seizures*, there is a split-second loss of muscle tone and the person falls to the ground.

The *major motor* seizures are tonic (simultaneous contraction of flexor and extensor muscles leading to rigidity) and clonic (alternate contraction of flexor or extensor muscles). In a *grand mal* seizure, there is tonic-clonic motor movement with uncontrolled activity of the skeletal muscles, loss of consciousness, tongue biting in some instances, and incontinence. This drastic and extremely vigorous activity leads to exhaustion. Coma ensues, followed by a deep sleep.

Diagnosis

Diagnosis of epilepsy is based on a thorough history and neurological examination, including a full description of an aura, if present, and the seizure. The physical examination helps rule out any metabolic disease that could precipitate seizures. Skull x-ray studies and computerized axial tomograms (CAT scan) help to identify any structural defects. Changes in the brain's electrical activity are recorded on the electroencephalogram (EEG), and this record is the most useful aid in diagnosis.

Treatment

The first rule of treatment is to protect the affected person from injury, next to treat any underlying disease. Treatment of the underlying disorder may reduce the frequency of seizures. Once the underlying disease is treated, the aim of treatment is to bring the seizures under control with the least possible disruption of the person's life-style and a minimum of side effects. This is accomplished primarily through anticonvulsant drug therapy. With proper drug management, 60% to 80% of persons with epilepsy can obtain good seizure control.[9]

Anticonvulsant drug therapy. At the start of anticonvulsant drug therapy, a medication is prescribed that usually is effective in treating the given type of seizure. The dose is gradually increased until the drug has its maximum effect or toxicity occurs. If control is not achieved, the dose is decreased just enough to prevent toxic effects, and another drug is added in similar fashion. It is desirable to use as few drugs as possible, to promote compliance and reduce side effects. Table 42-2 summarizes the principles of anticonvulsant drug therapy.

Most anticonvulsant drugs are taken orally, to be absorbed through the intestinal mucosa and metabolized by the liver. Liver damage that is present will affect drug tolerance as will other factors that alter absorption, distribution, metabolism, and excretion of the drug. Plasma levels are measured to determine absorption, compliance in taking medications, and possibly drug toxicity, but these levels do not indicate whether there is seizure control or not.

Drug toxicity is manifested in CNS symptoms of diplopia, ataxia, extreme drowsiness, and mental dullness. These symptoms should not be mistaken for the side effects of drowsiness, rash, and stomach upset, often seen during the first days of administration. Drug dosage is generally not reduced unless side effects interfere with functional activities. Gin-

---

Table 42–2   Principles of Anticonvulsant Drug Therapy

General Treatment	1. Treat underlying disease first, if any
	2. Aim is clinical control of seizures with the least curtailment of patient's life, and a minimum of side effects
Pharmacological Treatment	1. Start with a drug that normally is effective in this kind of seizure; titrate until maximum effect is reached, or toxicity occurs; if unable to control with one drug, add another
	2. Use as few drugs as possible; this helps compliance, and keeps unwanted side effects down
Plasma Levels	Plasma levels do NOT indicate whether there is seizure control or not; they indicate compliance, absorption, and possibility of drug toxicity

Courtesy: Marilyn Weber, R.N., M.S., Clinical Coordinator Epilepsy Clinic, Mt. Sinai Hospital, Milwaukee, Wisconsin.

Table 42-3 Anticonvulsant Drugs Used in Treatment of Specific Types of Epilepsy

Type of Seizure	Drug	Therapeutic Range (mcg/ml plasma)	Usual Adult Maintenance Dose (mg/day)
Partial seizures with complex symptomatology (temporal lobe)	phenytoin (Dilantin)	10 to 20	300
	phenobarbital	20 to 40	100
Generalized seizures tonic-clonic (grand mal)	primidone (Mysoline)	8 to 12	750
	phenobarbital derived from primidone	20 to 40	N.A.
Partial seizures with elementary symptomatology	carbamazepine (Tegretol)	6 to 10	800
Generalized seizures absence myoclonus	ethosuximide (Zarontin)	50 to 100	750
	trimethadione (Tridione)	700 or higher (as dimethadione)	800
Generalized seizures akinetic myoclonus	clonozepam (Clonopin)	0.015 to 0.030	10 to 20
Other generalized and partial seizures(?)	sodium valproate (Depakene)	30 to 100	1000

Courtesy: Marilyn Weber, R.N., M.S., Clinical Coordinator, Epilepsy Clinic, Mt. Sinai Hospital, Milwaukee, Wisconsin.

gival hyperplasia may occur in children with the continued use of phenytoin (Dilantin). Phenytoin is a suspected teratogenic agent. Nevertheless, it is often necessary to continue use of the drug during pregnancy, to prevent seizures.

The specific drug to be prescribed varies according to the type of seizure being treated. Drugs used to treat generalized seizures may aggravate or be ineffective with focal seizures. Drugs used to treat tonic-clonic and partial seizures with complex and elementary symptomatology are phenytoin (Dilantin), phenobarbital, primidone (Mysoline), and carbamazepine (Tegretol). Ethosuximide (Zarontin) and trimethadione (Tridione) are used to treat absence focal seizures (petit mal), and clonazepam (Clonopin), akinetic and myoclonic seizures. Other generalized and partial seizures may be treated with sodium valproate (Depakene). The most widely used anticonvulsant drugs are summarized in Table 42-3.

Determining the proper dose of the anticonvulsant drug(s) is a long and tedious process, which can become very frustrating to the person with epilepsy. Consistency in taking the medication is essential. Anticonvulsant drugs should never be discontinued rapidly, but the dose should be slowly decreased.

Status Epilepticus

A clonic-tonic seizure that does not stop spontaneously or in which the person passes from one seizure to another without regaining consciousness is called *status epilepticus*. It is a medical emergency and if not promptly treated may lead to respiratory failure and death.

The main causes of status epilepticus are patient failure to take the prescribed dose of medication,[8] and severe neurological or systemic disease in a person with no previous history of epilepsy. If status epilepticus is due to neurological or systemic disease, the cause needs to be identified and treated immediately, since the seizures probably will not respond until the underlying disturbance is corrected. When status epilepticus is the result of discontinuing medication, the drug regimen should be reinstituted as soon as possible. The prognosis is related to the underlying cause more than to the seizures themselves.

In summary, seizures are symptoms of an underlying disorder. Epilepsy, the most common type of seizure, is classified as partial or generalized. Specific drugs are used to treat each classification.

:Consciousness and Unconsciousness

In order to understand alterations in consciousness, the reader must first gain an understanding of the reticular activating system (RAS). The RAS controls overall CNS activity, including sleep and wakefulness. The RAS is not a discrete anatomical structure, but a diffuse formation that extends from the lower brain stem upward through the mesencephalon (midbrain) and thalamus and is distributed throughout the cerebral cortex. The RAS is divided into two areas, the bulboreticular facilitory area and the bulboreticular inhibitory area.

The *bulboreticular facilitory* area is located in the uppermost and lateral parts of the medulla, and all of the pons, mesencephalon, and diencephalon. The facilitory area is intrinsically active. If no inhibitory signals are being transmitted from other parts of the body, continuous nerve impulses will be transmitted both downward to the motor areas of the cord and upward toward the brain, producing immediate marked activation of the cerebral cortex. There are two positive feedback loops: (1) to the cerebral cortex and back to the reticular formation, and (2) to the peripheral muscles and back to the reticular formation. Stimulation of the facilitory area causes an increase in muscle tone throughout the body or in localized areas. Thus, once the RAS becomes activated, the feedback impulses from both the cerebral cortex and the periphery maintain the excitation. After prolonged wakefulness, the neurons in the RAS gradually become fatigued or less excitable. When this happens, neuronal mechanisms give way to lower-level functioning and sleep.

The lower three-fourths of the medulla is known as the *bulboreticular inhibitory* area. Stimulation of this area causes a decrease in muscle tone throughout the body. When both the bulboreticular inhibitory area and bulboreticular facilitory area are functioning normally, the motor function of the spinal cord is neither excited nor inhibited. If excitation of the inhibitory area from the basal ganglia, cerebral cortex, and cerebellum is stopped or reduced, that area becomes less active and facilitation then predominates.[10]

Unconsciousness can be due to many causes, so that there is variation from case to case in onset, duration, and extent of damage. Coma may have a metabolic, a supratentorial, or a subtentorial origin.

In metabolic coma, the metabolism of the cerebral cortex and brain stem is disrupted by toxins, by drugs, by anoxia, or by hypoglycemia.

As was described in Chapter 40, the tentorium, a tough dural fold, divides the cavity of the skull into the anterior and middle fossae above and the posterior fossa below. There is a large opening, the tentorial hiatus, through which the nerve pathways pass. Subtentorial or infratentorial coma may result from direct pressure or destruction of the brain stem in the posterior fossa, which interrupts the RAS. However, a more common cause of coma is a supratentorial mass, which indirectly involves the brain stem. In supratentorial coma, a mass (edema, brain tumor, blood clot) expands, creating increased pressure and displacing cerebral tissue away from the mass and toward a less dense area. Above the tentorium, there is a shift of tissue from one cavity to another and downward through the tentorial incisura, commonly called *herniation*. In turn, the herniation may produce compression of adjacent vessels and tissues with resultant ischemia and edema.

If the supratentorial lesion is near the midline, there may be central displacement, which causes expansion and edema of the diencephalon. If the supratentorial mass is lateral, the herniating tissue compresses the third cranial nerve, causing unilateral pupillary dilatation. Arterial occlusion produces ischemia, edema, and infarction. If the cerebrospinal fluid pathway is blocked and fluid cannot leave the ventricles, the mass will expand, as will the downward displacement of tissue through the tentorial notch. The result of this displacement is brain stem ischemia and hemorrhage extending from the diencephalon to the pons. If the lesion is a rapidly expanding one, displacement and obstruction will occur quickly, leading to irreversible infarction and hemorrhage. Loss of brain function advances in a rostral–caudal direction.

Diencephalon

Disruptions affecting the diencephalon, midbrain, pons, and medulla usually cause a predictable pattern of change in the level of consciousness (Table 42-4). The highest level of consciousness is seen in an alert person who is oriented to person, place, and time, and is totally aware of the surroundings. The first symptoms of diminution in level of consciousness are decreased concentration, agitation, dullness, and lethargy. With further deterioration, the person may become obtunded and may respond

Table 42-4 Rostral–Caudal Progression of Coma

Area Involved	Levels of Consciousness	Pupils	Muscle Tone	Respiration
Diencephalon (Thalamus/ Hypothalamus)	Decreased concentration, agitation, dullness, lethargy Obtundation	Respond to light briskly Full range of eye movements only on "doll's eyes" or caloric test	Some purposeful movement in response to pain; combative movement Decorticate	Yawning and sighing → Cheyne–Stokes
Midbrain	Stupor → coma	Midposition fixed (MPF)	Decerebrate	Neurogenic hyperventilation
Pons	Coma	MPF	Decerebrate	Apneustic
Medulla	Coma	MPF	Flaccid	Atactic

only to vigorous shaking. Early respiratory changes include yawning and sighing with progression to Cheyne–Stokes breathing (Chap. 18). This is indicative of bilateral hemisphere damage with danger of tentorial herniation. While the pupils may respond to light briskly, the full range of eye movements is seen only when the head is passively rotated from side-to-side (oculocephalic reflex or "doll's eyes" maneuver) or when the caloric test (injection of hot or cold water into the ear canal) is done to elicit nystagmus. In the "doll's eyes" test, the eyes move in the direction of rotation rather than holding their position as occurs normally. There is some combative movement as well as purposeful movement in response to pain. As coma progresses, the bulboreticular facilitory area becomes more active as fewer inhibitory signals descend from the basal ganglia and cerebral cortex. This results in decorticate posturing with flexion of the upper extremities and adduction and extension of the lower extremities.

Midbrain

With progression continuing in rostral–caudal fashion, the midbrain becomes involved. Cheyne–Stokes respiration changes to neurogenic hyperventilation. Respirations often exceed 40 per minute owing to uninhibited stimulation of both the inhibitory and expiratory centers. The pupils are fixed in midposition and no longer respond to stimuli. There is increased muscle excitability with decerebrate posturing, in which the arms are rigid and extended with the palms of the hand turned away from the body.

Pons

As coma advances to involve the pons, the pupils remain in midposition and fixed, and the decerebrate posturing continues. Breathing is apneustic, with sighs evident in mid-inspiration, and with prolonged inspiration and expiration owing to excessive stimulation of respiratory centers.

Medulla

With medullary involvement, the pupils remain fixed in midposition. Respirations are atactic, that is, totally uncoordinated and irregular. Apnea may occur because of the loss of responsiveness to carbon dioxide stimulation. Complete ventilatory assistance should be considered for any person with atactic breathing. Since the medulla has bulboreticular inhibitory neurons but no facilitory neurons, the hyperexcitability that gave rise to the decorticate and decerebrate posturing disappear, giving way to flaccidity.

In progressive brain deterioration, the patient's neurological capabilities appear to fall off in stepwise fashion. Similarly, as neurological function returns, there appears to be step-wise progress to higher levels of consciousness.

Brain Death

As we have learned to maintain circulation of oxygenated blood artificially, the definition of death has had to be re-examined. In 1968, criteria of irreversible coma were published by a Harvard Medical School Ad Hoc Committee.[11] The criteria include the following: (1) unresponsiveness, (2) no spontaneous respirations for a period of 3 minutes without assistance, (3) absence of CNS reflexes and ocular movements and presence of fixed dilated pupils, (4) flat EEG for at least 10 minutes, (5) the same findings during a repeat examination 24 hours later, and (6) no evidence of use of hypothermia or CNS depressants that may alter these findings.

Since that time, several other criteria have been proposed which modify the Harvard criteria. All have as their fundamental assumption the irreversibility of coma, and absence of responsiveness and respirations. All the criteria rely on tests of brain stem function and of cranial nerve reflexes. Yet it should not be overlooked that there are legal and moral aspects of brain death and they must be taken into consideration.

In summary, coma may be metabolic, supratentorial, or subtentorial in origin. The symptoms involved in the rostral-caudal progression of decreasing levels of consciousness are affected by facilitory and inhibitory areas of the reticular activating system.

:Study Guide

After you have studied this chapter, you should be able to meet the following objectives:

: : Describe the effects of contrecoup injury.

: : Compare the symptoms of concussion with those of contusion.

: : Explain why it is important to determine whether or not a head injury has resulted in chronic subdural hematoma.

: : List the constellation of symptoms involved in the postconcussion syndrome.

: : Explain the significance of unilateral pupillary dilatation with reference to intracranial pressure.

: : Describe the importance of measuring vital signs in assessment of increasing intracranial pressure.

: : Trace the sequence of events that occur in meningitis.

: : Describe the symptoms that are indicative of encephalitis.

: : State four or more causes of seizure activity other than epilepsy.

: : Describe the symptoms related to focal/partial epilepsy.

: : Compare minor motor seizures with major motor seizures.

: : Describe the precautions to be followed in prescribing anticonvulsant drugs.

: : Characterize *status epilepticus*.

: : Relate the activity of the bulboreticular facilitory area to level of consciousness.

: : Trace the progression of symptoms from consciousness to unconsciousness.

: : State the Harvard criteria of irreversible coma.

:References

1. Tindall GT, Fleischer AS: Head injury. Hospital Medicine 12, No. 5:89–110, 1976
2. Ransoff J, Koslow M: Guide to diagnosis and treatment of cerebral injury. Hospital Medicine 14, No. 5:127–143, 1978
3. Jeannett B, Teasdale G: Management of head injuries. Philadelphia, FA Davis, 1981
4. Jimm CR: Nursing assessment of patients for increased intracranial pressure. J Neurosurg Nurs 6, No. 1:27–37, 1974
5. Murphy FK, Mackowiak P, Luby J: Management of infections affecting the nervous system. In Rosenberg RN (ed): The Treatment of Neurological Diseases. New York, SP Medical & Scientific Books, 1979
6. Robbins SL, Cotran RS: Pathologic Basis of Disease, ed 2. Philadelphia, WB Saunders, 1979
7. Hawken M: Seizures: Etiology, classification, intervention. J Neurosurg Nurs 11, No. 3:166–170, 1979
8. Bruya MA, Bolin RH: Epilepsy: A controllable disease. Part 1. Classification and diagnosis of seizures. Am J Nurs 76, No. 3:388–397, 1976
9. Hawken M, Ozuna J: Practical aspects of anticonvulsant therapy. Am J Nurs 79, No. 6:1062–1068, 1979
10. Guyton AC: Textbook of Medical Physiology, ed 6. Philadelphia, WB Saunders, 1981
11. Black PM: Criteria of brain death. Review and comparison. Postgrad Med 57, No. 2:69–74, 1975

:Suggested Readings

Allen N: Prognostic indicators in coma. Heart Lung 8, No. 6:1075–1083, 1979

Blacker HM: Closed head injury. Primary Care 3, No. 2:231–239, 1976

Caronna JJ: Assessment and management of coma. Consultant 19, No. 1:175–184, 1979

Cooper P: Treatment of head injuries. In Rosenberg RN (ed): The Treatment of Neurological Diseases. New York, SP Medical & Scientific Books, 1979

Gifford RRM, Plant MR: Abnormal respiratory patterns in the comatose patient caused by intracranial dysfunction. J Neurosurg Nurs 7, No. 1:58–63, 1975

Hanlon K: Description and uses of intracranial pressure monitoring. Heart Lung 5, No. 2:277–282, 1976

Lovely MP: Identification and treatment of status epilepticus. J Neurosurg Nurs 12, No. 2:93–96, 1980

Mitchell P, Mauss N: Intracranial pressure: Fact and fancy. Nursing '76 6, No. 6:53–57, 1976

Norman SE, Browne TR: Seizure disorders. Am J Nurs 81, No. 5:984–993, 1981

Plum F, Posner JB: Diagnosis of Stupor and Coma. Philadelphia, FA Davis, 1973

Sklar FH: Treatment of increased intracranial pressure. In Rosenberg RN (ed): The Treatment of Neurological Diseases. New York, SP Medical & Scientific Books, 1979

Swift N: Head injury. Essentials of excellent care. Nursing '74 74, No. 9:27–33, 1974

Tucker CA: Complex partial seizures. Am J Nurs 81, No. 5:996–1000, 1981

43

Mary Wierenga

Alterations in Motor Function

Effective motor function requires not only that muscles move but that the mechanics of their movement be programmed in a manner that provides for smooth and coordinated movement. In some cases, purposeless and disruptive movements can be almost as disabling as the relative or complete absence of movement. This chapter discusses normal motor activity and its alterations as manifested in stroke, Parkinson's disease, and spinal cord injury.

:Control of Motor Function

Control of motor activity is achieved through the interaction of three systems: the cerebral cortex, the cerebellum, and the basal ganglia. These systems initiate and regulate the two types of motor pathways by which the cerebral cortex exerts influence on the spinal cord and the lower motor neuron pathways. Many fibers from the motor area of the cerebral cortex travel directly to the brain stem or spinal

cord. These fibers decussate, or cross over, to the opposite side of the nervous system in the *pyramids* of the medulla. These fibers make up the *pyramidal* system. Other fibers from the cortex project to the *cerebellum* and *basal ganglia* before they descend and innervate the motor neurons. These fibers do not decussate in the pyramids and are considered to be outside (extra) the pyramidal tract, hence the name *extrapyramidal* system. The pyramidal and extrapyramidal tracts have opposing effects on muscle tone. The *pyramidal system* is largely incitatory in nature; it initiates muscle movement. The *extrapyramidal* tract serves to smooth and coordinate muscle movement; it is largely inhibitory in nature. Spinal cord reflex is either facilitated or inhibited by these two levels of control (Table 43-1).

The motor neurons that have their origin in the cortex of the brain and whose fibers remain within the CNS are called upper motor neurons (UMN). The motor neurons that are located in the ventral horns of the cord and that send projections to the motor fibers

Table 43-1   Characteristics of Pyramidal and Extrapyramidal Motor Control

Feature	Pyramidal	Extrapyramidal		Peripheral
Nomenclature	(1) Voluntary motor pathway (2) Upper motor neuron (UMN) pathway (3) Corticospinal pathway	(1) Involuntary motor pathway (2) Extracorticospinal		(1) Final common pathway (2) Lower motor neuron (LMN) pathway
Location	From the Betz cells of the frontal lobe motor strip to the anterior horn cell of the spinal cord	Motor cortex with projections into basal ganglia, and communication with the reticular formation	Posterior fossa of cerebellum	From the ventral horn cells of the spinal cord to the muscles
Function	Initiates and transmits impulses for smooth voluntary movement to spinal cord	(1) Inhibits muscle tone throughout the body (2) Initiates and regulates gross intentional movements	(1) Coordination of movements by monitoring and making adjustments in motor activity elicited by other parts of the nervous system (2) "Dampen" muscle movement	Transmits impulses from the spinal cord to the muscles for voluntary movement
Disruption	Hyperactive reflexes and spastic paralysis on the contralateral side— hemiplegia	Muscle rigidity and incoordination Loss of discrete movement Abnormal posture	Incoordination, intention tremors, ataxia, overshooting; inability to progress in orderly sequence from one movement to another	Hypoactive reflexes and paresis or flaccid paralysis, usually monoplegia
Extent of damage	Small amount of damage in important area (*e.g.*, internal capsule) causes extensive decrease in function	If part of basal ganglia left intact, gross postural and "fixed" movements can still be performed; widespread damage leads to muscle rigidity throughout the body	Depends on the extent of damage to the cerebellum	Extensive damage (several levels) before there is significantly decreased function

are called lower motor neurons (LMN). The cranial nerves synapse with UMN in the brain or brain stem and are also LMN (Fig. 43-1).

Pyramidal tract.   The neuronal bodies for the pyramidal or corticospinal tract are found in the large pyramidal (Betz) cells of the motor cortex, which is located in the posterior portion of the frontal lobe in the precentral gyrus. Specific areas in this part of the brain are assigned to certain muscle groups on the *opposite* side of the body. The pattern for this motor activity is often depicted in the shape of a *homunculus*, as described in Chapter 40. The distortion in shape has a purpose—it represents, by the size of its various segments, body areas according to their motor function. Those that have minimal motor function (*e.g.*, the trunk) have minimal representation; those that have maximal motor function (*e.g.*, the hands) have maximal representation.

The voluntary motor tracts travel downward through the internal capsule where they are pulled closer together (following the shape of the homunculus) in preparation for the descent into the brain stem and spinal cord. The majority of nerve pathways decussate in the medulla, moving to the opposite side of the cord to innervate the opposite side of the body. The Betz cells on the right side of the motor cortex control hand movement on the left side of the body. As the pathway descends from the motor area, it sends collaterals to the other parts of the central nervous system, basal ganglia, cerebral cortex, cerebellum, and spinal cord, which help to maintain smooth, voluntary movement.

Disruption of pyramidal tract function.   The motor cortex, the pyramidal tract, or both are frequent sites of damage especially by stroke (discussed later in this chapter). With damage to the pyramidal tract there is disruption of voluntary motor movement, although the LMN pathway is not directly affected. The reflex arc of the spinal cord remains intact but is not controlled by the higher centers.

There are two common sites where damage to the pyramidal tract can occur: in the motor cortex, or in the internal capsule as it courses through the brain toward the spinal cord. For example, damage to a small area of the motor cortex causes a loss of voluntary motor activity in the represented muscles. On the other hand, even minimal damage to an important structure, such as the internal capsule, which carries both sensory and motor fibers, causes extensive dysfunction because all the fibers innervating one side of the body and the basal ganglia are located in this area. If the basal ganglia are not damaged,

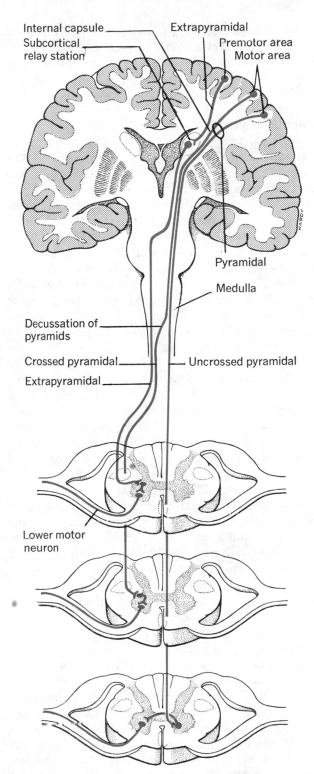

Figure 43–1.   Motor pathways among the cerebral cortex, one of the subcortical relay centers, and lower motor neurons in the spinal cord. Decussation (crossing) of fibers means that each side of the brain controls skeletal muscles on the opposite side of the body. (Chaffee EE, Lytle IM: Basic Physiology and Anatomy, 4th ed, p 244. Philadelphia, JB Lippincott, 1980)

gross postural and fixed movements will be intact but discrete function on the opposite side of the body will be lost. Thus, even though the damage may be seemingly insignificant in both areas, the resulting dysfunction may be quite different.

Lower motor neurons. The LMN is best understood when compared to the UMN or voluntary motor pathway. The LMN begins in the ventral horn cell of the spinal cord and its fibers project to the muscles. In contrast to UMN injury, which causes hyper-reflexia and hypertonicity, injury to the LMN interrupts the reflex, causing hyporeflexia, and when damage is extensive, flaccidity. With LMN dysfunction and flaccid paralysis, muscle atrophy becomes prominent. Because of nerve branching, dysfunction becomes discernible only when several LMN pathways are damaged. Monoparesis (weakness of one extremity) and monoplegia (paralysis of one extremity) are the most common dysfunctions arising from LMN damage.

Extrapyramidal tract. The extrapyramidal tract arises from the motor cortex and is indirectly routed through the brain with projections into the *basal ganglia* and the *cerebellum*. From the basal ganglia and the cerebellum, the fibers communicate with the next level of control, the reticular formation of the brain stem. The extrapyramidal system is usually considered a functional rather than an anatomical unit because of its many projections. In contrast to the more direct route of the pyramidal tract, the extrapyramidal tract reaches the spinal cord only after many detours and indirect routing. The final pathway is primarily the reticulospinal tract.

Basal ganglia. The basal ganglia are the several large masses that lie caudal to the thalamus and project around the internal capsule. The term corpus striatum (striped body) is sometimes used interchangeably with basal ganglia. The major components of the basal ganglia are the caudate (tailed) nucleus, the putamen, and the globus pallidus (pale body). The globus pallidus and the putamen make up the lenticular nucleus. Although not specifically a part of the basal ganglia, the subthalamic nucleus and substantia nigra are closely related on the basis of function. Neurons arising in the substantia nigra transmit dopamine, an inhibitory neuromediator, to the striatum.

The extrapyramidal tract fibers from the basal ganglia inhibit muscle tone throughout the body by transmitting inhibiting signals. These fibers, which

regulate gross intentional movements of the body that are normally performed subconsciously, provide the muscle tone needed for movement.

Cerebellar pathway. The cerebellum has both voluntary and involuntary components. It is responsible for muscle synergy (correlated action) throughout the body. The cerebellum monitors and makes corrective adjustments in the motor activity elicited by other parts of the brain. The cerebellum receives information continuously from the periphery of the body to assess the status of each body part—position, rate of movement, forces acting on it, and so on. The cerebellum compares what is actually happening to what is intended to happen and transmits appropriate corrective signals back to the motor system, instructing it to increase or decrease the activity of various muscles. In this way, the cerebellum coordinates the action of muscle groups and regulates their contractions so that smooth and accurate movements are performed. Voluntary movements can be performed without cerebellar intervention but the movements will be clumsy and uncoordinated. An extensive feedback system (both input and output) allows the cerebellum to make corrections rapidly while the motor movement is taking place.

A second function of the cerebellum is to "dampen" muscle movement. All body movements are basically pendular (like a pendulum). As movement begins, momentum develops and must be overcome before movement can be stopped. Because of momentum, all movements have a tendency to overshoot if they are not dampened. In the intact cerebellum, subconscious signals stop movement precisely at the intended point. In providing for this type of control, the cerebellum predicts the future position of moving parts of the body; the rapidity with which the limb is moving is detected from incoming proprioceptive signals as well as the projected time for the course of movement. This allows the cerebellum to inhibit agonist muscles and excite antagonist muscles when movement approaches the point of intention.

The cerebellum functions much the same way in involuntary, postural, and subconscious movements as it does in voluntary movement but through different pathways. Extrapyramidal movements, which originate in the cerebral cortex, send collaterals to the cerebellum. As the muscle movement occurs, messages from the muscles, joints, and periphery are sent back to the cerebellum, which provides the same "error" control for involuntary movement as it does for voluntary movement.

Disruption of extrapyramidal tract function.   Damage to the basal ganglial component of the extrapyramidal tract does not cause paralysis, as does damage to the pyramidal and lower motor neuron tracts. Disruption of these extrapyramidal fibers results instead, in muscle rigidity and incoordination. Remembering that the pyramidal and extrapyramidal tracts have opposing effects on muscle tone, one can understand that damage to either tract may disrupt the delicate balance that assures smooth muscle movement. If the damage is in the primary motor cortex, there may be no change in muscle tone because the pyramidal and extrapyramidal systems are affected equally. Usually, however, the lesion is large and involves extensive motor areas as well as the basal ganglia, which normally transmit inhibitory signals through the extrapyramidal system. In this case, loss of extrapyramidal inhibition leads to overactivity of the facilitory area with resultant increase in muscle tone.

There are several forms of disrupted motor activity that occur in impairment of the basal ganglial portion of the extrapyramidal tract. *Chorea* is characterized by quick, jerky, and purposeless movements, and is usually associated with damage to the basal ganglia. These random, uncontrolled contractions of different muscle groups interrupt normal progression of movement. *Athetosis* involves continuous, slow, writhing, worm-like movements, which exhibit a high degree of spasticity, and which make normal, voluntary movement difficult to perform. *Hemiballismus* consists of continued, wild, violent movements of large body parts.

Disruptions of the cerebellar system.   There are several types of disruption of motor activity that occur in impairment of the cerebellar portion of the extrapyramidal tract. The most common dysfunction is an uncoordinated movement of muscles, called *ataxia*. The loss of equilibrium is due to a lack of muscle posture manifested in a staggering, unsteady gait. If there is a lesion in one of the cerebellar hemispheres, the person will fall toward the side on which the lesion is situated. *Dysmetria* is characterized by an inability to predict and measure the end-point of a movement, resulting in movement past the point of intention, called past-pointing or overshooting. In this situation, the movement begins too early or too late, disrupting the normal orderly "progression of movement"; the condition is called *dysdiadochokinesia*. Similarly, a failure in progression of word formation resulting in explosive, slurred, almost unintelligible speech is called *dysarthia*. Failure of the cerebellum to dampen motor movement may give rise to *tremors*, in contrast to *resting* tremors seen in dysfunction of the basal ganglia portion of the extrapyramidal tract. When the cerebellum cannot dampen motor activity appropriately, overshooting occurs. Eventually, consciousness centers of the cerebrum recognize the overshooting and initiate movement in the opposite direction to bring the part into the intended position. But again, by virtue of momentum, overshooting and correction occur. The part may oscillate several times, causing intention tremors, before correction is made.

Nystagmus is the rapid, involuntary, horizontal, vertical, or rotatory movement of the eyeball. This cerebellar nystagmus is probably also a result of failure to dampen movements. The tremor is evident when the person attempts to look at a fixed point, especially on the side on which the disturbance is located.

In summary, movement is controlled by three interrelated motor systems: (1) the cerebral cortex, which is responsible for initiating voluntary motor activity; (2) the basal ganglia, which are responsible for maintaining posture; and (3) the cerebellum, which is responsible for coordinating movement. These three systems make up the pyramidal and extrapyramidal tracts, which affect motor movement through the spinal cord and the lower motor neuron (LMN) pathway.

Injuries or lesions to these areas tend to produce the following neurological deficits: (1) injury to the pyramidal tract results in paralysis of voluntary motor movement; (2) injury to the basal ganglia of the extrapyramidal tract results in increased muscle tone, postural deficits, and abnormal body positions; and (3) injury to the cerebellum of the extrapyramidal tract results in incoordination. Damage to the LMN results in monoparesis or flaccid monoplegia. Table 43-1 summarizes the characteristics of the three motor systems.

:Cerebral Circulation

Knowledge of normal cerebral circulation is essential to an understanding of vascular disorders. Blood transports oxygen, nutrients, and metabolic substances to the brain and removes waste products from the brain; thus, it is critical that blood supply to the brain be maintained. Arterial blood is supplied to the brain by the two internal carotid arteries (anteriorly) and the two vertebral arteries (posteriorly), which originate in the arch of the aorta (Fig. 43-2). The internal carotid artery branches into several

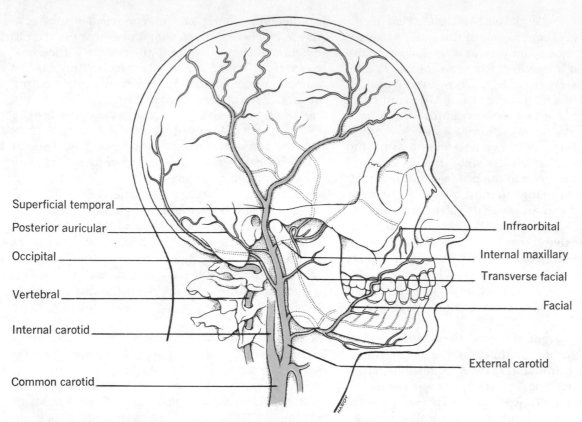

Superficial temporal

Posterior auricular

Occipital

Vertebral

Internal carotid

Common carotid

Infraorbital

Internal maxillary

Transverse facial

Facial

External carotid

Figure 43–2.   Branches of the right external carotid artery. The internal carotid artery ascends to the base of the brain. The right vertebral artery is also shown as it ascends through the transverse foramina of the cervical vertebrae. (Chaffee EE, Lytle IM: Basic Physiology and Anatomy, 4th ed, p 338. Philadelphia, JB Lippincott, 1980)

arteries: the ophthalmic, posterior communicating, the anterior communicating, the anterior cerebral, and the middle cerebral arteries (Fig. 43-3). The two vertebral arteries arise from the subclavian artery, ascend into the cranium through the foramen magnum, and join to form the large basilar artery. The basilar artery divides to form the posterior cerebral arteries. Branches of the basilar and vertebral arteries supply the medulla, pons, cerebellum, midbrain, and part of the diencephalon. The posterior cerebral arteries supply the temporal and occipital lobes.

Anastomotic connections and collateral circulation

There are two defense mechanisms that help protect the brain against ischemia: the collateral circulation, and autoregulation of blood flow. The internal carotid arteries and the vertebral arteries communicate at the base of the brain through the *circle of Willis*, ensuring continued circulation should blood flow through one of the main vessels be disrupted. There

are extensive anastomotic channels in the brain. Under normal circumstances, the anastomotic channels in the circle of Willis are not patent. If blood flow is occluded, however, these connections become patent, and can maintain blood supply to the affected area. There are no significant anastomotic connections other than in these large cerebral vessels and the small capillary vessels. Occlusions of adjacent or terminal arteries from the large cerebral vessels may result in neural damage because the anastomotic connections may not be adequate to allow blood to reach the ischemic area in sufficient quantity and with sufficient rapidity to meet the high metabolic needs of the occluded area.

The brain is amazingly able to regulate its own blood supply. Cerebral blood flow is constant within a mean blood pressure range of 60 mm Hg to 140 mm Hg. In persons with hypertension the pressure may be as high as 180 mm Hg to 200 mm Hg, but the cerebral blood flow remains constant.

The remarkable vasodilation mechanism of the brain operates when a high carbon dioxide concen-

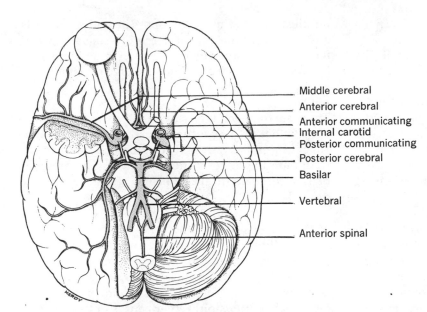

Middle cerebral
Anterior cerebral
Anterior communicating
Internal carotid
Posterior communicating
Posterior cerebral
Basilar
Vertebral
Anterior spinal

Figure 43–3.   The circle of Willis as seen at the base of a brain removed from the skull. (Chaffee EE, Lytle IM: Basic Physiology and Anatomy, 4th ed. Philadelphia, JB Lippincott, 1980)

tration, a high hydrogen ion concentration, or a low oxygen tension is present in the blood. High concentrations of hydrogen ion or carbon dioxide depress neural activity, and through vasodilation these substances are quickly removed. The brain utilizes oxygen at the rate of 3.5 ml of oxygen per 100 grams of brain tissue per minute.[1] If its blood flow should become insufficient, the vasodilation mechanism will immediately respond, bringing blood flow and oxygenation back to near-normal.

:Stroke

A cerebral vascular accident (CVA) is a sudden, severe episode of neurological symptoms caused by a deficit in blood supply to areas of the brain. It is manifested in any combination of the following symptoms: hemiplegia—paralysis of one side of the body; hemiparesis—weakness of muscle groups; aphasia—lack of sensory input; incontinence; perceptual deficits; and behavioral aberrations.

Stroke is one of the most common disorders of the cardiovascular system, ranking second only to heart attack. It was estimated that in 1978 172,500 Americans died of stroke and that another 750,000 persons experienced a CVA.[2] The incidence of first stroke increases with age from 0.25 per 1000 in the 35-to-44-year-old age group to 20 per 1000 in the 75-to-84-year-old age group and 40 per 1000 in those 85 years of age or older.[3] Stroke is more frequent in men than in women, and more frequent in black than in white persons.

As indicated above, stroke is more likely with advancing age. However, the exceptions to this generalization are embolic stroke and some types of hemorrhagic stroke, which are more frequent in younger persons. Stroke is also linked with atherosclerosis, obesity, cigarette smoking, physical inactivity, positive family history, elevated serum glucose, elevated serum lipids, increased blood volume or viscosity, anemia, and use of oral contraceptives.[3]

Prevention

Efforts to prevent stroke should be directed toward identifying and treating persons who have hypertension, transient ischemic attacks (TIAs), and cardiac disorders, all of which may be contributory to stroke.

Hypertension.   Hypertension, a major cause of hypertensive and other nonembolic forms of stroke, is a significant but treatable risk factor. In extreme hypertension, there may be hemorrhage into the meninges, or into the subdural, extradural, and subarachnoid spaces. In the present discussion, the term "hemorrhage" refers to intracerebral or intracranial bleeding into the brain substance, while the phrase "primary cerebral hemorrhage" excludes causes of hemorrhage other than hypertension (arteriovenous malformation, trauma, hemorrhagic tendency, tumor). The incidence of primary cerebral hemorrhage is as high as 25 per 100,000 of the population.[3]

Transient ischemic attacks (TIAs).   An early warning indication of impending stroke is TIAs. Many TIAs take the form of transient focal neurological deficits of vascular origin. Focal deficits are symptoms suggestive of the locus of the attack. Episodes of TIA may last for as little as a few minutes to as long as a day, and leave no residual damage. They are frequently called "angina of the brain." If the same set of symptoms occurs with each episode of TIA, the pathologic process probably involves one vessel. If the symptoms are variable, different vessels may be involved. Early diagnosis may permit surgical or medical intervention and thereby prevent extensive damage.

In contrast to a transient ischemic attack, a neurological deficit that continues to progress or worsen over a period of 1 or 2 days is called a *stroke-in-evolution*. It is a gradually evolving stroke occurring in a person with a history of TIAs, and is most likely due to thrombosis. A *completed stroke* may be described as follows: there has been maximum neurologic deficit due to thrombosis, to embolism, or (rarely) to hemorrhage; the patient's condition has stabilized or is improving; and there is residual neurologic damage. Recovery may take place over days, weeks, or months, and may be only partial.

Cardiac disorders. Various cardiac conditions predispose to formation of emboli. An embolus is a clot or other plug in a blood vessel. Most cerebral emboli have their origin in a thrombus in the left heart, from which they have broken away and been transported by the circulatory system to the cerebrum.

Stroke is associated with myocardial infarction, heart failure, and cardiac arrhythmias, all of which contribute to decreased cardiac output, in turn leading to cerebral embolism and ischemia. It can be expected that recent advances in the diagnosis and treatment of heart disease will favorably alter the incidence of embolic stroke.

Subclavian steal syndrome. Although relatively rare, accounting for only 4% of all cerebrovascular diseases and 17% of extracranial carotid disorders, subclavian steal should be considered when there is a complaint of dizziness and lightheadedness,[4] because, with the vascular surgery that is now available to redirect the blood flow, the prognosis for recovery is excellent.

When the subclavian artery is occluded near its origin, the blood flows from the vertebral artery (reverse or retrograde flow), draining from the basilar artery and the circle of Willis into the arm.[5] (The blood is "stolen" from the subclavian artery.) This subclavian steal syndrome is another cause of cerebral ischemia. Its symptoms include dizziness,

lightheadedness, and syncope; the radial pulse is absent or diminished; and there is usually a difference of 20 mm Hg or more in blood pressure between the affected and the unaffected arms.

Causes

There are three main processes affecting the cerebral vessels that may eventually lead to stroke: hemorrhage, embolism, and thrombosis. They vary in their rapidity of onset and prognosis. The presence of a concomitant disease will also affect the outcome of stroke.

The most frequently fatal stroke is rupture of the vessel wall—intracerebral *hemorrhage*. With rupture there is hemorrhage into the brain substance or subarachnoid space resulting in edema, compression of the brain contents, or spasms of the adjacent vessels. The most common predisposing factor is hypertension. Other causes of hemorrhage are aneurysm, trauma, erosion of vessels by tumors, vascular malformations, and blood dyscrasias. A cerebral hemorrhage occurs suddenly, usually when the person is active. The person may complain of a severe headache and stiff neck (nuchal rigidity) because blood has entered the cerebrospinal fluid (CSF). Focal symptoms depend on which vessel is involved. There is usually contralateral hemiplegia, with initial flaccidity progressing to spasticity. The hemorrhage and resultant edema exert great pressure on the brain substance, and the clinical course progresses rapidly to coma and frequently to death.

As has been described, an *embolus* is a clot that occludes a vessel. Although most cerebral emboli originate in a thrombus in the left heart, they may also originate in an atherosclerotic plaque in the carotid arteries. The embolus travels quickly to the brain and becomes lodged in a small artery through which it cannot pass. Therefore, this embolic stroke also has a sudden onset with immediate maximum deficit. The middle cerebral artery is the most frequent site of embolus formation. Cardiac arrhythmias are frequently noted and serve as a source of emboli. If there is a history of formation of numerous small emboli, the pattern of symptoms will vary depending on which vessels are involved. There may be more extensive tissue death due to emboli than occurs in the more slowly progressing thrombosis, because in the former there is no opportunity for collateral circulation to develop. Nevertheless, the damage is less than occurs in cerebral hemorrhage. If coma ensues, it will not be as deep as hemorrhagic coma, and recovery is more likely.

A *thrombotic* stroke has a much slower onset than embolic stroke, evolving over minutes or hours. The arterial lumen gradually becomes occluded due to atherosclerosis. Usually, thrombosis is seen in older people, and evidence of arteriosclerotic heart disease is frequently present, as is diabetes mellitus. The thrombotic stroke is not associated with activity, and may occur in a person at rest. Consciousness may or may not be lost, and improvement may be rapid.

Regardless of the cause, strokes disrupt the flow of oxygen, nutrients, and metabolic substances to the brain and the removal of waste products from the brain. With failure of cerebral blood flow there is not only cerebral anoxia, but also edema and congestion in the surrounding area, compressing the tissue and further impairing function. Consequently, as the edema subsides, in a few hours or several days, improvement may be noted. It is possible that the dysfunction may have been due in part to the edema and not to the stroke.

If there is generalized anoxia throughout the brain, symptoms of diffuse cerebral damage will be seen: drowsiness, disorientation, confusion, stupor, finally loss of consciousness. In most cases, the anoxia is localized, and specific neurological deficits related to the involved area of the brain are noted.

Localized effects by blood vessels. As stated earlier, arterial blood is supplied to the brain from the aortic arch by the two internal carotid arteries (anteriorly) and the two vertebral arteries (posteriorly). The carotid arteries are subject to development of atherosclerotic plaques at their site of origin from the aortic arch and at the bifurcations of the common carotid arteries and the proximal portions of the internal carotid arteries. The symptoms of stroke from this cause vary depending on the extent of collateral circulation that is present.

Anterior cerebral artery. The internal carotid divides into branches, of which the two largest are the anterior and middle cerebral arteries. The *anterior cerebral artery* supplies the medial portions of the frontal and parietal lobes, and the corpus callosum. Since the prefrontal area anterior to the motor strip in the frontal lobe is responsible for many thought processes, the characteristic signs of damage to this area are distractability and inability to plan in an orderly fashion. Confusion is the primary symptom when the frontal lobe is affected, as are other mental changes frequently classified as typical of dementia. The frontal lobe also contains the neurons that are concerned with motor function; therefore, contralateral paresis or paralysis, especially of the leg, may be seen. There also may be some sensory deficit due to parietal lobe involvement. Urinary incontinence often occurs.

Middle cerebral artery. The *middle cerebral artery* supplies most of the lateral surface of the cerebrum, and the deeper structures of the frontal, parietal, and temporal lobes, including the internal capsule and basal ganglia. Many major strokes involve the middle cerebral artery, so that a stroke having its origin at this site is likely to cause extensive damage. Among the symptoms that stem from middle cerebral artery stroke are (1) contralateral (motor and sensory loss) paralysis, especially of the arm (the leg area is supplied by the anterior cerebral artery); (2) homonymous hemianopia (contralateral blindness), if the stroke involves the optic nerve; (3) aphasia, if the stroke involves the dominant hemisphere; or (4) agnosia (lack of ability to recognize sensory stimuli), if the stroke involves the nondominant hemisphere.

Posterior cerebral artery. The *posterior cerebral artery* supplies the occipital lobe and the anterior and medial portions of the temporal lobe. If occlusion interrupts the blood supply to deeper structures, there may be mild contralateral hemiparesis (weakness on one side of the body), cerebellar ataxia (incoordination), and third nerve palsy. Visual disturbances of hemianopia, visual aphasia, or alexia (word blindness—an inability to recognize words as symbols of ideas) may occur. If both occipital lobes are involved, there may be cortical blindness (the cortical visual center cannot function).

The cerebellum and brain stem are supplied by branches of the basilar and vertebral arteries. The vertebral arteries may develop plaques at the sites of origin from the subclavian arteries and the first portion of the arteries before they enter the vertebral foramina. Ischemia owing to disruption of the *vertebral-basilar circulation* may produce a variety of symptoms. These include visual disturbances, such as diplopia due to involvement of the oculomotor, trochlear, and abducens nerves; ataxia due to cerebellar involvement; vertigo due to involvement of the vestibular nuclei; and dysphagia and dysphonia due to involvement of the glossopharyngeal and vagus nerves.

Diagnosis

Accurate diagnosis is based on a complete history, and a thorough physical and neurological examination. A careful history, including TIAs, their rapidity of onset and focal symptoms, as well as of any other diseases that may be present, will help to determine the type of stroke that is involved. Several test procedures are essential to diagnosis: Arteriography will demonstrate the site of the deficit, and afford visualization of most intracranial vascular areas. The brain scan and the electroencephalogram (EEG) also aid in localizing the area. And computerized axial tomography (CAT or CT scan) has become an important tool in diagnosing stroke and in differentiating cerebral hemorrhage and intracranial lesions that may mimic stroke.[6]

Treatment

The treatment of stroke itself is largely symptomatic. A main goal is to prevent complications and to treat any underlying disease. There is some controversy over whether or not effort should be made to lower blood pressure after a stroke. A chief consideration is to maintain oxygenation of brain tissue, and the possibility exists that a rapid fall in blood pressure could compromise oxygenation. There is also controversy over the use of anticoagulants as a means of preventing further occlusion. Anticoagulants represent "a two-edged sword" because they could precipitate hemorrhage. Surgical attempts at restoring blood supply to the brain focus on removing any clots from the carotid or vertebral arteries, or bypassing occluded vessels.

Recovery

When the patient regains consciousness (if consciousness was lost), characteristically there will be contralateral hemiplegia, with either a speech disturbance or a spatial-perceptual deficit, depending on which side of the brain was affected, and possibly incontinence. The specific focal deficits depend on which vessel is involved.

Motor recovery.   Initially following a stroke, there is total *flaccidity*, characterized by a decrease or absence of normal muscle tone. There is a tendency toward foot drop, outward rotation of the leg, and dependent edema in the affected extremities. Putting the extremities through passive range of motion helps to maintain the joint function, and to prevent edema, shoulder subluxation (incomplete dislocation), and muscle atrophy. The smooth, sequential movement of the exercises may help to re-establish motor patterns.

Early motor recovery is seen with the beginning of *spasticity*—the resistance of muscle groups to passive stretch, with an increase of muscle tone throughout the body. Spasticity follows the decrease in cerebral edema and the initial flaccidity, since there is now less inhibition of muscle tone from the basal ganglia. With spasticity, the flexor

muscles are usually stronger in the upper extremities, the extensor muscles, in the lower extremities.[7] Involuntary muscle contractions are manifested in shoulder adduction, forearm pronation, finger flexion, and knee and hip extension. If spasticity has not begun within 6 weeks (certainly within 3 months), function will probably not return to that extremity. Passive range of motion should be continued and positioning should be directed toward keeping all joints in functional position.

Aphasia.   Aphasia, a defect or loss of the power of expression by writing, speech, or signs, is estimated to be present in 40% of cases of stroke.[8] Confusion, anxiety, or memory loss may be present and, if not detected and treated, will seriously hinder rehabilitation.

Aphasia is a general term that encompasses varying degrees of inability to comprehend, integrate, and express speech. This generalization may lead to misinterpretation. Aphasia may be more accurately described as an acquired neurological disorder of *language* abilities due to damage in the CNS.[8] The term "language" implies a higher integrative function of perception, integration, and formulation of verbal stimuli, whereas a speech disorder is essentially a neuromuscular problem. For example, a person with dysarthia—an imperfect articulation of speech—still retains some language ability.

Just as there is confusion about the definition of aphasia, there is confusion about the terms of classification. There are two categories of asphasia: expressive–receptive and fluent–nonfluent, and both will be described next.

Motor, or *expressive*, aphasia is the loss of the ability to express thoughts and ideas in speech or writing. The person with expressive aphasia may be able to utter two or three words, usually words having an emotional overlay, with difficulty. Automatic speech and social phrases are usually easier to articulate. Although comprehension is usually intact, in speech some words may be omitted or inappropriate words used. *Jargon* aphasia is the utterance of nonexistent words, which the person is unable to recognize as such, and believes to be correct and appropriate.

Sensory, or *receptive*, aphasia is the inability to comprehend written or spoken words. Receptive aphasia is also called Wernicke's aphasia or auditory aphasia. Some persons manifest elements of both receptive and expressive aphasia, called *mixed* aphasia. When all language ability is lost—both receptive and expressive—the aphasia is said to be *global* or *total*. Most aphasias are partial, however, and a thorough speech evaluation is essential to a determination of the type and extent of aphasia and the therapy needed.

One of the most common characteristics of aphasia is the distorted spontaneous or conversational speech, which is usually classified as fluent (many) or nonfluent (few) words. Although the terms fluent and nonfluent have been in use for years, there has been a recent re-emphasis on them. *Fluency* refers to the characteristics of speech and not to content or ability to comprehend. Fluent output requires little or no effort, is articulate, and is of increased quantity. It is rambling, wordy, yet meaningless—what might be called empty speech. There are three categories of fluent aphasia: Wernicke's, anomic, and conduction aphasia.[8] *Wernicke's* aphasia is characterized by an inability to comprehend not only the speech, reading, and writing of other persons but also those of oneself. *Anomic* aphasia is speech that is nearly normal, but in which the person has difficulty selecting appropriate words. Inappropriate word use in the presence of good comprehension is called *conduction* aphasia.

Nonfluent aphasia presents opposite problems: poor articulation, poor modulation, dysarthria, and sparse output of words with considerable effort and limited to short phrases or single words. The words are substantive and have considerable meaning. Nonfluent aphasia may also be called *Broca's* aphasia. If the aphasia-producing lesion affects the anterior and posterior speech areas, a mixed or global aphasia may result, with problems of nonfluent aphasia and the comprehension difficulties of Wernicke's aphasia.

There is a correlation between the anatomical location of cerebral damage and the aphasia syndrome, which was recognized by Broca and Wernicke over a century ago. Although exceptions exist, most persons with nonfluent aphasia have lesions anterior to the Rolandic fissure, known as anterior Broca aphasia, and people with fluent aphasia have a lesion posterior to the fissure, known as posterior Wernicke's aphasia.[9]

Cause.   The most common cause of aphasia is vascular disease of the middle cerebral artery of the dominant cerebral hemisphere. In close to 90% of the population, the left hemisphere is dominant.

:Parkinson's Disease

As stated earlier, the motor system is composed of two antagonistic components, the excitatory pyramidal and the inhibitory extrapyramidal. These components form a single complex system, which is under cortical control but is modulated by the basal ganglia and the cerebellum. In addition, the basal ganglia along with the cerebellum are believed to control certain acquired motor skills that are usually performed without conscious awareness once they have been learned.

Disruption of the extrapyramidal system causes problems associated with inhibition of impulses, gross intentional movements, and body posture. In Parkinson's disease, the chief symptoms are characteristic of damage to the extrapyramidal tract: (1) increase in muscle tone and rigidity; (2) tremor, usually at rest; (3) akinesia (absence of spontaneous movement); and (4) postural difficulties due to an uncontrollable gait. The symptoms are progressive.

Clinical picture

The classical picture of a person with an advanced case of Parkinson's disease demonstrates the extrapyramidal nature of the symptoms. Tremor, rigidity, and akinesia are the three cardinal symptoms. Tremor is an early symptom and usually occurs at rest (resting tremor). The rhythmic alternating flexion and contraction of the muscles resembles pill rolling; in fact, it is often referred to as a pill-rolling tremor. The rigidity, a generalized hypertonicity of muscle, results in jerky, "cogwheel" motions in which considerable energy is needed to move muscle groups. Flexion contractions may result. In addition, there is less spontaneous movement (bradykinesia, slowed voluntary movement) and loss of unconscious associative movements. People with Parkinson's disease have difficulty initiating walking. When they walk, they take small, shuffling steps, lean forward, the head bent, without swinging their arms, and stop only with difficulty, as they move faster and faster (propulsion).

The characteristic facial appearance is stiff and masklike. The mouth may be open, with saliva drooling from the corners because the person cannot move the saliva to the back of the mouth and swallow it. The speech is slow, monotonous, without modulation, and poorly articulated. Autonomic symptoms of constipation, urinary incontinence, and lacrimation may be present. Although the person with Parkinson's disease may appear to be affected intellectually, there is no loss of intellectual function. There may be, however, occasional depression. There are several stages in the progression of Parkinson's disease. The symptoms usually are noted first on one side of the body and progress to bilateral involvement, with early postural changes in 1 to 2 years following onset. Postural changes and gait disturbances continue to become more pronounced until the person has significant disability and requires constant care.

Etiology

The etiology of Parkinson's disease is unknown but appears to be related to (1) small strokes known as lacunar infarcts (*arteriosclerotic* parkinsonism), (2) encephalitis (*postencephalitic* parkinsonism), (3) side effects of medications such as reserpine and the phenothiazines (*drug-induced* parkinsonism), (4) poisoning from magnesium, carbon monoxide, or mercury (*toxic* parkinsonism), and rarely (5) compression of the midbrain (*traumatic* parkinsonism). In the majority of cases, no cause can be found and the disease is classified as *idiopathic*. The level of the neurotransmitter dopamine is decreased in the substantia nigra and corpus striatum. Administration of L-dopa, a precursor of dopamine which, unlike dopamine, crosses the blood-brain barrier, has demonstrated significant improvement in clinical symptoms.

Treatment

Prior to the discovery of L-dopa, anticholinergics were the mainstay of treatment. Today, anticholinergics are used primarily in mild cases or when L-dopa is not tolerated. Although the exact mechanism is not known, research indicates that striated structures receive antagonistic cholinergic and dopamine inputs, and the balance between these two inputs determines motor control of the striatum.[10]

Since dopamine transmission is disrupted, it appears that there is a cholinergic preponderance, which is decreased with anticholinergic drugs, and this brings about improvement of the symptoms. The dopamine postsynaptic receptors are located on cholinergic cells.[11] They can inhibit the uptake and storage of dopamine, thus potentiating the postsynaptic efficacy of the neurotransmitter. This information also explains why cholinergics tend to exaggerate Parkinson's symptoms.

Trihexyphenidyl hydrochloride (Artane) is a widely used anticholinergic in Parkinson's disease. Other anticholinergics are procyclidine (Kemadrin) and benztropine mesylate (Cogentin). The anticholinergics lessen the tremors and rigidity and afford some functional improvement. Their potency seems to decrease over time, however, and increasing the dosage merely increases the side effects such as blurred vision, dry mouth, bowel and bladder problems, and some mental changes.

L-dopa. The evidence of decreased dopamine in the striatum in Parkinson's disease led to the administration of large doses of L-dopa (L-dihydroxyphenylalanine), which is able to be absorbed from the intestinal tract, crosses the blood-brain barrier, and is converted to dopamine by centrally acting dopa decarboxylase. The main problem with L-dopa, or the synthetic compound levodopa, is that the large dose that is needed to relieve symptoms has many side effects. Patients are started on very small doses of L-dopa, and the dose is gradually increased until therapeutic levels are reached. Nevertheless, side effects are seen in almost all of these patients. These may be relatively mild, such as nausea and vomiting; or there may be much more severe effects, ending in cardiac arrhythmia and death. Other adverse effects of L-dopa include depression, orthostatic hypotension, and involuntary movements of the tongue and lips. Most will disappear with reduction of the dose.

The large L-dopa dose is necessary because most of L-dopa is converted to dopamine (which does not cross the blood-brain barrier) by *peripheral* decarboxylase before it can cross the blood-brain barrier.[12] *Carbidopa*, a dopa-decarboxylase inhibitor, can be given to increase the amount of L-dopa entering the brain, and thus decrease the dose of L-dopa. With carbidopa, the patient does not have to eliminate vitamin B_6 from the diet. Vitamin B_6, a cofactor of dopa decarboxylase, has an adverse effect on L-dopa but not when administered with carbidopa.

:Spinal Cord Injury (SCI)

There are approximately 250,000 persons with spinal cord injury (SCI) in the United States.[13] In SCI, there is no sensory or motor function below the spinal cord level of the lesion, although there may be reflex activity. A *quadriplegic* has suffered an injury to the cervical (or upper thoracic) area of the spinal cord that involves all four extremities. There may be some function in the upper extremities, depending on the level of the lesion and the area innervated by that spinal cord level. The innervation can be determined by dermatome testing. Below the level of the lesion, there is no sensory input for heat, cold, or pain to warn of impending danger, nor is there any voluntary motor movement. There may be an increase in muscle tone in extensor spasms and hyperactive deep tendon reflexes. High lesions in the cervical or upper thoracic spinal cord usually cause some difficulty with sitting balance and respiratory function. Reflex emptying of bowel and bladder may be established. People who are paraplegic have sustained an injury to the lower thoracic, lumbar, or sacral portion of the spinal cord. The paralysis is in the lower extremities, usually involving the bowel and bladder but sparing respiratory function.

Etiology

Trauma to the spinal cord may be due to external or internal stressors. An external stressor is a knife, a bullet, or any other instrument that affords direct entry into the spinal cord from the outside. Internal stressors are much more common, and consist of damage to the vertebral column in which there has not been entry into the spinal canal, such as fracture, dislocation of the vertebral column, or such violent agitation that the cord suffers injury. Severe flexion–extension, such as is caused by a whiplash or a blow to the head, causes squeezing or shearing of the cord. Motor vehicle accidents are one of the major causes of SCI. Other causes are diving and skiing accidents. The greatest number of SCIs occur in young adult males.

A review of the spinal cord demonstrates that the spinal cord, like the brain, has extensive protective mechanisms—the bony protection of the vertebral column, the meninges, and the CSF. These mechanisms protect the structures responsible for innervation of the body, exclusive of the head. In addition to initiating the spinal reflex response, data originating in sensory endings are relayed to the brain stem and cerebellum, where they are utilized in various circuits, including those that influence motor performance. Sensory information is also relayed to the thalamus and cerebral cortex, where it becomes part of the conscious experience, with the possibility of immediate or delayed behavioral response. Motor neurons in the spinal cord are excited or inhibited by impulses originating at various levels of the brain from the medulla to the cerebral cortex. Vascular supply of the spinal cord comes mainly from the vertebral arteries. The anterior spinal artery from the vertebral arteries supplies the ventral and lateral portion of the spinal cord, including the anterior horns, lateral spinothalamic tracts, and pyramidal tracts. The posterior spinal artery supplies the posterior horns.

Disruption of the spinal cord. Damage to the spinal cord is frequently due to a sudden narrowing of the spinal canal in which the cord is "caught" between the lamina of a lower vertebra and the body of a higher one. Squeezing or shearing of the spinal cord causes destruction of gray matter and hemorrhage of varying degree. The anterior spinal artery and vertebral artery hemorrhage, causing ischemic necrosis, edema, and hematoma formation. The maximum effect is at the level of injury and one to two segments above and below the lesion.

The highest area of blood flow is in the gray matter. Within minutes of the SCI, hypoxia of the gray matter stimulates the release of catecholamines in large quantities. The mechanism of SCI is not well understood but is probably due to either direct vascular injury or norepinephrine-induced vasoconstriction. In severe SCI, the blood flow to the region may cease for long intervals. Researchers have used norepinephrine blocking agents such as reserpine, cooling, and steroids as measures to prevent additional ischemic damage with varying degrees of success. The duration of compression due to hematoma formation is extremely important in predicting the potential for improvement.

Although various terms are used to describe SCI, such as concussion, contusion, and compression, these terms are less useful than describing the effect of SCI. Injury to the spinal cord may result in complete, partial, or no permanent damage. The terms *severed* and *transected* spinal cord are often used, but rarely is the cord completely severed or transected. More appropriate terms are *complete SCI*, that is, loss of all motor and sensory function below the level of the lesion, and partial or *incomplete* SCI, in which some degree of motor and sensory function is retained. The following section discusses complete SCI.

Spinal shock and reflex recovery. Hematoma formation causes spinal shock, which lasts from 2 to 6 weeks, until the hematoma has dissolved. In spinal shock, there is a temporary decrease in neuronal excitability. Apparently, the motor neuron pools are dependent on excitation, usually supplied by the internuncial system, and when this is no longer present, the motor neurons are depressed.[14] This causes an acute disruption of the corticospinal pathway with paralysis of voluntary movement, and also temporarily abolishes spinal reflexes. This temporary loss of spinal reflexes is known as *spinal shock*. The resulting muscular flaccidity involves the loss of all motor, sensory, and reflex activity below the level of the lesion. Until spinal shock is resolved, the extent of damage cannot be totally determined. Several autonomic functions are also disrupted in spinal shock, resulting in retention of urine and feces, loss of vasomotor tone, and thermoregulatory sweating below the level of the lesion.

After a few weeks, flaccidity disappears and slowly gives rise to reflex activity initiated with a positive Babinski reflex. The reflex recovery follows a pattern: (1) return of the Babinski reflex, (2) minimal reflex activity, (3) flexor spasms, (4) alternate flexor–extensor spasms, and (5) after 6 months, dominant extensor spasms. The reflex spasms are due to the heightened sensitivity of the isolated segment of the cord, which has been released from control of the higher centers. These flexor and extensor spasms may be evoked by a variety of stimuli in the anesthetic area, occasionally even being stimulated by bedclothes or a draft of air. At the same time, bowel and bladder function improves and, in most lesions except those in the sacral area, automatic control of these functions can be developed.

After 1 year, the clinical picture of spinal cord injury demonstrates complete paralysis below the level of the lesion, and loss of motor and sensory function. In addition, the deep tendon reflexes are hyperactive, and bilateral positive Babinski reflexes are present. There is reflex sweating below the level of the lesion but this sweating is not under thermoregulatory control. In higher spinal cord injuries, there is bowel and bladder reflex emptying. With lower lesions, especially those affecting the sacral area, there may not be reflex bowel or bladder emptying.

Alterations in function

Cervical.   In the past, a person who experienced a high cervical lesion (C 1,2,3), did not survive the initial injury, but with the emergency transportation and treatment now available, this is no longer always the case. The main difficulty related to cervical lesions is that there is complete respiratory paralysis, and respiratory assistance is required. In lesions of C_3 to C_5, the phrenic nerve innervating the diaphragm is involved. Lesions between C_4 and T_{12} (thoracic) give rise to respiratory problems due to paralysis of the intercostal muscles, but respirations can be maintained without assistance. Colds and upper respiratory infections need to be vigorously avoided.

A lesion of C_4 results in a lack of voluntary movement in the trunk and the upper and lower extremities. But if C_4 is spared, the deltoids and the biceps are functional. A lesion at C_6 leaves the radial wrist extensors intact, and some flexion movements remain due to gravity. Triceps, finger flexors, and extensors are intact if the damage is at C_7. How much function will remain can be determined by assessing the area innervated by the spinal segment (dermatome).

Thoracic–lumbar.   Full innervation of upper extremity muscles and varying degrees of innervation of back, abdominal, and intercostal muscles are present with lesions at the thoracic level. In lower thoracic and upper lumbar lesions, full abdominal and upper back control is achieved. In lower lumbar lesions, hip flexors and quadriceps muscles are innervated.

Autonomic nervous system responses in SCI

Spinal cord injury interrupts autonomic nervous system function. Problems are particularly severe in quadriplegics because the preganglionic neurons of the sympathetic nervous system are located in the thoracic and lumbar areas of the spinal cord, and the communication between higher centers and these neurons is interrupted in high SCI. This leads to problems with temperature regulation, cardiovascular difficulties, bowel and bladder incontinence, and disturbances in sexual functioning. On the other hand, the preganglionic neurons of the parasympathetic nervous system are located either in the cranial nerves or in the sacral segment of the cord. In any SCI, the cranial portion of the parasympathetic nervous system remains under control of higher centers.

Thermoregulation.   Sweating below the level of the lesion is a cord reflex and does not contribute to thermoregulation. In high lesions, there is very little area for thermoregulation to take place, and excessive sweating is seen on the head and the neck. Excess body heat cannot be released effectively in hot weather, and a controlled environment is important to the patient's well-being.

Cardiovascular response.   In intact persons, customary changes in the internal environment do not cause changes in the blood pressure—it remains normal due to baroreceptor-mediated control by the autonomic nervous system. These mechanisms regulate heart rate, cardiac output, and adjustment of blood flow through peripheral and visceral vascular beds. In SCI, the baroreceptors become separated from the neural effector mechanism, so that blood pressure regulation and regional circulation become abnormal. For example, if a person with SCI is positioned so that the head is higher than the body, *postural hypotension* will result. There is a failure of compensatory mechanisms and effective vasoconstriction does not occur; there is peripheral pooling of blood, decreased venous return, and a lower cardiac output.

If lightheadedness or dizziness occurs, the person should be placed in a horizontal position. Ultimately, adaptation takes place and postural hypotension becomes less of a problem. A tilt table and support stockings can help prevent postural hypotension until adaptation is complete.

The adaptation mechanism is not fully understood. However, improvement in adaptation is thought to be related to (1) development of reflexes arising in the isolated spinal cord, (2) increased levels of urinary excretion of norepinephrine, (3) increased sensitivity of vascular beds to circulatory catecholamines, (4) increased blood volume, and (5) changes in baroreceptors and arterial PO_2 and PCO_2, which may stimulate reflex vasomotor constriction at the cord level.

Cardioacceleration normally is a result of both a reduction in vagal tone and an activation of sympathetic cardioacceleration stimulation. In the absence of sympathetic stimulation, the heart rate responds only to vagal reduction. There is also inadequate vasoconstrictor tone and cardiac output falls because of inadequate venous return.

Autonomic dysreflexia (hyperreflexia).   The parasympathetic section of the autonomic nervous system arises from the craniosacral area of the spinal cord, while the sympathetic nervous system arises from the thoracolumbar region of the spinal cord. In a spinal cord lesion above the level of sympathetic outflow—thoracic 6—stimulation of sensory receptors from a distended bladder or bowel sends impulses to the lower spinal cord. These impulses ascend the cord to the level of the lesion, where they are blocked. The autonomic reflexes, however, are intact, and a reflex arteriolar spasm takes place in the skin and viscera.

The increased sympathetic response causes the blood pressure to rise, and profuse sweating (nonthermoregulatory) occurs below the level of the lesion. The hypertension is recognized by the baroreceptors in the carotid sinus, aortic arch, and cerebral vessels. These receptors stimulate cranial nerve IX, the glossopharyngeal nerve, and cranial nerve X, the vagus nerve, to transmit afferent impulses to the vasomotor center of the medulla.[15] Normally, efferent impulses from the vagus would be relayed to the sinoatrial node of the heart in order to slow the cardiac rate, and other fibers would stimulate the splanchnic nerves to dilate the peripheral and visceral vasculature, and so lower the blood pressure. In the person with a spinal cord lesion, impulses along the tenth cranial nerve cause bradycardia, but impulses to the sympathetic motor preganglionic neurons in the thoracic and lumbar segments cannot go beyond the SCI. Therefore, compensatory vasodilation cannot occur below the level of the lesion and severe hypertension persists even though there is vasodilation above the level of the lesion. Vasodilation above the level of the lesion causes the skin of the neck and face to be hot and reddened, while at the level of the lesion it is pallid.

Sexuality.   The desire for sexual activity remains unchanged, although the hormonal level may be altered somewhat initially. Women may not menstruate for up to 7 months following injury; then they will revert to their normal pattern. Pregnant women with high lesions (quadriplegia) may not be aware that they are ready to deliver, and the pregnancy may stimulate an automatic reaction of dysreflexia. In the man, sexual function depends somewhat on the level of the lesion. A person with a high lesion will probably have reflexogenic erections. In lower lesions, especially those of sacral segments 2 through 4, reflex activity is absent. When reflex activity and erection are present, there is loss of coordination between erection and ejaculation, and semen may be forced back into the bladder retrogradely. Many men with SCI are sterile because of the lower temperature in the testicles.

Bowel and bladder function.   Renal disease is an important cause of death in SCI, and care must be taken to prevent infections in these patients. As with general muscle tone, the muscles of the bladder are flaccid immediately following the SCI. Overdistention of the bladder with resulting infection is a too-common problem. Following recovery from spinal shock, reflex bladder emptying may occur if the injury is not in sacral segments 2 to 4. Reflex bladder emptying is an automatic spinal cord reflex triggered by stimulation of the lower abdomen, inner aspects of the thighs, or the genitalia.

Bowel function responds much the same way as bladder function with initial flaccidity and sometimes reflex emptying after recovery from spinal shock. Extensive bowel-training programs promote utilization of reflex activity for bowel evacuation.

In summary, stroke, Parkinson's disease, and spinal cord injuries have been presented as examples of alterations in motor function. Each has different manifestations of motor damage, depending on whether the injury affects the pyramidal system, the extrapyramidal system, or the spinal cord.

:Study Guide

After you have studied this chapter, you should be able to meet the following objectives:

: : Describe the function of the pyramidal tract vs. the extrapyramidal tract.

: : Describe the effects of lower motor neuron injury.

:: Describe cerebellar control of motor activity and muscle movement.

:: Describe the effects of damage to the basal ganglial portion of the extrapyramidal tract.

:: Describe the disruptions that may occur when the cerebellar portion of the extrapyramidal tract is injured.

:: Describe the collateral circulation to the brain.

:: List the clinical manifestations of a CVA.

:: Characterize TIAs.

:: Compare embolus and thrombosis.

:: Describe the effects of a stroke involving the anterior, middle, and posterior cerebral arteries, respectively.

:: Compare the manifestations of motor aphasia with those of sensory aphasia.

:: Explain the symptoms of Parkinson's disease with reference to the extrapyramidal system.

:: Explain the rationale underlying the use of L-dopa in Parkinson's disease.

:: Describe the events that culminate in spinal shock.

:: Describe the effects of SCI on the cardiovascular system.

:: Explain the occurrence of hypertension following SCI.

:References

1. Guyton AC: Textbook of Medical Physiology, ed 6, p 347. Philadelphia, WB Saunders, 1981
2. Heart Facts. American Heart Association, Dallas, 1981
3. Sahs AL, Hartman EC, Aronson SM: Cause, Prevention, Treatment and Rehabilitation. London, Castle House Publications Ltd., 1980
4. DeLaria GA, Javid H: Evaluating subclavian steal syndrome. Consultant 20, No. 2:88–98, 1980
5. Burch GE, DePasquale NP: Axioms on cerebrovascular disease. Hospital Medicine 11, No. 6:8–22, 1975
6. Campbell JK: Use of computerized tomography and radionuclide scan in stroke. Current concepts of cerebrovascular disease. Stroke 12, No. 3:11–16, 1977
7. Bobath B: Adult Hemiplegia: Evaluation and Treatment, ed 2. London, William Heinemann Medical Books, 1978
8. Palmer EP: Language dysfunction in cerebrovascular disease. Primary Care 6, No. 4:827–842, 1979
9. Holland AL: Treatment for aphasia following stroke. Current concepts of cerebrovascular disease. Stroke 14, No. 2:5–8, 1979
10. Cotzias GG, Papavasilious PS, Genos SZ, Tolosa ES: Treatment of Parkinson's disease and allied conditions. In Tower DB (ed): The Nervous System. Volume 2. The Clinical Neurosciences. New York, Raven Press, 1975
11. Crawford I: Neurotransmitters: Relevance to neurologic disease and therapy. In Rosenberg RN (ed): The Treatment of Neurological Diseases. New York, S P Medical & Scientific Books, 1979
12. Stewart RM: Treatment of movement disorders. In Rosenberg RN (ed): The Treatment of Neurological Diseases. New York, S P Medical & Scientific Books, 1979
13. Report of the Panel on Stroke, Trauma, Regeneration, and Neoplasms to the National Advisory Neurological and Communicative Disorders and Stroke Council. U.S. Department of Health, Education, and Welfare, PHS, NIH Publication No. 79-1915, 1979, p 125
14. Newman PP: Neurophysiology. New York, S P Medical & Scientific Books, 1979
15. Feustel D: Autonomic hyperreflexia. Am J Nurs 76, No. 2:228–239, 1976

:Suggested Readings

Booth K: Subclavian steal syndrome: Treatment with proximal vertebral to common carotid artery transposition. J Neurosurg Nurs 12, No. 1:28–31, 1980

Cormarr AE: Sex among patients with spinal cord and/or cauda equina injuries. Medical Aspects of Human Sexuality 7, No. 3:222–238, 1973

Cormarr AE, Gunderson BB: Sexual function in traumatic paraplegia and quadriplegia. Am J Nurs 75, No. 2:250–256, 1975

Doolittle N: Arteriovenous malformations: The physiology, symptomatology, and nursing care. J Neurosurg Nurs 11, No. 4:221–226, 1979

Fischbach FT: Easing adjustment to Parkinson's disease. Am J Nurs 78, No. 1:66–69, 1978

Ginsberg MD, Reivich M: Cerebrovascular pathophysiology. In Tower DB (ed): The Nervous System. Volume 2. The Clinical Neurosciences. New York, Raven Press, 1975

Hirsch LF: Modern treatment of intracranial aneurysms. Postgrad Med 67, No. 3:153–160, 1980

Johnson M, Quinn J: The subarachnoid screw. Am J Nurs 77, No. 3:448–450, 1977

Jones HR: Disease of the vertebral system. Primary Care 6, No. 4:733–743, 1979

Kestler JP: Cardiac embolic cerebrovascular disease. Primary Care 6, No. 4:745–755, 1979

Larrabee JH: Physical care during early recovery. Am J Nurs 7, No. 8:1320–1329, 1977

Mesulam MM: Acute behavioral derangements without hemiplegia in cerebrovascular disease. Primary Care 6, No. 4:813–826, 1979

Norman S: Diagnostic categories for the patient with a right hemisphere lesion. Am J Nurs 79, No. 12:2126–2130, 1979

Norman S, Baratz R: Understanding aphasia. Am J Nurs 79, No. 12:2135–2138, 1979

Pacheco PM: Cerebral artery vasospasm and current trends of treatment. J Neurosurg Nurs 11, No. 3:171–172, 1979

Polhopek M: Stroke: An update on vascular disease. J Neurosurg Nurs 12, No. 2:81–87, 1980

Sahs AL: Medical management of vascular diseases of the brain. In Tower DB (ed): The Nervous System. Volume 2. The Clinical Neurosciences. New York, Raven Press, 1975

Smith J, Bullough B: Sexuality and the severely disabled person. Am J Nurs 75, No. 12:2194–2198, 1975

Wallhagen MI: The split brain: Implications for care and rehabilitation. Am J Nurs 79, No. 12:2118–2125, 1979

Webb PH: Neurological deficit after carotid endarterectomy. Am J Nurs 79, No. 4:654–658, 1979

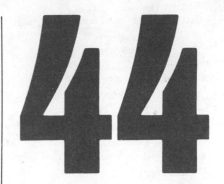

Janet Krejci

Chronic Organic Brain Syndrome

The term *chronic organic brain syndrome* (COBS) is usually used to denote any organomental deterioration. Any pathological process that affects the cerebral hemisphere can cause impairment of intellect, which is often referred to as dementia.

Based on community surveys, it is estimated that in the United States, 5% of persons above age 65—about 1 million people—have organic brain syndrome. These surveys also indicate that another 2 million persons (10% of that population group) have a mild form of COBS.[1] It is the most frequent diagnosis among elderly persons in state and county hospitals. COBS is believed to be the cause, whether direct or indirect, of between 90,000 and 97,000 deaths annually.[1] It has been suggested that life expectancy is considerably shortened by the presence of COBS.[2]

A widely held myth about COBS is that it is an inevitable accompaniment of aging. But the truth is that old age is not always accompanied by COBS; nor is COBS exclusively a disorder of the aged. As Comfort has stated: "Old people do not in fact become demented through any common or universal changes coupled to chronological age in the same way that loss of hair pigment is coupled."[3]

In other words, senility should not be equated with aging nor should the changes observed in COBS be considered normal. This is important, because behavior is often influenced by the manner in which an individual is treated. Once a person is diagnosed as having COBS, assumptions about the diagnosis are often communicated in subtle ways, and the person may, in turn, respond accordingly. This means that a person who *does not* have COBS may, if treated like one who *does* have COBS, develop certain behaviors that are consistent with it.

:Characteristics of COBS

The definitions of COBS vary: one dictionary describes it as "a deteriorated mentality," one writer as "any disorder caused by or associated with impairment of brain tissue."[4] Although general, this latter definition is workable, as it distinguishes COBS from functional disorders and stipulates that brain tissue is involved.

COBS is not a specific neurological diagnosis; rather, it can result from many neuropathological processes. Because it is usually slow to evolve, the earliest symptoms can pass almost unrecognized. There may be lapses in problem-solving ability or in the ability to grasp the meaning of a situation, or inflexibility in thought processes may be evident.

The person may carry out routine tasks adequately, but find it difficult to function well in intricate and demanding situations.

The constellation of symptoms associated with COBS is easily remembered by the acronym JAMCO: judgment, affect, memory, confusion, orientation. The syndrome is characterized by impairment of judgment and memory, a flat affect, confusion, and loss of orientation.

The *catastrophic reaction* is a phenomenon commonly seen in COBS. It is an adaptational response made by the person when faced with a task that seems overwhelming, possibly representing an unconscious attempt to defend the self against declining intellectual abilities.[5] On the basis of earlier experiences, the person may react by withdrawing from the situation or by becoming extremely agitated. Unfortunately, such a person may be offered little else but sedation through tranquilizers. The *sundown syndrome* is another behavioral manifestation of COBS, characterized by nocturnal awakening, confusion, agitation, and sometimes psychotic symptoms.[6]

Various primitive *reflexes*, such as the sucking and rooting reflexes, may return.[7]

Differentiation between chronic and acute brain syndromes and functional disorders

Certain conditions may mimic a COBS state, among which are two that merit discussion: acute or reversible brain syndrome, and functional disorders.

Acute brain syndrome. Acute brain syndrome may arise from disorders that cause *reduced cerebral blood flow*, interference with *glucose utilization*, *metabolic imbalances*, or other events that temporarily impede brain function. Among these are toxicity and primary disease states, such as diabetes, congestive heart failure, chronic obstructive lung disease, certain forms of cancer, kidney failure, and malnutrition. Needless to say, many of these conditions can be reversed if accurate diagnosis is made and the condition is properly treated and reversed; in fact, it is believed that 10% to 20% or more of those diagnosed as having COBS actually have treatable disorders.

There are useful guidelines for assessing acute states and differentiating them from COBS. In an acute process, the onset is likely to be abrupt, and one is more likely to see a fluctuating state of awareness, visual rather than auditory hallucinations, misidentification of significant others, and restlessness.[8] A person who already has COBS may also experience an acute process.

Functional disorders: depression as an example. Depression, a frequent problem among aging persons, can mimic COBS, and severe depression may eventuate in suicide.[9] *Pseudodementia* is the term that describes a depression that closely resembles a COBS state, manifesting symptoms of confusion, disorientation, and forgetfulness. Often there has been a recent memory deficit for both past and recent events, along with poor judgment. In response to questions, the person often replies merely, "I don't know." The symptoms are of shorter duration, and negativism is common.[4] The features of depression and COBS are summarized in Table 44-1.

Depression, unlike COBS, does have a specific treatment. Depression can accompany COBS and when treated can improve the patient's general condition even though the COBS remains.

Causes of COBS

COBS has several possible causes. Among them are multi-infarct dementia, Alzheimer's disease, Creutzfeldt–Jakob disease, Pick's disease, normal pressure hydrocephalus, and Wernicke–Korsakoff's syndrome. Each of these entities is briefly discussed in the section that follows.

Other processes that may give rise to dementia, such as neoplasms, infections, Huntington's chorea, and cerebral abscess, are not discussed here because of limitations of space.

Multi-infarct dementia. Dementia associated with vascular disease does not directly result from arteriosclerosis, but rather from infarction due to multiple emboli which disseminate throughout the brain[10]— hence the appellation multi-infarct dementia (MID). Although hypertension is often a precipitating factor, there is some concern about treating affected persons with antihypertensive medications for fear that too sharp a fall in blood pressure may further compromise cerebral perfusion.

Contrary to a widely held belief, MID is not the most common type of dementia. It is probably seen in only some 10% to 20% of all dementias.[10] The average age of onset for MID is 65, and men are affected more often than women. The duration of the disease is variable, but within about 4 years most patients die from a cerebral vascular accident or a superimposed infection, such as pneumonia. These persons may attempt suicide at some point during the course of the illness, because they frequently are acutely aware of their situation.

Memory impairment is often the first symptom of MID, followed by impairment in judgment. Some clinicians are of the opinion that more than half of these persons have an episode of delirium, possibly accompanied by hallucinations, as the first indication.[4] Catastrophic reaction and nocturnal confusion are common, also.[5]

Hachinski's Ischemia Scale is useful for differentiating MID from other dementias. On this scale, a point value is assigned to each of various disease manifestations—character of onset, history of stroke, focal neurologic symptoms, depression, history of hypertension, and others—and a high total point value is indicative of MID.[11]

Alzheimer's disease. Alzheimer's disease is by far the most frequent and best known of this group. It was first described in 1907 and is characterized by a gradual atrophy of the brain.

At present there is controversy over differentiating between what is sometimes called presenile dementia of Alzheimer's disease and the so-called senile dementia of Alzheimer's type. Most authorities agree that the two disorders are probably one and the same disease, comprising 65% of all dementias. The main difference between them is that of age. Alzheimer's disease occurs at an average age of 55, whereas senile dementia occurs at an average age of 75.

The cause of Alzheimer's disease is unknown. It affects women more often than men. Its onset is usually characterized by impairment of memory. There is a lack of insight. Usually, cognitive impairment follows within several years, and hyperexcitability, aphasia, apraxia, and agnosia may be associated findings. Gait disorders are prominent. The prognosis is extremely poor; the disease progresses relentlessly for some 5 to 10 years, ending in death.

Creutzfeldt–Jakob disease. Creutzfeldt–Jakob disease is an organic brain disease currently believed to be caused by a transmissible agent, possibly a virus. It is marked by degeneration of the pyramidal and extrapyramidal systems.

Creutzfeldt–Jakob disease is most readily distinguished by its rapid course, as the affected persons are usually severely demented within 6 months of onset. The disease is uniformly fatal, with death usually occurring within 7 months.[12] The early symptoms consist of abnormalities in personality and visual/spatial coordination. Extreme dementia and myoclonus follow as the disease advances.

Pick's disease. Pick's disease is a rare form of COBS. There is atrophy of the frontal, temporal, and parietal lobes of the brain. The neurons in the affected

Table 44-1 Diagnostic Features of Depression and Chronic Organic Brain Syndrome

Syndrome	Age at Onset	Mode of Onset	Contributing Factors	Brain Pathology	Characteristics	Course	Prognosis and Outcome
Depression	Any age; elderly are at special risk	Gradual or sudden; usually onset can be dated	Often a previous history of depression or significant losses	None	Transient memory problems with remote and present memory equally impaired Flat affect Low self-esteem Slowed psychomotor response Many "don't know" responses Occasional auditory hallucinations	Self-limiting with tendency to recur; rapid progression of symptoms	Dependent on response to treatment; usually recovery, sometimes suicide, especially in elderly males
Multi-infarct dementia	Range, 55 to 70 years; average 65 years	Gradual or acute; insidious with fluctuating states of awareness	Some familial tendency; life style consistent with atherosclerotic risk factors	Diffuse and/or focal changes due to atherosclerosis; thrombi may be present	Mental symptoms associated with hemiparesis Pathologic reflexes Pseudobulbar palsy and signs of cerebellar dysfunction	Downward course with intermittent and fluctuating progression of symptoms	Usually poor, but may be variable; death due to cerebral vascular accident, heart disease, or infection such as pneumonia
Alzheimer's disease	Range, 40 to 60 years; average 55 years	More abrupt than senile dementia	Multiple genetically determined factors	Cortical atrophy and loss of neurons	Memory loss Disorientation Agitation Language disturbance Lack of insight Deterioration of social behavior and personal habits	Rapidly progressive	Very poor; death usually due to infection or failure of other body systems
Senile dementia (of Alzheimer type)	Over 70 years; average, 75 years	Insidious	Same as Alzheimer's disease	Cortical atrophy and loss of neurons	Memory loss Disorientation Agitation Language disturbance Lack of insight Deterioration of social behavior and personal habits	Slow or rapid	Same as Alzheimer's disease

Disease	Age	Onset	Etiology	Pathology	Clinical features	Course	Prognosis
Creutzfeldt-Jakob disease	Middle years, earlier than Pick's; range, 20 to 68 years; average, 50 years	Rapid	Thought to be of slow virus etiology; mode of transmission unknown	Presence of status spongiosus (widespread vacuoles) in cerebral cortex and sometimes in basal ganglia	Cerebellar ataxia; Weakness of legs and complaints of neurasthenia and muscle wasting; Myoclonic fasciculations; Somnolence; Abnormalities in visual/spatial coordination	Rapidly progressive; complete dementia in 6 months	Very poor; death due to infection or cardiac or respiratory failure
Alcoholic encephalopathy, Wernicke-Korsakoff syndrome	40 to 80 years	Gradual	Alcoholic history	Wernicke's syndrome: lesions most pronounced in mammillary bodies, consist of small hemorrhages, congestion with brownish-gray discoloration; Korsakoff's syndrome: involves medial nucleus and sometimes posterior nucleus of thalamus	Confabulation; Loss of memory; Paresthesia, ataxia, weakness; Deterioration of psychomotor skills	Progressive	Poor unless abstinence from alcohol ingestion; administration of thiamin may arrest symptoms of Wernicke's syndrome
Pick's disease	As early as age 21; range, 40 to 60 years; average, 54 years	Slow and insidious	Familial incidence; hereditary mode of transmission of dominant type	Cortical atrophy of frontal and temporal lobes; presence of Pick bodies (round cytoplasmic inclusions) in nerve cells of affected brain areas	Speech disturbance, utterance of incomprehensible jargon; Lack of anxiety; Loss of initiative; Flat affect; Hypotonia; Incontinence	Progressive, more rapid than Alzheimer's disease	Very poor; death usually due to infection or general failure of body systems
Normal pressure hydrocephalus	Variable depending on primary etiology	Gradual	Idiopathic, or history of head trauma	Dilated ventricles	Amnesia and confusion; Mutism; Withdrawal; Gait disturbance; Urinary incontinence	Progressive	Poor in absence of intervention

areas contain cytoplasmic inclusions called *Pick bodies*.

The average age at onset of Pick's disease is 54 years. It is more common in women than in men. Behavioral manifestations may be noted earlier than memory deficits, taking the form of a striking absence of concern and care, a loss of initiative, echolalia (automatic repetition of anything said to the person), hypotonia, and incontinence.[13] The course of the disease is relentless, with death ensuing within 2 to 10 years. The immediate cause of death generally is infection.

Normal pressure hydrocephalus.

Normal pressure hydrocephalus (NPH) is in some cases reversible, or at least treatable. It is due to an obstruction of cerebral spinal fluid, with resulting dilatation of the ventricles. It can occur at any age, after head trauma, meningitis, or subarachnoid hemorrhage.

Gait disturbance is the cardinal sign of NPH, followed by incontinence of bowel and bladder. Severe dementia occurs in late stages. The person has a flat affect and tends to be withdrawn. Treatment of choice is the surgical creation of a shunt that routes the cerebrospinal fluid around the obstructed area and back into the circulation. The improved cerebral blood flow may bring some relief of symptoms.

Wernicke–Korsakoff's syndrome.

Wernicke–Korsakoff's syndrome is due to chronic alcoholism. Wernicke's disease is characterized by weakness or paralysis of the extraocular muscles, nystagmus, ataxia, and confusion. There may be signs of peripheral neuropathy. The person has an unsteady gait and complains of diplopia. There may be signs attributable to alcohol withdrawal—delirium, confusion, hallucinations, and so on. It is generally agreed that this disorder is caused by a deficiency in thiamin (vitamin B$_1$), and many of the symptoms are rapidly reversed when nutrition has been improved by supplemental thiamin.

In the Korsakoff component of the syndrome, there is severe impairment of recent memory. There is often difficulty in dealing with abstractions, and the person's capacity to learn is defective. Confabulation is probably the most distinguishing feature of the disease. Polyneuritis is also common. Unlike Wernicke's disease, Korsakoff's psychosis does not improve significantly with thiamin therapy. Features of Wernicke's disease and Korsakoff's syndrome may be found in one person.

Diagnosis and treatment

A detailed history given by both the affected person and the family members should be obtained in all cases of COBS—history of all drugs used and abused, recent significant losses of any kind, history of head trauma, premorbid personality, familial history of COBS, and history of psychiatric disorders, especially depression. A psychological assessment should be made also.

A "drug holiday"—a period during which any drugs being taken at the time treatment is started are temporarily discontinued—is suggested as a means of assessing the role of drugs in the patient's condition. It is estimated that 80% of demented elderly persons are receiving unnecessary tranquilizers, which may contribute to their bizarre behavior.[14] As drug absorption, distribution, metabolism, and excretion are all altered in the elderly, any drugs administered must be monitored very closely.

Reminiscence therapy is most useful with this population and worthy of mention. Many individuals afflicted with COBS are as a consequence of their illness near death. It has been said that Erikson's last stage, integrity versus despair, is the stage when one looks back and questions the meaningfulness of one's life.[15] Reminiscing allows one to do this. Even if this leads to the reliving of traumatic events, it is a necessary and natural phenomenon, and may lead to resolution of conflict.[8] This therapy is especially useful with COBS, for although memory is often impaired, remote memory is often retained the longest, so patients may participate in this activity with some satisfaction. Failing self-image can also be improved as patients can relive their productive, gratifying years with a caring listener. Reminiscing can be as simple as sharing old photographs on a one-to-one basis, or it can be more complex, such as a planned series of interactions that progress in subject matter from childhood to adulthood.

Family counseling is an important part of dealing with the situation, especially since family life may be totally disrupted by the patient and the problems. Obviously, if the COBS has a viral etiology, or if there is a familial history of COBS, the counseling would need to be directed accordingly. Psychosocial therapies should not be overlooked.

In summary, chronic organic brain syndrome is a significant health problem, particularly among the elderly. It is estimated that 80% of elderly persons at first admissions to psychiatric units are given a diagnosis of COBS and that it is the most frequent diagnosis among the elderly in state and county hospitals.

There are a number of antecedent conditions that may give rise to COBS, among which are multi-infarct dementia, Alzheimer's disease, Creutzfeldt–Jakob disease, Pick's disease, and Wernicke–Korsakoff's syndrome. Distinction should be made between chronic organic brain syndrome and both acute brain syndrome and functional disorders, of which depression is a representative example.

:Study Guide

After you have studied this chapter, you should be able to meet the following objectives:

: : Explain the special significance of diagnosis in COBS.

: : Explain how COBS can be differentiated from depression.

: : Explain the designation MID for dementia associated with vascular disease.

: : List the progressive stages in Alzheimer's disease.

: : Describe the symptoms of the Wernicke-Korsakoff syndrome.

:References

1. Report of the Panel on Inflammatory, Demyelinating and Degenerative Diseases to the National Advisory Neurological and Communicative Disorders and Stroke Council, p 61. U.S. Department of Health, Education, and Welfare, June 1, 1979. NIH Publication No. 79–1916

2. Karasu TB, Katzman R: Organic brain syndromes. In Bellak L, Katzman T (eds): Geriatric Psychiatry, p 129. New York, Grune & Stratton, 1976

3. Comfort A: The Practice of Geriatric Psychiatry, p 10. New York, Elsevier, 1980

4. Busse EW: Mental disorders in later life. In Busse EW, Pfeiffer E (eds): Mental Illness in Later Life, pp 91, 98. American Psychological Association, 1973

5. Slaby AE, Wyatt RJ: Dementia in the Presenium, pp 8, 160. Springfield, Charles C Thomas, 1974

6. Raskind M: Nocturnal Delirium, pp 4–5. New York, Biomedical Information Corp., 1979

7. Charatan FB: Chronic Organic Brain Syndrome, p 4. New York, Roering, 1979

8. Butler R, Lewis M: Aging and Mental Health, ed 2, pp 79, 269. St. Louis, CV Mosby, 1977

9. Burnside IM: Nursing and the Aged, p 173. New York, McGraw-Hill, 1976

10. Hachinski V et al: Multi-infarct dementia, Lancet 2:207–209, 1974

11. Hachinski V: Cerebral blood flow: Differentiation of Alzheimer's disease from multi-infarct dementia. In Katzman R et al (eds): Alzheimer's Disease: Senile Dementia and Related Disorders, pp 98–99. New York, Raven Press, 1978

12. Robbins SL, Cotran RS: Pathologic Basis of Disease, p 1549. Philadelphia, WB Saunders, 1979

13. Verwoerdt A: Clinical geropsychiatry, p 47–52. Baltimore, Williams & Wilkins, 1976

14. Poe W, Holloway D: Drugs and the Aged, p 83. New York, McGraw–Hill, 1980

15. Kimmel DC: Adulthood and Aging, p 406. New York, John C Wiley, 1974

:Suggested Readings

Barns EK et al: Guidelines to treatment approaches. The Gerontologist 13, No. 4:513–527, 1973

Bartol MA: Dialogue with dementia. Journal of Gerontological Nursing 5, No. 4:21–31, 1979

Bozian MW, Clark HM: Counteracting sensory changes in aging. Am J Nurs 80:473–476, 1980

Burnside IM: Alzheimer's disease: An overview. J Gerontol Nurs 5, No. 4:14–20, 1979

Butler RN: The role of NIA. In Katzman R et al (eds): Alzheimer's Disease: Senile Dementia and Related Disorders. Volume 7, Aging. New York, Raven Press, 1978

Butler RN, Lewis MI: Aging and Mental Health. St. Louis, C. V. Mosby, 1977

Charatan FB: Chronic Organic Brain Syndrome. New York, Roering, 1979

Comfort A: Practice of Geriatric Psychiatry. New York, Elsevier, 1980

Goldfarb AI et al: Hyperbaric oxygen treatment of organic mental syndromes in aged persons. J Gerontol 27, No. 2:212–217, 1972

Hachinski V: Multi-infarct dementia. Lancet 2:207–209, 1974

Hachinski V: Cerebral blood flow: Differentiation of Alzheimer's disease from multi-infarct dementia. In Katzman R et al (eds): Alzheimer's Disease: Senile Dementia and Related Disorders. Volume 7, Aging. New York, Raven Press, 1978

Harris R: The relationship between organic brain disease and physical status. In Gaitz C (ed): Aging and The Brain. London, Plenum Press, 1972

Hayter J: Patients with Alzheimer's disease. Am J Nurs 74:1460–1463, 1974

Karasu TB, Katzman R: Organic brain syndromes. In Bellak L, Karasu TB (eds): Geriatric Psychiatry. Baltimore, Williams & Wilkins, 1976

Kay DWK: Epidemiological aspects of organic brain disease. In Gaitz C (ed): Aging and The Brain. London, Plenum Press, 1972

Libow LS: Excess mortality and proximate causes of death. In Katzman R et al (eds): Alzheimer's Disease: Senile Dementia And Related Disorders. Volume 7, Aging. New York, Raven Press, 1978

McMordie WR, Blom S: Life review therapy: Psychotherapy for the elderly. Perspect Psychiatr Care 17, No. 4:162–164, 1979

Peck A et al: Mortality of the aged with chronic brain syndrome II. In Katzman R et al (eds): Alzheimer's Disease: Senile Dementia and Related Disorders. New York, Raven Press, 1978

Poe W, Halloway BS: Drugs and the Aged. New York, McGraw–Hill, 1980

Raskind MA: Nocturnal Delirium. New York, Biochemical Information Corp., 1979

Raskind MA, Storrie MC: The organic mental disorders. In Busse EW, Blazer DG (eds): Handbook of Geriatric Psychiatry. New York, Van Nostrand, 1980

Roth M: Epidemiological Studies. In Katzman R et al (eds): Alzheimer's Disease: Senile Dementia and Related Disorders. Volume 7, Aging. New York, Raven Press, 1978

Safford F: Developing A Training Program For Families of the Mentally Impaired Aged. New York, Isabella Geriatric Center, 1977

Scheinberg P: Multi-infarct dementia. In Katzman R et al (eds): Alzheimer's Disease: Senile Dementia and Related Disorders. Volume 7, Aging. New York, Raven Press, 1978

Schoenberg B: Neuroepidemiologic considerations in studies of Alzheimer's disease–senile dementia. In Katzman R et al (eds): Alzheimer's Disease: Senile Dementia and Related Disorders. Volume 7, Aging. New York, Raven Press, 1978

Sim M, Sussman I: Alzheimer's disease: Its natural history and differential diagnosis. J Nerv Ment Dis 135:489–498, 1962

Slaby AE, Wyatt RJ: Dementia In the Presenium. Springfield, Charles C Thomas, 1974

Wells CE: Chronic brain disease: An overview. Am J Psychiatry 135, No. 1:1–12, 1978

Index

pollen, allergy to, 56
polycystic disease, renal, 350
polycythemia, 275
polydipsia, 288
polygenic disorders, 71–72
polygenic inheritance, 72f
polygenic traits, 71
polymorphonuclear leukocytes (PMNs), 29
polyol, diabetes and, 465
polyp(s), precancerous, 91f
polypeptide(s), 66
polypeptide chain
    hemoglobin and, 263
    immunoglobulin structure and, 51f
polyploidy, 85
polysomy, 73
    X, 74–75
pons, 574
    coma progression and, 615
portal cirrhosis, 518–522
    manifestations of, 520t
portal hypertension, 519
postconcussion syndrome, 608–609
postnecrotic cirrhosis, 518
potassium
    balance of, alterations in, 298–303
    concentration of, ECG and, 302f
    dietary, renal failure and, 370
    effect on pH regulation, 317
    excess of, 301–303, 303t
    excretion of, chronic renal failure and, 367
    gains and losses of, 299
    level of, regulation of, 299
    membrane excitability and, 542
    regulation by kidney, 342
potassium in active transport, 13
potassium deficit, 299, 300t, 301
potassium-hydrogen ion exchange, 299
preeclampsia, 152
pregnancy, hypertension and, 152
premenstrual tension, 400
premotor cortex, 576
pressure, atmospheric, defined, 229
pressure waves, arterial, 141
priapism, 382
primary enzyme defects, 71
primary hypertension. See hypertension, primary
Prinzmetal's angina, 189
procallus, 37
procoagulation factors, 131
prolapse, uterine, 403
prophase, 83
prostaglandin(s), 32, 424
prostate
    benign nodular hyperplasia of, 388f
    cancer of, 389
    disorders of, 387–389
prostatitis, 387–388
    chronic, 388
protein
    adsorption of, 499
    dietary, renal failure and, 369
    metabolism of, 452
    structural defects of, 70
protopathic pathway, 566
pseudomembranous exudate, 33
pseudopodia of leukocytes, 30
pseudostratified columnar
    epithelium, 15

PTH (parathyroid hormone), calcium and phosphate and, 304
puberty
    male, 379
    oogenesis and, 396
pulmonary banding, 206
pulmonary capillary wedge pressure (PCWP), shock and, 168
pulmonary edema, acute, 218–220
pulmonary embolism, 125–126
    incidence of, 125f
pulse
    peripheral perfusion and, 116
    shock and, 168
pulse pressure, 142
pulsus paradoxus, 185
Purkinje system, 178, 196, 197
purulent exudate, 33
pyelonephritis, 353
pyramidal tract
    function of, disruption of, 619
    motor control and, 619–620
pyrogen(s), 40
pyuria, 351

radiation, body heat and, 39
    cancer caused by, 92
    cellular injury by, 22
    embryo development and, 75
    leukemia and, 42
    protection from, 97
    treatment of cancer by, 96
        adverse effects of, 96
radioimmunoassay, 432
radiosensitivity, 96
rales, 234
Ranvier, nodes of, 536
rapidly progressive glomerulonephritis, 357, 357f
RAS (reticular activating system), 554, 614
Raynaud's disease, 116–117
RBC (red blood cell count), 269
RDS (respiratory distress syndrome), 228
reagins, 55
receptors, hormone, 425–427
rectocele, 402
rectum, cancer of, 495–496
red blood cells
    alterations in, 268–275
    components of in transfusions, 273t
    development of, 269f
    lab tests of, 269
    normal, 268f
    standard laboratory values for, 269t
    structure of, 268
red blood cell count (RBC), 269
Reed-Sternberg (RS) cell, 63
referred pain, areas of, 596f
reflex(es), 550
    cough. See cough
    defecation, 479
    flexor-withdrawal, 563f
    spinal cord, 563–564
    stretch, 568
    visceral, hierarchy of, 585–586
refractory period, 542
regeneration, cellular, 34–35
renal colic, 355
renal disease. See kidney, disease of
renal failure

acute, 362–364
    causes of, 363t
    chronic. See chronic renal failure
renal phosphate buffer system, 315f
renin, endocrine function of kidney and, 343
renin-angiotensin-aldosterone
    mechanism, 143
    hypertension and, 150
repolarization, membrane, 542
reproductive system
    effect of chemotherapy on, 99
    female, 392f
        inflammations of, 404–407
    male, 374f
        excretory ducts of, 376f
reserve, respiratory, 229–230
respiration
    control of, 233
    control of pH and, 314–315
    defense mechanisms of, 243t
    failure of, 265–268
        in childhood, 242
        signs of, 242t
respiratory acidosis, 323–324, 324t
    thyroid hormone and, 436
respiratory alkalosis, 324–325, 325t
respiratory distress syndrome (RDS), 228
respiratory failure, 265–268
    causes of, 266t
    treatment of, 267
respiratory system, 224f
resting membrane potential, 541
reticular activating system (RAS), 554, 614
reticular fiber(s), 16
reticuloendothelial system, 31
reticulospinal system, pain and, 594
retinoblastoma, 91f
retinopathy, diabetic, 466–467
    lesions in, 467
retroversion of uterus, 401
RF (rheumatoid factor), 60
Rh blood types, 274–275
    babies and, 274
rheumatic fever, 199–200
    Jones criteria of diagnosis of, 199t
    treatment of, 200
rheumatoid arthritis, 60–62
    diagnosis of, 61
    diagnostic criteria for, 61t
    juvenile, 62
    pathologic changes in, 60
    treatment of, 62
rheumatoid factor (RF), 60
rheumatoid nodules, 61
rhinitis, allergic, 56
rhonchi, 234
ribonucleic acid
    defined, 8
    ribosomal, 8
    transfer, 8
ribosome(s)
    defined, 9
    ER and, 9f
rickets, renal, 368
risk factors
    atherosclerotic, 112–113
    suspected, atherosclerosis and, 113
    of venous thrombosis, 124t
RNA. See ribonucleic acid
rough ER, defined, 9